C0-CEC-742

Cardiovascular Pharmacology

Cardiovascular Pharmacology

Edited by

William W. Parmley, MD
Professor of Medicine
University of California, San Francisco
Chief, Division of Cardiology
Moffitt/Long Hospital

Kanu Chatterjee, MB, FRCP
Professor of Medicine
University of California, San Francisco
Associate Chief, Division of Cardiology
Moffitt/Long Hospital

Ͷ WOLFE

For full details of all Mosby–Year Book Europe, Ltd. titles please write to Mosby–Year Book Europe, Ltd. Lynton House, 7-12 Tavistock Square, London WC1H 9LB, England.

Library of Congress Cataloging-in-Publication Data

Cardiovascular pharmacology / edited by William W. Parmley, Kanu Chatterjee.
      p. cm.
    Includes bibliographical references and index.
    ISBN 1-56375-160-7
    1. Cardiovascular agents. I. Parmley, William W. (Willliam Watts),
1936–   . II. Chatterjee, Kanu. III. Title.
    [DNLM: 1. Cardiovascular Agents—therapeutic use. 2. Cardio-
vascular Diseases—drug therapy. QV 150 C2751 1993]
    RM345.C3763 1993
    615'.71—dc20
    93-7862

British Library Cataloguing-in-Publication Data.
A catalogue record for this book is available from the British Library.

ISBN: 1-56375-160-7

Editor: Elizabeth Greenspan
Editorial Assistant: David Yoon
Illustration Director: Carol Kalafatic
Illustrator: Nicholas Guarracino
Art Director: Kathryn Greenslade
Interior Design: Jeffrey S. Brown, Carol Drozdyk
Cover Design: Carol Drozdyk
Cover Illustration: Nicholas Guarracino

The right of William Parmley and Kanu Chatterjee to be identified as authors of this work has been asserted by them in accordance with the Copyright, Design and Patents Act 1988.

All rights reserved. No part of this publication may be reproduced, stored in a retrieval system, copied or transmitted, in any form or by any means, electronic, mechanical, photocopying, recording or otherwise, without prior written permission from the Publisher or in accordance with the pro-visions of the Copyright Act 1988, or under the terms of any license per-mitting limited copying issued by the Copyright Licensing Agency, 33-34 Alfred Place, London, WC1E 7DP.

Any person who does any unauthorized act in relation to this publication may be liable to criminal prosecution and civil claims for damage.

Permission to photocopy or reproduce solely for internal or personal use is permitted for libraries or other users registered with the Copyright Clear-ance Center, provided that the base fee of $4.00 per chapter plus $.10 per page is paid directly to the Copyright Clearance Center, 21 Congress Street, Salem, MA 01970. This consent does not extend to other kinds of copying, such as copying for general distribution, for advertising or promotional pur-poses, for creating new collected works, or for resales.

Copyright © 1994 Mosby–Year Book Europe, Ltd.
Published in 1994 by Wolfe Publishing, an imprint of Mosby–Year Book Europe, Ltd.

Originated in Hong Kong by Mandarin Offset

Produced in Hong Kong by Imago Publishing

Printed and bound in Hong Kong, 1994

10 9 8 7 6 5 4 3 2 1

PREFACE

The continuing development of therapeutic agents in medicine makes pharmacology one of the most dynamic and challenging areas of knowledge for the practicing physician. Cardiovascular disease is still the number one cause of mortality in the United States. Pharmacologic agents in cardiovascular disease, therefore, are one of the most important forms of therapy used by physicians today. Because there are so many drugs available, it is frequently difficult to put these agents into clinical perspective. One of the major advantages of this pharmacology book is that the chapters are written by clinicians for practicing physicians. Thus, there is a heavy emphasis on the clinical application of these agents rather than a dry, detailed description of all of the agents and the studies done with them. Each of the chapters has been written with this goal in mind. We trust that the clinical flavor of this text will be especially valuable to those who actively care for patients. In addition, there are useful examples of drug interactions in a chapter designed to discuss the common drug interactions that occur when a variety of cardiovascular drugs are given together. We hope that this book will assist the practitioner to better care for patients with cardiovascular disease.

William W. Parmley, MD

CONTENTS

CONTRIBUTORS

Jonathan Abrams, MD
Professor of Medicine (Cardiology)
University of New Mexico School of Medicine
Albuquerque, New Mexico

Neal L. Benowitz, MD
Professor of Medicine
Chief, Division of Clinical Pharmacology and Experimental Therapeutics
University of California, San Francisco
San Francisco General Hospital Medical Center
San Francisco, California

Shlomo Charlap, MD
Assistant Professor of Medicine
Downstate Medical Center
Physician in Charge, Coronary Care Unit
Long Island College Hospital
Brooklyn, New York

Kanu Chatterjee, MB, FRCP
Professor of Medicine
University of California, San Francisco
Associate Chief, Division of Cardiology
Moffitt/Long Hospital
San Francisco, California

James H. Chesebro, MD
Professor of Medicine
Harvard Medical School
Associate Director for Research, Cardiac Unit
Massachusetts General Hospital
Boston, Massachusetts

Arnold M. Chonko, MD, FACP
Professor of Medicine
Division of Nephrology and Hypertension
Director, Renal Dialysis Program
University of Kansas School of Medicine
Kansas City, Kansas

William P. Fay, MD
Assistant Professor of Internal Medicine
University of Michigan Medical Center
Ann Arbor, Michigan

William H. Frishman, MD
Professor and Associate Chairman
Department of Medicine
Albert Einstein College of Medicine
Montefiore Medical Center
Bronx, New York

Valentin Fuster, MD
Mallinkrodt Professor of Medicine
Harvard Medical School
Chief, Cardiac Unit
Massachusetts General Hospital
Boston, Massachusetts

CONTRIBUTORS

Jared J. Grantham, MD, FACP
Professor of Medicine
Division of Nephrology and Hypertension
Director, Division of Nephrology
University of Kansas School of Medicine
Kansas City, Kansas

John H. Ip, MD
Division of Cardiology
Mount Sinai Medical Center
New York, New York

Ik-Kyung Jang, MD
Assistant Professor of Medicine
Harvard Medical School
Massachusetts General Hospital
Boston, Massachusetts

John P. Kane, MD, PhD
Professor of Medicine, Biophysics, and Biochemistry
Director, Metabolic Clinic
University of California, San Francisco
San Francisco, California

Mary J. Malloy, MD
Clinical Professor of Medicine and Pediatrics
Director, Pediatric Lipid Clinic
Cardiovascular Research Institute
University of California, San Francisco
San Francisco, California

William W. Parmley, MD
Professor of Medicine
University of California, San Francisco
Chief, Division of Cardiology
Moffitt/Long Hospital
San Francisco, California

Mark Sale, MD
Assistant Professor of Medicine and Pharmacology
Georgetown University Medical Center
Washington, DC

Bramah N. Singh, MD, PhD
Chief of Cardiology
Veterans Affairs Medical Center, West Los Angeles
Professor of Medicine
University of California, Los Angeles
Los Angeles, California

Raymond L. Woosley, MD, PhD
Professor of Pharmacology and Medicine
Chair, Department of Pharmacology
Georgetown University Medical Center
Washington, DC

Basic Principles Of Clinical Pharmacology

1

Mark Sale
Raymond L. Woosley

Fundamental to the rational use of any drug is an understanding of the basic principles of pharmacology. One of the basic principles of pharmacology is that most drug effects, both beneficial and toxic, are due to the interaction of the drug molecule (or its metabolite) with a receptor. Specifically, the drug effect will depend on which receptors are occupied and the magnitude of the effect on the fraction of time that the receptor is occupied by the drug molecule. The fraction of time the receptor is occupied will, in turn, depend mathematically on the concentration of drug in the local environment. The concentration of drug in the local environment will, in turn, depend mathematically on certain physiologic parameters (volume of distribution and clearance among them) and on the dose (Fig. 1.1). Pharmacodynamic models can be used to predict drug effects. In general, these models are more accurate when based on drug concentrations than when based on drug dose. The usual example of this is theophylline. The correlation between concentration and drug effects is stronger than the relationship between dose and drug effects. More often than not the local environment of the receptor cannot be sampled directly. However, predictions of this concentration can be made using pharmacokinetic models. Thus, while admittedly complex, an integrated pharmacokinetic–pharmacodynamic approach to dose–response relationships is beginning to receive wider attention. In theory, pharmacokinetic–pharmacodynamic applications are powerful, allowing prediction of drug concentration, of onset and offset of drug effect, of the magnitude of the response, and of the dose necessary to achieve the desired effect. While these goals may be realized occasionally, more often the variability between patients precludes predictions of drug effects that are accurate enough to be the sole basis of clinical decisions. Therefore, these models should be viewed as adjuncts to other sources of clinical information. Nonetheless, knowledge of the factors that influence a drug's disposition in the body (pharmacokinetics) and drug action (pharmacodynamics) can simplify the approach to therapeutics and help provide an optimum benefit-to-risk ratio for the patient, especially at the initiation of therapy.

Dose—Response Relationships

The response to increasing doses of a drug is usually graded, asymptotically approaching a maximum (Fig. 1.2). In some cases a sigmoid relationship is apparent (Fig. 1.3). Both of these dose–response relationships are usually described by the same mathematics that describe ligand–receptor binding. In biochemistry it is called the Michaelis-Menton equation. In pharmacodynamics the same relationship is called the E_{max} or, when appropriate, the sigmoid E_{max} equation. The application of nonlinear regression analysis to dose–response curves can often be a fruitful approach to exploring relationships in addition to concentration–effect relationships. These may include many clinically relevant effects such as age–response relationships. These parameters of the equation can also be used to describe both the efficacy (maximum effect) and the potency (dose that elicits 50% of the maximum effect) of drugs. The mathematical basis of the E_{max} equation is discussed in the appendix.

In cases where the response is "all-or-none" (presence or absence of effect) or in which dose–response curves are flat, the relationship between dose and response is best described by probability statistics (e.g., the cumulative frequency of patients responding at a given dose or concentration).

Figure 1.1 Sequence of steps from drug dose to effect, illustrating the levels at which mathematical modeling can be used to describe and predict concentration and effects.

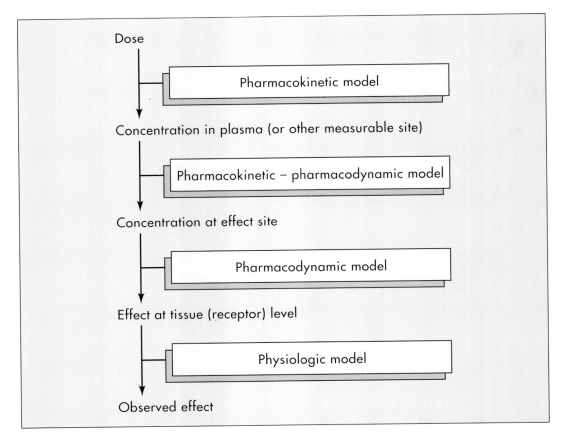

Dose

Pharmacokinetic model

Concentration in plasma (or other measurable site)

Pharmacokinetic – pharmacodynamic model

Concentration at effect site

Pharmacodynamic model

Effect at tissue (receptor) level

Physiologic model

Observed effect

Receptors

It was inferred at the turn of the century that the response to a drug is mediated by interaction of the drug with specific cellular binding sites—receptors. Since then, technological advances, notably affinity chromatography and photoaffinity labelling, have allowed characterization of the receptor macromolecules themselves and the steps involved from initial recognition between a receptor and a ligand (drug or endogenous substance) to the expression of effect.

Ligand-binding studies have also aided our current understanding of receptor localization, specificity and structure–activity relationships, and receptor dynamics. Recent advances in molecular biology have made it possible to express the genes encoding specific receptors in high concentrations in cell culture. Site-directed mutagenesis then makes it possible to study the components of receptor recognition and activation.

Receptors are heterogeneous, ranging from enzymes (digitalis glycosides bind to Na^+,K^+-adenosine

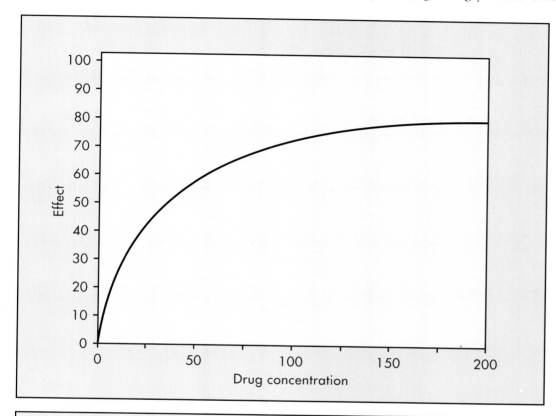

Figure 1.2 Typical dose/concentration response curve for E_{max} model. The largest effect that can be elicited by the drug is 100. A dose/concentration of 50 will elicit an effect of 50% of that.

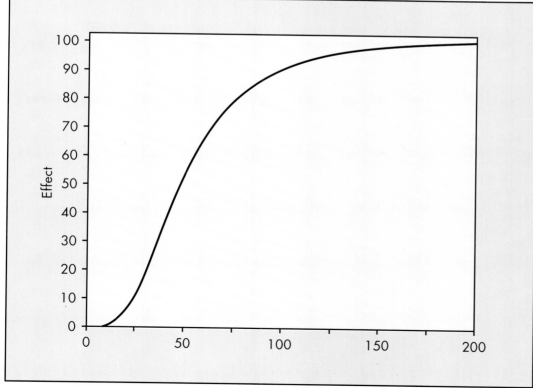

Figure 1.3 Typical dose/concentration response curve for sigmoid E_{max} model. The largest effect that can be elicited is again 100, with a dose/concentration of 50 giving rise to an effect of 50% of the maximum effect. The drugs depicted in this figure and in Figure 1.2 have the same efficacy and potency.

triphosphatase [ATPase]) to nucleic acids (with which many antineoplastic agents interact). But ligand–receptor interactions generally result in either changes in ion permeability or changes in some biochemical function such as activation of a cyclic nucleotide-dependent protein kinase, or both. To date, the best-studied receptor system is that of the adenylyl cyclase-coupled β-adrenergic receptor. The current concept of this receptor system comprises three components: (1) the hormone receptor and (2) a "coupling" protein or G protein regulated by guanine nucleotides (e.g., guanosine triphosphate [GTP], guanosine diphosphate [GDP]) that couples ligand–receptor binding to activation of (3) adenylyl cyclase (converts adenosine triphosphate [ATP] to cyclic adenosine monophosphate [cAMP]) (Fig. 1.4).

The ligand–receptor activation process can be modeled to various degrees of sophistication, the simplest model being that of an equilibrium between two receptor states: resting/closed and activated/open. One theory proposes that the relative affinity of a ligand for these two receptor states will determine its biologic activity. For example, agonists (agents that elicit a response) shift the equilibrium in favor of the activated state (i.e., they promote the interaction of the receptor with the coupling protein), while antagonists (agents that prevent a response to agonist) show equal affinity for both receptor states and do not alter their equilibrium. A partial agonist (for example, a β-blocker with intrinsic sympathomimetic activity) may be thought of as having an only somewhat greater affinity for the activated state. Thus, it will cause only a slight shift of the equilibrium in favor of the activated state.

An important concept is that the drug effect usually depends on either the number of receptors occupied or the number unoccupied. Thus, it depends not only on the fraction of receptors occupied (and thus on the drug concentration) but also on the number of receptors available. The receptor population is not fixed, and the number of receptors self-regulates in response to the degree of their stimulation. Thus, phenomena related to an attenuated or augmented response (tolerance, tachyphylaxis, desensitization, or supersensitivity to the drug) can be due wholly or in part to changes in receptor density. For example, β-adrenergic receptor density increases ("up-regulation") during chronic treatment with propranolol.

The effect appears to persist as long as propranolol is administered and for some time after discontinuation, providing a possible explanation for the delayed supersensitivity to β-adrenergic stimulation seen after stopping propranolol therapy.[1] Clinically, this may manifest as worsened angina, arrhythmias, and so forth. Chronic receptor stimulation (for example, the use of sympathomimetics in the treatment of allergic rhinitis) may lead to a reduction ("down-regulation") in receptor density, and therefore to a loss of efficacy. Treatment with antagonists possessing partial agonist activity also leads to receptor down-regulation and may contribute to their efficacy.

Another mechanism of receptor sensitivity control may be modification of receptor coupling to a regulatory protein, so that ligand–receptor binding is divorced from the sequence of events leading to effect. Such a mechanism may be important in instances of acute desensitization to agonist.

Structure–Activity Relationships

The therapeutic usefulness of most drugs depends on their specificity, which in turn implies interaction with a receptor. The ability of a drug to interact with a receptor depends on its having the correct physical, chemical, and spatial configuration. Minor modifications in structure can yield compounds with widely differing potencies or loss of efficacy. The screening of a series of chemical compounds related in structure to a known active compound can produce information on chemical relationships crucial to pharmacologic activity and can also provide clues to receptor configuration.

The specificity of a drug for a particular receptor also determines biologic activity. For example, chlorpromazine, procaine, and diphenhydramine all have a large cyclic hydrocarbon and a tertiary amino group in their molecular structure. All three drugs possess antihistaminic, local anesthetic, and antiarrhythmic effects. The extent to which these agents interact with the receptors involved in transducing these effects determines their relative potencies. Additionally, other chemical groupings provide the molecules with still other properties. Thus, of the three, diphenhydramine is the most effective antihistamine, procaine the best local anes-

Figure 1.4 Schematic diagram of the components of hormone-responsive adenylyl cyclase system. Association of H with R forms HR, which interacts with N, resulting in the exchange of GDP for GTP. R and N-GTP dissociate, allowing N-GTP to activate AC. The activation process results in hydrolysis of N-GTP to N-GDP. (R = β-adrenergic receptor; N = guanine nucleotide regulatory protein; AC = adenylyl cyclase; H = hormone or agonist) (Modified from Lefkowitz RJ, Michel T: Plasma membrane receptors. J Clin Invest 72:1185, 1983)

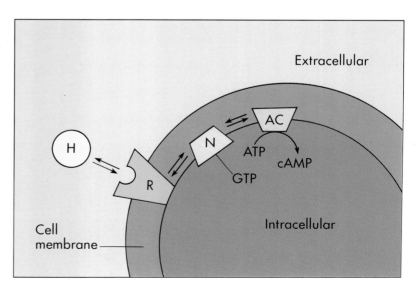

thetic, and chlorpromazine possesses antiemetic and neuroleptic activity.

In many cases, specificity extends to steric requirements. Thus, only the L-enantiomer of norepinephrine, and not the D-isomer, elevates blood pressure; the L-enantiomer of verapamil has more potent hypotensive and negative chronotropic effects than D-verapamil.[2] However, not all drugs interact with specific receptors. For example, by generation of a nitric oxide free radical, nitrate vasodilators may initiate vascular smooth muscle relaxation mediated by increases in cyclic guanosine monophosphate (cGMP).[3] Osmotic diuretics depend on their physical properties for therapeutic benefit. While these have a specific site of action, no interaction with a specific receptor is required. These, however, are the exception.

THERAPEUTIC WINDOW

The therapeutic window for a drug encompasses the range of doses or plasma concentrations (when there is a reliable correlation with pharmacologic effect) that elicit a therapeutic effect in most patients with adverse effects in only a few. Alternatively, the therapeutic window may be considered the range of doses or concentrations where the efficacy/toxicity ratio is the most favorable. At some appropriately chosen low dose, most patients will not respond at all. Increasing doses will result in a larger fraction of patients showing a desired therapeutic response, and this will be paralleled by an increasing number of patients who develop unwanted adverse effects. The wider the margin between the doses or concentrations that produce efficacy and those associated with adverse effects, the less rigidly the dose (concentration) must be controlled in order to obtain optimal efficacy and minimal toxicity, and the wider the therapeutic window. Conversely, a narrow therapeutic window requires careful dose adjustment in order to avoid toxic effects.

The therapeutic window also depends on the definition of efficacy. For example, in one study 90% of episodes of recurrent nonsustained ventricular tachycardia in patients undergoing tocainide therapy could be suppressed at plasma concentrations of 2.8 to 10 μg/ml (mean 6 μg/ml) while 90% suppression of ventricular extrasystoles required 9 to 13 μg/ml

(mean 11 μg/ml) (Fig. 1.5).[4] However, both of these (recurrent ventricular tachycardia and ventricular extrasystoles) are only surrogate markers for the clinical endpoint of interest, life-threatening arrhythmias. The concentration principle required to suppress life-threatening arrhythmias has not been adequately determined.

One aim of studying pharmacokinetics is to assist in the achievement and maintenance of plasma concentrations within the therapeutic window. This is especially important when dealing with cardiovascular agents since their *therapeutic ratio* (the plasma concentration that elicits toxic effects compared to the concentration that produces a desired therapeutic effect) is usually low.

ABSORPTION
Factors Influencing Absorption

Following administration (aside from intravenous injection), a drug must first be absorbed from the gut, oral mucosa, muscle, and so forth and must enter the systemic circulation before it can reach its site of action. Several factors influence the rate and extent of absorption from these sites, including the physicochemical properties of the drug, the surface area available for absorption, and regional blood flow. In general, lipid-soluble drugs penetrate cell membranes more readily than hydrophilic agents; a nonionized drug permeates more readily than an ionized drug. Since many drugs are either weak acids or weak bases, differences in the pH of the gastrointestinal tract (strongly acid stomach, nearly neutral small intestine) will determine the extent of ionization and thus the rate of absorption following oral administration. For practical purposes, however, the greatest amount of absorption occurs in the small intestine by virtue of the large surface area available.

Gastrointestinal pathology can influence the amount of drug absorbed. Diarrhea or extensive small bowel resection, both of which reduce intestinal transit time, can result in markedly diminished absorption, especially of sustained-release preparations that are designed to allow prolonged absorption.

The same principles apply to other routes of administration. For example, following intramuscular

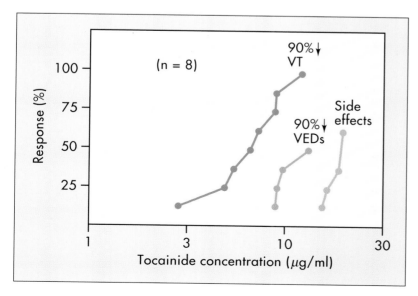

Figure 1.5 Relationship between drug plasma concentration and therapeutic or adverse effects in treatment of ventricular ectopic depolarizations (VEDs) and ventricular tachycardia (VT) with tocainide. (Modified from Roden DM, Reele SB, Higgins SB et al: Tocainide therapy for refractory ventricular arrhythmias. Am Heart J 100:15, 1980)

injection, absorption is more rapid from deltoid than from gluteal muscle since the former has a higher blood flow. Drugs that are insoluble at tissue pH, or those in an oily vehicle or microcrystalline suspension, will form a depot, releasing the drug slowly, which may allow less frequent injections.

Bioavailability

Bioavailability is the proportion of an administered dose reaching the systemic circulation. By definition, following intravenous injection a drug is 100% bioavailable. Thus bioavailability after, for instance, oral administration is determined by comparison of the areas under the plasma concentration time curves following oral and intravenous dosing. Bioavailability can be lowered by incomplete absorption due to problems in the drug's formulation or to the presence/absence of food. In addition, concomitant administration of agents that alter gastric pH (e.g., antacids) or motility (e.g., narcotic analgesics and atropine-like drugs which slow gastric emptying, or metoclopramide, which speeds it) can alter bioavailability. Efficient presystemic extraction by the bowel wall, or more usually the liver (first-pass effect), will lower systemic availability and have the same effect as when absorption from the gut is reduced.

The time course of absorption may also be important in instances where rapid attainment of a therapeutic plasma concentration is desirable following the initial (or single) dose. Although either rapid absorption or slow absorption can result in the same amount of drug becoming available systemically (equal area under the concentration–time curve), therapeutic concentrations are achieved sooner if absorption is rapid (Fig. 1.6). For some drugs (e.g, tocainide or mexiletine), it is possible to avoid rapid absorption and the resulting high peak plasma con-

centrations by giving the drugs with food. This can reduce the incidence of dose-related side-effects but efficacy is unaltered since the extent of absorption is unchanged.

DISTRIBUTION

Having entered the systemic circulation, the drug distributes throughout the body, carried by the extracellular (vascular and interstitial) water in which it is dissolved. As in the case of absorption from the site of administration, the drug's passage into various body tissues depends on the lipid solubility of the drug, its degree of ionization, the vascularity of the tissue, and the size of the drug molecule, or drug–protein complex when the drug is bound to plasma protein. Lipid-soluble drugs readily diffuse across capillaries and all biologic membranes (including the blood–brain and blood–cerebrospinal fluid barriers), while hydrophilic drugs depend on the permeability characteristics of the capillaries for their access to extravascular sites. The capillaries in the liver and kidney are particularly permeable to all but highly protein-bound drugs, while those of the brain are virtually impermeable to water-soluble molecules of any size. Since quantification of the amount of drug in the body spaces is usually not feasible, the plasma concentration usually serves as the most accessible surrogate to the drug concentration at the effect site, and therefore as a surrogate for drug effect.

Volume of Distribution

At any time following administration, the drug concentration in plasma will be defined by the amount of drug in the body and the volume in which it is distributed. Intracellular protein binding or tissue se-

Figure 1.6 Plasma concentration over time with rapid or slow absorption of drug. Bioavailability in both cases is 100%, because the area under each of the two curves equals that under the the intravenous dose curve. However, therapeutic effect in the two situations may differ greatly.

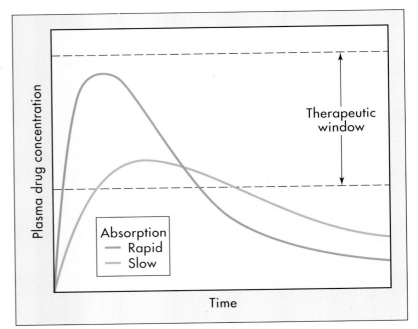

questration will result in only a small amount of drug left in the extracellular water. Thus, when most of the drug is located outside the plasma, the plasma concentration will be low. In this case, the calculated variable, the (apparent) volume of distribution, will be large, since it is estimated by the ratio of the amount of drug given to the plasma concentration. Therefore, usually the larger the calculated volume of distribution, the smaller the fraction in plasma. However, the apparent volume of distribution should not be ascribed to actual anatomic volumes. For instance, the volume of distribution of mexiletine is about 600 to 700 l,[5] far in excess of total body water. There are two possible reasons for such a large volume of distribution. The most common reason, as mentioned above, is extensive tissue (usually adipose) binding. The second is high presystemic extraction by the gut wall or liver. Either of these leaves little drug in the plasma, giving rise to a large calculated volume of distribution.

There are substances, however, that are confined to certain physiologic volumes and may be used as reference materials in pharmacokinetic studies. For example, certain dyes remain confined to plasma, inulin distributes throughout the extracellular water, and antipyrine occupies total body water. The corresponding volumes of distribution for these agents for a 70-kg individual are 3 l, 13 to 16 l, and 40 to 46 l, respectively. In general, however, the volume of distribution relates to the extent of tissue localization of a drug rather than to any actual physiologic volume.

METABOLISM AND ELIMINATION

As soon as a drug enters the circulation it is available for elimination. This usually occurs either by metabolic modification of the drug or by excretion via the kidneys (Fig. 1.7). The removal of a drug from the body is quantified as its clearance, and it is expressed as the volume of plasma from which the drug is completely removed per unit time (e.g., ml/min). This is entirely analogous to creatinine clearance. Total body clearance is the sum of clearance at all sites of elimination.

Hepatic Clearance

The liver is the most important site of drug metabolizing activity in the body. Hepatic extraction may include biotransformation (metabolism), biliary excretion, and drug binding to intracellular proteins. Hepatic clearance is influenced by two independent variables: the activity of drug metabolizing enzymes and liver blood flow. The relative importance of these two factors varies from drug to drug. For a drug with a low hepatic extraction ratio, increases in enzyme activity result in important changes in pharmacokinetic variables (increases in clearance and a shortened elimination half-life). However, increases in hepatic blood flow will not increase clearance, as the metabolic capacity of the liver is already maximal.

FIGURE 1.7 DISPOSITION OF CARDIOVASCULAR DRUGS

Drug	Inactivation or Major Route of Elimination (%)	Oral Bioavailability (%)	Active Metabolites	Protein Binding (%)
Quinidine	Liver (50–90) Kidney (10–30)	70	Probable	50–95
Procainamide	Kidney (30–60) Liver (40–70)	75[*]	Yes	15
Disopyramide	Kidney (36–77) Liver (11–37)	80	Yes	20–60[†]
Lidocaine	Liver	35	Yes	40–70[†]
Phenytoin	Liver	70–100[*,†]	No	90
Mexiletine	Liver	90	No	70
Tocainide	Liver Kidney	100	No	50
Flecainide	Liver	95	No	40
Encainide	Liver	26[‡]; 89[*,§]	Yes[‡]	
Lorcainide	Liver	80–100	Yes	85
Propafenone	Liver	10–50[*,†]	Yes	90
Bretylium	Kidney	20	No	?(low)
Amiodarone	Liver	20–50	Yes	?(high)
Verapamil	Liver	20	Yes	90
Nifedipine	Liver	45–60[*]	No	90
Diltiazem	Liver	38–90[†]	Yes	80
Propanolol	Liver	30–40[*]	Yes	95
Metoprolol	Liver	50[*]	No	12
Timolol	Liver	75[*]	No	10
Nadolol	Kidney	20	No	30
Pindolol	Liver (60) Kidney (40)	90	No	57
Digoxin	Kidney	60–75	No	20
Digitoxin	Liver	?(100)	No	95

[*]Inherited differences in metabolism
[†]Dose- or concentration-dependent

[‡]In "extensive metabolizers"
[§]In "poor metabolizers"

On the other hand, for a drug with a high extraction ratio, increased metabolizing activity has little effect, as nearly all the drug is already being removed from the blood presented to the organ. Conversely, changes in hepatic blood flow affect high-extraction drugs. In this case the metabolic capacity is not maximal and the delivery of more drug to the site of clearance will result in a higher clearance. Thus, changes in liver blood flow do not alter the disposition of phenytoin (a low extraction drug), while enzyme induction does not have a large effect on the disposition of lidocaine (a high extraction drug).

Some drugs are so extensively cleared by the liver after absorption from the gut and prior to entering the general circulation (the first-pass effect) that oral use is not feasible. One example is lidocaine, which, although well absorbed, is only about 35% systemically bioavailable after oral administration. Increasing the oral dose to attain therapeutic plasma levels results in a corresponding increase in the levels of lidocaine's metabolites. These levels, unfortunately, result in unacceptable central nervous system side-effects, precluding the use of large oral doses of lidocaine.

POLYMORPHIC DRUG METABOLISM

In recent years, physicians have become aware of genetic factors controlling the variability in hepatic drug metabolism. The best studied enzymes are the P450 cytochromes and hepatic N-acetyltransferase (NAT). NAT is inherited as an autosomal dominant trait resulting in 55% of whites being phenotypic rapid acetylators and 45% slow acetylators. Drugs such as hydralazine and procainamide must be given at higher doses to rapid acetylators to maintain therapeutic effects. Furthermore, acetylator phenotype can influence the rate of development of a lupus-like syndrome with these drugs. Although the lupus syndrome can occur in either phenotype, higher doses or greater duration of exposure are required in rapid acetylators.

Hepatic P450 enzymes oxidize many drugs as a first step in their elimination. Although there are several discrete P450s, the best characterized is the one responsible for the metabolism of the antihypertensive debrisoquine. Seven percent of the U.S. population inherit two of the four known mutant alleles for the gene that controls expression of this P450. This P450, termed P4502D6, is responsible for the metabolism of over 40 known drugs and when absent leads to pharmacokinetic differences in the handling of timolol, metoprolol, encainide, flecainide, propafenone, mexiletine, and many others. It is not possible to generalize about the clinical relevance of defective metabolism of these drugs because some have active metabolites and chirally specific actions and metabolism. However, defective metabolism in this relatively large portion of the population, termed polymorphic metabolism, alters the dose–response relationships for most of these drugs and influences their clinical use.[6]

Enzyme Induction/Inhibition

Certain agents (enzyme inducers) can promote synthesis of microsomal enzymes, resulting in increased drug-metabolizing capacity. In some cases, the increased activity results in more rapid clearance of the drug itself, and tolerance to the drug develops as a consequence. However, some drugs are able to induce enzymes for which they themselves are not substrates. Concomitantly administered agents that happen to be substrates for the induced enzyme may then be subject to increased hepatic metabolism. Enzyme induction is most likely to have important consequences for the disposition of drugs with a normally low hepatic extraction ratio.

A number of agents can inhibit drug-metabolizing enzymes, increasing the systemic availability of drugs normally highly extracted by the liver. For instance, cimetidine increases the availability and prolongs the half-life of lidocaine[7] and propranolol.[8] Propranolol, both by reducing hepatic blood flow and by inhibiting microsomal enzymes, decreases the clearance of lidocaine.[9]

Obviously, careful observation of the patient is necessary whenever multiple medications are prescribed, but especially when stopping or starting a drug that alters the metabolism of other agents. Some drugs with known or proposed enzyme induction or inhibition effects in man are listed in Figure 1.8.

Unexpected toxicity or loss of therapeutic effect is likely, and may not be immediately apparent. For example, amiodarone, the concentration of which in the liver is about 1000 times that in the plasma, inhibits the hepatic clearance of many other drugs.[10] Since the elimination half-life of amiodarone ranges from 2 to 15 weeks, it may take months before normal hepatic clearance of other drugs is restored after stopping amiodarone.

Renal Clearance

Metabolic products are usually more polar and thus more water-soluble than the parent compound, facilitating excretion via the kidneys by either passive glomerular filtration or active tubular secretion.

The kidneys are by far the most important route of excretion of unchanged drug or drug metabolites. In some cases, excretion by the kidneys is the major route of elimination and the means of terminating a drug's effect. In other cases, the kidneys simply excrete the inactive metabolites of a drug, usually produced by the liver.

Elimination by glomerular filtration is a passive process, dependent on the extent of plasma protein binding and blood flow. Since only free drug can pass the glomerular membrane, a highly protein-bound drug that is not actively secreted into the urine will be eliminated slowly. If this is the main route of elimination and the volume of distribution is large (i.e., little drug in plasma), a prolonged half-life can result. For example, diazoxide is 90% bound to albumin and eliminated by glomerular filtration with a half-life of about 30 hours. Changes in protein binding that result in an increase in free drug concentration will also increase renal elimination and shorten the elimination half-life.

While glomerular filtration always occurs, tubular secretion is an active process and may or may not occur, depending on the particular drug. When renal clearance exceeds clearance due to filtration, tubular secretion can be inferred. As free drug is carried across into the tubular lumen, more free drug dissociates from the protein–drug complex to restore the equilibrium. Protein binding, therefore, does not limit tubular secretion as it does glomerular filtration.

Tubular reabsorption can also be important in reducing the renal clearance of drug. Since the nonionized form of a weak acid or base can diffuse readily from the tubular urine (which has become more concentrated by the removal of salt and water) back across the tubule cells into plasma, an alkaline urine will promote excretion and prevent reabsorption of a weak acid, while an acid urine will diminish excre-tion and favor reabsorption. The opposite relationship is true for weak bases. For example, the half-life of mexiletine, a weak base, is approximately 9 hours when the urine is alkaline and 3 hours when acidic.[11]

Protein Binding

In plasma, most drugs are reversibly bound to plasma proteins, including albumin, alpha-1-acid glycoprotein (AAG), lipoproteins, and/or gamma globulins. This rapidly establishes an equilibrium between bound and unbound drug. Although the most abundant protein, albumin, avidly binds acidic drugs, many cardiovascular agents are basic and bind preferentially to AAG.[12] AAG is an "acute phase" protein whose concentration increases dramatically in response to stresses such as myocardial infarction, fever, and surgery. Increased levels have also been reported in chronic inflammatory diseases such as rheumatoid arthritis, inflammatory renal disease, and Crohn's disease. An increase in the level of AAG will shift the equilibrium toward the AAG-drug complex, reducing the concentration of free drug. This has been responsible for reports of high concentrations of quinidine,[13] disopyramide,[14] and lidocaine[15] that lack the expected toxicity because of lower than anticipated free fractions.

The degree of protein binding has implications for both drug disposition and drug effect. Only the unbound, free drug is able to cross cell membranes or bind to receptor sites, thereby eliciting a pharmacologic effect. A decrease in protein binding, as a result of disease or displacement by another drug, will increase the free fraction, which in turn increases the amount of drug available for equilibration with extravascular sites. This will increase the volume of distribution and may alter clearance as described below.

Changes in protein binding are most likely to be clinically important for those drugs that are highly protein bound. For example, for a drug that is 98% bound to plasma protein, a decrease in binding to 96% will double the free fraction from 2% to 4%. For a drug that is 60% bound, a similar decrease in

FIGURE 1.8 SOME DRUGS THAT ALTER DRUG METABOLISM

Hepatic Enzyme Inducers	Hepatic Enzyme Inhibitors
Phenytoin	Cimetidine
Phenobarbital	Allopurinol
Rifampin	Disulfiram
Ethanol	Anabolic steroids
Carbamazepine	Chloramphenicol
Glutethimide	Metronidazole
Griseofulvin	Quinacrine
	Isoniazid
	Estrogens/oral contraceptives
	Amiodarone
	Fluoxetine
	Erythromycin
	Ketoconazole

binding will result in only an increase of one twentieth (from 40% to 42%) in the free fraction. In the latter case, clinically important consequences of the change in protein binding are unlikely. In the former case, the clinical significance will depend on the total amount of drug present in the plasma and whether the increase in free fraction results in a corresponding increase in free drug concentration. This, in turn, depends on whether the increase in free fraction is accompanied by an increase in clearance.

Some drugs are cleared slowly, and drug–protein dissociation during a single pass through a metabolizing or eliminating organ is small. For example, phenytoin is one such "low-extraction" drug that is extensively protein-bound. A decrease in phenytoin binding to albumin, as occurs in the presence of uremia or displacement by salicylate, results in an increase in the free fraction and, transiently, the free concentration. Since the clearance of low-extraction drugs is related directly to the free fraction, an increase in the phenytoin free fraction results in increased clearance. As more free drug is cleared, the equilibrium is shifted toward free drug, and the total plasma phenytoin concentration falls. Thus, while the same amount of free drug is available to exert pharmacologic activity as before, reliance on total plasma concentration could be misleading. Both efficacy and toxicity may appear at lower than usual total plasma concentrations.

If the same decrease in protein binding occurs in the case of a highly extracted drug, such as lidocaine or propranolol, the net result may be different. Since both free and protein-bound drug are cleared, changes in binding do not affect clearance. Since clearance remains constant, the total concentration at steady state will remain the same. However, since the free fraction has increased, and less drug is protein-bound, the free concentration will also be increased.

In such a case, exaggerated pharmacologic activity, possibly resulting in unexpected toxicity, may occur at total plasma concentrations within the usual therapeutic range. In summary, there are few clinically relevant drug interactions that are due to displacement interactions at protein binding sites.

Plasma protein binding can therefore serve as a drug storage site, "protecting" drugs from passive elimination processes in the liver and kidneys, or it can act as a delivery system for drugs that are highly cleared by the liver or kidneys as a result of active transfer processes.

Concentration-Dependent Binding

For most drugs, the fraction of drug bound to protein, at least for doses in the therapeutic range and well beyond, remains constant. However, some drugs (e.g., disopyramide) show nonlinear, saturable protein binding in the range of concentrations attained during routine clinical use (Fig. 1.9). Thus, as the total plasma concentration increases, so does the free fraction. For example, doubling the total disopyramide concentration from 2 μg/ml to 4 μg/ml may increase the free disopyramide concentration as much as sixfold.[16] Saturable effects, including binding and clearance, can make drugs quite difficult to use since a small percentage increase in the dose of a drug may result in a much larger increase in free concentration and thus the drug effects.

PHARMACOKINETICS

Pharmacokinetics describes the relationship of the processes of absorption, distribution, and elimination of a drug with time. The fate of a drug in the body

Figure 1.9 Saturable protein binding of disopyramide. As the total disopyramide concentration increases, so does the free fraction (unbound/total drug). These are the extremes of values obtained in a population of 12 subjects. (Modified from Meffin PJ, Robert EW, Winkle RA et al: Role of concentration-dependent plasma protein binding in disopyramide disposition. J Pharmacokinet Biopharm 7:29, 1979)

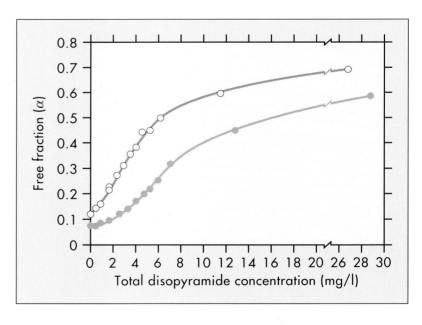

can be approximated by mathematical models that in turn are useful in determining appropriate dosing schedules.

Concept of Compartments

The various spaces into which the drug distributes are viewed as "compartments," or discrete volumes containing a certain mass of drug, with rate constants for entry and exit of drug from each of these compartments. Entry and exit of drug occur from a central compartment, which in practical terms may be thought of as the plasma (and perhaps highly perfused tissues such as brain, lung, heart, and kidneys, depending on the rapidity of distribution to these tissues relative to others). The drug may distribute more slowly into various tissues, which can then be regarded as peripheral compartments, with rate constants of entry to and exit from the central compartment (Fig. 1.10). Mathematically, the rate constant is a constant of proportionality that describes the rate of drug movement out of a compartment. The rate of drug movement out of a compartment is equal to the rate constant times the amount of drug (or the concentration of drug) in that compartment. The usual analogy is a bucket with a hole near the bottom. When there is a large amount of water in the bucket (a high concentration of drug), the water (drug) moves out very quickly. As the amount of water in the bucket (drug in the compartment) falls, the movement is slower. Although the postulated compartments may correspond to drug distribution and elimination from discrete tissue groups, such physiologic processes cannot in general be inferred from the model. It is important to recognize that the purpose of partitioning a drug into compartments is simply to allow convenient mathematical description of the time course of drug disposition.

The simplest case is that of rapid intravenous injection of a drug that is not distributed to other compartments. In this case, a semilogarithmic plot of plasma concentration against time yields a straight line (Fig. 1.11).

Such a linear relationship describes a first-order process; the amount of drug cleared from the plasma depends, at any instant, on the amount remaining in the plasma. Thus, plasma concentration decreases by a constant fraction with each unit of time. The most useful unit of time is that required for the plasma concentration to decrease by half, and is termed the "elimination half-life."

Following intravenous administration of a drug, a plot of the logarithm of plasma concentration against time (semilog plot) often shows an initial curvature. This departure from linearity represents the initial dilution of drug within the plasma and its distribution to other tissues. Once distribution is complete, drug

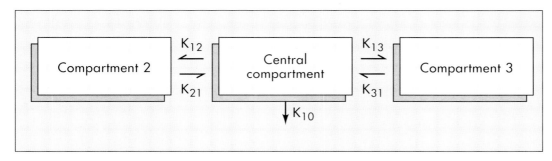

Figure 1.10 Schematic diagram of a multicompartment open model, in this case three compartments. Rate constants for drug transfer between compartments are the K values. Note that drug input and output occur only via the central compartment.

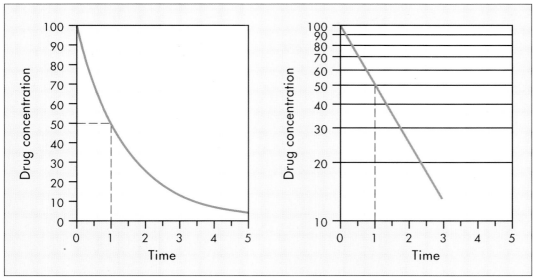

Figure 1.11 Drug concentration with time during first-order elimination for a single compartment plotted on an arithmetic scale (left) and on a semilog scale (right).

in both the central and peripheral compartments is in equilibrium. The curve can be dissected into two straight lines rather than one straight line; the first represents the distribution half-life, and the second, described above, is terminal elimination (Fig. 1.12).

This concept of mass-action compartments wherein drug is distributed can be extended to multicompartment models. The semilog plot of plasma concentration with time following a single intravenous dose will then be described by a polyexponential equation, with rate constants for entry to and exit from each compartment. Modern computers and methods of nonlinear regression can fit very complex models with any number of compartments. However, it is rare to find a pharmacokinetic profile that requires more than two compartments for an adequate description. A notable exception is amiodarone.

If the drug is administered by some route other than intravenously, it first will have to be absorbed into the circulation. A semilog plot of plasma concentration against time shows an initial increase in concentration as drug is absorbed, followed by equilibration of drug between central and peripheral compartments, and a linear elimination phase with a slope identical to the slope that would have been evidenced had the drug been administered intravenously. Absorption, like elimination, is usually a first-order process; a constant fraction of the total drug present is absorbed per unit time. As the amount of drug remaining to be absorbed diminishes, so does the rate of absorption. However, sustained-release preparations, in which drug slowly dissolves out of a wax or polymer matrix, are designed to be roughly analogous to a constant-rate infusion. This is termed zero-order absorption: a constant amount of drug is absorbed per unit time, independent of the amount of drug left to be absorbed.

It should also be mentioned that pathways of elimination (e.g., biotransformation, renal tubular secretion) may become saturated at high doses of drug, and elimination may change from a first-order to a zero-order process. This is the case for elimination of propranolol,[17] phenytoin,[18] and possibly diltiazem,[19] which exhibit first-order elimination at low doses and zero-order elimination at high doses, leading to disproportionately large increases in plasma concentration with increasing dose (Fig. 1.13).

The mathematical relationships describing the above processes provide the basis for constructing dosing schedules and are of practical utility in understanding and interpreting plasma drug concentration information.[20,21] These relationships are considered in the appendix to this chapter.

Multiple Doses

Most drugs are given as multiple doses in order to maintain an effective plasma concentration. In practice, there will be fluctuation about a mean plasma concentration between doses. The degree of the fluctuation will depend on the length of the dosing interval relative to the elimination half-life. If the dosing interval is short relative to the half-life, the fluctuation will be small, but the degree of accumulation will be large. Conversely, a long dosing interval combined with a short half-life will result in wide fluctuation but little accumulation. By definition, the plasma

Figure 1.12 Semilogarithmic plot of drug concentration against time, two-compartment model. The initial rapid fall in plasma concentration primarily reflects distribution.

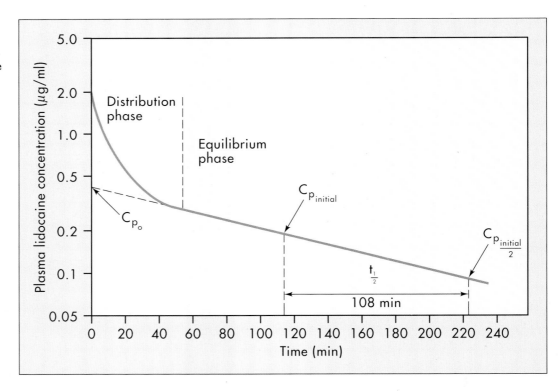

concentration of a drug administered at intervals corresponding to its half-life will show a twofold fluctuation between minimum and maximum plasma concentration. Whether a twofold fluctuation in drug concentration is acceptable will depend in large part on the width of the therapeutic window (Fig. 1.14).[22]

Steady State

By definition, following multiple dosing or continuous infusion a drug will reach "steady state" when the rate of entry into the body equals the rate of elimination. An important concept is that the time taken to reach steady state or to eliminate the drug

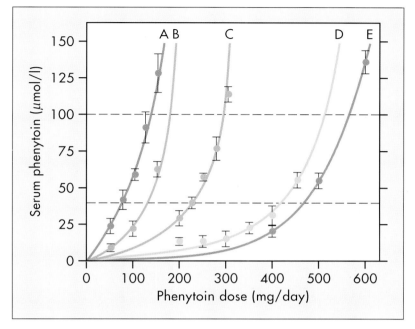

Figure 1.13 Effect of increasing phenytoin dose on plasma phenytoin concentration. The five curves represent five different patients. Dashed lines indicate therapeutic window. At low doses, increasing the dosage produces a proportional increase in plasma concentration. At high doses, as elimination pathways become saturated, increased dosage produces a disproportionately large increase in plasma concentration. (Modified from Richens A, Dunlop A: Serum phenytoin levels in the management of epilepsy. Lancet 2:247, 1975)

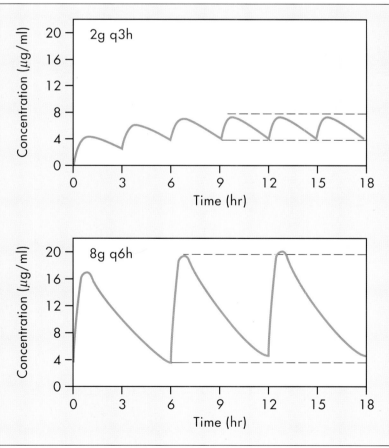

Figure 1.14 Relationship among the elimination half-life, the width of the therapeutic window, and the frequency of dosing for a rapidly absorbed and eliminated drug (in this case, procainamide). These computer simulations of plasma concentrations show that frequent dosing is required when the therapeutic window is narrow (4 μg/ml to 8 μg/ml; top panel) to avoid excessively high or low values. If the therapeutic window were wider (e.g., 4 μg/ml to 20 μg/ml; bottom panel), larger doses could be given less frequently. Since elimination half-life (139 minutes) is not changed, the time to reach steady state conditions is the same. (Modified from Roden DM, Woosley RL: Application of pharmacologic principles in the evaluation of new antiarrhythmic agents. In Morganroth J, Moore EN (eds): Sudden Cardiac Death and Congestive Heart Failure: Diagnosis and Treatment, pp 13–30. Dordrecht, Netherlands, Martinus Nijhoff, 1983)

completely is dependent only on the elimination half-life of the drug or active metabolites. Figure 1.15 illustrates the relationship between half-life and drug accumulation/elimination. It is evident that after approximately five half-lives, either process is virtually complete. Neither increasing the dose nor increasing the rate of administration will hasten achievement of the plasma concentration plateau; such maneuvers simply increase the final plasma concentration achieved (Fig. 1.16). Loading doses (see below) may allow one to reach an effective concentration sooner but do not alter the time required to reach steady state.

It also follows that factors that influence the elimination half-life also will affect the time taken to reach steady state. For instance, a reduction in liver blood flow due to diminished cardiac output or treatment with β-blockers or cimetidine can prolong the half-life of drugs that are extensively metabolized in the liver. Renal dysfunction can slow clearance and thus prolong the half-life of drugs eliminated by the kidneys. In either case it will take correspondingly longer to reach steady state, so that premature dose escalation based on the usual time taken to achieve plateau plasma levels would lead to excessive accumulation of drug. Chronic administration of drug can also be associated with changes in elimination kinetics, especially for those drugs eliminated mainly by the liver and those with hemodynamic effects that reduce splanchnic blood flow.

Loading Dose

In many instances, it is not feasible to wait four to five half-lives before effective plasma concentrations are attained. In such cases, a loading dose can be employed to initially increase plasma concentration rapidly, followed by maintenance doses to keep the plasma concentration within the therapeutic range. It will still take five half-lives to achieve steady state concentration, but an effective plasma concentration will be attained sooner. The price paid is an increased risk of reaching toxic plasma levels if the initial dose is misestimated. In addition, should the maintenance dose be too high or too low, side effects or loss of efficacy, respectively, will develop after an apparently beneficial effect due to the loading dose. Recognition that these changes in drug response are due to such simple pharmacokinetic phenomena is often delayed, or the connection is never made. If a drug is given intravenously, greater control of plasma drug concentration can be achieved by combining bolus injection(s) with rapid or maintenance infusions (Fig. 1.17).

ACTIVE METABOLITES

Although in most cases drugs are metabolized to compounds with little, or clinically inconsequential pharmacologic activity, in some instances metabolites can contribute significantly to the efficacy or toxicity

FIGURE 1.15 RELATIONSHIP BETWEEN HALF-LIFE AND EXTENT OF COMPLETION OF A FIRST-ORDER PROCESS

Number of half-lives elapsed	Amount of Drug Excreted (%)*
1	50
2	75
3	87.5
4	93.8
5	96.9
6	98.4
7	99.2

*Or accumulated to steady state.

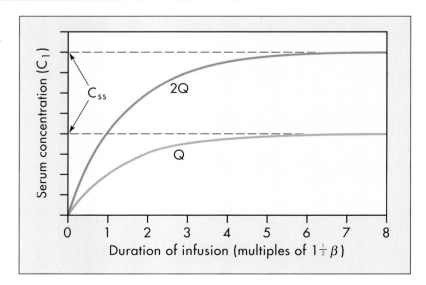

Figure 1.16 Plasma concentration against time for constant infusion of a drug at rates Q and 2Q. Note that plateau concentration is reached at the same time, independent of Q, but the plateau concentration achieved depends on Q.

observed after administration of parent drug. For instance, the monoethylglycine xylidide metabolite (MEGX) of lidocaine possesses some antiarrhythmic activity and the glycine xylidide metabolite potentiates the convulsant properties of both lidocaine and MEGX.[23] Certain metabolites of quinidine may be antiarrhythmic and may contribute to QT prolongation seen during therapy.[24] N-acetylprocainamide (NAPA), the major metabolite of procainamide, can be antiarrhythmic in its own right with electrophysiologic and clinical effects distinct from procainamide. Investigation of this metabolite has provided insight into the apparent great variability in response to procainamide. In a comparison of intravenous procainamide (before NAPA could be produced) with oral NAPA, about half the patients responded to procainamide but not NAPA, while some responded to both, and some to neither.[25] Therefore, NAPA may or may not contribute to the antiarrhythmic actions of procainamide. However, high concentrations of NAPA can certainly contribute to toxicity, including

torsade de pointes, a syndrome of polymorphic ventricular tachycardia occurring in a setting of marked prolongation of QT interval. The acetylator phenotype, which markedly influences the response to procainamide and other drugs, including hydralazine and isoniazid, which serve as substrates for N-acetyltransferase, is genetically determined and bimodally distributed. In white and black populations, the distribution between slow and fast acetylators is approximately equal, while Asians are virtually all (90%) rapid acetylators. Procainamide-induced lupus occurs more frequently and earlier in slow acetylators. Unfortunately, there is no simple way of predicting acetylator phenotype, so it may be wise to monitor both parent drug and metabolite levels on at least one sample in patients receiving these drugs. A NAPA/procainamide ratio greater than 1:1 when dosing is at steady state (and renal failure is absent) indicates a rapid acetylator phenotype. The clinician should be aware that the patient may be responding to parent drug and/or metabolite.

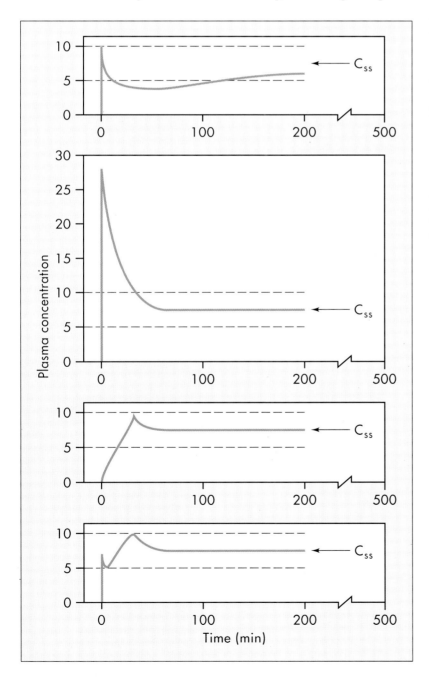

Figure 1.17 Alternatives for loading and maintenance (infusion) regimens after intravenous administration of a drug with half-life of 100 minutes. Dashed lines indicate therapeutic window; C_{ss} = drug concentration when a steady state is achieved. Dose regimens (top to bottom panels): single dose, adjusted to avoid peak levels in toxic range, later results in subtherapeutic levels; single dose large enough to ensure therapeutic levels throughout results in early plasma levels in toxic range; rapid infusion followed by maintenance infusion (double infusion technique) results in delay in achieving therapeutic levels; rapid injection followed by double infusion results in early therapeutic levels with plasma concentration maintained within the therapeutic window. (Modified from Woosley RL, Shand DG: Pharmacokinetics of antiarrhythmic drugs. Am J Cardiol 41:986, 1978)

As discussed above, the clinical implications of polymorphic metabolism will depend on the relative potencies and pharmacokinetics of the parent drug and metabolites. For example, in extensive metabolizers (EM) for P4502D6 (approximately 93% of patients) the plasma concentration of propafenone was 1.1 ± 0.6 ng/ml/mg daily dose, but for poor metabolizers (PM) the concentration was 2.5 ± 0.5 ng/ml/mg daily dose during effective therapy. Figure 1.18A demonstrates the relationship between plasma concentration and prolongation of QRS intervals, a measure of sodium channel blocking activity in a group of patients treated with propafenone. Figure 1.18B demonstrates the relationship in EM and PM and the clearly different concentration response relationships for the two groups of patients. These data indicate that the major metabolite, 5-hydroxypropafenone, contributes to the antiarrhythmic activity of propafenone. However, the parent compound but not 5-hydroxypropafenone has β-blocking activity. Therefore, EM and PM patients have similar degrees of sodium channel blockade but very different degrees of β-blocking activity.[26]

EFFECT OF DISEASE ON DRUG DISPOSITION

Drug disposition is usually determined at a fairly early stage in the development of a drug, usually using healthy young men as study volunteers. Unfortunately, the disposition of a drug in the patients for whom it is intended is often markedly different (Fig. 1.19), and other disease processes and concomitant drug therapy can further complicate matters. Although the choice of initial dosage regimens in individual patients with hepatic or renal disease is often empiric, some knowledge of the impact of various disease states on drug disposition can be a valuable adjunct to patient observation.

Liver Disease

Chronic liver disease has the most impact on drugs that are normally cleared mostly by the liver. Both drug metabolizing activity and hepatic blood flow may be reduced, with portosystemic shunting diverting portal blood (and unchanged drug) directly to the

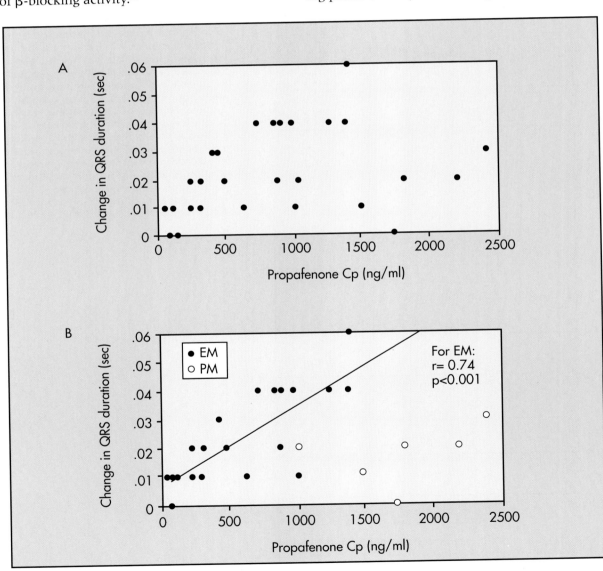

Figure 1.18 Change in QRS duration as a function of plasma concentration of propafenone. **A** Data for all patients. **B** Data for PMs (closed circles) and EMs (open circles), with linear regression fit for EMs. (C_p = plasma concentration) (Modified from Siddoway LA, Thompson KA, McAllister CB et al: Polymorphism of propafenone metabolism and disposition in man: Clinical and pharmacokinetic consequences. Circulation 75:785, 1987)

systemic circulation. These changes reduce hepatic clearance, and thus raise plasma concentrations of unchanged drug. For most drugs, reduction in dosage or increase in dosage interval is necessary to avoid toxicity. For a drug with active metabolites, the net effect would depend on the pharmacokinetics and pharmacodynamics of the metabolites compared to the parent drug. In cases where therapeutic benefit is largely derived from active metabolites, another agent, not subject to hepatic metabolism, might be considered. Aside from changes in drug disposition, there is some evidence of pharmacodynamic change for certain drugs in patients with hepatic disease. For example, the central nervous system effects of chlorpromazine are exaggerated in such patients, particularly in the presence of hepatic encephalopathy.[27]

Cardiac Failure

The decreased cardiac output and increased sympathetic tone in patients with congestive heart failure result both in diminished blood supply to the gut, liver, and kidneys, and in poor peripheral perfusion. These changes have implications for drug absorption, distribution, and elimination.

Delayed and incomplete absorption of drugs in patients with cardiac failure can be expected. For instance, cardiac patients may absorb approximately one-half as much quinidine as normal subjects, and take twice as long to reach peak plasma concentration.[28] However, because of the reduced volume of distribution, plasma concentrations attained by cardiac patients may be higher than those in control subjects (Fig. 1.20).

A decreased volume of distribution in cardiac failure has also been described for disopyramide[29] and lidocaine.[30] Cardiac failure may also result in significant changes in drug clearance, both for drugs whose clearance depends mainly on organ blood flow and those whose clearance is determined by drug metabolizing enzyme activity. Perfusion of the liver and kidneys is decreased, and a decrease in drug metabolizing enzyme activity has been found in liver biopsy specimens from patients with congestive cardiomyopathy. A direct relationship between plasma clearance of lidocaine and cardiac output has been described, with a 39% decrease in lidocaine clearance among heart failure patients compared to normal subjects.[30]

Depending on the relative magnitude of changes in clearance and volume of distribution, the elimination half-life may be unaffected or prolonged. Despite changes in clearance, the mean elimination half-lives of lidocaine,[30] procainamide,[31] and quinidine[28] appear similar in patients with and without heart failure, while those of disopyramide[29] and mexiletine[32] appear to be prolonged, with a proportionately longer time to reach steady state.

FIGURE 1.19 ANTIARRHYTHMIC DRUG ELIMINATION HALF-LIVES (MEAN OF REPORTED VALUES, HOURS)

	Normal Volunteers	Patients With Chronic Arrhythmias
Tocainide	11	14
N-acetylprocainamide	6.5	10
Mexiletine	10.5	12.5
Aprindine	22	48
Flecainide	14	20.3

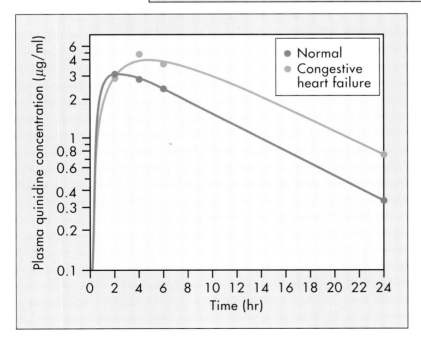

Figure 1.20 Plasma quinidine concentrations in normal subjects and in congestive heart failure patients following oral administration of 600 mg quinidine sulfate. The data points are the mean levels in ten subjects. (Modified from Crouthamel WG: The effect of congestive heart failure on quinidine pharmacokinetics. Am Heart J 90:335, 1975)

It is clear that drug therapy in patients with cardiac failure mandates the use of initial low doses with escalation under careful supervision. Prolongation of elimination half-life may also warrant less frequent dosing and less frequent changes of dose since the length of time to steady state plasma concentration is increased.

Renal Disease

Obviously, renal disease will have the most impact on those drugs eliminated mainly by the kidneys (see Fig. 1.7). However, renal disease can also affect protein binding[33] (hypoalbuminemia; presence of binding inhibitors or altered affinity of protein for drug), drug metabolism (diminished activity of some enzyme systems including *N*-acetyltransferase), and urinary pH (alkalinization can alter tubular reabsorption of drugs and the degree of ionization of weak bases, resulting in diminished excretion).

It is difficult to predict the interplay and relative contribution of these various effects to changes in drug disposition. However, for drugs that are mainly eliminated by renal excretion, one can expect decreased clearance and prolongation of elimination half-life, often in direct proportion to the decrease in creatinine clearance. For example, the half-life of digitoxin, elimination of which involves mainly extrarenal pathways, does not change in renal failure, while the half-life of digoxin, which is largely eliminated by the kidneys, increases with severe renal failure from 36 hours to about 4 days. The active metabolite of procainamide, NAPA, and the lidocaine analogue, tocainide, are eliminated by the kidneys and can accumulate to toxic levels in renal failure.[34,35] Obviously, if accumulation to toxic levels is to be avoided, less drug must be administered by either increasing the dosing interval or decreasing the dose administered.

Acute Myocardial Infarction

The patient with acute myocardial infarction (MI) presents a special challenge with respect to drug therapy. Altered hemodynamics and increased levels of AAG can markedly affect the disposition of any drug administered following myocardial infarction.

Lidocaine is one of the most frequently administered and probably the most extensively studied drug in the setting of acute MI. Administration of lidocaine to patients suspected of having sustained an infarction results in a broad range of plasma levels with accumulation of lidocaine in plasma during a constant infusion in those patients with confirmed infarction (Fig. 1.21). These changes can be largely explained by an increase in plasma protein binding as a result of increased levels of AAG.[15] Although the total plasma concentration rises parallel to AAG concentration, the free fraction declines, and free lidocaine concentration remains fairly constant. Therefore, higher than usual plasma concentrations may be well tolerated in acute myocardial infarction (concentrations greater than 6 μg/ml, normally considered toxic, have been reported to be well tolerated several days after myocardial infarction) and indeed may be necessary to maintain adequate free lidocaine levels for antiarrhythmic effect. Similar high plasma concentrations of drug when administered to patients with myocardial infarction have been reported for quinidine[13] and disopyramide.[14] In addition to increased total plasma concentration of drugs binding to AAG, the changes in drug disposition described for lowered cardiac output and renal impairment may also apply following myocardial infarction.

A further consideration in drug therapy following myocardial infarction is that the usual temporal relationship between drug administration and effect may be altered. The heart is normally a highly perfused organ so that most drugs in plasma rapidly equilibrate with myocardial tissue. However, in infarction, the areas of poorly perfused myocardium appear to

---

FIGURE 1.21 EFFECTS OF TIME ON TOTAL AND FREE PLASMA LIDOCAINE CONCENTRATIONS, AAG, AND PERCENT FREE LIDOCAINE IN EIGHT PATIENTS WITH MYOCARDIAL INFARCTION ON A CONSTANT 2 MG/MIN INFUSION (MEAN AND RANGE)

	Time (hr)			
	12	24	36	48
Total lidocaine (μg/ml)	3.15 (1.9–4.1)	3.38 (1.7–4.5)	3.61 (1.6–4.7)	4.23* (2.7–6)
Free lidocaine (μg/ml)	0.99 (0.67–1.25)	0.99 (0.58–1.48)	1.02 (0.54–1.28)	1.11 (0.84–1.43)
AAG (mg/dl)	95 (57–127)	101 (61–137)	108 (78–136)	120*† (91–152)
Free lidocaine (%)	0.31 (0.25–0.39)	0.30 (0.22–0.34)	0.29 (0.22–0.39)	0.27† (0.21–0.32)

*p < 0.03 at 12, 24, and 36 hr
†p < 0.03 at 12 and 24 hr

(From Routledge PA, Shand DG, Barchowsky A et al: Relationship between alpha-1-acid glycoprotein and lidocaine disposition in myocardial infarction. Clin Pharmacol Ther 30:154, 1981) accumulate (and eliminate) drug far more slowly than does the rest of the heart.[36] Thus, such areas function as peripheral, rather than central, pharmacokinetic compartments and, depending on the drug's effector site, there may be a corresponding delay between drug administration and pharmacologic effect.

Age

Drug disposition in both the elderly and the very young can vary widely from that in the young adult population in which it is usually defined. Deterioration of renal and hepatic function, or immaturity of these processes, can result in significant changes in the pharmacokinetic variables. For example, the half-life of inulin (eliminated by glomerular filtration) in an infant is approximately three times that in an adult. In addition, the extremes of age may be associated with changes in sensitivity to drugs. For example, elderly patients have a reduced response to β-receptor agonists and antagonists. The likely explanation in this case is a reduction in the number of β-receptors with age.[37] On the other hand, an increased sensitivity to benzodiazepines[38] and coumarin anticoagulants[39] has been noted in elderly patients. Unfortunately, few drugs have been systematically evaluated in either the very young or the elderly, and information has often been gained through anecdotes or adverse clinical experiences, sometimes at considerable human expense (e.g., chloramphenicol and the "gray baby" syndrome).

THERAPEUTIC DRUG MONITORING

The usefulness of drug plasma concentrations as a means of guiding therapy presupposes a correlation between pharmacologic effect and plasma concentration of a drug. In addition, it presupposes that the plasma concentration correlates better with pharmacologic effect than does dose. While this is generally true, there are instances when plasma concentration can be misleading. For example, a pharmacologic effect may persist even after drug has been eliminated from plasma. Often, this may be accounted for by the presence of an active metabolite (e.g., propafenone), or some irreversible action of the drug that requires physiologic regeneration for termination of effect (e.g., depletion of catecholamine stores by reserpine). In some cases there may be a temporal delay between plasma concentration and effect that may be the result of the drug's receptor site residing in a poorly perfused tissue, or a tissue into which drug only diffuses slowly (e.g., digoxin diffuses slowly into myocardial tissue so that its cardiac effects are not apparent for an hour or more after intravenous administration) (Fig. 1.22).[40]

Further complications are poorly defined therapeutic ranges (the usually quoted therapeutic range for quinidine is derived using a nonspecific assay and is based mainly on 30-year-old data on conversion of atrial fibrillation[41]) and great interpatient variability in response. Part of this variability is explained by the fact that the free, unbound drug is considered pharmacologically active, while most therapeutic ranges are based on total plasma concentration of

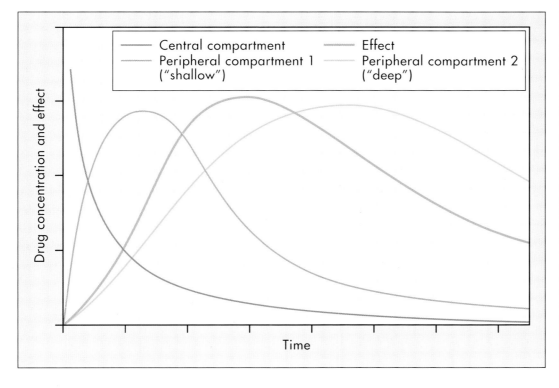

Figure 1.22 The relationship between changes in response and changes in concentration of drug throughout various body compartments of a three-compartment pharmacokinetic model. Note that the effect curve is not in phase with drug concentration in any kinetic compartment and is least well represented by that in the central (plasma) compartment. Such a relationship is illustrative of data obtained after intravenous digoxin administration, where the effect curve could reflect shortening of the QS$_2$ interval or reduction in the left ventricular ejection time. (Modified from Whiting B, Kelman AW: The modelling of drug response. Clin Sci 59:311, 1980)

the drug (free drug plus that quantity bound to plasma protein). The extent of binding to plasma protein varies considerably. A range of 51% to 87% among normal subjects has been quoted for quinidine[42]; it is likely that variability among patients is greater. The situation could be improved by monitoring free drug rather than total plasma drug concentration, since this should correlate better with pharmacologic effect. For example, acute ECG changes due to intravenous quinidine[43] and disopyramide[44] correlate well with free, but not total, drug levels. Unfortunately, free levels of drug are rarely measured, partly because they are often too low for accurate measurement by conventional methods. It also should be mentioned that drug concentrations in whole blood or serum are not equivalent to plasma concentration. The ratio of blood to plasma concentration is related to the hematocrit, the affinity of the drug for blood cells, and the protein binding. Determination in serum carries the potential of loss of drug adsorbed to clots. Finally, drugs frequently exert their effects in peripheral compartments; thus the plasma sample will best reflect the peripheral compartment concentration after the distribution phase has passed.

The specificity of the drug assay also should be taken into consideration when interpreting drug level data. Is the assay specific for unchanged drug, or does it also include metabolites that may themselves possess pharmacologic activity and distinct pharmacokinetics? Newer, more specific assays, measuring parent drug alone, may not correlate well with a therapeutic range based on older, nonspecific assays or, more importantly, with drug action.

Data on drug concentration in plasma can only be useful if accompanied by some knowledge of the dosing history, when the sample was obtained relative to the dosing interval, clinical response, concomitant medication, and other disease processes. Only then can the measured concentration be evaluated in a meaningful way. Finally, drug levels are only an adjunct to clinical judgment. Some patients respond (or even develop side effects) at low concentrations, while others may require high concentrations to achieve efficacy and tolerate these concentrations without side effects.

Conclusion

Currently available cardiovascular agents are limited by side effects and the potential for exacerbating the condition being treated. In addition, altered disposition of drug as a result of changes in protein binding or concomitant disease processes, active metabolites, drug interactions, and poorly defined therapeutic ranges with great interpatient variability are some of the factors that complicate therapy. The optimal use of these drugs requires an understanding of their pharmacokinetics and pharmacodynamics. The considerations presented here can serve only as a first approximation in determining a suitable drug regimen. Clinical observation then allows at least some appreciation of how a particular patient handles a drug. With an understanding of basic pharmacologic principles, the patient's response to and disposition of drug at other doses can then be predicted at the initiation of therapy and adjusted intelligently during therapy. A grasp of such principles is invaluable in both the choice of drug and the establishment of an optimum benefit-to-risk ratio for the patient.

Appendix: Mathematical Considerations
Pharmacokinetic Model

A number of simple mathematical relationships describe the fate of drug in the body. Following intravenous administration, the plasma concentration of a drug (C_p) declines with time (t) from its initial concentration (C_0) at a rate proportional to C_p:

$$\frac{dC_p}{dt} = -k_e C_p \tag{1}$$

where k_e is the proportionality or rate constant of elimination. Integrating equation (1) gives

$$C_p = C_0 e^{-k_e t} \tag{2}$$

and taking logarithms

$$\log_e C_p = \log_e C_0 - \frac{k_e t}{2.303}$$

Thus, a semilogarithmic plot of C_p against t yields a straight line with y-intercept $\log C_0$ and slope $-k_e/2.303$. Since the elimination half-life ($t_{1/2}$) is, by definition, the time taken for C_p to be reduced to $C_p/2$, substituting into equation (2) yields

$$\frac{C_p}{2} = C_p e^{-k_e t_{1/2}}$$

from which it can be shown that

$$t_{1/2} = \frac{0.693}{k_e} \tag{3}$$

Note that these considerations should apply equally well to absorption kinetics, when absorption is a first-order process. Then k is the absorption rate constant, and $t_{1/2}$ is the absorption half-life. The semilogarithmic plot also allows calculation of volume of a distribution (V_d), since

$$V_d = \frac{D}{C_0}$$

where D is the administered dose.

Since total clearance (Cl) is the volume of plasma from which drug is completely removed per unit time,

$$Cl = k_e V_d \qquad (4)$$

Combining equations (3) and (4),

$$t_{1/2} = \frac{0.693 V_d}{Cl}$$

Thus, elimination half-life depends on both the volume of distribution and the clearance. In multicompartment models similar considerations apply. For intravenous injection with distribution and elimination phases.

$$C_p = Ae^{-\alpha t} + Be^{-\beta t}$$

where the first term may be viewed as corresponding to the distribution process, while the second term describes elimination. Both terms contribute to the calculation of C_0 and k_e while several volumes of distribution can be defined. Equilibrium volume of distribution (often designated V_{dss}) will be the sum of all the compartment volumes in which the drug is distributed. Both the volume of the central compartment, and V_{dss} are important in determining intravenous dose requirements.

Constant Infusion

If a drug is administered by constant infusion at rate Q into a simple one-compartment model then, assuming first-order elimination, C_p changes with time:

$$\frac{dC_p}{dt} = \text{infusion rate} - \text{elimination rate}$$

$$= \frac{Q}{V_d} - k_e C_p$$

Integrating gives

$$C_p = \frac{Q}{k_e V_d}(1 - e^{-k_e t})$$

As t approaches infinity, $(1 - e^{-k_e t})$ approaches 1, and

$$C_p = \frac{Q}{k_e V_d} = C_{ss} \qquad (5)$$

where C_{ss} is the plasma concentration at steady state. Stated another way, at steady state, drug input equals drug output:

$$\frac{Q}{V_d} = k_e C_{ss}$$

Since

$$k_e = \frac{Cl}{V_d}$$

substitution into equation (5) yields

$$C_{ss} = \frac{Q}{Cl} \qquad (6)$$

Multiple Doses

Multiple doses, whether intravenous, oral, or intramuscular, generally can be thought of as extensions of the case above. Thus, following oral administration, and assuming constant-rate absorption over the dosing interval (as an approximation to the more usual first-order kinetics of absorption):

$$Q = \text{amount of drug absorbed / dose interval}$$

$$= \frac{fD}{\tau}$$

where f is the fraction bioavailable, D is the dose, and τ is the dose interval. Substituting in equation (6) for Q

$$C_{ss} = \frac{fD}{Cl\tau}$$

Recall that if a drug is completely bioavailable, $f = 1$.

Although the arguments presented here adequately describe the kinetics of many drugs, they are, of course, a very simplified approach to complex physiologic processes, more detailed analyses of which are always possible.

Pharmacodynamic Model

The relationship between drug dose or concentration and effect is termed pharmacodynamics. As in the case of pharmacokinetics, we often attempt to describe this relationship using equations. The primary reason these equations are used is that they have been found empirically to describe the observations. At best, both pharmacokinetic and pharmacodynamic equations are greatly simplified models of physiology. While the basis for pharmacokinetic models has become the compartment, with drug movement between compartments described by first-order differential equations, the basis for pharmacodynamic models is often the same equation that describes enzyme kinetics or binding of a ligand to a receptor.

The correlate of drug effect will again be the concentration of drug–receptor complex. The drug effect will be assumed to be proportional to the drug–receptor complex concentration. We will assume that the total number of receptors remains constant, which is usually true over short periods. A dynamic equilibrium will be established between unoccupied receptors, free drug, and drug–receptor complexes (Fig. 1.23).

The rate of formation of the drug–receptor complex will be proportional to the concentration of drug, and to the concentration of free receptor, assuming that they combine in a one-to-one ratio. The rate of degradation of the drug–receptor complex will be proportional to the concentration of drug–receptor complex; if there is twice as much drug–receptor complex, twice as much will break down into free drug and unoccupied receptor in a given time period. At steady state, the formation of drug–receptor complexes will equal the breakdown of drug–receptor complexes, or

$$C_D R_F K_1 = R_D K_2$$

where C_D is the concentration of free drug, R_F is the concentration of free receptor, and R_D is the concentration of drug–receptor complex. Solving for concentration of drug–receptor complex,

$$R_D = \frac{C_D R_F K_1}{K_2} \qquad (7)$$

We will define K_2/K_1 to be K_d for the dissociation constant.

The total receptor concentration R_T will equal the concentration of occupied receptors, plus the concentration of free receptors.

$$R_T = R_D + R_F$$

Solving for R_F and substituting into equation (7),

$$R_D = \frac{C_D(R_T - R_D)}{K_d}$$

Solving for R_D,

$$R_D = \frac{C_D R_T}{K_d + C_D}$$

If the drug effect E is proportional to the concentration of drug–receptor complex, this equation will be multiplied by a constant:

$$E = \frac{K R_T C_D}{K_d + C_D}$$

As we do not generally know the total concentration of receptors, this can be combined with the constant.

$$E = \frac{K C_D}{K_d + C_D}$$

If all the receptors were occupied, we would have the maximal effect, or the constant times the total concentration of receptors. This constant ($K R_T$) will be called $E_{\max}$ for maximal possible effect. When the concentration of drug is equal to K_d, the expression will reduce to

$$E = \frac{E_{\max}}{2}$$

Therefore, this constant (K_d) is called C_{50}, or the concentration that produces half of the maximal effect. The final expression drug effect then is:

$$E = \frac{E_{\max} C_D}{C_{50} + C_D}$$

$E_{\max}$ thus describes the maximal effect that the drug can elicit, and C_{50} is a measure of the potency of the drug.

It may happen that more than one drug molecule must occupy a receptor site for activation. In the case of two receptor sites, the rate of formation of drug–receptor complex will be proportional to the square of the concentration of drug. This is because two independent events must occur: the binding of the first molecule and the binding of the second molecule. The rules of probability state that the probability of two independent events occurring is equal to the product of the probability of each. Therefore, at equilibrium,

$$C_D{}^2 R_F K_1 = R_D K_2$$

Following through the same algebra gives the expression

$$E = \frac{E_{\max} C_D{}^2}{K_d + C_D{}^2}$$

The exponent 2 gives rise to the sigmoidosity of the relationship. This is often called a sigmoid $E_{\max}$ function. In order for the constant K_d to be equal to the concentration that elicits 50% of the maximal effect, this must also be raised to the power n. The general equation for $E_{\max}$/sigmoid $E_{\max}$ model, then, is

$$E = \frac{E_{\max} C_D{}^n}{C_{50}{}^n + C_D{}^n}$$

In general it is not true that n represents the number of drug molecules that must bind to the receptor. Often, n is found not to be an integer, and occasionally it is found to be less than one. The simpler $E_{\max}$ model is a special case of the sigmoid $E_{\max}$, with the exponent equal to 1.

Figure 1.23 An equilibrium is established between drug, free receptors, and drug–receptor complexes. The rate of formation of drug–receptor complex will be proportional to the concentration of both drug and receptor; the rate of dissociation of drug–receptor complex will be proportional to the concentration of the complex.

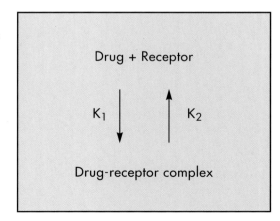

Cardiovascular Pharmacology

REFERENCES

1. Raftery EF: Cardiovascular drug withdrawal syndromes. A potential problem with calcium antagonists? Drugs 28:371, 1984
2. Giacomini JC, Nelson WL, Theodore L et al: The pharmacokinetics and pharmacodynamics of D- and DL-verapamil in rabbits. J Cardiovasc Pharmacol 7:469, 1985
3. Murad F, Rapoport RM, Fiscus R: Role of cyclic-GMP in relaxations of vascular smooth muscle. J Cardiovasc Pharmacol 7(Suppl 3):5111, 1985
4. Roden DM, Reele SB, Higgins SB et al: Tocainide therapy for refractory ventricular arrhythmias. Am Heart J 100:15, 1980
5. Prescott LF, Clements JA, Pottage A: Absorption, distribution and elimination of mexiletine. Postgrad Med J 53(Suppl 1):50, 1977
6. Buchert E, Woosley RL: Clinical implications of variable antiarrhythmic drug metabolism. Pharmacogenetics 2:2, 1992
7. Bauer LA, Edwards WAD, Randolph FP, Blouin RA: Cimetidine-induced decrease in lidocaine metabolism. Am Heart J 108:413, 1984
8. Feely J, Wilkinson GR, Wood AJJ: Reduction of liver blood flow and propranolol metabolism by cimetidine. N Engl J Med 304:692, 1981
9. Bax NDS, Tucker GT, Lennard MS, Woods HF: The impairment of lignocaine clearance by propranolol-major contribution from enzyme inhibition. Br J Clin Pharmacol 19:597, 1985
10. Marcus SL: Drug interactions with amiodarone. Am Heart J 106:924, 1983
11. Kaye CM, Kiddie MA, Turner P: Variable pharmacokinetics of mexiletine. Postgrad Med J 53(Suppl 1):56, 1977
12. Piafsky KM: Disease-induced changes in the plasma binding of basic drugs. Clin Pharmacokinetics 5:246, 1980
13. David BM, Whifford EG, Ilett KF: Disopyramide binding to alpha-1-acid glycoprotein: Sequential effects following acute myocardial infarction. Clin Exp Pharmacol Physiol 9:478, 1982
14. Kessler KM, Kissane B, Cassidy J et al: Dynamic variability of binding of antiarrhythmic drugs during the evolution of acute myocardial infarction. Circulation 70:472, 1984
15. Routledge PA, Shand DG, Barchowsky A et al: Relationship between alpha-1-acid glycoprotein and lidocaine disposition in myocardial infarction. Clin Exp Pharmacol Ther 30:154, 1981
16. Meffin PJ, Robert EW, Winkle RA et al: Role of concentration dependent plasma protein binding in disopyramide disposition. J Pharmacokinet Biopharm 7:29, 1979
17. Wood AJJ, Carr RK, Vestal RE et al: Direct measurement of propranolol bioavailability during accumulation to steady state. Br J Clin Pharmacol 6:345, 1978
18. Richens A, Dunlop A: Serum phenytoin levels in the management of epilepsy. Lancet 2:247, 1975
19. McAllister RG, Hamann SR, Blouin RA: Pharmacokinetics of calcium-entry blockers. Am J Cardiol 55:30B, 1985
20. Greenblatt DJ, Koch-Weser J: Clinical pharmacokinetics, Part II. N Engl J Med 293:964, 1975
21. Woosley RL, Shand DG: Pharmacokinetics of antiarrhythmic drugs. Am J Cardiol 41:986, 1978
22. Roden DM, Woosley RL: Application of pharmacologic principles in the evaluation of new antiarrhythmic agents. In Morganroth J, Moore EN (eds): Sudden Cardiac Death and Congestive Heart Failure: Diagnosis and Treatment, pp 13–30. Dordrecht, Netherlands, Martinus Nijhoff, 1983
23. Narang PK, Crouthamel WG, Carliner NH, Fisher ML: Lidocaine and its active metabolites. Clin Pharmacol Ther 25:654,1978
24. Holford NHG, Coates PE, Guentert TW, Riegelman S, Sheiner LB: The effect of quinidine and its metabolites on the electrocardiogram and systolic time intervals: Concentration-effect relationships. Br J Clin Pharmacol 11:187, 1981
25. Roden DM, Reele SB, Higgins SB et al: Antiarrhythmic efficacy, pharmacokinetics and safety of N-acetylprocainamide in human subjects: Comparison with procainamide. Am J Cardiol 46:463, 1980
26. Lee JT, Kroemer HK, Silberstein DJ et al: The role of genetically determined polymorphic drug metabolism in the beta-blockade produced by propafenone. N Engl J Med 322:1164, 1990
27. Maxwell JD, Carrella M, Parkes JD et al: Plasma disappearance and cerebral effects of chlorpromazine in cirrhosis. Clin Sci 43:143, 1972
28. Crouthamel WG: The effect of congestive heart failure on quinidine pharmacokinetics. Am Heart J 90:335, 1975
29. Landmark K, Bredesen JE, Thaulow E et al: Pharmacokinetics of disopyramide in patients with imminent to moderate cardiac failure. Eur J Clin Pharmacol 19:187, 1981
30. Thomson PD, Melmon KL, Richardson JA et al: Lidocaine pharmacokinetics in advanced heart failure, liver disease, and renal failure in humans. Ann Intern Med 78:499, 1973
31. Kessler KM, Kayden DS, Estes D et al: Procainamide pharmacokinetics/pharmacodynamics in acute myocardial infarction or congestive heart failure. Circulation 70(Suppl II):II-446, 1984
32. Leahey EB Jr, Giardina EGV, Bigger JT Jr: Effect of ventricular failure on steady state kinetics of mexiletine. Clin Res 26:239A, 1980
33. Reidenberg MM, Drayer DE: Alteration of drug-protein binding in renal disease. Clin Pharmacokinet 9(Suppl):18, 1984
34. Drayer DE, Lowenthal DT, Woosley RL et al: Cumulation of N-acetylprocainamide, an active metabolite of procainamide, in patients with impaired renal function. Clin Pharmacol Ther 22:63, 1977
35. Weigers U, Hanrath P, Kuck KH et al: Pharmacokinetics of tocainide in patients with renal dysfunction and during hemodialysis. Eur J Clin Pharmacol 24:503, 1983
36. Wenger TL, Browning DJ, Masterton CE et al: Procainamide delivery to ischemic canine myocardium following rapid intravenous administration. Circ Res 46:789, 1980
37. Vestal RE, Wood AJJ, Shand DG: Reduced β-adrenoreceptor sensitivity in the elderly. Clin Pharmacol Ther 26:181, 1979
38. Reidenberg MM, Levy M, Warner H et al: Relationship between diazepam dose, plasma level,

age, and central nervous system depression. Clin Pharmacol Ther 23:371, 1978

39. Husted S, Andreasen F: The influence of age on the response to anticoagulants. Br J Clin Pharmacol 4:559, 1977

40. Whiting B, Kelman AW: The modelling of drug response. Clin Sci 59:311, 1980

41. Sokolow M, Ball RE: Factors influencing conversion of chronic atrial fibrillation with special reference to serum quinidine concentration. Circulation 14:568, 1956

42. Kates RE, Sokoloski TD, Comstock TJ: Binding of quinidine to plasma proteins in normal subjects and in patients with hyperlipoproteinemias. Clin Pharmacol Ther 23:30, 1978

43. Woo E, Greenblatt DJ: Pharmacokinetic and clinical implications of quinidine-protein binding. J Pharmaceut Sci 68:466, 1979

44. North FC, Mitchell LB, Wyse DG, Duff HJ: Electrophysiologic responses to free and total disopyramide concentrations in patients with inducible sustained ventricular tachycardia. Circulation 70:II-442, 1984

GENERAL REFERENCES

Benet LZ, Massoud N, Gabertoglio JG (eds): Pharmacokinetic Basis for Drug Treatment. New York, Raven Press, 1984

Holford NHG, Sheiner LB: Understanding of dose-effect relationship: Clinical application of pharmacokinetic-pharmacodynamic models. Clin Pharmacokinet 6:429, 1981

Kupersmith J: Monitoring of antiarrhythmic drug levels: Values and pitfalls. Ann NY Acad Sci 432:138, 1984

Lefkowitz RJ, Michel T: Plasma membrane receptors. J Clin Invest 72:1185, 1983

Molinoff PB: α- and β-Adrenergic receptor subtypes. Properties, distribution and regulation. Drugs 28(Suppl 2):1, 1984

Sweeney GD: Variability in the human drug response. Thromb Res 30(Suppl IV):3, 1983

Williams RL: Drug administration in hepatic disease. N Engl J Med 309:1616, 1983

Woosley RL, Roden DM: Importance of metabolites in antiarrhythmic therapy. Am J Cardiol 52:8C, 1983

Diuretics

Arnold M. Chonko

Jared J. Grantham

Many cardiovascular diseases interfere with the normal renal excretion of sodium, chloride, and water, leading to their retention in an expanded extracellular fluid compartment. Diuretic drugs promote the renal loss of solutes and water and by these actions they can be extremely useful in the treatment of edematous states.

The principal mechanisms and clinical utility of diuretics are best understood in the context of the perturbed physiology of renal salt and water handling that occurs in various cardiovascular abnormalities. But first a brief review of normal renal salt and water handling is in order.

REVIEW OF RENAL PHYSIOLOGY: SALT AND WATER HANDLING

Figure 2.1 is a schematic diagram of the mammalian nephron and the various transport processes that occur along its course. Each kidney is composed of about 1 million nephrons. Renal plasma flow averages about one tenth of the cardiac output under usual circumstances (500 ml/min).[1]

Renal blood flow is critically dependent on cardiac output and systemic arterial blood pressure. In the range of mean arterial pressures from 80 to nearly

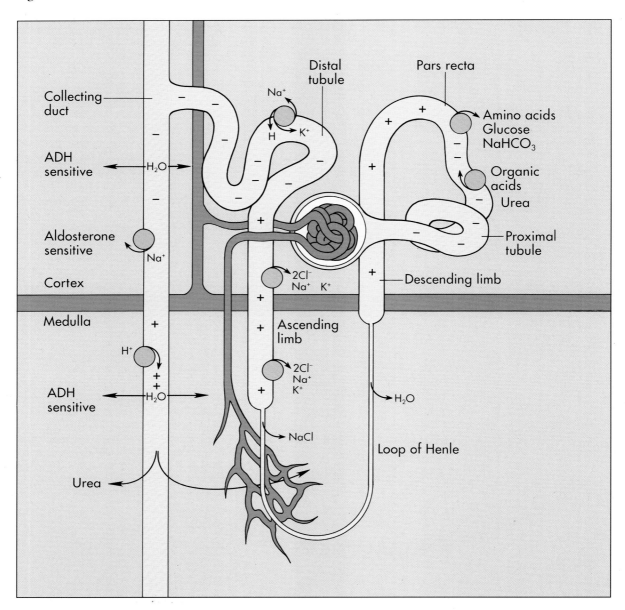

Figure 2.1 Sites of tubule salt and water absorption. Sodium is reabsorbed with inorganic anions, amino acids, and glucose in the proximal tubule against an electrical gradient that is lumen negative. In the late part of the proximal tubule (pars recta), sodium and water are reabsorbed to a lesser extent and organic acids (hippurate, urate) and urea are secreted into the urine. The electrical potential is lumen positive in the pars recta. Water, not salt, is removed from tubule fluid in the thin descending limb of Henle's loop, but in the ascending portion salt is reabsorbed without water, rendering the tubule fluid hypos-motic with respect to the interstitium. Sodium, chloride, and potassium are reabsorbed by the medullary and cortical portions of the ascending limb; the lumen potential is positive. Sodium is reabsorbed and potassium and hydrogen ions are secreted in the distal tubule and collecting ducts. Water absorption in these segments is regulated by antidiuretic hormone (ADH). The electrical potential is lumen negative in the cortical sections and positive in the medullary segments. Urea is concentrated in the interstitium of the medulla and assists in the generation of maximally concentrated urine.

can be lowered to less than 1 mEq/l in these segments. Urine is also maximally concentrated in collecting ducts in response to maximal plasma levels of antidiuretic hormone. Potassium is also secreted by the collecting ducts.

It is important to recognize that sodium and water excretion can be regulated by separate mechanisms. Sodium excretion is dependent on GFR, aldosterone, and atrial natriuretic factors (and other unknown natriuretic factors).[6] The osmotic concentration of the urine depends primarily on the GFR and the plasma antidiuretic hormone level. As shown in Figure 2.2, only about 1% of the filtered sodium and water normally remain at the end of the renal tubules.

Principles of Diuretic Action
Types of Diuresis
There are two general types of diuresis: solute and water diuresis (Fig. 2.3). Solute diuresis develops when the transtubular reabsorption of solute is impaired and the solute entering the tubule lumen by glomerular filtration is not absorbed to a normal extent. Inhibition of salt transport in the renal tubule diminishes osmotic water absorption, and a solute diuresis ensues. Salt absorption can be inhibited in two ways. First, a substance such as mannitol may be

freely filtered into the urine; however, mannitol is not absorbed by tubules and the impermeant solute reduces the osmotic absorption of water.[3,7] Agents that act principally as nonabsorbable filtered solutes are known collectively as osmotic diuretics. Solute diuresis can also result from inhibition of active salt reabsorption in the tubule cell (see Fig. 2.3). Pharmacologic agents interact with the machinery of transport to slow the absorption of solute and, secondarily, the osmotic absorption of fluid. Most potent diuretic drugs interfere with solute movement across urinary plasma membranes.

Water diuresis without a corresponding increase in solute loss may be induced by pharmacologic means (see Fig. 2.3). Agents that block the cellular action of vasopressin may cause water loss without a concurrent increase in solute excretion.

Cellular Mechanisms of Diuretic Action
In general, sodium and chloride enter renal cells from the urine by association with special transport proteins in the urinary membrane. The movement of these ions is dissipative, that is, down electrochemical gradients. The gradient for the entry of sodium is established at the basolateral membrane where the cation is pumped out of the cells by the sodium pump, also known as the Na^+,K^+-ATPase pump.

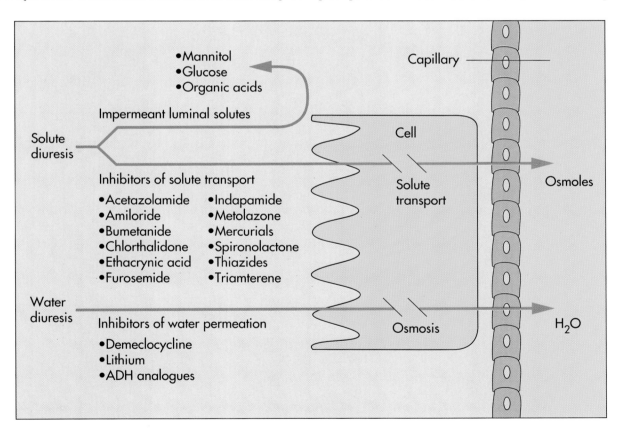

Figure 2.3 Principles of diuretic action. See text for details. (Modified from Grantham JJ, Chonko AM: Diuretics. In Brenner BM, Stein JH (eds): Topics in Nephrology, pp 178–209. New York, Churchill Livingstone, 1978)

Chloride appears to move into the cell coupled to the downhill movement of sodium and leaves the cells across the basolateral membrane down an electrochemical gradient.

Diuretics act primarily from the urine side to interfere with the coupling of sodium and other solute movement from urine to cytoplasm. It is clear that the loop diuretics (furosemide, ethacrynic acid, and bumetanide) act to block sodium, potassium, and chloride cotransport (Fig. 2.4). In the cortical distal tubule and collecting tubules amiloride and triamterene inhibit sodium entry into the cells from the lumen (Fig. 2.5).

Acetazolamide does not interact with sodium directly in the lumen membrane, but this carbonic anhydrase inhibitor effectively acts from the urinary side by diminishing first the absorption of bicarbonate from the urine, and secondarily that of sodium.[3,8]

Spironolactone acts primarily from the basolateral side of the tubule cells (see Fig. 2.5). It competes with aldosterone for cellular receptors, and in this way the effect of the hormone is diminished. Aldosterone potentiates sodium absorption by increasing the movement of sodium from urine to cytoplasm and by increasing the activity of the sodium pump.

There are several interesting consequences of the site and mechanism of action of pharmacologic diuretics. Since most act primarily from the urine side, they must either be filtered or secreted into the urine to be effective. Many of the drugs are highly protein bound and are not filtered appreciably. The concentration of the diuretics in the urine by the combined processes of water absorption and tubular diuretic secretion leads to relatively high levels in the tubule fluid. This feature accounts for the apparent selective action within the kidney that spares other organs from the effects of the agents.

Recent work has revealed a powerful endogenous diuretic synthesized and stored in the atria of humans and other animals. This new diuretic is referred to as atrial natriuretic factor, cardionatrin, or atriopeptin, depending on the laboratory of record.[6] It is a polypeptide substance that is released from the atria in response to extracellular fluid volume expansion. The atrial factor decreases intrarenal vascular resistance and increases GFR. In addition, the peptide may decrease tubular sodium chloride reabsorption in the medullary collecting duct.[9] The diuresis caused by the peptide is very impressive in experimental animals. The possible role of this substance in the regulation of body salt and water balance is under intensive study.

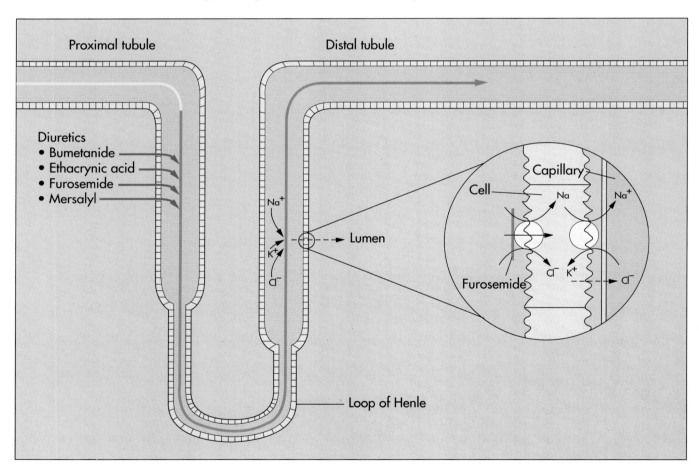

Figure 2.4 Mechanism of action of "loop" diuretics. The diuretics are secreted by proximal tubules and interfere with the luminal uptake of sodium, potassium, and chloride by cells of the ascending limb of Henle's loop. (Modified from Grantham JJ, Chonko AM: Diuretics. In Brenner BM, Stein JH (eds): Topics in Nephrology, pp 178–209. New York, Churchill Livingstone, 1978)

Action of Diuretics on Nephron Segments

The nephron loci at which diuretic drugs exert their major inhibitory actions on salt and water transport are shown in Figures 2.4 through 2.6.

GLOMERULUS

Heretofore, it had been impossible to separate the glomerular from the tubular effects of diuretic drugs; however, Deen and associates[10] and Savin and Terreros[11] have devised experimental techniques that allow for a direct examination of glomerular filtration. From these studies, it appears that physiologic and pharmacologic substances may alter the GFR directly by changing either the rate of renal plasma flow, by means of afferent and efferent arteriolar constriction or dilation, or by changes in the ultrafiltration coefficient (K_f) of the filtration barrier. Diuretic drugs set into motion a cascade of secondary events

such as renin release and, in turn, generation of angiotensin, aldosterone, antidiuretic hormone, and intrarenal prostaglandins. These substances may exert significant influences on the glomerular filtration barrier. There are currently no reports to indicate that diuretics have direct effects on the hydraulic permeability of the glomerular filtration barrier.

PROXIMAL TUBULE

The proximal tubule is a segment in which diuretics of even minor action could exert profound effects on urinary salt excretion since approximately 60% of the glomerular filtrate is reabsorbed here. Mannitol and other "osmotic" agents have only a small diuretic effect in the proximal tubule, and none of the clinically useful pharmacologic agents have a detectable effect in this segment.

Other diuretics (furosemide, ethacrynic acid, thiazides) can potentially inhibit salt and water absorp-

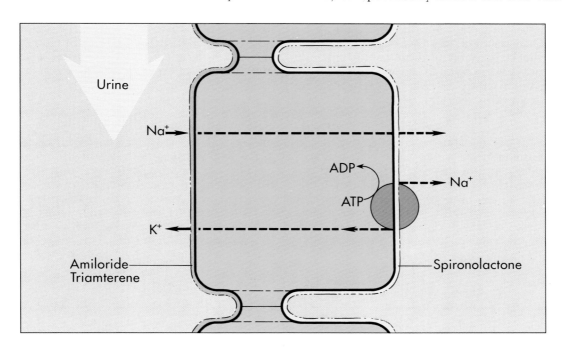

Figure 2.5 Mechanism of action of distal and collecting tubule diuretics. Spironolactone interferes with the effect of aldosterone to increase the rate of sodium–potassium exchange at the basolateral surface. Amiloride and triamterene interact with lumen membrane transporters to prevent the entry of urinary sodium into the cytoplasm. The net effect of all these drugs is to decrease sodium absorption and potassium secretion.

Figure 2.6 Sites of the renal tubule where diuretics have their major effect.

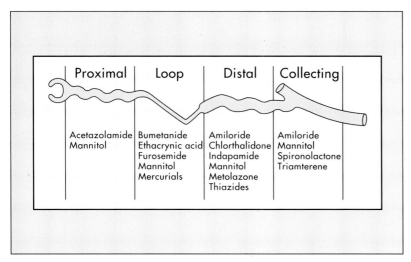

Proximal	Loop	Distal	Collecting
Acetazolamide	Bumetanide	Amiloride	Amiloride
Mannitol	Ethacrynic acid	Chlorthalidone	Mannitol
	Furosemide	Indapamide	Spironolactone
	Mannitol	Mannitol	Triamterene
	Mercurials	Metolazone	
		Thiazides	

tion proximally, but in sustained states of plasma volume contraction caused by these agents, the proximal tubules absorb proportionately *more* salt and water than normal. This paradoxic feature of many diuretics is a reflection of the so-called braking phenomenon observed with the chronic use of diuretics.

Acetazolamide causes diuresis by inhibiting the absorption of bicarbonate from the proximal tubule fluid. When bicarbonate absorption is impaired this impermeant anion obligates sodium and water to be held in the urine. Acetazolamide is the drug with the most dependable proximal site of action, but its effect leads to metabolic acidosis due to bicarbonaturia.

LOOP OF HENLE

No diuretics are known to be effective in the initial portion of the ascending limb of Henle's loop. The medullary and cortical portions of the ascending limb are the site of action of several potent diuretics: bumetanide, furosemide, ethacrynic acid, and mercurials.[2,12,13] Each agent causes a diuresis typified by chloruresis. Current evidence favors the view that the diuretics block the entry of these solutes into the cell at a common cotransport carrier located at the urinary plasma membrane (see Fig. 2.4). Thiazides do not appear to act in this segment.

DISTAL CONVOLUTED TUBULE

Thiazide derivatives inhibit salt transport in this segment of the nephron, but the cellular mechanism of action is unknown. Metolazone and indapamide act here as well. Amiloride and triamterene inhibit salt and water transport in the distal convoluted tubule by blocking luminal sodium channels. The action of aldosterone in this segment is competitively inhibited by spironolactone (see Fig. 2.5).

COLLECTING SYSTEM

The collecting system is crucial in the context of all diuretic action, for any inhibitory action of diuretics proximal to the collecting segments can be outweighed by enhanced salt and water absorption in these terminal segments. Amiloride inhibits sodium absorption by interfering with the transport of sodium across the urinary membrane (see Fig. 2.5). This action reduces the activity of the basolateral sodium pump, which in turn decreases potassium secretion.

The action of aldosterone can be inhibited with spironolactone but the diuretic effectiveness of spironolactone depends on whether aldosterone has a significant primary or secondary role to increase sodium reabsorption.

The collecting system is the principal segment where vasopressin mediates increased water absorption. Inhibition of the antidiuretic hormone effect leads to a water diuresis. Lithium in therapeutic doses for the treatment of manic-depressive illnesses causes nephrogenic diabetes insipidus. The cellular basis for the inhibitory effect of lithium on the vasopressin response is not clear. Demeclocycline also blocks the renal tubular action of vasopressin.[14,15]

RENAL HANDLING OF DIURETIC DRUGS

Most clinically useful diuretic drugs are organic anions at physiologic pH, are highly bound to serum proteins, are not freely filtered into the urine and, following gastrointestinal absorption or parenteral administration, are actively transported (secreted) into the urine by the proximal tubules.[2,16] Certain endogenous organic anions such as uric acid, lactic acid, and β-hydroxybutyric acid and certain common drugs such as penicillin, probenecid, and cephalo-

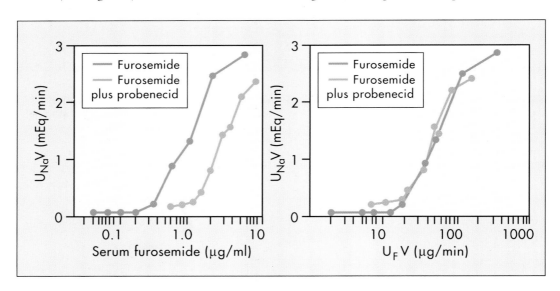

Figure 2.7 The acute effect of probenecid to diminish urinary furosemide excretion in human volunteers. **Left** Relationship between serum furosemide concentrations and the sodium excretion rate. **Right** Relationship between the urinary excretion rate of furosemide and the sodium excretion rate. Note that probenecid delays the entry of furosemide into the urine but does not interfere with the natriuretic effect of furosemide once the drug reaches the urine. (Modified from Chennavasin P, Seiwell R, Brater DC et al: Pharmacodynamic analysis of the furosemide-probenecid interaction in man. Kidney Int 16:187, 1979)

sporin antibiotics are also secreted into the urine at this nephron locus.[17]

Amiloride and triamterene, organic cations at physiologic pH, are highly protein bound and appear in the urine in very high concentrations.[18,19] They are secreted by the organic cation transport system also located within the basolateral membrane of proximal tubule cells. Thus, most diuretic drugs enter the urine via glomerular filtration and proximal tubule transport into the urine, from which they exert their inhibitory effect on salt and water transport in nephron segments farther downstream.

The potent diuretic drugs are organic anions that must be present in the urine to effect a solute diuresis. Hook and Williamson[16] showed that probenecid blocked the acute natriuresis and chloruresis usually caused by furosemide (see Fig. 2.4). Chennavasin and colleagues[20] found that probenecid delayed entry of the diuretic into the urine (Fig. 2.7). In the presence of probenecid, furosemide enters the urine primarily by filtration rather than by tubular secretion. Since furosemide is highly protein bound, glomerular filtration is a rather inefficient way to excrete the drug. Consequently, low levels of furosemide are excreted in the urine for longer periods in the presence rather than the absence of probenecid. How furosemide recirculates in the renal plasma when its tubular secretion is blocked by probenecid is shown in Figure 2.8. The relatively short natriuresis and chloruresis caused by furosemide is prolonged by probenecid. Similar findings have been observed with probenecid and chlorothiazide in humans.[17,21]

Azotemic subjects are relatively resistant to diuretics. Furosemide is not excreted as promptly nor is the natriuresis as great in azotemic patients as in normal subjects, even though less of the drug is bound to plasma proteins in azotemia and a larger fraction of plasma furosemide is filtered into the urine.[22,23] The mechanism of impaired natriuresis in azotemia is unknown.

Inhibitors of prostaglandin synthesis (nonsteroidal anti-inflammatory drugs) may diminish the response to diuretics.[24,25] Indomethacin, a prototypical chemical, decreases the diuretic response to furosemide in humans without affecting the total amount or the rate of diuretic excretion in the urine. The inhibitors of prostaglandin synthesis may interfere with the tubular effects of urinary furosemide (and related "loop-impairing" diuretics such as bumetamide or ethacrynic acid). Prostaglandin inhibitors also alter renal hemodynamics, and this effect may also play a role in the blunted natriuresis seen with these drugs.

RENAL COMPENSATORY RESPONSES TO DIURETICS: THE BRAKING PHENOMENON

Every perceptive clinician has noted that the diuresis induced by any drug is inherently self-limited. Diuresis sufficient to decrease the plasma volume causes the compensatory increase of solute and water absorption in portions of the nephron that are not pharmacologically inhibited by the drug. In other words, when a diuretic blocks solute and water transport across one particular nephron segment, the fractional reabsorption of glomerular filtrate can increase across other segments of the nephron located proximal and/or distal to the inhibited segment.

Intrarenal adjustments in response to diuretics tend to slow down or "brake" the urinary excretion of salt. This "braking phenomenon" is illustrated schematically in Figure 2.9. A normal subject given a

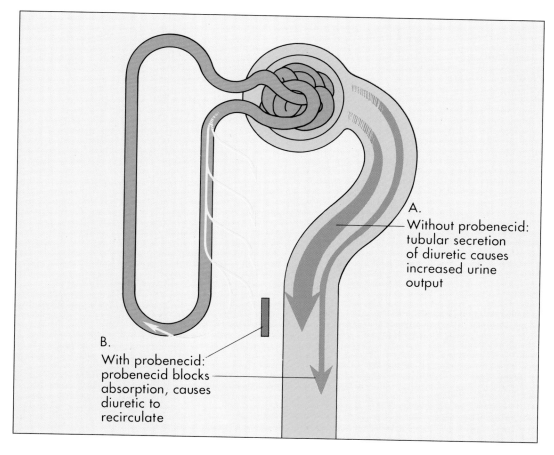

A.
Without probenecid: tubular secretion of diuretic causes increased urine output

B.
With probenecid: probenecid blocks absorption, causes diuretic to recirculate

Figure 2.8

Schematic representation of the renal clearance of furosemide **A** without and **B** with probenecid administration. Furosemide is primarily secreted into the urine under normal conditions. When probenecid is administered, furosemide secretion is blocked and the diuretic recirculates in the plasma and enters the urine more slowly via glomerular filtration. (Modified from Chonko AM, Grantham JJ: Treatment of edema states. In Narins RG, Kleeman CR (eds): Clinical Disorders of Fluid and Electrolyte Metabolism, 4th ed. New York, McGraw-Hill, 1986)

potent "loop diuretic" and a fixed daily salt intake quickly develops negative salt balance. During the first few days of diuretic administration body weight declines as the extracellular fluid volume decreases. After the initial diuresis the amount of salt appearing in the urine progressively diminishes so that within a few days the urinary salt losses fall to levels equal to the oral salt intake—a point of salt balance. At this point there is increased fractional reabsorption of salt in the proximal tubules and distal nephron sufficient to offset the saluretic action of the diuretic in the loop of Henle. The braking phenomenon to diminish the net excretion of salt in response to loop inhibition is mediated by increased absorption of salt proximally due to multiple factors that are operative at this nephron locus and increased salt absorption in the

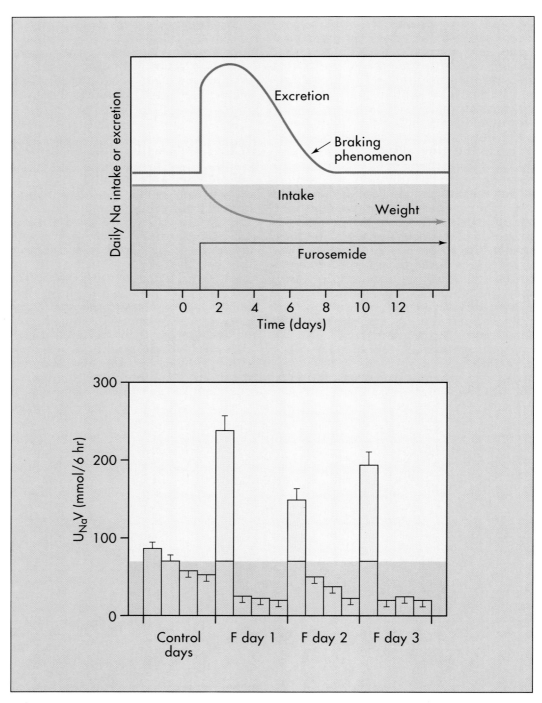

Figure 2.9 Illustration of the "braking phenomenon" that accounts for how salt (and fluid) balance is established during the administration of furosemide. **Top** Relationship between sodium intake and excretion, before and after daily furosemide administration. Note that the urinary excretion of sodium exceeds dietary intake for several days during which time the person loses 1 to 2 kg of weight. After 7 to 8 days, the urinary excretion of sodium once again equals the daily intake of sodium as "hyperabsorption" of filtered sodium occurs across tubule segments not blocked by furosemide. **Bottom** Relationship between sodium intake and excretion in human volunteers taking furosemide (F) and adhering to a constant intake of sodium. Note that the urine excretion of sodium exceeds intake only for several hours each day when furosemide is being excreted in the urine; the remainder of each day the urine sodium excretion is diminished to levels below the control excretory values (gray area) as tubule segments hyperabsorb glomerular filtrate in response to mild plasma volume contraction. The net effect of pulse use of furosemide is to defeat the goal of producing a persistent decrease in ECF volume. (Modified from Grantham JJ, Chonko AM: Diuretics. In Brenner BM, Stein JH (eds): Topics in Nephrology, pp 178–209. New York, Churchill Livingstone, 1978; and Wilcox CS, Mitch WE, Kelly RA et al: Response of the kidney to furosemide: I. Effects of salt intake and renal compensation. J Lab Clin Med 102:450, 1983)

distal nephron due to stimulation of aldosterone by volume contraction. The braking phenomenon conceptually appears to be the mirror image of the so-called escape phenomenon seen in patients on a high salt intake and exogenous mineralocorticoid.[3]

Recent work in normal humans has confirmed the braking phenomenon hypothesis.[26] Although furosemide is the only diuretic that has been tested experimentally in humans, it is reasonable to assume that the braking phenomenon plays a role in reestablishing salt and water balance in association with the use of most, if not all, clinically effective diuretics. The mechanism of the diuretic braking phenomenon with prolonged furosemide administration appears to be related to enhanced sodium reabsorption in the thiazide-sensitive nephron segment, most likely the distal convoluted tubule.[27]

The braking phenomenon has led to some misunderstanding among clinicians about the effectiveness of diuretics. Most clinicians judge the effectiveness of a diuretic by the volume of urine that is excreted after the drug is given. If a drug is given in a dosage interval that ensures a persistent tubular effect, then the volume of urine and the amount of sodium excreted will fall to a level nearly equal to the oral intake in a few days. The patient will notice that the drug no longer causes an increase in urine formation, and the physician may conclude incorrectly that the drug is no longer effective. Very often this scenario leads to the physician choosing a drug with a short duration of action but one that causes an impressive urine response after each use. This, of course, simply leads to a "roller coaster ride" when one considers the fluctuations that will occur in the plasma volume in response to pulses of increased urine formation. The only way intermittent diuresis with a short-acting diuretic can cause persistent plasma volume contraction is for the patient to maintain a low dietary intake of sodium chloride (see Fig. 2.9).[26] Otherwise, the use of pulse doses of short-acting diuretics pleases the patient and the physician but not the cardiovascular system.

CLINICAL USE OF DIURETICS IN DISEASE STATES (FIGURE 2.10)
Congestive Heart Failure

In congestive heart failure, it is the heart that fails not the kidneys. As shown in Figure 2.11, a failing heart has a higher than normal left ventricular end-dias-

---

FIGURE 2.10 COMPARISON OF VARIOUS DIURETICS

Drug	Protein Binding (%)	Major Excretory Routes	Normal Dose Interval (hr)	Dose Adjustment with Decrease GFR (ml/min) >50	10–50	<10	Comments and Extrarenal Effects
Acetazolamide	90–95	Renal	6	6	12	Avoid	Decreases aqueous humor formation in the eye; diuresis ceases with development of metabolic acidosis
Amiloride	65–75	Renal	24	?	?	?	Blocks potassium excretion; tendency to induce hyperkalemia
Bumetanide	95–97	Renal/hepatic	6	6	Unchanged		Similar to furosemide except greater potency
Chlorthalidone	76	Renal/hepatic	24	24	24	48	Tendency for exaggerated urine potassium loss if patient fails to restrict sodium intake
Ethacrynic acid	90	Renal	6	6	6	Avoid	Potential for ototoxicity due to effects on cochlear endolymph solute transport
Furosemide	91–99	Renal	6	6	6	6	Increases renal blood flow venous capacitance
Indapamide	71–79	Renal	24	24	24	Avoid	Has direct arterial vasodilatory action
Mannitol	92	Renal	6	6	Avoid	Avoid	Avoid in renal failure
Mercurials		Renal	24	24	Avoid	Avoid	Relatively potassium sparing; replaced by newer drugs
Metolazone	95	Renal/hepatic	24	24	Unchanged		Appears to be useful when GFR <30 ml/min
Spironolactone	98	Hepatic	6	6–12	12–24	Avoid	Blocks potassium excretion; tendency to induce hyperkalemia
Thiazides	65–95	Renal	12	12	12	Avoid	Usually not useful when GFR <30 ml/min
Triamterene	70–80	Renal/hepatic	12	12	12	Avoid	Blocks potassium excretion; hyperkalemia; can cause nephrolithiasis; folic acid antagonist

tolic volume for a given ventricular performance. The failure of cardiac output to increase with effort results in underperfusion of tissues, causing symptoms of increased fatigue and dyspnea on exertion. The initial response of the cardiovascular system to an added hemodynamic burden or insult to myocardial contractility is to recruit several compensatory mechanisms: an increase in catecholamine release, an increase in renal tubule sodium and water retention (designed to enhance the cardiac output via the Frank-Starling phenomenon), or development of myocardial hypertrophy. Thus, the renal response can be viewed as a protective mechanism in the course of pump failure (Fig. 2.12; see Fig. 2.11). As the cardiac output decreases, the kidney responds with increased retention of fluid. In consequence, the venous return to the heart is increased and the myocardium is stretched farther (i.e., increased preload) to permit an increased stroke volume and cardiac output. Ultimately plasma volume expansion leads to pulmonary vascular congestion and translocation of fluid from the pulmonary capillaries into the alveoli (pulmonary edema).

Diuretics are beneficial by virtue of their ability to reduce both the plasma volume and the venous return to the heart (i.e., decreased preload) so that the symptoms of dyspnea caused by pulmonary con-gestion are ameliorated. Diuretics do not necessarily improve myocardial performance by a direct mechanism (see Fig. 2.11); nevertheless, diuretics may improve myocardial performance indirectly by relieving pulmonary vascular congestion and improving blood oxygenation.

Bumetanide, furosemide, and ethacrynic acid may be particularly useful in the treatment of acute pulmonary edema in the setting of acute myocardial infarction since these drugs may provide a beneficial extrarenal hemodynamic effect (i.e., augmented peripheral venous capacitance within minutes of intravenous administration) (Fig. 2.13). The augmentation occurs independently of the diuretic effects of these agents.[28,29] This phenomenon may not take place in conditions of acute pulmonary edema associated with chronic cardiomyopathic disease. In fact, transient hemodynamic deterioration has been reported following intravenous administration of furosemide in patients with chronic heart failure.[30] An increase in mean arterial pressure, systemic vascular resistance, and left ventricular filling pressure, along with decreased cardiac output, were observed. The precise mechanism for this transient increase in left ventricular outflow resistance, which causes worsening of left ventricular pump function, remains unclear; however, there was evidence for activation of the neurohumoral

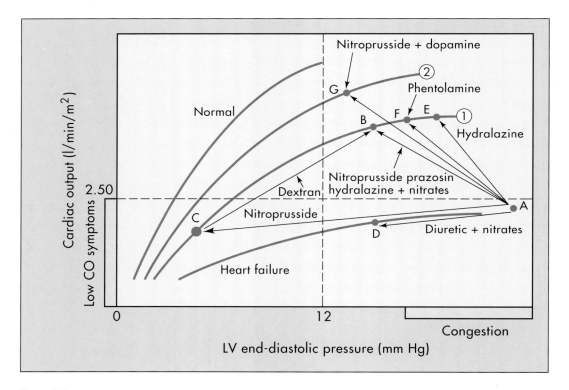

Figure 2.11 The relationship between cardiac output (CO) and left ventricular end-diastolic pressure (LVEDP) in a normal subject (left curve) and patients with congestive heart failure (right curves). The horizontal broken line indicates the lower limits of normal for CO and the vertical broken line indicates the upper limit of normal of LVEDP. Congestion indicates pulmonary venous congestion. Point A indicates the inefficient relationship between cardiac output and LVEDP ("cardiac preload") in a person with severe congestive heart failure. Intermediate curves (1) and (2) show the improved relationships between CO and LVEDP after administration of various vasodilator drugs such as hydralazine, nitrates plus hydralazine, prazosin, nitroprusside, and nitroprusside plus dopamine (an inotropic drug). Note that diuretic therapy alone (point D) or in combination with venodilators such as nitroglycerin relieves pulmonary venous congestion but does not usually improve the cardiac output significantly. (Modified from Mason DT, Awan NA, Joye JA et al: Treatment of acute and chronic congestive heart failure by vasodilator-afterload reduction. Arch Intern Med 140:157, 1980)

axis since plasma renin activity, plasma norepinephrine, and argine vasopressin levels increased concomitantly. The clinical relevance of these transient effects remains to be elucidated (see Fig. 2.13).[28–30]

ACE inhibitors reduce both preload and afterload and can increase cardiac output while simultaneously lowering pulmonary vascular congestion. Inhibition of angiotensin-converting enzyme (ACE) has been shown in several well-controlled trials to improve the disordered hemodynamics, alleviate the symptoms, and improve survival in patients suffering from congestive heart failure.[31–35] When administered with a diuretic, the ACE inhibitor minimizes the loss of serum potassium and blunts the reflex renin-angiotensin stimulating effect of diuretic therapy.

The most limiting feature of ACE inhibitors is the tendency to produce hypotension in patients with low cardiac output. However, this untoward effect can be minimized by starting with low doses (6.25 mg of captopril twice daily or 2.5 mg of enalapril once daily) and titrating upward. It is best to withhold diuretics, if possible, for 48 hours prior to the start of ACE inhibition therapy for treatment of left ventricular dysfunction. Edwards demonstrated that angiotensin II preferentially constricts the efferent arterioles of the renal microvasculature.[36] It has become clear that individuals with a stimulated renin-angiotensin axis with poor renal perfusion due to congestive heart failure, bilateral renal artery stenosis, or renal artery stenosis in a solitary kidney can experience sudden declines in glomerular filtration rate with the start of ACE inhibition.[37,38] Fortunately, in these situations the azotemia usually reverses with discontinuation of the ACE inhibitor therapy. Conversion from ACE inhibitors to other vasodilator drugs is indicated if renal dysfunction does not reverse with lessened diuretic therapy in patients with congestive heart failure. ACE inhibitors can also cause angioedema (idiosyncratic reaction), chronic cough (increased kinin accumulation), and hyperkalemia in patients with renal insufficiency (diminished aldosterone effect).[38,39]

Diuretics may also lower arterial blood pressure and improve cardiac hemodynamics by lessening car-

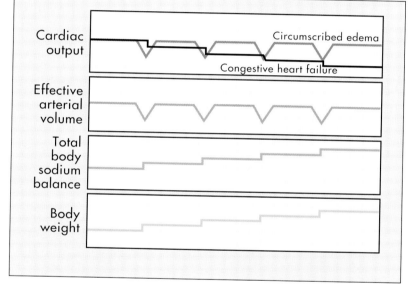

Figure 2.12 The authors' hypothesis for edema formation and maintenance in conditions of circumscribed edema versus congestive heart failure. In congestive heart failure (heavy line, top) a decrease in cardiac output decreases effective arterial volume; in circumscribed edema (light line, top) effective arterial volume is decreased because fluid is translocated into tissues as a result of venous or lymphatic obstruction or a local increase in capillary hydrostatic pressure. In both cases the renal response of increased sodium (and water) retention restores effective arterial volume at the expense of net increases in total body sodium and body weight. (Modified from Chonko AM, Grantham JJ: Treatment of edema states. In Narins RG, Kleeman CR (eds): Clinical Disorders of Fluid and Electrolyte Metabolism, 4th ed. New York, McGraw-Hill, 1986)

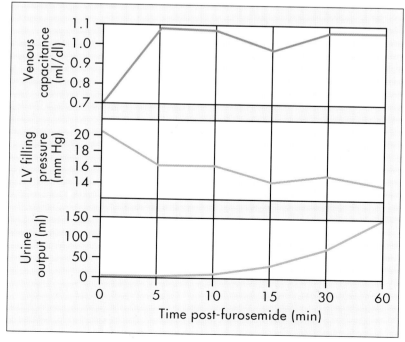

Figure 2.13 The beneficial hemodynamic effects of intravenous furosemide administration in a patient with acute myocardial infarction and pulmonary edema. Temporal changes in calf venous capacitance (top), mean left ventricular filling pressure (middle), and urine output (bottom) are illustrated. Note that the decrease in the ventricular filling pressure and the simultaneous increase in calf venous capacitance preceded significant increased urine output during the initial 15-minute interval after furosemide. (Modified from Dikshit K, Vyden JK, Forrester JS et al: Renal and extrarenal hemodynamic effects of furosemide in congestive heart failure after acute myocardial infarction. N Engl J Med 288:1087, 1971)

diac afterload. Diuretics should be used as adjunctive therapeutic agents in the treatment of chronic congestive heart failure. Therapeutic measures that directly improve myocardial performance should also be employed. Digitalis has a positive inotropic effect; vasodilators reduce left ventricular afterload and decrease pulmonary venous pressure.

Some patients with congestive heart failure appear to be refractory to the effects of furosemide. This may be due to impaired intestinal absorption, but refractoriness may be observed even when the drug is administered intravenously.[40,41] This "unresponsivity" is not due to lack of entry of furosemide into the urine; rather, the poor diuretic response is more likely related to avid absorption of glomerular filtrate at nephron sites not blocked by furosemide (probably the proximal tubule and the late portions of the nephron). An inappropriate braking phenomenon is likely operative in this state (see Fig. 2.9). Although combined therapy with multiple diuretic drugs that work at several loci within the nephron (e.g., combining furosemide with thiazide derivatives concomitantly blocks the loop of Henle and distal convoluted tubule) may be useful, often it is more beneficial to use vasodilator drug therapy to effect an enhanced cardiac output and renal blood flow.

Some patients are resistant even to high-dose intravenous therapy with a loop diuretic given several times daily. The limiting factor in achieving appropriate diuresis in most of these patients is a decrease in delivery of sodium chloride to the diuretic-sensitive sites because of the combination of a fall in glomerular filtration rate and a rise in proximal tubule reabsorption. In certain cases, the addition of either acetazolamide or corticosteroids can be helpful.[42,43] Acetazolamide decreases proximal tubule transport while corticosteroids cause renal vasodilation and raise the glomerular filtration rate. Brater and associates have advanced the notion that a continuous intravenous infusion of a loop diuretic such as bumetanide is more effective and less toxic than conventional intermittent bolus therapy in patients with refractory edema and chronic renal insufficiency.[44,45] A similar benefit may occur in selected diuretic-resistant patients with cardiac (or hepatic) disease.

Cirrhosis and Ascites

Diuretics must be used cautiously to treat edema and ascites in cirrhotic patients who are highly susceptible to vascular collapse. The cornerstone of therapy is sodium restriction. Modest diuresis can be accomplished without complications in seriously ill patients with abdominal discomfort due to tense ascites. The rate of maximal ascites reabsorption is about 900 ml/d.[46] Therefore, in patients with ascites and no peripheral edema, a diuresis that exceeds a net fluid loss of 900 ml/d may lead to rapid depletion of the plasma volume, vascular collapse, and renal hypoperfusion. Functional acute renal failure, the so-called hepatorenal syndrome, has resulted from the overaggressive use of diuretic agents in cirrhotic patients.[46,47]

Physicians favor spironolactone in the initial therapy of the cirrhotic patient who continues to accumulate ascites and edema while adhering to a sodium-restrict-ed diet. Up to 75% of patients respond to spironolactone without other diuretic intervention.[48] Daily doses of 100 to 200 mg are usually successful with an upper limit of 400 mg/d. In refractory cases furosemide can be added in stepwise increased doses of 40 mg every 2 to 3 days, to a maximum dose of 120 mg/d.

Recently, high-volume paracentesis with removal of 3 to 5 l of ascitic fluid over several hours followed with intravenous infusion of albumin concentrates (averaging 60 to 80 g) has proved beneficial in patients with intense ascites refractory to diuretic therapy. Surprisingly, this procedure did not produce vascular collapse, electrolyte imbalance, or progressive azotemia if plasma volume was adequately replaced.[49–51] Whether the risk of infection and inconvenience of the paracentesis procedure will limit the effectiveness of such therapy remains to be elucidated. Follow-up treatment with spironolactone or amiloride may help delay reaccumulation of ascites.

Nephrotic Syndrome

Generalized edema is a cardinal feature of the nephrotic syndrome. Intrarenal factors unrelated to the systemic development of hypoalbuminemia may contribute to enhanced salt and water retention by the kidneys.[52] Of interest, the tubule hyperabsorption of glomerular filtrate appears to take place beyond the distal convolution. Thus, there may be several mechanisms operative in the pathogenesis of avid renal salt and water retention in the nephrotic syndrome. In this condition the arterial circulation is perceived by the kidney as "ineffective," and enhanced tubule absorption of glomerular filtrate occurs even when the creatinine clearance is normal.

It appears that patients with edema formation due to nephrotic proteinuria represent a heterogeneous population in regard to the "adequacy of filling" of their plasma volumes.[53,54] In one study the relationship between plasma renin activity and urine sodium excretion in nephrotics suggested two different pathophysiologic forms.[54] One group had persistently elevated plasma renin and aldosterone levels and appeared "vasoconstricted." These persons had normal creatinine clearance rates, were normotensive, and often achieved complete remission with corticosteroid therapy. A second group had decreased plasma renin and aldosterone levels and appeared "hypervolemic." These persons had decreased creatinine clearance rates, were hypertensive, and did not respond to corticosteroids. The former, as opposed to the latter group, would probably be more prone to vascular collapse if aggressive pharmacologic diuresis were instituted.

Dietary limits are important in the management of the nephrotic syndrome. Sodium restriction, preferably to 40 to 60 mEq/d (1000 to 1500 mg), is effective in arresting or slowing the rate of edema formation in most persons and, in conjunction with cautious use of diuretics, can often lead to resolution of edema. Protein supplementation to intakes of 2 to 3 g/kg/d, particularly with proteins of high biologic quality (i.e., rich in essential amino acids), can induce a positive nitrogen balance and support hepatic albumin synthesis. As an initial diuretic, a thiazide is a safe choice. If the edema is massive and resistant to therapy, and the patient does not have a symptomatic reduction in plasma volume, bumetanide, furosemide, or ethacrynic acid may be substituted or added to the thiazide. In hypokalemic patients, amiloride, triamterene, or spironolactone may be added to the diuretic regimen.

Some nephrotics are resistant to the effects of potent diuretic drugs. The natriuretic response to appropriate urinary levels of furosemide may be reduced in comparison to normal persons. An exaggerated braking phenomenon probably accounts for the hyperabsorption of glomerular filtrate across non-inhibited portions of the nephron.

In refractory patients, combination therapy with metolazone and spironolactone has been useful.[55] Infusion of colloid ("salt-poor" albumin) in combination with diuretic agents is beneficial in mobilizing huge collections of edema. Unfortunately, such measures provide only temporary benefit since the infused protein is rapidly lost into the urine.

Idiopathic Edema

Idiopathic edema is a common disorder of women characterized by cyclical episodes of sodium retention and edema formation in the absence of cardiac, endocrine, hepatic, or renal disease.[56,57] The etiology of this disorder remains unclear. Exaggerated orthostatic pooling of blood, exaggerated renal response to estrogen or to sympathetic nerve discharge, hypoalbuminemia, or alteration in peripheral capillary permeability have each been proposed to explain the tendency to retain salt. It has been suggested that the major cause of idiopathic edema is prolonged use of diuretics (and perhaps laxatives).[58,59] The intermittent use of potent loop-acting diuretics in the setting of wide variations in daily sodium, water, and carbohydrate intake may be particularly responsible. Many women with idiopathic edema appear to be extraordinarily conscious of their appearance and exhibit a dietary pattern of intermittent "starvation" followed by salt and carbohydrate "refeeding"; this sequence of events is known to precipitate the renal retention of sodium and water. The initial edema formation in this syndrome may be "refeeding" edema, which then is exacerbated by diuretic intake. In patients who have intermittent reductions in potassium intake and continue to take diuretic drugs chronically, potassium depletion may develop. Potassium depletion can potentiate the common clinical symptoms of this syndrome, which include weakness, malaise, irritability, abdominal bloating, and increased thirst. Idiopathic edema may be treated most effectively by withdrawing all diuretics and instituting a moderate dietary sodium and water restriction (87 mEq sodium and 1500 ml water per day). Dietary counseling to avoid a pattern of intermittent starvation and gluttony and the institution of an exercise program (daily swimming or bicycling) are also important therapeutic measures. Patients who stop diuretics and follow the dietary restrictions but do not become edema-free within 4 weeks should be reexamined for the presence of occult thyroid or cardiac disease. Cautious use of angiotensin-converting enzyme inhibitors has been associated with weight loss and symptomatic improvement in patients with idiopathic edema.[60] Sowers and associates have described several women who benefitted from the oral administration of the dopamine agonist, bromocriptine.[61] It appears that idiopathic edema is truly a syndrome with variable causes and responses to therapy.

Essential Hypertension

Diuretics are useful drugs for the treatment of hypertension.[62,63] The major mechanism by which diuretics lower the mean arterial blood pressure in patients with hypertension is related to the contraction of the extracellular fluid volume induced by these drugs, particularly when the patient adheres to a sodium-restricted diet (about 2 g of sodium or 87 mEq of sodium per day).[62,63] It is common for persons to lose 1 to 2 l of extracellular fluid (about 300 ml of plasma) in response to the start of therapy with a thiazide diuretic. Of interest, the patient's peripheral vascular resistance often rises in response to the initial plasma volume depletion. However, a major decrease in venous return to the heart (decreased preload) leads to a decreased cardiac output such that the net effect of the diuretic therapy is to lower the net product of cardiac output and peripheral vascular resistance, the mean arterial blood pressure.

It appears that over the long term, continued diuretic therapy in conjunction with moderate dietary salt restriction produces a favorable readjustment in the basic hemodynamic relationships in persons with hypertension; namely, the peripheral resistance falls and the cardiac output rises, but the former more so than the latter, so that the arterial blood pressure falls toward the normal range. The mechanisms responsible for the significant fall in peripheral vascular resistance induced in patients who take diuretic drugs for several months remain to be elucidated. Several hypotheses have been advanced, including readjustment of baroreceptor sensitivity, depletion of sodium from critical peripheral vascular receptor sites for endogenous vasopressors, such as angiotensin II and norepinephrine, and redistribution of calcium ions to critical intracellular sites within vascular smooth muscle cells.[64] There is little evidence in support of the notion that thiazide or loop diuretics have direct vasodilatory actions on the peripheral arterial vasculature. For instance, the blood pressure does not fall in nephrectomized patients taking thiazide or loop diuretics who are maintained on dialysis. An exception to this rule is indapamide, a new thiazide derivative that clearly possesses direct arteriolar vasodilating properties.[65]

We favor the use of long-acting thiazide (or related) diuretics to reduce elevated blood pressure unless the patient's GFR is below 40 to 50 ml/min, a point where a "loop diuretic" is indicated in order to induce and maintain a diuresis. Shorter-acting "loop diuretics" are potent agents, but they are excreted rapidly from the body and produce a sawtoothed pattern of natriuresis and antinatriuresis as the braking phenomenon supervenes in persons with a normal GFR. A long-acting diuretic such as trichlormethiazide or metolazone can be taken once per day, which enhances patient compliance and provides a smoother course of natriuresis and diuresis since the drug is slowly excreted into the urine over the course of the day.

Another potential benefit of thiazide diuretics in

hypertensive patients relates to their effect to lower the urine calcium level and place the patient in a favorable calcium balance provided that calcium intake is adequate (800 to 1000 mg/d). Resnick and co-workers[66] and McCarron[67] have found that certain populations with "essential hypertension," particularly black persons and elderly persons, may ingest lower amounts of calcium in their diets and have lower amounts of serum ionized calcium (and presumably intracellular calcium) than nonhypertensive age-matched controls. Thiazide diuretics may be particularly useful as therapy for hypertension in these persons owing to the anticalciuric effects of these agents. Since loop diuretics such as bumetanide, ethacrynic acid, and furosemide all enhance calciuria, it may not be wise to use these diuretics as first-step agents for the treatment of hypertension, particularly if the patient has a normal GFR.

Since potent diuretics can cause renal magnesium and potassium wasting and induce carbohydrate intolerance and hyperlipidemia, some investigators have questioned whether diuretic drugs should be instituted as first-step therapy for patients with mild or borderline hypertension (systolic BP 140 to 150 mm Hg and diastolic BP 90 to 100 mm Hg), particularly since these patients often respond to monotherapy with adrenergic blocking drugs, angiotensin-converting enzyme inhibitors or calcium channel blocking drugs that do not cause kaliuresis or magnesiuresis (and may not cause hyperlipidemia as consistently as potent diuretics).[68,69] However, persons who do not favorably respond to monotherapy with adrenergic blockade (i.e., do not normalize their blood pressure) can be given diuretics as a second step since subtle plasma volume expansion often occurs with the adrenergic blockers and negates their antihypertensive effects.[69] Direct vasodilators such as hydralazine and minoxidil consistently induce renal salt retention and necessitate the addition of a diuretic drug in order to maintain blood pressure control.[70]

Recent concerns about the unfavorable impact of left ventricular cardiac hypertrophy on the survival of patients with essential hypertension has led to a further reevaluation of the general use of diuretic drugs as first-line therapy for all patients with hypertension. Diuretic drugs in general (with the possible exception of indapamide) do not reverse left ventricular cardiac hypertrophy in clinical trials and animal experiments despite their beneficial reduction of arterial blood pressure. In contrast, calcium channel blockers, angiotensin-converting enzyme inhibitors, and centrally acting adrenergic inhibitors (α-methyldopa having been the first drug to display this property) have been shown to reverse left ventricular hypertrophy in clinical trials and animal experiments. These latter drugs may offer an important advantage over diuretics in the treatment of the patient with hypertension and left ventricular cardiac hypertrophy.[71–73]

CLINICAL COMPLICATIONS OF DIURETIC DRUGS (FIGURE 2.14)

An understanding of the braking phenomenon is important when one considers the clinical complications commonly induced by diuretic drugs. Many of these complications derive from the increased absorption of glomerular filtrate mediated by plasma volume contraction in portions of the nephron not affected directly by the diuretic. The absorption of most filtered solutes is affected by the state of expansion or contraction of the extracellular fluid (ECF) volume. Therefore, most of the important complications of diuretics can be explained within the framework of our understanding of segmental nephron absorptive characteristics.

ECF volume depletion is a common complication of the potent loop-acting diuretics.[3–5] Patients are protected to some extent against ECF volume depletion by the braking phenomenon. Those patients most prone to develop ECF volume depletion have gastrointestinal tract complications such as nausea, vomiting, or diarrhea and are unable to ingest appropriate amounts of salt and water to correct the major

FIGURE 2.14 COMPLICATIONS OF DIURETIC THERAPY

Fluid, Electrolyte, and Acid-Base Disorders
    Extracellular fluid volume depletion
    Potassium depletion
    Metabolic alkalosis
    Hyponatremia
    Hypercalcemia
    Metabolic acidosis
Metabolic Disorders
    Hyperuricemia
    Hyperglycemia
    Hyperlipidemia
    Gynecomastia/sexual dysfunction
    Osteomalacia
Toxic Disorders
    Ototoxicity
    Hypersensitivity

portion of the ongoing daily urinary losses. In patients with underlying renal insufficiency, ECF volume depletion can lead to the development of overt uremia, although in many persons a picture of prerenal azotemia results.

Recent experiments in rodents indicate that 30% to 60% of the elevated plasma urea concentration that occurs in the animal during diuretic induced sodium depletion is accounted for by an enhanced urea appearance rate. Thus, both plasma volume contraction and enhanced urea production combine to produce a "prerenal" azotemic picture in patients who are too vigorously treated with diuretic drugs.[74]

ECF volume contraction is important in maintaining another complication of diuretic treatment, the genesis and maintenance of metabolic alkalosis. Both ECF volume depletion and the metabolic alkalosis respond to replenishment of the ECF with isotonic saline and/or discontinuation or dose reduction of the diuretic drugs.

Potassium depletion has received extensive attention in the recent medical literature.[75–81] Some investigators believe that concern about this complication is exaggerated.[77,78] Certainly severe potassium depletion may cause malfunction of other organ systems, including cardiac muscle irritability, particularly in conjunction with digitalis therapy[80]; decreased striated muscle blood flow and predisposition to rhabdomyolysis[82]; and sluggish pancreatic insulin release and carbohydrate intolerance.[84] Inhibition of potassium absorption in the proximal tubule may contribute to urinary potassium loss, but most diuretics promote urinary potassium loss by an indirect action on the distal convoluted and cortical collecting tubules. Urinary potassium secretion is strongly dependent on the rate of urine flow, high levels of sodium in the final urine, high levels of impermeant anions in urine (i.e., carbenicillin), and elevated plasma levels of aldosterone.

In patients taking diuretics, exaggerated kaliuresis usually does not occur if an appropriate decrease in volume of the ECF compartment is achieved. Urinary potassium loss and potassium depletion are most pronounced in those patients who take diuretics and ingest large loads of solute and water! In these patients supplemental intake of potassium chloride may be necessary, although restriction of dietary sodium intake (about 87 mEq/d) is the most appropriate way to abolish excessive urinary potassium wasting.

Spironolactone, triamterene, and amiloride block potassium secretion in the distal and collecting tubules. These agents are effective when used in combination with the more potent agents that act in the loop of Henle and distal tubule in order to reduce the urinary loss of potassium.[85] Antikaliuretic drugs should not be used routinely in patients with renal insufficiency since life-threatening hyperkalemia and metabolic acidosis may develop.[86,87]

Metabolic alkalosis is often seen in the setting of total body potassium depletion during the use of diuretics.[88,89] Potassium depletion causes increased secretion of hydrogen ion by renal tubules together with an increased excretion of ammonium as the chloride salt. Consequently, for each equivalent of ammonium excreted one equivalent of bicarbonate is

"generated" for the plasma compartment in place of chloride. Owing to contraction of the ECF volume the metabolic alkalosis is "maintained" by increased reabsorption of sodium bicarbonate. "Contraction" metabolic alkalosis can also result from the intense renal loss of sodium chloride caused by potent loop diuretics. In most cases of diuretic-induced metabolic alkalosis, reduction of the dose of diuretic will correct the alkalosis, although potassium supplementation in excess of normal dietary intake is sometimes required.[90]

Hyponatremia is seen relatively frequently in patients taking diuretics. Fichman and co-workers[91] studied 10 patients with severe, symptomatic hyponatremia due to thiazides. All of the patients were potassium-depleted. Their plasma antidiuretic hormone activity was paradoxically elevated, and this may have contributed to the hyponatremic state.

Diuretics active in the ascending loop of Henle impair the generation of dilute urine by blocking sodium chloride absorption. Hyponatremia develops in patients who drink water at a rate faster than the ascending limb can generate dilute urine. Potent loop diuretics also cause contraction of the extracellular fluid compartment and release of antidiuretic hormone to further the development of hyponatremia.[92]

Captopril, an oral drug that inhibits the enzyme responsible for the conversion of angiotensin I to angiotensin II, has been shown to correct the hypotonic, hyponatremic state that often develops in patients with severe congestive heart failure who require potent diuretic therapy.[93,94] A combination of captopril and furosemide was superior to either drug used alone for the production of a sustained diuresis, which led to a rise in the serum sodium concentration in most patients.

Most diuretics acutely increase the renal excretion of calcium, phosphorus, and magnesium. In general, the increased rate of elimination reflects the natriuretic or chloruretic potency of the particular diuretic. The chronic administration of diuretics causes the calciuria and phosphaturia to return to (or fall below) the control values. There have been no reports of sustained diuretic-induced phosphaturia or calciuria that have resulted in overt phosphate or calcium depletion syndromes as long as the patient is able to ingest adequate amounts of calcium and phosphorus. On the contrary, long-term thiazide administration may lead to overt hypercalcemia.[95] Thus, it would seem that compensatory mechanisms, perhaps related to increased proximal tubule reabsorption due to ECF volume contraction, may counteract the acute phosphaturic and calciuric effects of certain diuretics.

Thiazide diuretics decrease calcium excretion with acute and chronic use by augmenting calcium reabsorption in the distal tubule.[94,95] This property of the thiazides is central to their use in the treatment of calcium renal lithiasis.[98,99] By contrast, furosemide and ethacrynic acid increase calcium excretion on acute and chronic administration and are useful in the treatment of acute hypercalcemic conditions. Since overt calcium depletion has not resulted from long-term therapy with these drugs, it is likely that extrarenal mechanisms such as increased gastrointestinal calcium absorption must compensate for the increased calcium losses into the urine. When using furosemide to induce calciuresis in the treatment of hypercalcemia, isotonic saline solution must be given in generous amounts to match or slightly exceed the urine loss of sodium chloride.[100]

Thiazides and furosemide chronically increase renal magnesium wasting; however, the long-term consequences of this effect remain uncertain. Some investigators suggest that occult magnesium depletion accounts for a significant percentage of diuretic-related cardiac arrhythmias.[82]

Metabolic acidosis may occur as a complication of acetazolamide or spironolactone therapy. Acetazolamide induces renal sodium bicarbonate wasting, which halts when the plasma bicarbonate level falls to 18 to 19 mEq/l. Amiloride, spironolactone, and triamterene may also produce hyperchloremic metabolic acidosis.[86,87] The elevated potassium levels reduce ammonia extraction by renal tubules and decrease net ammonium chloride excretion into the urine. Reducing body potassium stores (with polystyrene sulfonate resin [Kayexalate]) may improve the acidosis.[101]

Hyperuricemia is common in patients treated with diuretics. Plasma uric acid is filtered by the glomeruli. Uric acid also enters the urine by secretion in proximal tubules. Urinary uric acid is also reabsorbed by these same proximal segments and in the last analysis an amount of uric acid equal to 8% to 12% of the filtered uric acid appears normally in the final urine.[17] The renal excretion of uric acid is decreased by plasma volume contraction and increased by plasma volume expansion. Diuretics elevate plasma uric acid levels by increasing tubular reabsorption of the anion in consequence of plasma volume contraction. Simultaneous replacement of urinary salt losses during the administration of a diuretic prevents the fall in uric acid clearance that occurs when volume contraction is allowed to develop, proving that the hyperuricemia is secondary to ECF volume contraction.[102]

Reduction in diuretic dose often corrects the hyperuricemia. However, such a reduction in dose may not be feasible in certain patients with avid salt retention. We find that addition of a uricosuric drug, such as probenecid, is beneficial since the diuretic effect is delayed when probenecid diminishes the rapid excretion of the diuretic into the urine (see Figs. 2.7 and 2.8). Both the natriuretic effect of the diuretic and the uricosuric effect of the probenecid are preserved when these drugs are administered together. An alternative strategy is to use the xanthine oxidase inhibitor allopurinol to reduce the plasma uric acid level. Because this drug may cause hepatitis, exfoliative dermatitis, and cataracts, it seems prudent to use allopurinol only in those patients with gouty arthritis or nephropathy. Sustained plasma uric acid elevations up to 14 mg/dl have no apparent deleterious effects on renal function[103]; however, levels higher than this may warrant treatment, particularly if the GFR is less than 50 ml/min.

Hyperglycemia has been reported with the use of chlorothiazide, furosemide, and ethacrynic acid.[104–106] The mechanism(s) by which the thiazide derivatives and the loop of Henle agents induce glucose intolerance remains controversial, but potassium loss may be the most important factor relating the development of overt glucose intolerance with the use of potent diuretic drugs. Long-term studies of nondiabetic hypertensive patients taking diuretics indicate that less than 5% have overt glucose intolerance.[107] There may be more risk of decreasing glucose control, however, in insulin-dependent diabetics who require potent diuretics to control hypertension or edema formation. Hyperglycemia has not been reported with use of potassium-sparing diuretics.

During the past few years several investigators have found that glucose intolerance and/or hyperinsulinemia are commonly present in persons with high blood pressure.[108,109] More recently, it has also been demonstrated that resistance to insulin-stimulated glucose uptake is present in patients with hypertension. Moreover, hypertensive persons treated with hydrochlorothiazide, in contrast to those treated with the angiotensin-converting enzyme inhibitor captopril, had increased basal insulin concentration and an enhanced late insulin response to a glucose challenge.[110] Hydrochlorothiazide therapy was also associated with an adverse effect on blood lipids, whereas captopril therapy was not found to adversely affect blood lipids in the short term. These findings have led several investigators to recommend that diuretics be used in low dose for the treatment of hypertension.[111]

Hyperlipidemia is observed with the use of diuretics. Grimm and associates[112] reported that hydrochlorothiazide or chlorthalidone increased plasma total cholesterol, very-low-density and low-density lipoprotein cholesterol, and plasma triglyceride concentrations, with triglyceride concentrations showing the largest increase. High-density lipoprotein cholesterol remained stable during thiazide diuretic treatment. Although the magnitude of the increase in plasma lipid content appears to be related to the dose of the thiazide diuretic drugs, the mechanism responsible for the increased lipid levels remains unclear. Furosemide and spironolactone administered under similar conditions also increase serum cholesterol and triglyceride levels.[113] The clinical significance of these observations remains controversial at present. Indapamide does not alter lipids in an unfavorable manner.[114]

Gynecomastia, irregular menses, and impotence have been associated with the use of spironolactone.

Ototoxicity has been reported following the use of furosemide and ethacrynic acid; reversible hearing loss associated with high-dose therapy has been reported in patients with renal insufficiency.[115]

Hypersensitivity reactions also have been reported with diuretic drug use, particularly the thiazides and furosemide. These reactions include rash, leukopenia, thrombocytopenia, necrotizing vasculitis, and acute hypersensitivity pneumonitis. The common ground for these reactions may be the presence of sulfur within the ring structure of the thiazides and furosemide. Amiloride, triamterene, and ethacrynic acid do not contain sulfur and can be substituted for the former drugs if an idiosyncratic reaction develops.

75. Morgan DB, Davidson C: Hypokalemia and diuretics: An analysis of publications. Br Med J 280:905, 1980

76. Holland OB, Nixon JV, Kuhnert L: Diuretic-induced ventricular ectopic activity. Am J Med 70:762, 1981

77. Harrington JT, Isner JM, Kassirer JP: Our national obsession with potassium. Am J Med 73:155, 1982

78. Freis ED: Critique of the clinical importance of diuretic-induced hypokalemia and elevated cholesterol level. Arch Intern Med 149:2640, 1989

79. Struthers AD, Whitesmith R, Reid JL: Prior thiazide diuretic treatment increases adrenaline-induced hypokalemia. Lancet 1:1358, 1983

80. Kaplan NM: Our appropriate concern about hypokalemia. Am J Med 77:1, 1984

81. Knochel JP: Diuretic-induced hypokalemia. Am J Med 77:18, 1984

82. Hollifield JW: Potassium and magnesium abnormalities: Diuretics and arrhythmias in hypertension. Am J Med 77:28, 1984

83. Knochel JP, Schlein EM: On the mechanism of rhabdomyolysis in potassium depletion. J Clin Invest 51:1750, 1972

84. Fajans S, Floyd JC, Knopf RF et al: Benzothiadiazine suppression of insulin release from normal and abnormal islet cell tissue in man. J Clin Invest 45:481, 1966

85. Schnaper HW, Freis ED, Friedman RG et al: Potassium restoration in hypertensive patients made hypokalemic by hydrochlorothizide. Arch Intern Med 149:2677, 1989

86. Gabow PA, Moore S, Schrier RW: Spironolactone-induced hyperchloremic acidosis in cirrhosis. Ann Intern Med 90:338, 1979

87. Greenblatt DJ, Koch-Weser J: Adverse reactions to spironolactone. JAMA 225:40, 1973

88. Seldin DW, Rector FC Jr: The generation and maintenance of metabolic alkalosis. Kidney Int 1:306, 1972

89. Kurtzman NA, White MG, Rogers PW: Pathophysiology of metabolic alkalosis. Arch Intern Med 131:702, 1973

90. Garella S: Saline-resistant metabolic alkalosis or "chloride-wasting nephropathy." Ann Intern Med 73:31, 1970

91. Fichman MP, Vorherr H, Kleeman CR et al: Diuretic-induced hyponatremia. Ann Intern Med 75:853, 1971

92. Ashraf N, Locksley R, Arieff AI: Thiazide-induced hyponatremia associated with death or neurologic damage in outpatients. Am J Med 70:1163, 1981

93. Dzau VJ, Hollenberg NK: Renal response to captopril in severe heart failure: Role of furosemide in natriuresis and reversal of hyponatremia. Ann Intern Med 100:777, 1984

94. Packer M, Medina N, Yushak M: Correction of dilutional hyponatremia in severe chronic heart failure by converting-enzyme inhibition. Ann Intern Med 100:782, 1984

95. Higgins BA, Nassim JR, Collins J et al: The effect of bendrofluazide on urine calcium excretion. Clin Sci 27:457, 1964

96. Breslau N, Moses AM, Weiner IM: The role of volume contraction in the hypocalciuric action of chlorothiazide. Kidney Int 10:164, 1976

97. Costanzo LS, Windhager EE: Calcium and sodium transport by the distal convoluted tubule of the rat. Am J Physiol 235:F492, 1978

98. Yendt ER, Gagne RJA, Cohanim M: The effects of thiazides in idiopathic hypercalciuria. Am J Med Sci 251:449, 1966

99. Yendt ER, Guay GF, Garcia DA: The use of thiazides in the prevention of renal calculi. Can Med Assoc J 102:614, 1970

100. Suki WN, Yium JJ, VonMinden M et al: Acute treatment of hypercalcemia with furosemide. N Engl J Med 283:836, 1970

101. Szylman P, Better OS, Chaimowitz C et al: Role of hyperkalemia in the metabolic acidosis of isolated hypoaldosteronism. N Engl J Med 294:361, 1976

102. Steele TH, Oppenheimer S: Factors affecting urate excretion following diuretic administration in man. Am J Med 47:564, 1969

103. Berger L, Yu T: Renal function in gout: IV. An analysis of 524 gouty subjects including long-term follow-up studies. Am J Med 59:605, 1975

104. Wilkins RW: New drugs for the treatment of hypertension. Ann Intern Med 50:1, 1959

105. Wolff FW, Parmley WW, White K et al: Drug-induced diabetes. JAMA 185:568, 1963

106. Weller JM, Borondy M: Effect of furosemide on glucose metabolism. Metabolism 16:532, 1967

107. Berglund G, Andersson O: Beta blockers or diuretics in hypertension? A six year follow-up of blood pressure and metabolic side-effects. Lancet 1:744, 1971

108. Ferrannini E, Buzzigoli G, Bonadonna R et al: Insulin resistance in essential hypertension. N Engl J Med 317:350, 1987

109. Swislocki ALM, Hoffman BB, Reaven GM: Insulin resistance, glucose intolerance and hyperinsulinemia in patients with hypertension. Am J Hypertens 2:419, 1989

110. Pollare T, Lithell H, Berne C: A comparison of the effects of hydrochlorothiazide and captopril on glucose and lipid metabolism in patients with hypertension. N Engl J Med 321:868, 1989

111. Kaplan N: How bad are diuretic-induced hypokalemia and hypercholesterolemia? Arch Intern Med 149:109, 1989

112. Grimm RH, Leon AS, Hunninghake DB et al: Effects of thiazide diuretics on plasma lipids and lipoproteins in mildly hypertensive patients. Ann Intern Med 94:7, 1981

113. Ames RP: The influence of non-beta-blocking drugs on the lipid profile: Are diuretics outclassed as initial therapy for hypertension? Am Heart J 14:998, 1987

114. Meyer-Sabellek W, Gotzen R, Heitz J et al: Serum lipoprotein levels during long-term treatment of hypertension with indapamide. Hypertension 7:170, 1985

115. David DS, Hitzig P: Diuretics and ototoxicity. N Engl J Med 284:1328, 1971

Digitalis, Catecholamines, and Other Positive Inotropic Agents

3

Kanu Chatterjee

It is now generally agreed that augmented contractility usually results from the increased availability of intracellular free calcium to the myocardial contractile proteins. Increased sensitivity of the filaments to calcium may also be associated with enhanced contractile force. The number of crossbridges formed between actin and myosin myofilaments appears to determine the amount of force developed during contraction. A regulating protein, tropomyosin, normally prevents interaction of actin and myosin. Binding of calcium to the subunit, troponin C of another regulatory protein, troponin, allows interaction of the myofilaments by reversing the inhibiting action of tropomyosin. The magnitude of developed force appears to depend on the number of troponin C subunits of troponin bound to calcium, which, in turn, is related to the intracellular free calcium concentration.[1-3]

Although the precise mechanism of increased intracellular calcium concentration necessary for increased contractility has not been totally clarified, it appears that a number of different mechanisms can enhance calcium concentration.[4] A transient increase in intracellular sodium is associated with increased calcium entry or calcium retention through the sodium–calcium exchange mechanism. Increased intracellular sodium concentration may result from inhibition of sodium efflux or enhanced sodium influx through the fast sodium channel. Higher extracellular concentration may promote calcium influx across the sarcolemmal membrane and enhance contractility. Increased calcium influx via the slow (calcium) channel, or due to increased sarcolemmal permeability to calcium, may also increase intracellular calcium concentration. Cytosolic calcium content may also increase due to augmented release of calcium from the sarcoplasmic reticulum or decreased calcium uptake by the sarcoplasmic reticulum.

Myocardial cyclic AMP (adenosine 3'5'-cyclic monophosphate) exerts an important regulatory influence on intracellular calcium concentration and contractile state. Cyclic AMP production is mediated by the membrane-bound enzyme adenylate cyclase, the activity of which is regulated by both stimulatory and inhibitory protein subunits.[5] The mechanism of action of the various agonists of the surface receptors to activate the adenylate cyclase appears to be mediated through these regulatory subunits.

Increased intracellular cyclic AMP content is associated with increased activation of the cyclic AMP-dependent protein kinase, which catalyzes the phosphorylation of proteins that regulate calcium fluxes across the sarcolemma, apparently through the slow calcium channels.[6] An increased release of calcium from the sarcoplasmic reticulum and augmented reuptake and storage of calcium in the sarcoplasmic reticulum may also occur as a result of increased intracellular cyclic AMP concentration.[7] Calcium flux into or out of the sarcoplasmic reticulum is partly mediated by the phosphorylation of a protein, phospholamban, which appears to regulate an adenosine triphosphate (ATP)-dependent calcium pump in the sarcoplasmic reticulum.[8]

Increased cyclic AMP concentration may also result from its decreased degradation, which is primarily mediated by the enzyme phosphodiesterase.[9] Thus, inhibition of the activity of phosphodiesterase enhances cyclic AMP content, which in turn is associated with increased intracellular calcium concentration. Furthermore, the inhibition of phosphoprotein phosphatase necessary for dephosphorylation of the phosphorylated proteins may produce effects similar to those of increased cyclic AMP.[10]

Although an increase in intracellular calcium content is the final mechanism for a positive inotropic effect of most pharmacologic agents, evidence exists that enhanced contractility may also occur from the increased sensitivity of contractile elements to calcium, without an increase in intracellular concentration. The classification of inotropic drugs based on the potential mechanisms as proposed by Katz[4] is shown in Figure 3.1.

Digitalis Glycosides

In 1785, William Withering, in his accounts of foxglove, reported the beneficial effects of digitalis in dropsy, although apparently he did not recognize that dropsy might have resulted from heart failure.[11] In 1911, McKenzie observed that digitalis can slow the ventricular response in the presence of atrial fibrillation.[12] Thus, the potential beneficial cardiovascular effects of digitalis have long been acknowledged. However, the drug's physiologic and pharmacologic effects, and its pharmacokinetics and potential clinical applications, have only recently been elucidated.

Pharmacology

A number of cardiac glycosides are presently in clinical use. Digitoxin, gitalin, and digitalis are derived from the leaves of the foxglove plant (Digitalis purpurea); digoxin, lanatoside C, and deslanoside from Digitalis lanata; and ouabain from seeds of Strophanthus gratus. Presently, however, digoxin is the most commonly used cardiac glycoside.

Cardiac glycosides combine a steroid nucleus with an unsaturated lactose ring at the 17 position with a series of sugars attached to carbon 3 of the nucleus (Fig. 3.2).[13] The steroid and lactose part without the sugars, which appears essential for the activity, is called genin or aglycone. The sugar molecules influence the pharmacokinetic properties, including absorption, half-life, and metabolism.

Digoxin

Digoxin (12-hydroxydigitoxin) is relatively well absorbed from the gastrointestinal tract. However, its absorption may be influenced by a number of factors. Altered gastrointestinal motility due to foods or drugs may cause variable absorption. In general, decreased motility is associated with enhanced absorption, and increased motility with reduced absorption. Concurrent administration of nonabsorbable substances, such as cholestyramine, colestipol, kaolin, pectin, and antacids, retards absorption of digoxin from the gastrointestinal tract.[14] Antacids containing magnesium trisilicate may bind digoxin and prevent its absorption. Sulfasalazine and neomycin also interfere with the absorption of digoxin. Absorption of digoxin is passive and primarily occurs in the small intestine and colon; minimal absorption has been observed in the stomach.[15] Cardiac glycosides with a greater number of hydroxyl groups are less well absorbed.[16] Hydrolysis of digoxin and its derivatives is nearly complete at a pH of 1, but these drugs are stable above pH 3. Digoxin may, therefore, be hydrolyzed to a considerable extent into its active and inactive metabolites in patients with peptic ulcer with high gastric acidity and markedly delayed gastric emptying.

Although decreased plasma digoxin levels following oral administration have occasionally been observed in patients with congestive heart failure,[17] pharmacokinetic studies with the use of tritiated digoxin have failed to demonstrate any decrease in bioavailability and absorption of digoxin solution or digoxin tablets, even in patients with severe right-sided heart failure.[18] No significant differences in the plasma concentration curves were observed either before or after treatment of severe right-sided heart failure, suggesting that absorption of digoxin is not retarded in the presence of congestive heart failure.

Different preparations of digoxin tablets were reported to have dissimilar bioavailability (the percentage of orally administered drug entering the systemic circulation unaltered).[19] Dissolution rate of digoxin appears to be the major determinant of bioavailability. Digoxin solution (elixir) is better

---

FIGURE 3.1 CLASSIFICATION OF INOTROPIC DRUGS BASED ON THEIR MECHANISMS OF ACTION

Drugs That Increase Cytosolic Calcium
Drugs that, by increasing intracellular sodium, promote calcium entry or retention by sodium/calcium exchange
    Drugs that inhibit sodium efflux (digitalis)
    Drugs that promote sodium influx via the fast (sodium) channel (veratrum alkaloids)
Drugs that directly increase calcium influx across the sarcolemma
    Drugs that increase extracellular calcium (parathyroid hormone)
    Drugs that promote calcium influx via the slow channel (calcium) (Bay-K-8644, possibly α-adrenergic agonists)
    Drugs that increase sarcolemmal calcium permeability (ionophores, e.g., A23187)
Drugs that inhibit calcium efflux across the sarcolemma (hypothetical)
Drugs that increase the movement of calcium from the sarcoplasmic reticulum into the cytosol
    Drugs that increase calcium efflux from the sarcoplasmic reticulum
    Drugs that decrease calcium uptake from the sarcoplasmic reticulum

Drugs That Increase Cyclic AMP Levels
Drugs that increase cyclic AMP production (β-adrenergic agonists, glucagon)
Drugs that decrease cyclic AMP breakdown (methylxanthines, bipyridines)

Drugs That Modify Myofibrillar Proteins
Drugs that increase calcium sensitivity of the contractile proteins (AR-L 115 BS, possibly α-adrenergic agonists)
Drugs that modify myosin isozyme composition (thyroxine)

(Reproduced by permission from Katz AM: Discussion section. Article by Endoh M, Yanagisawa T, Taira N, Blinks JR: Effects of new inotropic agents on cyclic nucleotide metabolism and calcium transients in canine ventricular muscle. Circulation 73(Suppl III):III-117, 1986)

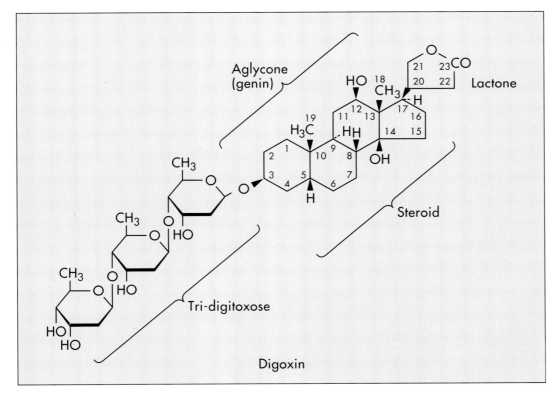

Figure 3.2 Structure of digoxin (glycoside). (Modified from Katzung BG, Parmley WW: Cardiac glycosides and the drugs used in treatment of congestive heart failure. In Katzung BG (ed): Basic and Clinical Pharmacology, p 144. Los Altos, CA, Lange Publications, 1984)

absorbed than tablets. However, digoxin tablets with a dissolution rate greater than 65% have an absorption equivalent to that of oral solution.[20] The bioavailability of the presently available digoxin tablets is more predictable, due to the Food and Drug Administration's implementation of minimal dissolution rates of 55% or greater at 1 hour. The new gelatin capsule of digoxin (Lanoxicaps) increases bioavailability to 90% to 95%.[21] The absolute bioavailability is the percentage of the unchanged drug that is absorbed after oral administration, compared with the same dose of the drug administered intravenously. The average absolute bioavailability of digoxin tablets appears to be between 60% and 80%. With absorption of 70%, a 0.5-mg oral dose of digoxin is equivalent to 0.35 mg of digoxin given intravenously. This ratio of 1.5 to 1 between oral and intravenous digoxin is similar to that reported after biologic titration.[22]

Clinical response is an important consideration in determining the dose and route of administration in individual patients. In addition abnormalities in absorption and concomitant drug therapy should be taken into account during oral digoxin therapy. Absorption characteristics of digoxin in patients with malabsorption syndromes have not been clarified. It appears, however, that when the dissolution rate of digoxin at 1 hour is high (greater than 65%), absorption of digoxin is adequate even in the presence of malabsorption states.[23]

Digoxin can be detected in plasma within 30 minutes following oral administration, but the peak levels occur between 30 and 60 minutes and a plateau is observed within 6 hours.[24] When digoxin tablets are given after meals, the peak plasma concentrations occur approximately 45 minutes later without significantly affecting the total bioavailability or the peak concentrations. When digoxin is administered in solution, absorption is not affected by food.[25] After intravenous injection, the pharmacologic effects of digoxin occur within 15 to 30 minutes and reach a peak within 1 to 5 hours.[26]

Digoxin is not extensively metabolized in humans. After absorption, digoxin is bound to plasma proteins to only a modest extent (approximately 25% or less). Plasma protein binding is even less in the presence of renal impairment.[27] Tissue proteins also bind digoxin; the concentration of the glycoside in human cardiac tissue may be as high as 30 times that in the plasma.[26] The plasma-to-myocardial ratio is remarkably constant; thus, the pharmacodynamic effects can generally be predicted from the serum concentrations. Digoxin is also readily bound to skeletal muscle, but adipose tissue contains little digoxin. Thus, lean body weight provides a more appropriate basis for determining its volume of distribution, which is large (5 to 8 l/kg). Although digoxin concentration in skeletal muscle is lower than that in kidney or heart, the total digoxin content of skeletal muscle is significantly greater because of its proportionately larger mass in the body.

The time course of digoxin distribution in the body is well characterized by a two-compartment model.[28] The half-time of distribution from the vascular compartment to the peripheral sites is about 30 minutes.

Myocardial uptake of digoxin is influenced by the serum concentrations of sodium and potassium. Studies with radiolabeled (^{3}H) digoxin have demonstrated that hyponatremia and hyperkalemia reduce the myocardial concentration of digoxin and that hypokalemia increases the digoxin concentration in the myocardium.[29,30] Myocardial uptake during alterations in the serum concentrations of sodium and potassium correlates with the binding of digoxin to the Na$^+$,K$^+$-ATPase and provides an explanation for the hypokalemia-induced potentiation of digitalis toxicity. The binding of digitalis glycoside to Na$^+$,K$^+$-ATPase in intact cells is stimulated by intracellular Na$^+$. The conditions that enhance sodium influx also promote glycoside binding to Na$^+$,K$^+$-ATPase. Concomitant administration of quinidine not only increases the serum digoxin concentration but also enhances the myocardial concentration of digoxin; however, the myocardial concentration of digoxin remains proportional to the serum digoxin concentrations.[31]

Digoxin is eliminated primarily by renal excretion; 60% to 90% of the administered dose is excreted unchanged in the urine and only a small fraction (15% to 20%) appears in the stool. Renal elimination of digoxin is primarily by glomerular filtration, although the saturable tubular secretion process also contributes.[32] That digoxin serum levels may rise when tubular secretion is blocked by concomitant administration of spironolactone has been demonstrated.[22] The rate of digoxin excretion appears to be independent of the route of administration. The elimination half-life of digoxin in healthy persons with normal renal function is approximately 36 hours. Tubular reabsorption of digoxin has also been demonstrated. Tubular reabsorption can reduce renal clearance of digoxin in patients with cardiovascular disorders and prerenal azotemia.[27] Intestinal reabsorption of digoxin via the enterohepatic circulation is limited and represents approximately 6.5% of the administered dose.[33]

To initiate digitalization, an initial loading dose of 0.5 to 0.75 mg can be administered; this is followed by 0.25 to 0.5 mg at 6-hour intervals until digitalization is achieved. When *rapid digitalization* is required, digoxin is administered intravenously, with an initial 0.5 to 1.0-mg dose followed by 0.25 to 0.5 mg at 6-hour intervals until digitalization is achieved. If rapid digitalization is not required, one does not need to administer a loading dose; daily oral administration of 0.25 to 0.5 mg of digoxin produces digitalization of most adult patients within 7 to 10 days. The usual oral maintenance dose is 0.125 to 0.25 mg daily; however, the dose needs to be adjusted according to renal function. When gelatin capsules (Lanoxicaps) are used, rapid digitalization can be obtained by administering 0.4 mg orally initially, then four doses of 0.2 mg every 4 hours, not exceeding a total of 1.6 mg. For slow digitalization, 0.1 to 0.4 mg is administered daily for 7 days. The oral maintenance dose of gelatin capsules is 0.1 to 0.2 mg daily.

Digitoxin

Digitoxin is almost completely absorbed from the gastrointestinal tract. Since it is less polar than other glycosides, binding to plasma proteins is very high and almost 97% of digitoxin is bound to plasma albumin.[34] Consequently, the renal clearance of digitoxin is lower and the half-life of elimination of digitoxin (4 to 6 days) is influenced very little by renal function. Displacement of digitoxin from its binding sites with plasma proteins can occur with the concomitant use of a number of drugs,[35] however, the clinical relevance of such interactions remains unclear.

Digitoxin is almost completely metabolized in the liver to inactive metabolites. Although conversion to digoxin occurs in the liver, the concentration of digoxin formed is too small to be clinically important. The inactive metabolites formed are excreted mainly by the kidneys. The plasma half-life of digitoxin is 4 to 6 days, considerably longer than that of digoxin. Drugs like phenylbutazone and phenobarbital, which enhance hepatic drug-metabolizing enzymatic activity, have been shown to accelerate digitoxin metabolism.[36] Enterohepatic recirculation occurs and approximately 25% of the metabolic end-products are excreted in the feces. The enterohepatic recycling can be partly interrupted by nonabsorbable resins such as cholestyramine that bind digitoxin in the gastrointestinal tract, and thus the digitoxin clearance rate may increase.

For rapid digitalization, the initial oral dose of digitoxin is 0.6 mg, followed by 0.4 mg 4 to 6 hours later, and then 0.2 mg every 6 hours until the full digitalization dose has been administered. The daily oral maintenance dose of digitoxin ranges from 0.05 to 0.2 mg.

Other Cardiac Glycosides

OUABAIN

This cardiac glycoside possesses very high polarity and is available only in the injectable form. It is excreted almost exclusively through the kidney. The onset of action is within 5 to 10 minutes and the peak effect is observed within 30 minutes to 2 hours. The plasma half-life is approximately 21 hours when renal function is normal; impaired renal function, however, will retard the excretion of ouabain. When very rapid pharmacohemodynamic effects are desired, ouabain is used occasionally in preference to other glycosides. The digitalizing dose is between 0.25 and 0.5 mg.

DESLANOSIDE

Deslanoside (Cedilanid-D) is structurally similar to digoxin, but its gastrointestinal absorption is unreliable and less than that of digoxin because of additional glucose residue attached to the terminal sugar. The onset of action when the drug is administered intravenously is within 10 to 30 minutes and the peak effect tends to occur within 1 to 2 hours. Renal excretion is the principal means of elimination and the plasma half-life is approximately 36 hours. Elimination of deslanoside is also influenced by renal function; slower elimination occurs with depressed renal function. Clinical use of deslanoside is extremely limited except for occasional emergency digitalization, when it can be administered intravenously in two doses of 0.6 to 0.8 mg each.

The pharmacokinetics of the cardiac glycosides is summarized in Figure 3.3.

Mechanisms of Action of Cardiac Glycosides: Positive Inotropic Effect

An increase in the amount of intracellular calcium available to react with the contractile proteins appears to be essential for the positive inotropic effect of the cardiotonic digitalis glycosides. However, the precise mechanism governing the increased availability of intracellular calcium still remains controversial. Using the photoactive calcium-sensitive protein aequorin, an increase in the intracellular calcium transient in response to acetylstrophanthidin has been demonstrated.[37] It is generally accepted that the cardiac glycosides interact with the Na+,K+-ATPase and that this enzyme represents the receptor for the cardiac glycosides. Various potential reactions that

FIGURE 3.3 THE PHARMACOKINETIC VALUES AND DIGITALIZING AND MAINTENANCE DOSES OF CARDIAC GLYCOSIDES

	Digoxin	Digitoxin	Ouabain	Deslanoside
Gastrointestinal absorption	60%–85%	90%–100%	Unreliable	Unreliable
Onset of action	15–30 min	1/2–2 h	5–10 min	10–30 min
Peak effect	1–5 h	4–12 h	1/2–2 h	1–2 h
Plasma half-life	36 h	5–7 days	21 h	36 h
Plasma concentration (ng/ml)				
Therapeutic	0.8–1.6	14–26		
Toxic	>2.4	>34		
Principal elimination route	Renal	Hepatic–renal	Renal	Renal
Total digitalizing dose (mg)				
Oral	1.0–1.5	1.3–1.6		
Intravenous	0.75–1.5	1.2–1.6	0.25–0.5	1.2–1.6
Daily oral maintenance dose (mg)	0.125–0.5	0.05–0.2		

(Modified from Moe GK, Farah AE: Digitalis and allied cardiac glycosides. In Goodman LS, Gilman A (eds): The Pharmacological Basis of Therapeutics, 5th ed, p 653, New York, Macmillan, 1975)

might contribute to increased intracellular calcium are illustrated in Figure 3.4.[13] Inhibition of Na^+, K^+-ATPase may reduce the transport of sodium out of the cell (*1*, Fig. 3.4) resulting in an increase in intracellular sodium. This increase in sodium may retard the normal release of calcium from the cell via the Na^+/Ca^{2+} exchange mechanism (*1a*, Fig. 3.4), which results in an increase in intracellular calcium. Facilitation of the entry of calcium into the cell through the voltage-dependent calcium channel during the plateau phase of the action potential is another possibility (*2*, Fig. 3.4). A third potential mechanism for increased intracellular calcium is the enhanced release of stored calcium from the sarcoplasmic reticulum (*3*, Fig. 3.4). Substantial evidence now exists for the inhibition by cardiac glycosides of the sarcolemmal sodium pump, the magnesium (Mg^{2+}) and ATP-dependent, sodium- and potassium-activated transport enzyme complex known as Na^+,K^+-ATPase.[30] The effects on the sodium pump of therapeutic doses of cardiac glycosides, which only increased contractility without inducing toxic arrhythmias, were evaluated by measuring isotonic fluxes.[29,30] The uptake of the K^+ analog, rubidium-86 ($^{86}Rb^+$), as a measure of monovalent cation transport, was determined in the myocardial biopsy specimens before and after administration of cardiac glycosides. Contractile state was assessed by measuring the maximum rise of left ventricular pressure at the onset of systole (left ventricular maximal rate of rise of pressure, LV dP/dt_{max}), which increased by 29% ± 3% after the administration of a subtoxic dose of ouabain. It was accompanied by a 21% ± 6% reduction of $^{86}Rb^+$ uptake (sodium pump inhibition). Toxic doses of digoxin caused a greater reduction of rubidium uptake, by 59%, at the onset of digoxin-toxic arrhythmias. The relative sensitivities of canine Purkinje fibers and myocardial cells to inhibition of the sodium pump after acute toxic doses of digoxin have been evaluated.[30] At the onset of overt toxicity, the reduction in $^{86}Rb^+$

uptake in myocardial tissue was 44% ± 0%, and in Purkinje fibers 76% ± 3%, suggesting a greater inhibition of the sodium pump by digoxin in Purkinje fibers. Studies using synchronously beating monolayers of cultured chick embryo ventricular cells have demonstrated sodium pump inhibition by cardiac glycosides.[30] Inhibition of $^{42}K^+$ or $^{86}Rb^+$ uptake associated with inhibition of sodium efflux was observed concurrently with an increase in inotropy, following exposure to ouabain. It has been suggested that mechanisms other than sodium pump inhibition may be involved in producing the positive inotropic effects of cardiac glycosides at low doses.[38–40] Indeed, with a very low dose of ouabain, positive inotropic effects associated with stimulation of the sodium pump have been observed.[38] It has been suggested that a stimulatory effect on the sodium pump is mediated by endogenous catecholamines.[30] Ouabain increases endogenous norepinephrine release in perfused organ preparations,[41] and with low concentrations it inhibits norepinephrine reuptake in guinea pig myocardium.[42] Sodium pump stimulation, as evidenced by rubidium uptake, is not observed in the presence of propranolol.

The potential mechanisms for increased intracellular calcium concentration following inhibition of sodium pump have also been extensively investigated. Most studies indicate that there is an increase in the "rapidly exchangeable calcium pool," often combined with an increase in both calcium "influx" and calcium "efflux."[30] An increase in the intracellular calcium transient by digitalis has also been shown in studies using the aequorin method,[37,43] microelectrode measurements,[44,45] and the intracellular calcium optical indicator.[46] Enhanced inward calcium current via the calcium channels is a potential mechanism for the increased intracellular calcium and the positive inotropic effect. However, such mechanisms for the positive inotropic effects of digitalis have not been established. It does appear that digitalis increases

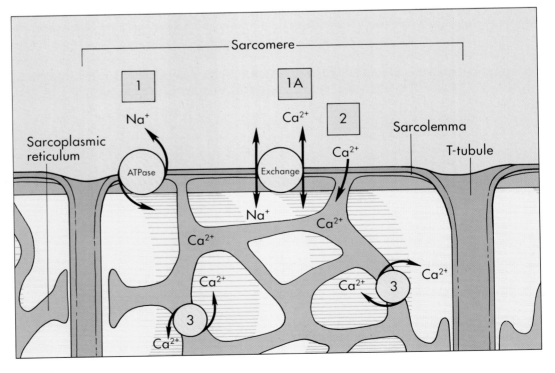

Figure 3.4 Schematic diagram to illustrate the possible sites of action of digitalis. The potential mechanisms are inhibition of sodium pump (1) and activation of the Na^+/Ca^{2+} exchanger (1a). It may also act on the ionic channel permeable to calcium (2) and the sarcoplasmic reticulum (SR; 3). (Modified from Katzung BG, Parmley WW: Cardiac glycosides and the other drugs used in the treatment of congestive heart failure. In Katzung BG (ed): Basic and Clinical Pharmacology, p 145. Los Altos, CA, Lange Publications, 1984)

intracellular calcium directly or through increased release of catecholamines.[47–49]

Considerable evidence now suggests that the inhibition of sodium transport out of the cells, associated with an increase in the intracellular sodium concentration, causes a secondary increase in the intracellular pool. This apparently is mediated by activation of the transsarcolemmal sodium-calcium exchange system. With the use of sodium-sensitive microelectrodes, an increase in intracellular sodium concentration has been reported in response to cardiac glycosides, which increased contractility.[44,50,51] The transsarcolemmal sodium gradient has marked effects on the rapidly exchangeable component of the intracellular calcium pool.[29,30] Thus, it appears that the positive inotropic effects of cardiac glycosides are related to the inhibition of the sodium pump, which causes a transient increase in intracellular sodium.[52] The increase in intracellular sodium results in enhanced calcium exchange, leading to a positive inotropic effect. However, other mechanisms such as increased release or decreased uptake of endogenous norepinephrine might also be contributory.

Electrophysiologic Effects

The electrophysiologic effects of digitalis have been reviewed in a number of recent publications.[29,30,53–56] Digitalis exerts its electrophysiologic effects directly, as well as through interaction with the autonomic nervous system. Direct actions initially cause a prolongation of the cellular action potential, with an increase in membrane resistance. This is followed by a period of shortening of the action potential, accompanied by a decrease in membrane resistance, probably due to increased intracellular calcium, which increases membrane potassium conductance. Reduction of the action potential's duration may contribute to the shortening of atrial and ventricular refractoriness.

Indirect actions of cardiac glycosides on the cardiac conduction system appear to be mediated through the autonomic nervous system. In patients with heart failure, digitalis frequently slows the sinus rate, presumably because of decreased sympathetic tone resulting from improved cardiac function. The sympathoinhibitory effect of digitalis in heart failure, however, probably results from activation of low or high pressure baroreceptor mechanisms, rather than from an enhanced inotropic state. In the absence of heart failure, digitalis usually does not produce any change in heart rate or may even cause a slight increase in sinus rate. Therapeutic doses of digitalis appear to exert a predominant vagotonic effect on the atrial myocardium and specialized conduction tissues.[30–57] In the intact animal with preserved autonomic function, these indirect cholinergic effects are manifested by abbreviation of the atrial refractory period and enhanced conduction.[48] In conscious humans, however, no change, or even an increase in atrial refractory period, has been observed following intravenous administration of digitalis.[57] Atrial conduction velocity may not change or may not even increase.

Reduction of atrioventricular (AV) nodal conduction is one of the major therapeutic effects of digitalis.

In both experimental animals and in human subjects, digitalis decreases AV nodal conduction and prolongs the nodal effective refractory period. AV nodal effects of digitalis appear to result primarily from its cholinergic and antiadrenergic actions, although a slight direct depression of the AV nodal conduction has been demonstrated in transplanted denervated hearts.[58] However, neither a significant reduction in conduction nor an increase in refractoriness of the AV node occur after vagal blockade or in transplanted hearts after acute administration of therapeutic doses of digitalis.

It appears that the electrophysiologic effects of digitalis in Purkinje fiber and ventricular myocardium, which consist of slight prolongation of the action potential, are related to its direct actions on the transmembrane potential and are not mediated by the autonomic nervous system.[30]

In experimental animals, prolongation of the action potential duration, which apparently results from increased slow inward current, correlates with the ST segment and T wave changes in the electrocardiogram. The prolongation of the action potential duration may result from increased slow inward current.[58] Prolonged exposure to higher concentrations of digitalis may shorten the action potential duration of the Purkinje fibers and ventricular muscle, primarily due to abbreviation of phase 2 of the action potential. This effect explains the shortening of the QT interval during digitalis therapy and decreased ventricular effective refractory period. The shortening of the action potential duration is accompanied by reduction of the maximum diastolic potential action potential amplitude, and conduction velocity. Decreased action potential duration following prolonged exposure to digitalis has been attributed to a decrease in membrane resistance, possibly due to a rise in potassium conductance.

Interaction with the Autonomic Nervous System

With therapeutic concentrations of digitalis, the predominant effect is activation of the parasympathetic nervous system, and with toxic concentrations there also may be stimulation of the sympathetic system. Digitalis may increase vagal activity by several mechanisms. The therapeutic concentration of digitalis can modify the activity of the arterial baroreceptors, the cardiopulmonary receptors, the efferent vagal nerve pathways, and the end-organ responses to vagal stimulation.[56] Digitalis can activate arterial baroreceptors and chemoreceptors and other afferent nerve fibers in the nodose ganglion. Experiments using isolated carotid sinus or aortic arch and monitoring changes in hemodynamic and electrical activity have indicated that digitalis causes excitation of baroreceptors in the carotid sinus and aortic arch. Direct application of digitalis to the epicardium or selective injection into the left anterior descending coronary artery causes hypotension and bradycardia.[59,60] In normal subjects, decreases in forearm blood flow and increases in forearm vascular resistance in response to lower body negative pressure were significantly greater after administration of lanatoside C, suggesting that digitalis augmented the tonic inhibitory influence of the cardiopulmonary receptors.[61] Thus, it appears that digitalis sensitizes baroreceptors and cardiopulmonary receptors so that the afferent input to the central nervous system is enhanced. This results in increased vagal activity and possibly withdrawal of sympathetic activity.

Digitalis also influences the effects of the sympathetic nervous system. However, higher concentrations of digitalis are required to produce sympathetic effects than parasympathetic effects. Various experiments have shown that with high concentrations of digitalis in the brain, the efferent sympathetic outflow is increased.[49] A relatively large concentration of digitalis can induce neuronal release of catecholamines and prevent catecholamine reuptake. These peripheral effects and effects on the central nervous system may result in increased cardiac and systemic sympathetic tone.

The interactions of digitalis with the autonomic nervous system are important in determining its clinical effects. With therapeutic levels of digitalis, parasympathetic effects dominate; with larger toxic concentrations, sympathetic effects may be manifest.

Enhanced parasympathetic activity can potentially produce negative inotropic effects and decrease the cardiac response to its direct positive inotropic effects. Furthermore, the magnitude of increase in cardiac output due to the positive inotropic effects may be curtailed due to a concomitant reduction in heart rate. In patients with heart failure, vagal tone is reduced and the sympathetic tone is enhanced. Thus, direct actions of digitalis may be more prominent in the presence of heart failure. Reduction of the ventricular response in atrial flutter or fibrillation results primarily from its parasympathetic nervous system-mediated effects on the AV node. Conversion of supraventricular tachycardia to sinus rhythm by digitalis alone is in some instances most likely related to its vagotonic effect. The electrophysiologic effects of digitalis are influenced by end-organ autonomic tone. In patients with atrial fibrillation, the ventricular response following digitalis is slower at rest, when vagal tone is high; during exercise, when vagal tone is decreased and sympathetic activity is increased, the ventricular response is considerably faster.

Physiologic, biochemical, and histochemical studies have provided evidence for the vagal innervation of the ventricles, particularly in the interventricular septum in the region of the bundle branches.[62–64] Experimental studies have also suggested that vagal stimulation decreases β-adrenergic–mediated cardiac catecholamine release from the heart.[65,66] Such vagally mediated antiadrenergic effects have the potential to exert beneficial antiarrhythmic effects.

Interaction with the autonomic nervous system may also contribute to the development of digitalis-induced arrhythmias. Large concentrations of digitalis enhance sympathetic tone, both by effects on the central nervous system, which increase efferent nerve activity, and by increasing catecholamine release or decreasing catecholamine reuptake. However, antiadrenergic drugs are usually not very effective in the control of arrhythmias resulting from digitalis toxicity.

Clinical Applications

The management of heart failure and the management of arrhythmias are the two major indications for digitalis therapy. Changes in cardiac function and systemic hemodynamics are related to the positive inotropic and peripheral vascular effects of digitalis. That digitalis augments myocardial contractility has been demonstrated in a number of experimental and clinical studies.[67] In isolated papillary muscle preparations, changes in contractility were assessed by determining the velocity of muscle shortening at varying loads, that is, the force–velocity curve, which shifted upward and to the right after strophanthidin.[68] The maximum velocity of shortening as well as the maximum developed isometric force increased. The time required to develop peak tension also decreases following digitalis. In papillary muscles obtained from cats with experimentally produced heart failure, similar changes in indices of contractility have been reported after digitalis.[69]

Chronic digoxin therapy increases the left ventricular rate of rise of pressure (dP/dt), velocity of circumferential fiber shortening, and excursion of left ventricular systolic diameter in normal, conscious, chronically instrumented dogs.[70] Echocardiographic studies in normal subjects have also demonstrated increased ejection fraction and mean rate of shortening of left ventricular dimensions after chronic digitalis administration.[71] The force–velocity curve in human subjects shifts upward and to the right, as in papillary muscle preparations after ouabain.[68] In both normal subjects and in patients with heart failure, digitalis decreases the QS_2 interval, left ventricular ejection time, and pre-ejection period. These findings suggest that digitalis enhances contractility of both normal and failing myocardium.

In normal subjects, and in the absence of depressed ventricular systolic function, cardiac output may not increase, despite an increased contractility, because of the counterbalancing effects of digitalis on the other determinants of cardiac output. A reduction in heart rate and the vagally mediated negative inotropic effects may potentially curtail the expected increase in cardiac output resulting from its direct positive inotropic effect. The most important counteracting mechanism, however, is the increase in systemic vascular resistance, which increases the resistance to left ventricular ejection and decreases stroke volume.

Digitalis-induced constriction of isolated arterial

and venous segments, increased arterial and venous tone in intact animals, and increased systemic vascular resistance in normal humans have been demonstrated.[72,73] Increased systemic vascular tone results from its direct effects on the smooth muscle of peripheral vascular beds and also from activation of the sympathetic nervous system. Increased mesenteric vascular resistance, which may decrease splanchnic blood flow, constriction of hepatic veins leading to the pooling of blood in the portal venous system, and decreased venous return to the heart have been reported.[73,74] Increased coronary vascular tone in response to digitalis has been observed both in experimental animals and in patients with coronary artery disease.[75,76]

Activation of the sympathetic nervous system is an important mechanism of digitalis-induced peripheral vasoconstriction. Stimulation of the α-receptors, mediated through the central nervous system, appears to be the predominant mechanism.[77] Digitalis-induced vasoconstriction is blocked by the α-blocking agent phenoxybenzamine, providing evidence for the participation of α-receptors in promoting peripheral vascular tone.[75]

Systemic and regional vasoconstriction appear to be more pronounced after a rapid bolus injection of digitalis.[76] Clinical studies have demonstrated that a 10-second infusion of digitalis increased systemic and coronary vascular resistance significantly and caused transient deterioration of myocardial lactate metabolism. A 15-minute infusion of the same dose of digitalis was not associated with any significant change in systemic or coronary vascular resistance or in myocardial lactate metabolism. Thus, when intravenous administration of digitalis is required, a slow infusion is preferable to avoid these potentially deleterious peripheral vascular effects.

In patients with chronic heart failure associated with depressed left ventricular systolic function, cardiac output generally increases.[78] Peripheral vascular responses to digitalis in heart failure also appear to be different from those in normal subjects. Reduction in both arteriolar and venous tone, instead of an increase, has been observed in heart failure.[72] In heart failure, decreased peripheral vascular tone appears to result primarily from sympathoinhibitory responses to digitalis. Sympathetic neural recordings revealed that after the administration of deslanoside, muscle sympathetic nerve activity decreased in heart failure, along with decreased forearm vascular resistance, decreased right atrial and pulmonary capillary wedge pressure, and increased cardiac output.[79] The mechanisms of sympathoinhibitory effects of digitalis in heart failure have not been entirely clarified, but improved cardiac function due to enhanced contractility does not appear to be contributory—a greater increase in contractility and better hemodynamic changes in response to dobutamine, a potent inotropic agent, are not associated with any decrease in muscle sympathetic nerve activity.[79] Mechanical and nonmechanical activation of afferent arterial and cardiopulmonary baroreflex mechanisms appears important for digitalis-induced sympathoinhibition in heart failure. This presumably results from sensitization of tonically active, inhibitory low or high pressure baroreceptors. Such mechanisms are also supported by observations that digitalis rapidly normalizes baroreflex-mediated vascular responses to orthostatic stress in patients with heart failure.[80] In normal subjects, adminstration of deslanoside causes no changes in forearm vascular resistance or muscle sympathetic nerve activity despite an increase in arterial systolic mean and pulse pressure, suggesting that digitalis may produce sympathoexcitatory responses in the absence of heart failure.[79]

Increased cardiac output in patients with heart failure following digitalis therapy may be accompanied by improved renal hemodynamics and increased diuresis. However, digitalis has been shown to inhibit renal tubular reabsorption of sodium. A direct infusion of ouabain into the renal artery has been reported to inhibit renal Na^+,K^+-ATPase and impair concentrating and diluting function.[81] Suppression of the renin–angiotensin system consequent on an increase of intracellular calcium by digitalis may have an important influence on renal hemodynamics.[82] However, the major mechanism for increased diuresis after digitalis in heart failure appears to be an improvement in cardiac function and increased cardiac output.

ACUTE MYOCARDIAL INFARCTION

Despite the demonstration in experimental and clinical studies that digitalis may increase myocardial contractility in the acute phase of myocardial infarction, the role of digitalis therapy in the management of pump failure in patients with acute myocardial infarction in sinus rhythm is limited. Increased contractility of the nonischemic and border zones following digitalis has been reported after coronary artery ligation in the dog.[83,84] Systolic shortening of ischemic epicardial and endocardial myocardial layers in dogs increases after ouabain; however, systolic shortening of the infarcted segments remains unchanged. Increases in left ventricular dP/dt and stroke work index and a reduction in left ventricular filling pressure have also been observed in patients with acute myocardial infarction.[85] In most investigations, however, no significant increase in cardiac output or decrease in left ventricular filling pressure occurred, suggesting that despite enhanced contractile function, overall cardiac pump function remained unchanged.[86,87] In patients with heart failure, variable and inconsistent changes in cardiac output and left ventricular filling pressure have been observed

(Fig. 3.5).[88,89] Although a significant increase in left ventricular stroke work index was reported in the majority of these clinical studies, cardiac output and stroke volume usually remained unchanged. Similarly, inconsistent changes in pulmonary capillary wedge pressure and left ventricular end-diastolic pressure have been observed in response to digitalis.

It has also been demonstrated in patients with acute myocardial infarction that when hemodynamic improvement occurs with digitalis, its magnitude is inversely related to the severity of heart failure.[90] Patients without heart failure responded with a significant increase in cardiac output; in patients with heart failure or shock, there was no change in either cardiac output or left ventricular filling pressure. Stroke work index also increased significantly only in those patients who had no clinical heart failure. Therefore, in patients with severe pump failure or cardiogenic shock, digitalis does not appear to produce any beneficial hemodynamic effects.[90–92] Digitalis also appears to be a relatively weaker inotropic agent compared with others presently available. Dobutamine, a β-receptor agonist, produces a much greater increase in cardiac output and a greater reduction in pulmonary capillary wedge pressure than digitalis (see Fig. 3.5).[89] The onset of the hemodynamic response of intravenous digitalis is also considerably slower than that of dobutamine.

Increased contractility and systemic vascular resistance following digitalis can potentially increase myocardial oxygen requirements. A concomitant increase in coronary vascular tone may decrease coronary blood flow; thus, the potential exists for precipitation or enhancement of myocardial ischemia with digitalis. In patients with chronic coronary artery disease without heart failure, coronary blood flow and myocardial oxygen consumption usually remain unchanged despite increased contractility.[93,94] However, coronary blood flow and myocardial oxygen consumption increase after intravenous ouabain in patients with acute myocardial infarction (Fig.

3.6).[90] In some patients angina and myocardial lactate production developed after ouabain, implying anaerobic metabolism and ischemia. In patients with chronic coronary artery disease, the left ventricular diastolic volume may decrease after digitalis; thus, decreased wall tension may prevent the expected increase in myocardial oxygen consumption. In the majority of patients with acute myocardial infarction and heart failure, left ventricular filling pressure and presumably left ventricular diastolic volume remain unchanged, providing a possible explanation for a net increase in myocardial oxygen consumption in these patients.

Whether digitalis, given in the acute phase of myocardial infarction, extends myocardial injury or not remains controversial. In experimental uncomplicated myocardial infarction, digitalis has been shown to increase the extent of myocardial injury.[95] Similarly, in patients without heart failure, increased creatine phosphokinase efflux, suggesting increased infarct size, has been observed after digoxin therapy.[96] However, in patients with heart failure and an elevated pulmonary capillary wedge pressure, decreased infarct size determined by creatine kinase (CK) curves has been reported.[97] Thus, the effects of digitalis on coronary hemodynamics, myocardial oxygen consumption, and extent of myocardial injury are likely to be variable and influenced both by the presence or absence of heart failure and by the magnitude of changes in the determinants of myocardial oxygen requirements and myocardial perfusion. Because of the lack of consistent beneficial hemodynamic effects, a slower onset of action, and the availability of more potent inotropic agents, digitalis is not the drug of choice for inotropic therapy of pump failure complicating acute myocardial infarction.

In some retrospective nonrandomized studies, continued digitalis therapy following acute myocardial infarction has been reported as an independent adverse risk factor for long-term survival.[98,99] During years of follow-up, the cumulative survival rate for

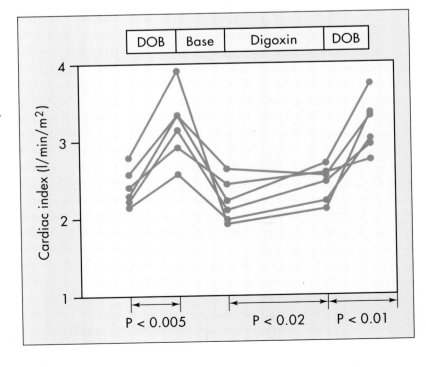

Figure 3.5 Changes in cardiac index in response to intravenous dobutamine (DOB) and digoxin in patients with acute myocardial infarction. With dobutamine there was a substanial increase in cardiac index; digoxin, however, produced insignificant changes. (Modified from Goldstein RA, Passamani ER, Roberts R: A comparison of digoxin and dobutamine in patients with acute infarction and cardiac failure. N Engl J Med 303:846, 1980)

patients treated with digitalis was 66%, compared with 87% for those not treated.[98] This adverse influence on late survival has been considered a result of increased arrhythmogenicity with digitalis in the presence of healed myocardial infarction. In canine hearts, the healed infarcted myocardium was found to be the site of origin of ventricular tachycardia due to digitalis toxicity.[100] Digitalis has been reported to be an independent risk factor for sudden death in postmyocardial infarction patients with depressed left ventricular systolic function.[101,102] Digitalis use, reduced ejection fraction, clinical heart failure, and high levels of ventricular premature ventricular depolarizations have also been identified by multivariate analysis as independent risk factors for adverse cardiac events and total mortality in postinfarction patients.[103–107] It has to be emphasized that digitalis therapy is usually instituted for the management of supraventricular arrhythmias and heart failure—the complications of acute myocardial infarction that are associated with a worse prognosis.[108] Some studies have reported that when the risks related to atrial arrhythmias and left ventricular failure are adjusted, no significant independent adverse influence of digitalis therapy is observed.[109] Thus, no conclusive evidence presently exists to suggest withholding long-term digitalis therapy if indicated in patients with healed myocardial infarction. Nevertheless, because of the potential increased risk of sudden death and total mortality, digitalis should be used in postinfarction patients only for the management of supraventricular arrhythmias. Digitalis therapy may be of benefit in postinfarction patients who develop established symptomatic chronic congestive heart failure associated with depressed systolic function.

CHRONIC HEART FAILURE

That acute digitalis therapy increases contractile function in patients with chronic heart failure in sinus rhythm has been demonstrated in clinical studies.[110] Increased contractile function was evident from the shortening of Q-A_2 intervals and the ratio of pre-ejection period to left ventricular ejection time.[110] An increase in the mean velocity of circumferential fiber shortening was also observed; the increase in fiber shortening occurred without any change in end-diastolic volume and despite an increase in arterial pressure and a decrease in heart rate.[111] An increase in the maximum velocity of fiber shortening (V_{max}) has been reported in patients with overt heart failure.[93] Thus, it seems well established that acute digitalis therapy enhances contractile function, and the positive inotropic effect appears to be more pronounced when left ventricular function is depressed. In patients in sinus rhythm, variable changes in left ventricular function have been reported during maintenance digoxin therapy. In some studies, an abbreviation of systolic time intervals, decreased heart size, and improvement in left ventricular segmental wall motion were observed during oral digoxin therapy.[112,113] A sustained increase in the velocity of fiber shortening and ejection fraction has been reported during maintenance digoxin therapy.[111] Even in normal subjects, a persistent improvement in left ventricular performance has been reported during long-term oral administration of digoxin.[114] However, other similar uncontrolled studies have failed to establish long-term beneficial effects of digoxin in patients in sinus rhythm; there were no significant changes in systolic time intervals.[114] Radionuclide angiographic studies also failed to demonstrate any sustained improvement in resting left ventricular function after maintenance digoxin therapy.[115]

Hemodynamic studies have demonstrated that, after acute administration of digitalis, cardiac output does not always increase. In an earlier review of the response of acute digitalis therapy in 117 patients, it was found that about 65% of patients had a significant increase in cardiac output and a decrease in left atrial and pulmonary arterial pressures.[114] Another 20% of patients had a modest increase in cardiac output. Systemic vascular resistance may increase in some patients after bolus intravenous administration of digoxin.[116] Slow infusion of digoxin, however, does not change systemic vascular resistance, and cardiac output tends to increase in most patients.[78] Changes in left ventricular function during exercise were assessed after acute and chronic digitalis therapy; in general, an improvement in exercise hemody-

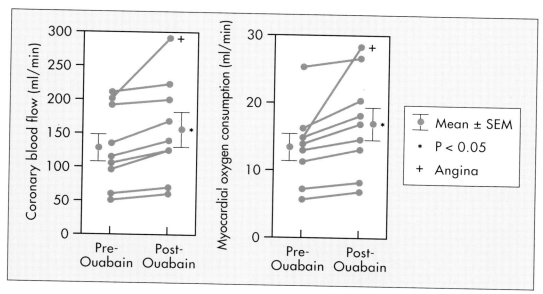

Figure 3.6 Ouabain-induced changes in coronary blood flow and myocardial oxygen consumption in patients with acute myocardial infarction. In most patients, coronary sinus blood flow and myocardial oxygen consumption increased, and occasionally the patient developed angina. (Modified from Forrester J, Chatterjee K: Preservation of ischemic myocardium. In Vogel JHK (ed): Advances in Cardiology, Vol II, p 158. Basel, S Karger, 1974)

namics and left ventricular performance was observed.[78,117] Withdrawal of chronic digoxin therapy has been shown to cause deterioration in hemodynamics and left ventricular function, both at rest and during exercise (Fig. 3.7). Hemodynamic improvement, however, is unlikely to occur in patients with severe chronic congestive heart failure (e.g., New York Heart Association [NYHA] class IV),[117] since the response to inotropic stimulation depends on the relative quantities of damaged myocardium devoid of contractile reserve.

Withdrawal of digitalis in patients with compensated heart failure causes variable changes in the clinical status.[118] Digitalis therapy could be discontinued without clinical deterioration in many patients: 48% to 100% of patients did not experience any symptomatic deterioration after withdrawal of digitalis. Results of diuretic therapy alone were compared with those of digoxin and diuretics, and no benefit from the addition of digoxin to diuretics was observed.[119–121] All these studies, however, were uncontrolled and frequently had a small sample size. Furthermore, heterogeneous patient populations were investigated, and frequently the appropriateness of digitalis therapy was not specified.

Placebo-controlled studies, however, have suggested that chronic digoxin therapy is likely to produce clinical improvement in most patients with congestive heart failure who have depressed left ventricular systolic function and an S_3 gallop (Fig. 3.8).[122,123] Clinical deterioration occurred in most patients when placebo was substituted for digoxin. In patients with normal systolic function or in those without S_3 gallop, maintenance digoxin therapy was not associated with any improvement. In one placebo-controlled study, chronic digoxin therapy was found to be of no clinical benefit in patients with stable chronic congestive heart failure. However, in this study most patients were elderly and only one patient had an S_3 gallop.[124]

Withdrawal of digoxin was also associated with a significant increase in left ventricular end-diastolic dimension and left ventricular ejection time and pre-ejection period and a decrease in the velocity of circumferential fiber shortening, indicating deterioration of left ventricular function.

In another prospective but nonrandomized study,[125] withdrawal of maintenance digoxin therapy did not result in any change in symptoms, exercise tolerance, radiologic or clinical findings of heart failure, or the radionuclide left ventricular ejection fraction. The effect of chronic digoxin therapy on exercise performance has been compared with that of xamoterol, a partial β_1-receptor agonist in a prospective randomized, controlled study in patients with mild chronic heart failure.[126] Compared with placebo, exercise performance improved with xamoterol but not with digoxin. Lack of improvement in exercise duration with chronic digoxin therapy has been reported in other prospective randomized, placebo-controlled studies.[127] The Captopril-Digoxin Multicenter Research Group compared the effects of captopril with those of digoxin in patients with mild to moderate heart failure in a double-blind, placebo-controlled study. Compared with placebo, the magnitude of increase in exercise duration with digoxin was not statistically significant and also there was no improvement in clinical class in the digoxin-treated patients. Captopril therapy resulted in significantly improved exercise duration and clinical class. Digoxin, however, increased left ventricular ejection fraction significantly compared with captopril and placebo. Furthermore, treatment failure, increased need for diuretic therapy, and hospitalizations had lower incidence compared with placebo in both digoxin-treated and captopril-treated groups. The relative

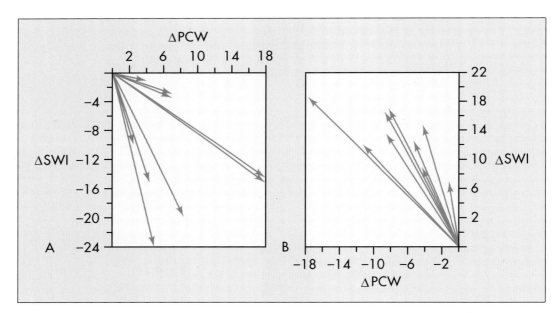

Figure 3.7 Changes in pulmonary capillary wedge pressure (ΔPCW) and stroke work index (ΔSWI) following withdrawal (**A**) and after rapid administration (**B**) of digoxin in patients with chronic heart failure in sinus rhythm. Discontinuation of chronic digoxin therapy was associated with decreased SWI and increased PCW pressure, and readministration of digoxin caused a decrease in PCW pressure and an increase in SWI. (Modified from Arnold S et al: Long-term digitalis therapy improves left ventricular function in heart failure. N Engl J Med 303:1443, 1980)

effectiveness of digoxin and enalapril, another converting enyme inhibitor, in improving clinical class and exercise duration in patients with mild to severe congestive heart failure has also been studied in a randomized double-blind trial.[128] Both enalapril and digoxin therapy resulted in a significant improvement in clinical class and exercise tolerance. In another multicenter, prospective, randomized trial, the magnitude of increase in exercise time on treadmill and percent fractional shortening of left ventricular dimension as determined by echocardiography were similar in treatment with enalapril and digoxin of patients with mild to moderate chronic congestive heart failure (New York Heart Association class II and III) in sinus rhythm. However, enalapril-treated patients experienced fewer adverse clinical events and had less fatigue during submaximal exercise.[129] In a multicenter, double-blind, placebo-controlled randomized study of patients with mild to moderate chronic heart failure in sinus rhythm not treated with converting enzyme inhibitors, withdrawal of digoxin resulted in worsening heart failure, requiring an increase in diuretics, emergency room care, increased frequency of hospitalization, and deterioration in treadmill exercise time.[130] In a similarly randomized trial in patients with chronic heart failure but already treated with angiotensin-converting enzyme inhibitors, withdrawal of digoxin was associated with a significantly higher frequency of deterioration of congestive heart failure symptoms, need for increased diuretics, emergency room care, and hospitalization. Withdrawal of digoxin also caused a significant decrease in exercise tolerance and left ventricular

ejection fraction.[131] In another double-blind placebo-controlled trial, digoxin was found to cause significant improvement in dyspnea, left ventricular fractional shortening as measured by M-mode echocardiography, heart failure score, and cardiothoracic ratio.[132] Unlike many other studies, in this study, digoxin doses were titrated to a therapeutic level.

Clinical efficacy, potential to improve ventricular function, arrhythmogenicity, and the impact on survival of digoxin therapy were compared with those of oral milrinone, a phosphodiesterase inhibitor, in a prospective randomized double-blind trial.[133] Exercise duration on a treadmill increased by similar magnitude with both digoxin and milrinone. Digoxin reduced the frequency of decompensation from heart failure from 47% with placebo to 15%; with milrinone, the frequency of decompensation decreased to 34%. However, clinical conditions deteriorated in a greater number of patients treated with milrinone (20%) than with digoxin (3%). Three-month mortality from all causes (according to the intention to treat) tended to be higher in patients treated with milrinone. Furthermore, increased ventricular arrhythmias occurred more frequently in patients receiving milrinone. Left ventricular ejection fraction increased with digoxin but remained unchanged with milrinone. Thus, digoxin therapy was as effective, if not more effective, than milrinone in these patient populations.

Concomitant digoxin and vasodilator therapy appears to be more effective than either therapy alone. In the Veterans Administration Heart Failure Trial,[134] the addition of hydralazine and isosorbide

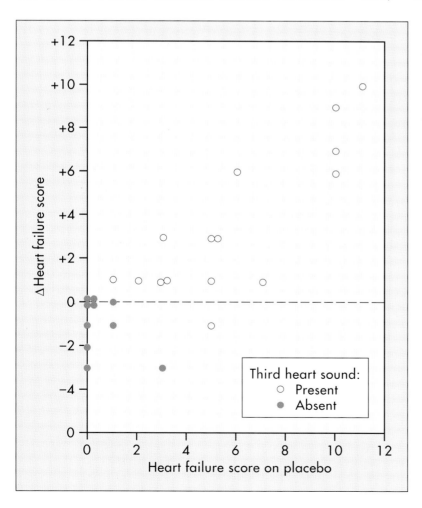

Figure 3.8 Changes in heart failure score while on maintenance digoxin treatment compared with score while on placebo in a group of patients with chronic heart failure. Heart failure scores were determined based on the results of clinical, radiologic, and noninvasive investigations. Patients with a third heart sound had improvement while on digoxin therapy. (Modified from Lee DC, Johnson RA, Bingham JB: Heart failure in outpatients: A randomized trial of digoxin versus placebo. N Engl J Med 306:699, 1982)

dinitrate to conventional treatment consisting of digitalis and diuretic therapy was associated with an improved survival. Similarly, in the CONSENSUS trial,[135] combined enalapril and digitalis and diuretic therapy was more effective at improving symptoms and survival in patients with severe chronic congestive heart failure than conventional therapy (digitalis and diuretics) was.

The comparative hemodynamic and neurohormonal effects of captopril and digoxin, given both separately and in combination, have been studied in patients with chronic heart failure.[136] Although both captopril and digoxin decreased pulmonary capillary wedge pressure and systemic vascular resistance significantly, only digoxin increased cardiac index and stroke work index. During maximal exercise, a significant reduction in systemic vascular resistance, and an increase in cardiac index were observed with captopril alone, whereas digoxin alone decreased pulmonary capillary wedge pressure and increased the stroke work index. The combination of captopril and digoxin caused a substantial reduction in pulmonary capillary wedge pressure and systemic vascular resistance, and an increase in the cardiac index both at rest and during exercise. A significant reduction in serum norepinephrine concentrations was observed with digoxin. Although in this study circulating norepinephrine levels remained unchanged with captopril, a significant reduction of norepinephrine has been observed during acute and chronic angiotensin-converting enzyme inhibitor therapy.[137,138]

It is apparent that digoxin usually improves left ventricular function in patients with chronic congestive heart failure, although significant symptomatic improvement may not be obvious in many patients. Digoxin appears to be more effective in patients with overt heart failure and significantly impaired left ventricular systolic function. In patients with very mild heart failure and relatively preserved systolic function, digoxin therapy is less likely to produce sustained benefit. Digoxin therapy, however, is likely to be beneficial in symptomatic patients with more than very mild heart failure, and should be considered in conjunction with vasodilators or angiotensin-converting enzyme inhibitors and diuretics. Digoxin therapy is of particular benefit in the treatment of heart failure associated with atrial fibrillation. Presently available data suggest that vasodilators and angiotensin-converting enzyme inhibitors improve the prognosis of patients concurrently treated with digitalis and diuretics; thus, digitalis and diuretic therapy alone should not be considered sufficient in the management of patients with chronic heart failure and vasodilators or angiotensin-converting enzyme inhibitors should be added whenever feasible and tolerated.

In isolated mitral stenosis with normal sinus rhythm, digitalis is of little value. However, digitalis is clearly indicated in the presence of atrial fibrillation and produces its salutary effect by decreasing the ventricular response, which allows decompression of the left atrium. Hypertrophic cardiomyopathy is another relative contraindication for digitalis therapy; left ventricular systolic function is normal or supernormal, and a further increase in contractile state with digitalis may be associated with increased left ventricular outflow obstruction. In occasional patients with hypertrophic cardiomyopathy, left ventricular systolic function declines and congestive symptoms develop; in these patients digitalis can be used to improve left ventricular performance. When atrial fibrillation develops, digitalis can be used cautiously to decrease the ventricular response, provided the presence of accessory pathways is excluded. However, β-adrenergic blocking agents or calcium channel blocking drugs (verapamil or diltiazem) are preferable in these patients to control the ventricular response.

Clinical experience suggests that patients with restrictive cardiomyopathy also do not derive significant benefit from digitalis therapy. Amyloid heart disease appears to predispose to digitalis intoxication. Little benefit is also expected in patients with cardiac tamponade or constrictive pericarditis.

ANGINA PECTORIS

Although in patients with cardiomegaly digoxin can decrease myocardial oxygen consumption by decreasing left ventricular volume, digoxin therapy is seldom indicated for treatment of angina pectoris. In patients with depressed left ventricular function, but without overt heart failure, the addition of digitalis to β-blocking drugs may improve exercise tolerance.[139] In patients with cardiomegaly and symptoms of heart failure, digoxin therapy occasionally decreases the frequency of angina.[122] However, nitrates and calcium channel blocking drugs are more appropriate pharmacologic agents for the treatment of angina in these patients.

In the absence of heart failure and depressed left ventricular function, digitalis does not produce any beneficial effects and may increase the frequency of anginal attacks.[140,141]

CHRONIC OBSTRUCTIVE PULMONARY DISEASE

Although digitalis exerts a positive inotropic effect in experimental animals with right-sided heart failure,[142] its role in the management of cor pulmonale secondary to obstructive lung disease has not been clarified. In the absence of right-sided heart failure, digitalis does not produce any beneficial effects.[143] Hemodynamic improvement can occur in some patients with overt heart failure due to cor pulmonale.[144] Acute digitalization, however, may increase pulmonary vascular resistance and cause deterioration of right ventricular performance. Furthermore, pulmonary disease may predispose to the development of digitalis toxicity. Patients with cor pulmonale with hypercapnia and hypoxemia appear to be more sensitive to digitalis during a strophanthidin test.[145] Arrhythmias suggestive of digitalis intoxication can develop in these patients with subtoxic serum concentrations of digoxin. Catecholamine release from cardiac adrenergic receptors and the adrenal glands in response to acute hypoxemia lowers the threshold for digitalis-induced arrhythmias.[146,147] Such mechanisms may explain the clinical observation that when systemic sympathomimetic amines are used for the treatment of chronic pulmonary disease, the addition of digitalis enhances the propensity to develop arrhythmias.

It appears that digitalis should be used with caution in patients with pulmonary disease who are hypoxemic. Furthermore, the hemodynamic and clinical benefits are marginal even in patients with right-sided heart failure. Thus, digitalis should be reserved only for those patients with cor pulmonale and right-sided heart failure unresponsive to alternative therapies (vasodilators and diuretics).

PROPHYLACTIC DIGITALIZATION

The value of long-term digitalis therapy in patients with aortic or mitral valve disease before the development of heart failure has not been established. In view of the potential risk of developing digitalis toxicity, prophylactic digitalis therapy is not indicated in these patients. Preoperative prophylactic digitalization has been advocated in patients undergoing aortocoronary bypass or major thoracoabdominal surgery to decrease the incidence of postoperative supraventricular tachyarrhythmias.[148] No conclusive evidence exists, however, for such beneficial effects; on the contrary, an increased incidence of tachyarrhythmias has been reported after coronary artery bypass surgery in digitalized patients.[149] Thus, there is little justification for routine preoperative digitalis therapy.

CARDIAC ARRHYTHMAS
Atrial Fibrillation

Atrial fibrillation with a rapid ventricular response is the most common indication for the use of digitalis. Decreased atrioventricular conduction resulting from the vagotonic effect of digitalis is associated with a decreased ventricular response. Increased ventricular filling associated with a slower ventricular rate improves hemodynamics. Conversion of atrial fibrillation to sinus rhythm with digitalis alone is not expected. In certain clinical circumstances (e.g., postoperative atrial fibrillation), addition of β-adrenergic blocking or calcium channel blocking drugs (verapamil or diltiazem) decreases the ventricular response more effectively because of the synergistic effects to decrease AV conduction. In atrial flutter, decreased AV conduction with digitalis is associated with increased AV block and a decreased ventricular response. Usually a relatively larger dose of digitalis is required to decrease AV nodal conduction in atrial flutter than in atrial fibrillation because of the relatively increased refractoriness of the AV node in the presence of atrial fibrillation. Digitalis may occasionally convert atrial flutter to fibrillation with a further decrease in ventricular rate. As in atrial fibrillation, the concomitant use of β-adrenergic blocking drugs or calcium antagonists may decrease the ventricular response more effectively. Digitalis is also effective in the control of paroxysmal atrial or AV nodal tachycardia. The oral or intravenous administration of digoxin may abruptly terminate such attacks probably as the result of its vagotonic effect. However, the calcium channel blocking agents verapamil and diltiazem and adenosine, which are more effective than digitalis in terminating supraventricular tachycardia, are the agents of choice.

Although digitalis is occasionally effective in controlling supraventricular tachycardia associated with the Wolff-Parkinson-White syndrome, it is not the drug of choice. Types Ia, Ic, and III antiarrhythmic drugs are more effective to control supraventricular tachyarrhythmias associated with the pre-excitation syndrome. Digitalis is contraindicated for the treatment of atrial fibrillation associated with the Wolff-Parkinson-White syndrome, since the ventricular rate may increase markedly.

DIGITALIS TOXICITY

Toxicity, which is occasionally life-threatening, is the major concern during digitalis therapy in patients with cardiovascular disorders. Withering stated, "The fox-glove, when given in very large and quickly repeated doses, occasions sickness, vomiting, purging, giddiness, confused vision, objects appearing green or yellow, increased secretion of urine, with frequent motions to part with it, and sometimes inability to retain it; slow pulse, even as low as 35 in a minute, cold sweats, convulsions, syncope and death." These clinical manifestations of severe digitalis toxicity, as observed by Withering more than 200 years ago, precisely outline both the cardiac and extracardiac manifestations of digitalis toxicity.

The true prevalence of digitalis toxicity is difficult to estimate. In Withering's era, the reported incidence was between 18% and 25%.[150] In hospitalized patients, adverse effects were observed in 19.8% to 21% of patients receiving digitalis.[151,152] Beller and co-workers reported a 23% incidence of definite digitalis toxicity in hospitalized patients.[153] Another 6% of patients had possible digitalis toxicity. Recent assessments have revealed a lower incidence, between 6% and 18%.[150,154] The apparent decreased prevalence might have resulted from increased knowledge of the pharmacodynamics and pharmacokinetics of presently available digitalis preparations and also from an increased awareness of the potential manifestations of digitalis toxicity.

Manifestations of Digitalis Toxicity

Manifestations of digitalis toxicity may be either extracardiac or cardiac. The extracardiac manifestations are often nonspecific and may be similar to those of congestive heart failure, making the diagnosis of digitalis toxicity difficult. In as many as 28% of patients, extracardiac symptoms may remain unsuspected as manifestations of digitalis toxicity. In almost 50% of patients, extracardiac symptoms do not precede cardiac arrhythmias related to digitalis toxicity.[155]

Extracardiac Manifestations

Gastrointestinal symptoms (anorexia, nausea, vomiting, and diarrhea) are relatively common extracardiac symptoms of digitalis toxicity. Anorexia is often the earliest symptom and is followed by nausea or vomiting. Abdominal pain and bloating may also occur. Digitalis administration has been associated with mesenteric infarction, which, in some instances, results in fatal hemorrhagic necrosis of the gut.[156] Additionally, the malabsorption syndrome has been reported in patients with heart failure treated with digitalis.[157] Neurologic manifestations are characterized by fatigue and by muscular weakness involving legs and arms. Visual disturbances usually manifest as hazy vision, difficulty in reading, alteration of the color of objects, photophobia, glittering moving spots, and flashes of yellow, red, green, or dark colors. Difficulties of red-green perception are more frequent visual disturbances. Ocular symptoms compatible with a diagnosis of retrobulbar neuritis have been reported as manifestations of digitalis toxicity. Transient psychosis, hallucinations, restlessness, insomnia, apathy, and drowsiness have also been observed. Frank delirium, often termed *foxglove frenzy* or *digitalis delirium,* may also occur. Digitalis therapy has been associated with painful gynecomastia in men and breast enlargement in women. Rarely, allergic skin lesions have been attributed to digitalis toxicity. Urticaria, scariatiniform rash, papules, vesicles, purpura bullosa, and angioneurotic edema associated with eosinophilia or thrombocytopenia have been observed. The mechanisms of all extracardiac manifestations[157] of digitalis toxicity have not yet been totally clarified. Digitalis has been demonstrated to increase visceral smooth muscle tone and prolong the transit time through the gastrointestinal tract. Rectal smooth muscles appear to be the most affected, and gastric smooth muscles the least sensitive to a digitalis-induced increase in tone. Decreased intestinal blood flow, resulting from vasoconstriction of the mesenteric and splanchnic circulations, has been implicated in many of the gastrointestinal symptoms of digitalis toxicity.[51] It has been demonstrated, however, that the emetic effects of digitalis are mediated by the area postrema at the base of the fourth cerebral ventricle.[51] Many of the extracardiac toxic effects of digitalis glycosides, including neurologic manifestations, appear to result from the excitation effects of digitalis on nerve cells in the cortical and medullary regions of the central nervous system. Perfusion of the lateral ventricles in experimental animals with ouabain causes a marked release of 5-hydroxytryptamine, suggesting that this compound plays a role in the genesis of digitalis glycoside-induced neurotoxicity. Digitalis may also increase the dopamine content of the central nervous system, which might contribute to its toxic effects. Although these experimental studies suggest that the effects of digitalis glycosides on the central nervous system,

mediated by an alteration in one or more neurotransmitters, may precipitate cardiac and noncardiac toxicity, further studies will be required to establish the precise mechanisms.

The mechanism for gynecomastia in men or breast enlargement in women is probably related to an elevation in the serum estrogen level and a decrease in serum luteinizing homone and plasma testosterone. The structural similarity between estrogens and digitalis glycosides and their metabolites might explain these endocrine side effects. The various extracardiac manifestations of digitalis toxicity are summarized in Figure 3.9.

Cardiac Adverse Effects

Cardiac arrhythmias are the most serious side effects of digitalis toxicity.[158,159] Almost all types of arrhythmias have been reported to occur with digitalis intoxication. It needs to be emphasized, however, that with rare exception arrhythmias identical to those induced by digitalis may also occur owing to underlying pathologic conditions. Digitalis-induced arrhythmias may not be clinically manifest and can remain "masked" until the dominant rhythm is slowed. Arrhythmias related to digitalis toxicity can be categorized according to the electrophysiologic mechanisms (Fig. 3.10).[158]

Digitalis-induced arrhythmias should be suspected "when there is the appearance of a slow heart rate in a patient with fast or normal heart rate, the appearance of a fast heart rate in a patient with a normal heart rate, the appearance of a regular rhythm in a patient with an irregular rhythm, and the appearance of a regularly irregular rhythm."[159] Arrhythmias considered most suggestive of digitalis toxicity are nonparoxysmal AV junctional tachycardia and paroxysmal atrial tachycardia with AV block. Bidirectional tachycardia, nonconducted premature atrial contractions, and double junctional rhythm are virtually diagnostic of digitalis toxicity. Regularization of rhythm in a patient with atrial fibrillation and ventricular tachycardia with exit block is also very suggestive of digitalis toxicity. Bigeminal ventricular

---

FIGURE 3.9 EXTRACARDIAC MANIFESTATIONS OF DIGITALIS TOXICITY

Gastrointestinal
Anorexia, nausea, vomiting, diarrhea, abdominal pain, bloating, malabsorption, mesenteric infarction

Neurologic
Fatigue, muscular weakness, visual disturbances, difficulties in red-green perception, symptoms of retrobulbar neuritis, insomnia, apathy, drowsiness, frank delirium ("foxglove frenzy," digitalis delirium)

Endocrine
Gynecomastia in men, enlargement of breasts in women

Dermatologic
Allergic skin lesions

rhythm and multiform premature ventricular contractions are quite common but are nonspecific.

Arrhythmias that are relatively unlikely to be due to digitalis toxicity are sinus tachycardia, paroxysmal AV junctional tachycardia without AV block, multifocal atrial tachycardia, parasystole, and nonparoxysmal ventricular (idioventricular) tachycardia. Mobitz type II AV block, complete infranodal AV block, bilateral bundle branch block, and atrial flutter or fibrillation with a rapid ventricular response are extremely rare manifestations of digitalis toxicity.

Sinoatrial (SA) and AV nodal block appear to result from the interaction of the "indirect" effects of digitalis mediated through the parasympathetic nervous system and its direct effects. Decreased conduction in the specialized conduction system may result not only in a bradyarrhythmia but also in a tachyarrhythmia.

Abnormal impulse initiation resulting from digitalis toxicity may also cause tachyarrhythmias. Depolarization during phase 4 of the action potential may enhance pulse initiation. The transient inward current induced by toxic concentrations of digitalis is oscillatory and causes the delayed afterdepolarization. The afterdepolarization, in turn, may induce a rate-dependent tachycardia referred to as a "triggered" arrhythmia.

Afterdepolarization occurs as a result of toxic inhibition of the "sodium pump." The accumulation of intracellular sodium is associated with increased intracellular calcium resulting from altered function of the Na^+–Ca^{2+} exchange mechanism and calcium release from intracellular stores. The increase in intracellular calcium triggers a transient inward current, the immediate cause of afterdepolarizations.

Experimental studies suggest that afterdepolarizations and triggered activity may be the basis of many digitalis-induced arrhythmias,[55] particularly repetitive ventricular responses and tachyarrhythmias.

Predisposing Factors for Digitalis Toxicity[158–161]

AGE Clinical observations suggest that elderly patients tolerate digitalis relatively poorly and develop digitalis toxicity more rapidly; in contrast, digitalis is well tolerated by younger persons. In infants, serum concentrations of digoxin of 2 to 3 ng/ml are not usually associated with any manifestations of digitalis toxicity. In comparison with adults, the absorption of digoxin in the newborn is not different but the volume of distribution is increased. In the premature infant, the rate of urinary excretion is decreased and the half-life of digoxin is increased. Experimental studies in animal models indicate that in young hearts a higher concentration of digitalis is required to induce depolarization of the cell membrane and afterdepolarization.[55] It has been suggested that the age-related changes in the sodium pump and its binding capacity for digitalis may account for the differences in tolerance to digitalis between the young and the elderly. The manifestations of digitalis toxicity in children are different from those in adults: in children, sinus bradycardia, sinoatrial block, and atrial or AV junctional rhythm are more common than the ventricular tachyarrhythmias.

After the administration of a similar dose of digoxin, the serum concentration of digoxin is higher in elderly patients than it is in younger patients. The higher serum concentration of digoxin in the elderly patient results from a decreased glomerular filtration rate and renal clearance and also from the decreased volume of distribution due to smaller skeletal muscle mass.

CARDIAC DISEASE Certain cardiac disorders have been suspected to predispose to cardiac digitalis toxicity. Patients with chronic obstructive pulmonary disease appear to be more susceptible to the development of arrhythmias due to ventricular automaticity. Hypoxia, hypokalemia, and therapy with sympathomimetic agents and methylxanthines contribute

FIGURE 3.10 ARRHYTHMIAS CAUSED BY DIGITALIS TOXICITY

1. Ectopic rhythm (re-entry, enhanced automaticity, or both)
   Atrial tachycardia with block
   Nonparoxysmal junctional tachycardia
   Reciprocation
   Ventricular tachycardia, flutter, fibrillation
   Bidirectional tachycardia
   Parasystolic ventricular tachycardia
   Atrial flutter, fibrillation
2. Depression of pacemakers with or without accelerated subsidiary pacemaker
   Sinus slowing
   Sinoatrial arrest
3. Depression of conduction
   Sinoatrial block, atrioventricular, exit block in association with
      Sinus rhythm
      Atrial tachycardia
      Atrial flutter
      Junctional rhythm
      Ventricular tachycardia
4. Ectopic rhythm with simultaneous depression of conduction junctional rhythm
   Ventricular tachycardia with decreased atrioventricular conduction
5. Atrioventricular dissociation with escape of subsidiary pacemaker
   Double junctional rhythm
6. Triggered automaticity
   Ventricular tachycardia triggered by supraventricular tachycardia
   Junctional tachycardia triggered by ventricular tachycardia

(Adapted From Fisch C, Knoebel SB: Digitalis cardiotoxicity. J Am Coll Cardiol, 5:91A, 1985)

to increased sensitivity. Patients with amyloid heart disease also appear to be prone to develop arrhythmias during digitalis therapy. Increased sensitivity to digitalis in ischemia or infarcted myocardium has been demonstrated in animal models.[100] The site of initiation of digitalis-induced ventricular tachycardia has been localized to the infarcted and peri-infarction zones. Patients with recent myocardial infarction, however, appear to tolerate the usual therapeutic doses of digitalis without an increase in the incidence of arrhythmias. The effect of digitalis therapy on long-term survival after myocardial infarction remains controversial. Some uncontrolled studies have suggested that the digitalis therapy may be an independent adverse risk factor for survival[98]; others have failed to demonstrate any increased risk of mortality in digitalis-treated patients.[162] Rather, the severity of the hemodynamic abnormality and the degree of depression of cardiac function influence the prognosis adversely.

RENAL FAILURE Decreased digitalis tolerance in patients with impaired renal function has been well documented. Serum digoxin level increases due to decreased renal excretion and volume of distribution. In the presence of renal failure, digoxin clearance parallels creatinine clearance. The precise mechanism for the decreased volume of distribution remains unclear; however a decrease in affinity of the receptor site for digoxin remains a possibility. In patients with severe renal failure, the loading and maintenance dose of digoxin should be reduced. In patients with end-stage renal disease, an intravenous dose of 0.7 mg resulted in a 24-hour level of digoxin ranging from 1.0 to 2.1 ng/ml, which did not produce digitalis toxicity.[161] Patients with severe renal failure in end-stage renal disease who weigh 40 kg need a maintenance dose of 0.0625 mg daily, while the 90-kg patient requires 0.1 mg daily to maintain a serum digoxin level in the therapeutic range. Hemodialysis removes only a small fraction of total body digoxin stores, about 4%. A supplemental digoxin dose after dialysis can increase the serum digoxin levels and cause toxicity. Elimination of digitoxin is less dependent on kidney function, since it is extensively metabolized in the liver.

SERUM POTASSIUM Hypokalemia predisposes to the toxic effects of digitalis. Decreased serum potassium levels following diuretic therapy, after dialysis, after administration of glucose, or due to gastrointestinal loss of potassium may induce ectopic arrhythmias after administration of relatively smaller doses of digitalis. Increased automaticity due to enhanced phase 4 depolarization occurs more frequently in the presence of low potassium concentrations. In animal models, lower doses of digoxin induce ventricular tachycardia in the presence of hypokalemia. Hypokalemia increases the uptake and bind-ing of glycosides to Na^+,K^+-ATPase. However, direct membrane effects of decreased renal excretion of digoxin induced by hyperkalemia or hypokalemia may also contribute to digitalis toxicity. A decreased serum potassium concentration may enhance digitalis-induced depression of AV nodal conduction. Hypokalemia might be contributory to digitalis-

induced ectopic atrial tachycardia with block and nonparoxysmal AV junctional tachycardia, which result from increased automaticity of ectopic pacemakers and depressed AV conduction. Severe hyperkalemia also depresses AV conduction and potentiates the effects of digitalis on AV conduction. In patients with atrial fibrillation treated with digitalis, hyperkalemia may precipitate complete AV block. The presence of AV junctional disease and the synergistic effects of digitalis and hyperkalemia on AV conduction may produce severe bradycardia or asystole.

SERUM CALCIUM That infusion of calcium in digitalized patients may induce ventricular tachycardia has been observed in clinical studies.[163] However, in experimental studies, no deleterious effects of hypercalcemia were observed in digitalized animals and there was no evidence for the additive effects of calcium and digitalis. Thus, unless the rate of infusion of calcium is very rapid or the serum concentration of calcium is very high, it is unlikely that moderate, transient hypercalcemia will enhance cardiac toxicity.

SERUM MAGNESIUM Hypomagnesemia can increase myocardial digoxin uptake, decrease the sodium pump activity, and increase the amplitude of digoxin-induced after-depolarizations.[164] Hypomagnesemia can exist with normal serum levels and can cause intracellular hypokalemia that is refractory to potassium replacement. Thus, decreased magnesium stores, like hypokalemia, can precipitate toxicity at therapeutic levels of digoxin. In experimental animals, hypomagnesemia enhances ouabain-induced automaticity in the presence of AV block and lowers the ouabain doses required to induce ventricular tachyarrhythmias.[165] Clinical studies, however, have failed to demonstrate any conclusive evidence for the relation between the hypomagnesemia and digitalis toxicity.[166] Nevertheless, arrhythmias attributable to digitalis toxicity may respond favorably to intravenous administration of magnesium,[167] which may result from its nonspecific antiarrhythmic effect.

ALKALOSIS In patients with metabolic alkalosis and normal potassium concentrations, therapeutic concentrations of digoxin may be associated with a greater incidence of arrhythmias than seen in patients without alkalosis.[168] The mechanism for this apparent increased sensitivity to digitalis associated with alkalosis remains unclear.

HYPOTHYROIDISM Decreased thyroid function increases serum digoxin levels by decreasing glomerular filtration rate and the volume of distribution of digoxin. The myocardium of the myxedematous patient appears to have reduced tolerance to digoxin, which is reversed with thyroid replacement.[169] Hyperthyroid patients tend to tolerate larger doses of digitalis and eliminate glycosides faster.

CARDIOPULMONARY BYPASS Sensitivity to the toxic effects of digitalis appears to increase in the first 24 hours after cardiopulmonary bypass.[170] Toxicity is not related to blood gas changes or serum electrolyte concentrations and is manifest at a relatively lower serum digoxin concentration.

DIGITALIS AND ELECTRIC SHOCK In animal studies, digitalis administration decreases the amount of electrical energy required to induce ventricular tachyarrhythmias. Synchronized direct-current shock frequently precipitates supraventricular and ventricular ectopic arrhythmias in digitalized patients. However, recent animal and clinical studies have documented that in the presence of therapeutic concentrations of digoxin, direct-current shock does not enhance the incidence of arrhythmias attributable to digitalis toxicity.[171,172] However, in patients with overt digitalis toxicity, electrical shocks at all energy levels may precipitate sustained ventricular tachycardia. Thus, the risk of arrhythmia after direct-current shock is increased only in the presence of overt digitalis toxicity and countershocks can be applied safely in therapeutically digitalized patients.

DRUG INTERACTION[161,172,173] Changes in serum digoxin levels due to interaction with other drugs may predispose the patient to digitalis toxicity. Digitalis–drug interactions are described elsewhere in these volumes. Concurrent administration of antacids, bran, kaolin pectate, cholestyramine, colestipol, activated charcoal, sulfasalazine, neomycin, or p-aminosalicyclic acid can decrease digoxin absorption.[173] Sudden withdrawal of these drugs without decreasing the oral dose of digoxin may enhance its absorption and increase its serum level, resulting in toxicity. Administration of certain antibiotics (e.g., erythromycin) may increase serum digoxin levels due to increased bioavailability resulting from decreased metabolism.

In clinical practice, interaction with certain antiarrhythmic drugs that increase serum digoxin levels appears to predispose to digitalis toxicity more frequently. Quinidine causes an increase in the serum digoxin level in over 90% of patients, and this can precipitate toxicity. The increase in digoxin level in individual patients is variable and ranges from none to sixfold, with an average increase of twofold. The magnitude of increase in the serum digoxin level is proportional to the quinidine dose. Both extracardiac toxicity and AV conduction delay may occur as a result of this interaction.[174] The mechanism for the increased serum digoxin level following quinidine therapy is not completely understood. A decrease in total body, renal, and nonrenal clearance and decreased volume of distribution of digoxin appear to occur after administration of quinidine. It has been proposed that the early rise in serum digoxin levels results from the displacement of digoxin from tissue stores.

The ratio of skeletal to serum digoxin concentration decreases, which suggests displacement of digoxin from skeletal muscle. The ratio of myocardial to serum digoxin, however, remains unchanged during this interaction. Studies in animals demonstrate that the increased serum digoxin level is not accompanied by a proportional increase in digoxin effect as measured by percent inhibition of rubidium myocardial uptake, implying that digoxin may be selectively displaced from active binding sites, since overall myocardial digoxin content increases appropriately.[175]

Since the digoxin blood level tends to increase with the first dose of quinidine, and a new digoxin steady state is achieved by the fifth day, it has been suggested that the dose of digoxin should be halved prior to the addition of quinidine.[173] It is, however, more important to assess the patient clinically and to monitor electrocardiographic changes until the new steady state is achieved during concurrent quinidine–digoxin therapy.

Serum levels of digitoxin may also increase when quinidine is added. Renal clearance of digitoxin declines and is accompanied by an increased serum level. The nonrenal clearance may also decrease, but the volume of distribution remains unchanged and the digitoxin half-life is lengthened.[172]

Amiodarone, another potent antiarrhythmic agent, increases serum digoxin levels by 25% to 70%, and this increase appears to be related to the dose of amiodarone administered.[173] Generally, toxic manifestations of this interaction consist of bradycardia and varying degrees of AV block, rather than tachyarrhythmia. Renal and nonrenal clearance is decreased without any significant change in the apparent volume of distribution of digoxin. Procainamide, disopyramide, mexiletine, flecainide, and ethmozine do not appear to change serum digoxin concentrations significantly. Propafanone, however, can increase serum digoxin concentration.

The calcium channel blocking agent verapamil interacts with digoxin and increases its serum concentration in approximately 90% of patients.[173] Decreased renal and nonrenal clearance and volume of distribution result in elevated serum digoxin levels; these mechanisms are very similar to the digoxin–quinidine interaction. An inhibition of the tubular secretion of digoxin appears to be the mechanism for decreased renal clearance, since creatinine clearance remains unchanged. The magnitude of increase in serum digoxin levels is related to the dose of verapamil. A marked increase in the serum level of digoxin with concomitant administration of verapamil may cause potentially fatal cardiac toxicity, usually in the form of bradycardia and asystole rather than tachyarrhythmias. Tiapamil, a congener of verapamil, causes an increase in serum digoxin levels similar to that of verapamil. Nifedipine and nicardipine, two related calcium channel blocking agents, do not appear to affect serum digoxin levels significantly, and diltiazem, with larger doses (180 mg/d), causes only a small (average 22%) and probably not clinically relevant increase. Similarly, little or no change in digoxin levels is observed with gallopamil and lidoflazine.[173] Other drugs that can increase serum digoxin levels are spironolactone (inhibition of active tubular digoxin secretion) and some antihypertensive agents (decreased renal blood flow and glomerular filtration rate).[29]

Thus, several commonly used drugs can raise the serum digoxin concentration and predispose to toxicity, and drug interactions should always be considered in patients who are on digitalis therapy.

Diagnosis

Digitalis toxicity should be suspected in any patient receiving digitalis who complains of new gastrointestinal, ocular, or central nervous system symptoms. The appearance of a new arrhythmia should also be considered a potential indication of digitalis toxicity. Some electrocardiographic changes are very suggestive of digitalis effect; frequently, there is ST segment sagging, most prominent in leads I, aV_L, V_5, and V_6. The T wave voltage is frequently reduced, and because of accelerated repolarization the QT interval may be shortened. These changes do not indicate toxicity and do not necessarily precede arrhythmias.

The serum digoxin level is often helpful in the diagnosis of suspected digitalis toxicity, although the level by itself does not confirm or exclude digitalis toxicity in individual patients. The digoxin concentrations are usually measured by the radioimmunoassay technique. The optimal time for measurement of serum digoxin is just prior to the next dose, or at least 6 hours after an oral dose and 4 hours after intravenous administration. False-positive assays can be encountered in certain clinical circumstances, which include spironolactone therapy, the presence of circulating, gamma-emitting radio-imagers, hyperbilirubinemia, and renal failure. In as many as 60% of patients with chronic renal failure, false-positive results can be observed and appear to be due to an endogenous circulating digoxin-like substance.[176]

To determine the therapeutic and toxic concentration of digoxin, correlations of the therapeutic and toxic manifestations to serum digoxin levels have been determined in normal volunteers and in patients with various cardiac disorders.[29] The mean serum digoxin level in the absence of toxicity was 1.4 ng/ml; in patients with toxicity, it was two to three times higher. The therapeutic range has been regarded as 0.5 to 2.0 ng/ml. However, considerable overlap exists between the digoxin levels in toxic and nontoxic patients. Approximately 10% of patients who have serum digoxin concentrations within the therapeutic range manifest cardiac toxicity; similarly, in about 10% of patients without toxicity, serum digoxin levels are between 2 and 4 ng/ml. Studies correlating noncardiac symptoms of toxicity and serum digoxin concentrations have also revealed considerable overlap among serum digoxin levels in patients with and without extracardiac manifestations of toxicity, even when the mean serum digoxin levels in the two groups differed significantly.[29] Nevertheless, the higher the serum digoxin levels, the higher is the likelihood of toxicity; the probability of toxicity with serum digoxin levels exceeding 3 ng/ml is 12 times higher than when the level is between 0 and 0.99 ng/ml.[177]

Serum concentrations of digoxin in relation to its inotropic and hemodynamic effects have been determined, and the inotropic effects do not appear to be greater with serum digoxin levels above 1 to 2 ng/ml.[29] Supplemental doses of digoxin given intravenously to patients on conventional maintenance digoxin doses do not cause any further hemodynamic improvement.[78] These findings suggest that doses sufficient to maintain digoxin concentrations in the range of 1 to 2 ng/ml may provide maximal or near-maximal therapeutic effects. As the risk of digitalis toxicity increases with higher serum digoxin concentrations, the risk-to-benefit ratio appears to be optimal, with digoxin levels ranging between 1 and 2 ng/ml.[29] Mean serum levels of digitoxin, as with digoxin, were considerably higher (34 to 96 ng/ml) in patients with toxicity than in patients without toxicity (16.6 to 31.8 ng/ml) in different studies,[29] but considerable overlap in digitoxin concentrations was also found between the two groups.

It is apparent that the determination of serum digitalis levels is useful in the diagnosis of digitalis toxicity. However, levels within the "therapeutic range" should not be considered to exclude toxicity when clinical suspicion is strong, particularly in the presence of circumstances that predispose to digitalis toxicity (e.g., hypokalemia, hypomagnesemia, and severe acid-base imbalance).

In addition, as an aid in the diagnosis of digitalis toxicity, monitoring serum digitalis concentrations may be helpful to ensure adequate digitalization in a patient with suboptimal clinical response. Digitalis assays are also useful in detecting noncompliance, malabsorption, drug interactions, or poor bioavailability in patients who do not demonstrate the expected clinical response while on maintenance digitalis therapy.

It has been suggested that the estimation of electrolyte contents of the saliva may be useful to determine the digitalis effect in individual patients.[178] Salivary potassium and calcium concentrations and the products of potassium and calcium concentrations in saliva were significantly higher in the presence of digitalis toxicity than in the absence of toxicity. The diagnostic value of this test was independent of the digitalis preparation used. It has been postulated that changes in the salivary electrolyte concentrations represent inhibition of monovalent cation transport. This test, however, has not been adequately evaluated, and its role in the diagnosis of digitalis toxicity remains uncertain presently.

Red blood cell sodium and potassium levels may also correlate with digitalis effect.[179] Digitalis-induced inhibition of the sodium pump of erythrocytes decreases the rate of potassium or rubidium uptake, decreases the intracellular potassium, and increases sodium concentrations. Thus, erythrocyte rubidium uptake, or the measurements of the intracellular concentrations of sodium and potassium of erythrocytes may aid in the diagnosis of digitalis toxicity. However, these tests have not been adequately evaluated and their clinical value has not been established. The acetyl strophanthidin test has been advocated to predict whether a given patient is overdigitalized or underdigitalized.[180] The appearance of arrhythmias following intravenous administration of acetyl strophanthidin, a short-acting digitalis-like drug, had been considered suggestive of cardiac toxicity; however, the predictive value of this test has not been determined.

Management

All patients with significant arrhythmias, with or without hemodynamic compromise, should be hospitalized for observation and electrocardiographic monitoring. Patients with minor noncardiac symptoms, or with insignificant arrhythmias (e.g., occasional ectopic beats or atrial fibrillation with a slow ventricular response) do not require hospitalization and can be managed effectively by stopping the drug. Depending on the initial serum concentration, discontinuing digoxin for 24 to 48 hours causes adequate reduction of digoxin level, with reversal of toxicity in patients with normal renal function. Digitoxin should be discontinued for several days because of its longer half-life. The electrocardiogram should be repeated to ensure disappearance of the arrhythmia.

GENERAL THERAPY General therapy of significant digitalis toxicity should include bed rest to avoid sympathetic stimulation and exacerbation of arrhythmias and discontinuation of digitalis, diuretics, and drugs that can potentially increase the serum digoxin level. Constant monitoring of cardiac rhythm is essential because multiple arrhythmias with variable hemodynamic consequences may occur over time. Serum electrolytes and digoxin concentrations should be determined and renal and hepatic function as well as blood gases and acid-base balance assessed. In patients with massive digitalis overdose, either deliberate or accidental, activated charcoal (50 to 100 g initially, then 20 g every 6 hours) may be administered to retard glycoside absorption. The corticosteroid-binding resin cholestyramine (4 to 8 g every 6 hours) may decrease the serum half-life of digitoxin significantly because it undergoes considerable enterohepatic circulation.[181] Colestipol appears to have a similar effect.[182] Digoxin has only minimal enterohepatic circulation, but cholestyramine may retard its initial absorption.

ATROPINE AND PACING[172] Rhythm disturbances that compromise cardiac function require immediate and active intervention. Sinus bradycardia, AV block, and sinoatrial exit block can often be treated effectively with atropine alone. However, atropine is not always effective, and transvenous ventricular endocardial pacing may be required. The risk of ventricular arrhythmias during placement or displacement of the pacemaker electrode catheter appears to be higher. In the presence of intact AV conduction, atrial pacing reduces the risk of pacemaker-induced ventricular tachyarrhythmias; however, digitalis increases AV nodal refractoriness and, hence, ventricular pacing is preferable. Overdrive pacing can occasionally result in "overdrive acceleration" of the underlying tachyarrhythmia.

ANTIARRHYTHMIC AGENTS[172] Phenytoin suppresses digitalis-induced enhanced automaticity and delayed afterdepolarization. It may also reverse digoxin-induced depression of AV and sinoatrial conduction. Decreased sympathetic outflow mediated by its effects on the central nervous system is considered as the mechanism of action.[183] Ventricular arrhythmias are particularly responsive to phenytoin (the other arrhythmias that may also respond are atrial tachycardia with block and nonparoxysmal junctional tachycardia). The inotropic effect of digitalis does not appear to be affected. It should be administered by slow intravenous infusion of 50 to 100 mg over 5 minutes, up to 15 mg/kg. Intravenous therapy should be followed by oral therapy (5 mg/kg daily) if the arrhythmia is controlled. Hypotension is the major complication of intravenous phenytoin therapy.

LIDOCAINE Lidocaine is useful for controlling digitalis-induced ectopic rhythms. It does not adversely affect sinus rate or atrial, AV nodal, or His-Purkinje conduction. It does not possess any significant myocardial depressant effect. Rarely, lidocaine can suppress the ectopic pacemaker focus in the presence of advanced AV block and precipitate ventricular standstill. Indications for lidocaine therapy are ventricular tachyarrhythmias and atrial tachycardia with block.[184]

β-ADRENERGIC BLOCKING AGENTS β-Adrenergic blocking agents are occasionally useful in controlling certain ectopic arrhythmias resulting from digitalis toxicity. The antiadrenergic effects decrease the automaticity and the direct effects shorten the refractory period of atrial and ventricular muscles and of the His-Purkinje fibers.[185] These potential beneficial effects, however, must be carefully weighed against the adverse effects, which include depression, sinoatrial and junctional pacemakers, and AV conduction. Thus, marked bradycardia or even asystole may result following the use of β-adrenergic blocking agents. Furthermore, their negative inotropic effects may cause hemodynamic compromise. Thus, in the presence of bradycardia, AV conduction abnormality, and heart failure, β-adrenergic blocking agents should not be used.

QUINIDINE, PROCAINAMIDE, AND DISOPYRAMIDE Quinidine, procainamide, and disopyramide should be avoided in the treatment of arrhythmias associated with digitalis toxicity. These agents can cause depression of AV and His-Purkinje conduction and precipitate asystole. Myocardial depressant effects may worsen heart failure.

BRETYLIUM Bretylium is also relatively contraindicated in digitalis toxicity. Initially, it can worsen tachyarrhythmias owing to release of stored catecholamines, which can enhance automaticity and delayed afterdepolarization and worsen hypokalemia.[186]

AMIODARONE Amiodarone has been effective, occasionally, in controlling digitalis-induced ventricular tachycardia. However, amiodarone given intravenously or orally decreases AV conduction and can induce advanced AV block in the presence of digitalis toxicity. It also increases the serum digoxin level: thus, amiodarone should be avoided in the treatment of digitalis toxicity.

VERAPAMIL Verapamil, a calcium channel blocking agent with negative inotropic and chronotropic properties, can worsen digitalis-induced AV block while suppressing delayed afterdepolarizations and triggered ectopy. It increases serum digoxin levels and can cause deterioration in heart failure. Thus, verapamil should not be used for treating supraventricular tachyarrhythmias associated with digitalis toxicity.

ELECTROLYTE REPLACEMENT Potassium replacement is often the initial therapy of choice for ectopic rhythms, particularly in the presence of hypokalemia. Potassium replacement is effective in treating ventricular ectopy and tachycardia, atrial tachycardia with block, and nonparoxysmal AV junctional tachycardia. Increased extracellular potassium following potassium replacement therapy enhances sodium pump activity, which is associated with decreased intracellular calcium and secondary afterpolarization. Potassium should be administered with caution in the presence of conduction disturbances and should not be used in the absence of hypokalemia. The actions of potassium and digitalis are additive on the conduction tissues, and marked conduction abnormalities may occur following potassium therapy in the presence of digitalis toxicity. Potassium therapy is also contraindicated in renal failure and in the presence of pre-existing hyperkalemia. Hyperkalemia decreases resting membrane potential and potentiates digoxin's effect on AV conduction. A given dose of potassium chloride can produce a greater than expected increase in serum potassium level in patients with digitalis toxicity due to inhibition of the sodium–potassium pump. When indicated, potassium can be administered intravenously at a rate of 0.5 mEq/min in a saline solution through a large vein.

Magnesium given intravenously suppresses digitalis-induced ventricular arrhythmias.[187] However, it may also induce advanced AV block, hypotension, and respiratory depression. It is contraindicated in patients with renal failure, hypermagnesemia, and AV block.

CAROTID SINUS MASSAGE Carotid sinus massage should not be attempted for diagnostic or therapeutic purposes in patients with supraventricular tachyarrhythmias due to suspected digitalis toxicity. In patients with digitalis toxicity, carotid sinus massage can precipitate ventricular asystole, advanced atrioventricular block, and malignant ventricular arrhythmias.[188]

CARDIOVERSION Cardioversion should be avoided, if possible, in patients with digitalis toxicity. Digitalis decreases the energy threshold for cardioversion-induced arrhythmias severalfold, and cardioversion can precipitate refractory ventricular tachyarrhythmias.[189] Release of catecholamines from cardiac nerve endings and alteration of membrane function leading to intracellular potassium egress might be the mechanism for the cardioversion-induced arrhythmias. Cardioversion, however, is recommended despite an increased risk of arrhythmias in patients in whom pharmacotherapy is ineffective and hemodynamic instability exists. Cardioversion therapy should be initiated at lower energy levels, which reduce the risk of developing arrhythmias. It needs to be emphasized that cardioversion does not enhance arrhythmias in the absence of overt digitalis toxicity.[190]

DIALYSIS Renal or peritoneal dialysis is ineffective in decreasing total body digoxin content. Adsorptive hemoperfusion has been reported to increase the rate of removal of digoxin in some patients with digoxin toxicity.[191] With adsorptive hemoperfusion, the patient's blood is passed over an adsorbing substance such as charcoal and the drug is directly bound to the absorbent, which removes the glycoside. However, it is less effective than other therapeutic measures, such as digoxin-specific antibodies.

DIGOXIN-SPECIFIC ANTIBODIES Digoxin-immune Fab is an antigen-binding agent and has emerged as an effective treatment for digitalis toxicity. In 1966, Buller and Chen demonstrated antibodies to digoxin in rabbits in response to immunization with a digoxin-albumin conjugate, and rabbit antiserum reversed manifestations of digitalis intoxication in experimental animals.[192] Subsequently, purified digoxin-specific antibodies were isolated from sheep antisera.[193] The whole heterologous antibodies, without purification, are likely to induce immediate and late hypersensitivity in humans, because of the presence of such foreign proteins. Digestion of the intact immunoglobulin (IgG) with papain yields two antigen-binding fragments (Fab) and one crystalline fragment (Fc), which contains the complement binding site. Digoxin-specific Fab can be isolated and purified from the papain-digested hyperimmune animal serum by the process of immunoadsorption. The purified Fab appears to possess the same affinity as the IgG for binding digoxin. Fab is less immunogenic than the IgG due to the absence of the Fc fragment. Because of the smaller size, these fragments distribute more rapidly and into a larger distribution of volume. The Fab-digoxin complex is also more rapidly excreted by glomerular filtration, while the IgG-digoxin complex is slowly degraded by the reticuloendothelial system.

Fab binds one molecule of digoxin, and the affinity of Fab for digoxin is greater than the affinity of digoxin for Na^+,K^+-ATPase. $F(ab)_2$, an antibody fragment that contains two Fab molecules held together by a disulfide bond, also has similar digoxin binding affinity and has been used for the treatment of digitalis toxicity.[194] Because of the higher binding affinity of the cardiac glycosides digoxin and digitoxin for Fab fragments, free cardiac glycosides rapidly bind with Fab and the concentrations of free glycosides decrease. Since the receptor–glycoside interactions are reversible, a concentration gradient is established as extracellular free digoxin concentrations decrease, causing a progressive efflux of cellular digoxin from its binding sites, which then bind to Fab fragments and become inactivated.

Following intravenous infusion of Fab, serum concentration of free (unbound) digoxin decreases to almost undetectable levels within a few minutes. Total serum digoxin concentrations, however, increase rapidly, usually exceeding pretreatment serum concentration of these glycosides 10- to 20-fold. Almost all of the glycosides in serum are inactive and bound to Fab during the first 12 hours after the administration of Fab. The onset of action of Fab is usually within 30 minutes. The elimination half-life is between 15 and 20 hours in patients with normal renal function. In patients with renal failure, the excretion of the Fab-digoxin complex is probably significantly delayed. In functionally anephric patients, the Fab-digoxin complex is cleared not by glomerular filtration and renal excretion but probably by the reticuloendothelial system. In patients with normal renal function, reinstitution of digoxin therapy should be delayed for 2 to 3 days until the Fab fragments are eliminated. In patients with impaired renal function a delay of 1 week or longer may be necessary.

Pharmacodynamic studies in experimental animal preparations have documented the efficacy of digoxin-specific antibodies and antibody fragments in reversing the physiologic and toxic effects of digoxin. Digoxin-induced inhibition of sodium and potassium transport in erythrocytes is reversed with digoxin antibody and antibody fragments.[193] Increased developed tension in isolated guinea pig atrial muscle strips with digoxin is reversed by antibody fragments.[193] The electrical inexcitability of canine Purkinje fibers exposed to toxic levels of digoxin can be reversed with digoxin antibodies with return of normal membrane properties.[195] Digoxin-induced increase in AV nodal effective and functional refractory period and conduction time are also rapidly reversed by digoxin antibodies.[195] Intact animal studies have shown that advanced cardiac toxicity is rapidly reversed with antibody fragments even after the administration of what are usually lethal doses for the animals.[196] The inotropic effects of digoxin are also reversed by Fab fragments and digoxin-specific antibodies.[197]

Several clinical studies have reported the efficacy of Fab fragments in the management of acute and chronic digoxin intoxication.[198–202] Extracardiac manifestations of digitalis toxicity are relatively less than cardiac manifestations in patients with acute digoxin intoxication. Many patients, particularly without pre-existing cardiac disorder, tolerate acute overdoses of digoxin well. Usual cardiac manifestations are sinus bradycardia, junctional rhythm, and varying degrees of AV block. However, ventricular tachyarrhythmias can occur that appear to be associated with a worse prognosis. Acute digoxin intoxication may be associated with hyperkalemia resulting from inhibition of the membrane-bound Na^+,K^+-ATPase pump, causing a net efflux of intracellular potassium and a rise in extracellular potassium. A serum potassium concentration higher than 5.5 mEq/l has been reported to be associated with a very poor prognosis (almost 100% mortality) in patients with acute digoxin intoxication treated conventionally.[203] It has also been reported that with supportive treatment, in patients with acute digoxin intoxication, the overall mortality is about 20%, irrespective of serum potassium concentrations.[204] Manifestations and diagnosis of chronic digoxin intoxication have been outlined previously. The cardiac and noncardiac manifestations of digitalis toxicity are reversed by Fab fragments in the vast majority of patients. Wenger and co-workers[202] reported a complete resolution of digitalis toxicity in 53 of 56 patients treated with Fab. Reversal of digitalis toxicity occurred even in patients with impaired renal function and in both hyperkalemic and normokalemic patients. Only 2 of 15 patients with pretreatment serum potassium concentrations higher than 5.0 mEq/l died despite Fab therapy. Serum potassium levels decreased significantly and digoxin-induced bradyarrhythmias and tachyarrhythmias reversed in almost all patients.

Treatment with digoxin-immune Fab should be considered in patients with potentially life-threatening digoxin or digitoxin intoxication. Digoxin overdose, with ingestion of 10 mg of digoxin by previously healthy adults or 4 mg by healthy children or when the steady-state serum digoxin concentrations are greater than 10 ng/ml, is often associated with cardiac arrest, and these patients should be considered for treatment with Fab. A serum potassium concentration exceeding 5 mEq/l is another indication of Fab treatment. Life-threatening arrhythmias such as ventricular tachycardia or progressive bradyarrhythmias, particularly when associated with compromised hemodynamics, are another indication for Fab therapy.

Commercially available digoxin antibody consists of ovine digoxin-specific antibody fragments (Fab) provided as a sterile lyophilized powder; each vial contains 40 mg of ovine Fab, 75 mg of sorbitol, and 28 mg of sodium chloride.

The dose of Fab is calculated to equal, in moles, the amount of digoxin or digitoxin in the patient's body. An estimate of total body load is based either on the known ingested dose or is estimated using a steady-state serum concentration. For *toxicity from an acute ingestion*, the total body load of digoxin will be approximately equal to the dose ingested.

To estimate total load from the steady-state serum concentration, the patient's serum digoxin concentration (SDC) in nanograms per milliliter is multiplied by the mean volume of distribution of digoxin in the body (5.6 l/kg times patient weight in kilograms) to give total body load in micrograms. This is divided by 1000 to obtain the estimated amount of digoxin in the body in milligrams. For *digitoxin* toxicity, total body load can be estimated by using the value 0.56 l/kg volume in place of the 5.6 l/kg for digoxin.

The dose of Fab (in milligrams) is calculated by multiplying the total body load (in milligrams) by 60 (approximate ratio of molecular weight of Fab to molecular weight of digoxin providing an equimolar dose of antibody fragments).

For digoxin:

Fab dose in mg = [(SDC)(5.6)(weight in kg) — 1000)](60)

For digitoxin:

Fab dose in mg = [(SDC)(0.56)(weight in kg) — 1000)](60)

The dose can be rounded to the nearest multiple of 40 mg so that the full contents of each vial are administered.

The contents of each of the required number of vials are initially dissolved in 4 ml of sterile distilled water, giving an isosmotic solution with a Fab concentration of 10 mg/ml. This solution of Fab should be further diluted with isotonic saline (0.9% sodium chloride) to give a final concentration of Fab of 5 mg/ml. The final diluted solution is administered through a 0.22-μm Millipore filter intravenously at a constant rate over 20 minutes. In life-threatening situations it may be administered via bolus injection without a filter. No obvious adverse reactions to Fab therapy have been observed in clinical studies. Some degree of deterioration in left ventricular function was suspected in some patients; however, no controlled hemodynamic studies are available to assess the results of Fab therapy on cardiac function. Deterioration of renal function, acute hypersensitivity reaction, and delayed serum sickness have not been observed in patients receiving Fab therapy.

Skin testing of patients has revealed an extremely low incidence of reactions, and skin testing is not routinely required. Skin testing may be appropriate for high-risk patients, that is, those with a previous history of known allergies or previous exposure to digoxin-specific antibodies. Injection of 0.1 ml of 1:100 Fab (prepared by diluting 0.1 ml of already prepared solution with 9.9 ml sterile isotonic saline) and observing for 20 minutes or alternatively injecting 0.1 ml (1 mg) of undiluted Fab and observing for 5 minutes will help screen for sensitivity to Fab. If no reaction occurs, then full treatment should be started. The therapeutic approach for the treatment of digitalis toxicity is outlined in Figure 3.11.

CATECHOLAMINES

A number of sympathomimetic amines are in clinical use, most commonly to correct hypotension or to increase cardiac output. Drugs such as norepinephrine, epinephrine, and isoproterenol, which contain O-dihydroxybenzene, also known as catechol, are frequently termed *catecholamines*.

The pharmacophysiologic effects of the sympathomimetic amines are mediated through their interaction with the adrenergic receptors. The response of the effector cells to catecholamines is related to activation of one of the two major types of receptors, α and β, as classified initially by Ahlquist in 1948,[205] based on the response to a number of sympathomimetic amines. Since then, subtypes of both α (α_1, α_2) and β (β_1, β_2) receptors have been identified along with their specific agonists and antagonists.[206] The distribution of the adrenoreceptors is widespread, and the effector cells may have α- or β-receptors or both. α_1-Adrenoreceptors are present in the postganglionic effector cells, and activation of α_1-receptors is associated with contraction of vascular and nonvascular smooth muscles. α_2-Adrenoreceptors were initially recognized only in prejunctional nerve terminals, where their stimulation causes inhibition of the neuronal release of the neurotransmitter.[207] Recently, however, it has been appreciated that in many tissues, including vascular smooth muscle, the α_2-receptors can also be postjunctional, and stimulation of these receptors is associated with vasoconstriction.[208] It appears that in various animal species α_1-receptors are present in the myocardium.[209] Subtypes of β-receptors have been recognized by the sensitivity of β-receptors of different organs to their agonists and antagonists: heart, small intestine, and pancreas contain β_1-receptors, and bronchi, vascular beds, and uterus contain β_2-receptors. β_2-Receptors are also found on prejunctional nerve terminals where their activation facilitates the release of neurotransmitters.[207] The activation of cardiac β_1-receptors is associated with increased contractility (positive inotropic effect), cardioacceleration (positive chronotropic effect), and enhanced AV nodal conduction (positive dromotropic effect). Vasodilation and decreased peripheral vascular tone result when β_2-adrenoreceptors are stimulated. Studies have indicated that a small proportion of the β-receptors in human myocardium are of the β_2-subtype.[210]

Normally, the adrenergic nervous system exerts an important physiologic role in regulating myocardial inotropic state and peripheral vascular tone. The inotropic state is modulated through the interaction of the myocardial β-receptors and the endogenous catecholamines. Norepinephrine released from the cardiac sympathetic nerve endings is the principal endogenous catecholamine involved in regulating the inotropic state; the circulating epinephrine released from the adrenal medulla and the norepinephrine released from noncardiac nerve endings appear to be of less importance. The influence of circulating catecholamines may become more important in patients with heart failure in maintaining the inotropic state.

FIGURE 3.11 MANAGEMENT OF DIGITALIS TOXICITY

General Therapy
Discontinue digitalis
Monitor cardiac rhythm
Determine electrolytes and serum digoxin concentration
Observe for hemodynamic compromise
In massive digitalis overdose, give activated charcoal or cholestyramine orally

Management of Arrhythmias
Potassium and magnesium replacement, indicated in the presence of hypokalemia and contraindicated in the presence of pre-existing hyperkalemia, bradycardia, and atrioventricular block
Phenytoin and lidocaine in ventricular arrhythmias in the presence of atrioventricular block
Atropine for sinoatrial and atrioventricular conduction anomalies
Pacemaker therapy for persistent bradycardia and atrioventricular block
Cardioversion with lowest effective energy for immediate therapy for ventricular tachycardia and fibrillation
Drugs to be avoided: procainamide, quinidine, disopyramide, β-blocking agents, isoproterenol, bretylium, amiodarone, and verapamil
Fab-digoxin therapy
Life-threatening arrhythmias (ventricular tachycardia)
Hyperkalemia (serum K^+ > 5.5 mEq/l)

Management of Hypotension and Low-Output State
Vasopressor to maintain arterial pressure
Fab-digoxin therapy
Control associated arrhythmias

Various abnormalities of catecholamine kinetics and metabolism, and of adrenoreceptors, have been recognized in heart failure. The arterial plasma norepinephrine concentrations are frequently elevated. In some patients, the dopamine level is also increased but the epinephrine level may remain within the normal range.[211] Although increased plasma norepinephrine concentrations result partly from decreased clearance, there is also increased "spill over" from the neuronal junctions, with suggests enhanced sympathetic activity in heart failure.[212] Changes in sympathetic activity, however, are not uniform in all vascular beds. Myocardial and renal norepinephrine release is significantly increased, despite decreased clearance, whereas pulmonary clearance and release may remain unchanged.[212,213] An increased concentration of circulating norepinephrine and increased myocardial norepinephrine release occur in the presence of depleted myocardial norepinephrine stores.[214] The ratio of tissue concentrations of dopamine/norepinephrine in the failing myocardium increases, and it has been suggested that in the failing heart the rate-limiting enzyme for norepinephrine synthesis may not be tyrosine hydroxylase, which is necessary for conversion of tyrosine to dopa, but may instead be dopamine β-hydroxylase, which is required for conversion of dopamine to norepinephrine.[215,216] The activity of tyrosine hydroxylase, normally a rate-limiting enzyme for norepinephrine production, may not change in heart failure. Similarly, neuronal reuptake and the activity of the enzymes catecholamine-orthomethyltransferase and monoamine oxidase necessary for the metabolism of catecholamines appear to be unaltered in heart failure. The precise explanation for decreased myocardial norepinephrine stores remains unclear; however, chronically enhanced cardiac sympathetic activity, as evident from increased myocardial norepinephrine release, has been suggested as the possible mechanism.[213] Decreased catecholamine sensitivity and reduced β-adrenoreceptor density have also been documented in failing human hearts.[217,218]

Changes in myocardial adrenergic function in heart failure may have considerable pathophysiologic and therapeutic implications.[219,220] Human atria and ventricles contain both β1- and β2-adrenoreceptors. Nonfailing human ventricles contain primarily β1-receptors. Of the total pool of β-adrenoreceptors, approximately 80% are of β1 type and 20% are of β2 type, although the range of the latter can vary from 0% to 35%. Atria, as compared with ventricles, may contain a higher percentage of β2-receptors, particularly in the region of the SA node, and the β2-selective agonists may exert more pronounced chronotropic response compared with β1-selective agonists. Binding of both subtypes of β-adrenore-ceptors with the neurotransmitters or hormones enhances inotropism via increasing the adenylate cyclase activity and generation of cyclic AMP. Generation of cyclic AMP following β1-receptor activation is much less than after activation of β2-receptors. Nevertheless, the increase in inotropism following β1-receptor stimulation is far greater than after β2-receptor stimulation, because the degree of inotropic stimulation is proportionate to the number of receptors present. Adrenergic function appears to be significantly altered in heart failure. Myocardial β-adrenergic receptors of

failing human ventricles are subsensitive to stimulation by isoproterenol, a nonselective β-adrenergic agonist. Maximal stimulation of inotropism and stimulation of adenylate cyclase by isoproterenol decrease markedly, which is related to a decrease in the total pool of β-adrenergic receptors. Decreased β-receptor density in heart failure results primarily from decreased β1-receptor subtype, which may be 60% to 70% lower than the receptor density of the nonfailing ventricles. In the failing human ventricles, β2-adrenergic receptor density appears to remain relatively unchanged; thus, β1/β2 subtype ratio changes from approximately 80:20 in nonfailing heart to 60:40 in failing heart. Although β2-receptor density is maintained in heart failure, the adenylate cyclase response to β2-selective agonists is attenuated, probably due to "uncoupling" of β-receptors from their pharmacologic pathway.

It has also been observed that the other components of the β-adrenergic receptor density and adenylate cyclase complex might be abnormal in patients with congestive heart failure. Abnormalities in the quantity or function of the guanine-nucleotide proteins have been observed in heart failure. A substantial decrease in the stimulating guanosine triphosphate (GTP) binding protein Gs has been observed in dogs with ventricular failure due to pressure overload and in patients with advanced congestive heart failure.[220] An increase in activity of the inhibitory G protein (G1) has also been observed and has been proposed for the uncoupling of the β2-receptor in the failing human heart.[219] Abnormalities of myocardial adrenergic function may have important therapeutic implications in the inotropic treatment of congestive heart failure. Because of the down-regulation of the β1-receptors, the selective β1-receptor agonists may be less effective in enhancing inotropism of the failing ventricles. Inotropic agents with β2-agonist properties such as dobutamine may have an advantage in the inotropic treatment of heart failure, since β2-receptor density tends to remain unchanged.

Although β-receptors are the predominant myocardial adrenoreceptors, α1-adrenergic receptors have also been demonstrated in mammalian myocardium, including human myocardium. However, the ratio of α- to β-receptor density in human myocardium is low, between 0.13 and 0.19.[221] Although activation of myocardial α1-receptors is associated with positive inotropic effects, its contribution compared with β-receptor activation for enhancing inotropy is likely to be minor because of their much lower density. The duration of action potential is prolonged and the development of contraction is relatively slow following α1-receptor stimulation.[222] The duration of contraction following β1-receptor stimulation is shorter and myocardial relaxation is faster.[223,224] α1-Receptor stimulation does not produce any myocardial relaxant effects.[222] Activation of myocardial β-receptors increases intracellular cyclic AMP concentration by stimulating the adenylate cyclase enzyme system. Cyclic AMP leads to activation of protein kinases and to phosphorylation of several proteins that apparently promote slow calcium inward current. This causes an increased release of calcium from the sarcoplasmic reticulum, either because it triggers calcium-dependent calcium release or because a greater filling of the sarcoplasmic stores with calcium occurs, which is then available for subsequent contractions.[223,224] In contrast to β-receptor stimulation, α_1-receptor stimulation does not produce any significant changes in cyclic AMP levels. Phosphodiesterase inhibition potentiates the effects of β-receptor agonists by raising cyclic AMP levels but has no effects on α-receptor agonists, providing further evidence for the noncyclic AMP-mediated mechanism of action of the myocardial α_1-receptor activation. It has been suggested that α_1-receptor stimulation results in hydrolysis or turnover of polyphosphoinositides (P1), which results in formation of inositol 1,4,5-triphosphate (IP3) and diacyl-glycerol (DAG).[225,226] It has been shown that IP3 increases cytosolic free calcium by triggering release of calcium from internal stores and is the proposed mechanism of the positive inotropic effect of the α-receptor activation.[225]

The cardiovascular effects of sympathomimetic drugs result from activation of the α- or β-receptors or both, and the net effects are determined by the predominance of α- or β-receptor stimulation, which varies with the type of sympathomimetic amine. It needs to be appreciated that most sympathomimetic drugs influence both α- and β-receptor activity, but relative activation of α- and β-receptors varies tremendously. Some drugs, such as phenylephrine, possess almost pure α-receptor stimulating activity, and others, such as isoproterenol, have almost pure β-receptor stimulating activity. Drugs such as dopamine stimulate dopaminergic receptors,

in addition to α- and β-adrenergic receptors. Drugs with both α- and β-receptor activity may produce variable responses on blood pressure, depending on the magnitude of α- and β-receptor activity. Stimulation of α-receptors increases blood pressure, and stimulation of β_2-receptors decreases blood pressure owing to reduction of systemic vascular resistance. A concomitant increase in cardiac output due to β_1-receptor stimulation may also modify the blood pressure response. Augmented contractility, increased heart rate, and decreased systemic vascular resistance may all contribute to an increased cardiac output following the use of sympathomimetic drugs possessing predominantly β-activity. On the other hand, drugs with predominant α-activity may cause a reduction in cardiac output owing to increased systemic vascular resistance, which also raises the resistance to left ventricular ejection.

The electrophysiologic effects of β_1-receptor agonists mediate their chronotropic and dromotropic effects and also their arrhythmogenicity. The sinus node discharge rate (automaticity) increases, resulting in an increased heart rate. The refractory period of the action potentials is abbreviated, and there is enhanced spontaneous phase 4 depolarization of the Purkinje cells, contributing to ventricular arrhythmias.[227] The electrophysiologic effects of different sympathomimetic drugs vary, and therefore their relative potency to induce tachycardia or arrhythmias is also variable. The expected hemodynamic effects of the various catecholamines in clinical use are summarized in Figure 3.12.

FIGURE 3.12 HEMODYNAMIC EFFECTS OF SYMPATHOMIMETIC DRUGS

| Drug | Receptor Activation | | | Hemodynamic Effects | | | | |
	α	β_1	β_2	SVR	MAP	CO	HR	PCWP
Norepinephrine	+++	+	−	↑↑↑	↑↑↑	↔↓↑	↔↑	↑↔
Isoproterenol		+++	+++	↓↓↓	↓↓	↑↑↑	↑↑↑	↓↓
Epinephrine	+++	+++	+++	↓	↑↔	↑↑	↑↑↑	↑↔
Dopamine	++	++	−	↓↔	↑↑	↑↑	↑	↑↔
	(and DA₁ and DA₂ receptors)							
Dobutamine	+	+++	+	↓	↔↓	↑↑↑	↔↑	↓↔
Phenylephrine	+++	+	−	↑↑↑	↑↑	↔↓	↓↔	↑↔
Methoxamine	+++	−	−	↑↑↑	↑↑↑	↔↓	↓	↑↔
Metaraminol	++	−	−	↑↑	↑↑	↔↓	↔↓	↑↔
Salbutamol	−	+	+++	↓↓	↓↔	↑↑	↔↑	↓↔
Pirbuterol	−	+	+++	↓↓	↓↔	↑↑	↔↑	↓↔
Prenalterol	−	++	+	↓	↔↓	↑	↔↑	↓↔
TA-064	−	++	+	↓	↔	↑	↔↑	↓↔
Butopamine	−	++	+	↓	↔	↑	↑	↓↔
Levodopa	+	+	+	↓	↔	↑	↔↑	↔
	(activation of DA₁ and DA₂ receptors)							
Ibopamine	−	+	+	↓	↔	↑	↑↔	↑↔
	(DA₁ and DA₂ receptor activation)							
Dopexamine	−	+	+	↓	↔↓	↑	↔	↓
	(DA₁ receptor agonist)							
Propylbutyl-dopamine	−	−	−	↓	↓	↑	↔	↓
	(activation of DA₁ and DA₂ receptors)							
Fenoldopam	−	−	−	↓	↔	↑	↔↑	↓
	(DA₁ agonist)							

(+ = Activation; − = No effect; ↑ = Increase; ↓ = Decrease; ↔ = No change; SVR = Systemic vascular resistance; MAP = Mean arterial pressure; CO = Cardiac output; HR = Heart rate; PCWP = Pulmonary capillary wedge pressure)

Clinical Applications in Cardiology

NOREPINEPHRINE

The use of norepinephrine is limited to correcting severe hypotension in some patients with cardiogenic or septic shock, usually when other vasopressor agents fail to maintain adequate arterial pressure. Its hemodynamic effects have been evaluated in patients with pump failure and shock complicating myocardial infarction.[228] In patients with cardiogenic shock, arterial pressure and systemic vascular resistance increase with little or no change in cardiac output. Although it has the potential to increase cardiac output by stimulating the β_1-adrenoreceptors, a concomitant increase in systemic vascular resistance resulting from α-receptor stimulation increases resistance to left ventricular ejection, which tends to decrease cardiac output. Furthermore, excessive tachycardia and ventricular arrhythmias may occur when larger doses are used. Renal, cerebral, hepatic, and skeletal muscle blood flow may decrease because of regional vasoconstriction.[229] Coronary blood flow and myocardial oxygen consumption may increase due to increased myocardial oxygen requirements resulting from increased afterload, inotropic state and heart rate, and the worsening myocardial oxygen balance may enhance ischemia and the extent of myocardial injury following acute myocardial infarction. This effect, however, may be partially offset by the increase in blood pressure and therefore coronary perfusion pressure with improved myocardial perfusion.

Norepinephrine is administered intravenously, and the infusion rate should be increased slowly, starting with a small dose, 0.025 to 0.1 µg/kg/min while monitoring changes in arterial pressure; the usual dose is 2 to 8 µg/min. The half-life of norepinephrine is approximately 2 minutes, and its pressor response usually disappears within 1 to 2 minutes after discontinuation of the infusion. Most of the infused norepinephrine is metabolized by catechol-amine-orthomethyl-transferase and monoamine oxidase and is excreted as inactive compounds. Only 4% to 16% of an administered dose is excreted unchanged in the urine.[229]

EPINEPHRINE

Epinephrine is a potent agonist at α_1-, α_2-, β_1-, and β_2-adrenergic receptors. At all doses, heart rate and myocardial contractility increase due to direct activation of myocardial β_1- and possibly β_2-adrenoreceptors. The changes in peripheral vascular resistance appear to be dose-dependent. At low doses (less than 0.1 µg/kg/min), systemic vascular resistance tends to fall because its β_2-adrenoreceptor-mediated vasodilatory effects predominate. Blood flow to skeletal muscle and splanchnic bed may increase with decreased flow to cutaneous and renal vascular beds. Low doses of epinephrine increase myocardial blood flow, presumably due to autoregulation rather than its direct effect on the coronary circulation. Higher doses of epinephrine also increase heart rate and myocardial contractility. However, vasoconstrictor responses mediated by activation of vascular α_1- and α_2-receptors override β_2-receptor-mediated vasodilator responses, resulting in increased systemic vascular resistance and arterial pressure. Myocardial blood flow may also increase owing to augmented perfusion pressure.

The principal therapeutic use of epinephrine is during resuscitation from cardiac arrest. Administration of epinephrine is associated with increased systolic and diastolic pressure and improved cerebral and coronary perfusion. Epinephrine is occasionally used to restore an idioventricular rhythm in patients with the Stokes-Adams syndrome before an artificial pacemaker is installed. However, isoproterenol is more effective than epinephrine for this indication. In some patients with low cardiac output and hypotension following cardiac surgery, epinephrine infusion is useful. However, excessive vasoconstriction and increased systemic vascular resistance may be associated with a decrease or no change in cardiac output. Furthermore, excessive tachycardia and arrhythmias limit its use. The usual dose of epinephrine, when given by intravenous infusion, is 0.25 to 0.30 µg/kg/min. The infused epinephrine is metabolized and disposed in the same way as norepinephrine.[229]

ISOPROTERENOL

Isoproterenol is a potent β-adrenoreceptor agonist that stimulates β_1- and β_2-adrenoreceptors equally. Myocardial contractility and heart rate increase due to activation of β_1-receptors, and systemic vascular resistance falls due to β_2-receptor-mediated vasodilatation. Marked reduction in systemic vascular resistance can produce significant hypotension and compromise myocardial perfusion due to decreased perfusion pressure. Decreased diastolic perfusion time due to excessive tachycardia may also impair myocardial perfusion. Myocardial oxygen requirements also increase concurrently, and myocardial oxygen balance may worsen. Thus, the potential exists for an increase in ischemia and the extent of myocardial injury, despite improvements in cardiac performance. At low doses, isoproterenol may increase coronary blood flow to the subendocardium and subepicardium; but at higher doses, subendocardial and subepicardial perfusion may decrease owing to decreased perfusion pressure and diastolic perfusion time.

Isoproterenol is also a potent arrhythmogenic agent, and ventricular tachyarrhythmias are common with larger doses of isoproterenol. Augmented cardiac output is usually distributed to skeletal muscles. Renal blood flow tends to increase in patients with cardiogenic shock, but there may be a redistribution of flow from the renal cortex to the medulla, causing no improvement in or a deterioration of renal function. These undesirable hemodynamic and metabolic effects of isoproterenol, along with its arrhythmogenicity, have restricted its use in most clinical situations. It is usually used in patients with bradycardia or complete AV block before a temporary pacemaker can be inserted. In patients with low cardiac output resulting from or associated with increased pulmonary vascular resistance, as in some patients following mitral valve surgery, isoproterenol infusion may improve hemodynamics. Isoproterenol is used frequently to maintain adequate heart rate and inotropic state of the denervated transplanted heart. The usual dose of isoproterenol when given by intravenous infusion is 2 to 5 µg/min. Its metabolism and excretion are similar to those of epinephrine and norepinephrine.[229]

Systemic and regional hemodynamic effects of dopamine are mediated through a number of mechanisms: activation of dopaminergic α- and β1-receptors and release of norepinephrine (tyramine-like effect). The subtypes of dopamine receptors, DA1 and DA2 (D1 and D2), have been identified by radioligand binding assays and by pharmacophysiologic studies. DA1 receptors are postsynaptic, and their stimulation is associated with dilatation of the renal, mesenteric, coronary, and cerebrovascular beds. Activation of DA2 receptors, which are located on postganglionic sympathetic nerves and autonomic ganglia, is associated with inhibition of norepinephrine release from the sympathetic nerve endings. The expected pharmacologic effects of activation of dopamine receptors are illustrated in Figure 3.13. The subtype DA2 receptors are also present in the emetic center of the area postrema and in the anterior lobe of the pituitary gland. Stimulation of DA2 receptors in these areas is associated with nausea and vomiting and decreased prolactin release, respectively.

The renal, peripheral vascular, and cardiac effects of dopamine appear to be dose-related.[230–232] With a dose of 0.5 to 2 µg/kg/min given intravenously, dopamine receptors are activated and some peripheral vasodilation along with increased renal flow, urine volume, and sodium excretion results. Dopamine-induced natriuresis has been observed in the absence of any increase in total renal blood flow, and a redistribution of medullary flow to the cortex has been proposed as the potential mechanism. If there is a reduction in arterial pressure, renal function may not improve because of reduced renal perfusion pressure. With a larger dose, 2 to 5 µg/kg/min, cardiac β1-receptors are stimulated and positive inotropic and chronotropic effects are manifested by an increase in cardiac output. Pulmonary capillary wedge pressure may decrease slightly or may remain unchanged, and there may not be any increase in arterial pressure. A larger dose, exceeding 5 to 10 µg/kg/min, is associated with peripheral vasoconstriction and increased systemic vascular resistance resulting from activation of the α-receptors. There is no further change in cardiac output as arterial pressure increases. Pulmonary capillary wedge pressure, pulmonary artery pressure, and pulmonary vascular resistance tend to increase.

It should be noted that in individual patients the hemodynamic responses expected in response to a given dose of dopamine may not occur. In some patients, with a very low dose of dopamine (e.g., 2 µg/kg/min), an increase in cardiac output due to increased contractility may be observed. At intermediate infusion rates, arterial and venous constriction may result from activation of α-adrenergic receptors, leading to increases in arterial and ventricular filling pressures. Increased filling pressures result primarily from increased venous return to the heart.

In patients with hypotension and low cardiac output, the addition of dobutamine to dopamine may allow maintenance of arterial pressure and cardiac output, and it is possible to use relatively lower doses of both dopamine and dobutamine, so that the potential adverse effects resulting from the adminis-

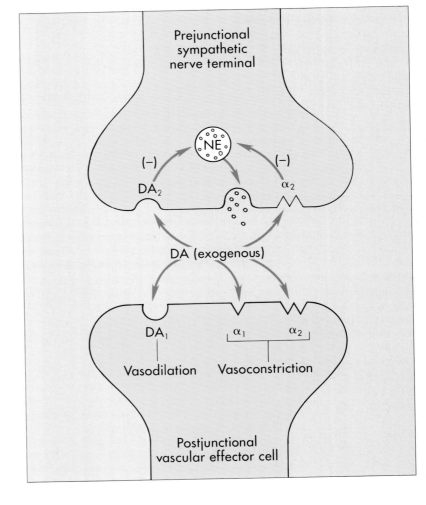

Figure 3.13 Location of the subtypes of dopamine and α-receptors. DA1 receptors, α1-receptors, and α2-receptors are located on postganglionic vascular effector cells and DA2 receptors are on the prejunctional sympathetic nerve terminal. With dopamine infusion, activation of DA1 receptors causes vasodilation and activation of DA2 receptors causes inhibition of norepinephrine (NE) release. A higher dose of dopamine simulates α1- and α2-receptors on the effector cells to cause vasoconstriction and prejunctional α2-receptors to inhibit release of norepinephrine. (Modified from Goldberg U, Razfers SI: Dopamine receptors: Applications in clinical cardiology. Circulation 72:245, 1985. Reprinted with permission of the American Heart Association, Inc)

tration of higher doses of these agents can be prevented. The increase in pulmonary capillary wedge pressure that tends to occur with high doses of dopamine can be avoided by maintaining adequate arterial pressure and cardiac output.[233]

Compared with isoproterenol, dopamine possesses lesser positive inotropic, chronotropic, and arrhythmogenic properties; as a result, the magnitude of increase in cardiac output with dopamine is less than that with isoproterenol, but excessive tachycardia and ventricular tachyarrhythmias are also less frequent.[229] Vasoconstriction and augmentation of peripheral vascular resistance with dopamine are less than with norepinephrine, and the magnitude of increase in arterial pressure is also less. However, dopamine induces fewer arrhythmias and fewer adverse hemodynamic and metabolic effects compared with norepinephrine, and it is preferable to norepinephrine for the treatment of hypotension.

In certain clinical situations, dopamine is preferable to other catecholamines. In patients with decreased urine output with or without heart failure, an infusion of low-dose dopamine may augment urine output. When hypotension results primarily from low systemic vascular resistance, as in septic shock, dopamine is effective in maintaining arterial pressure. Dopamine is also useful for correcting the hypotension accompanying a reduced cardiac output, particularly when pulmonary capillary wedge pressure is not markedly elevated. A rise in pulmonary capillary wedge pressure can often be prevented by the concomitant use of a venodilator such as nitroglycerin. Excessive vasoconstriction with larger doses of dopamine may be associated with undesirable systemic hemodynamic effects, which can be reduced by the simultaneous administration of vasodilator-like sodium nitroprusside and nitroglycerin.[234,235]

In experimental animals with acute myocardial ischemia, dopamine increased blood flow in the normal and moderately ischemic myocardial segments; in the severely ischemic zones, blood flow remained virtually unchanged. However, if excessive tachycardia developed in response to dopamine, an increase in paradoxical systolic bulging of the ischemic myocardial segments along with decreased myocardial blood flow and endocardial/epicardial flow ratio to the severely ischemic zones were observed.[236] Thus, the potential benefits of dopamine on the mechanical and metabolic function of severely ischemic myocardium were offset by tachycardia. In the absence of cardiac acceleration, dopamine may not increase ischemic zone ST segment elevation, despite augmented contractility.[237] Increased arterial pressure and therefore coronary artery perfusion pressure may improve perfusion of the ischemic myocardial zones. An increment in myocardial blood flow in the territory of a narrowed coronary artery during dopamine infusion has been reported.[238] With higher doses of dopamine, increased arterial pressure, heart rate, systemic vascular resistance, and contractility augment myocardial oxygen requirements, and the potential exists for enhancement of myocardial ischemia in patients with coronary artery disease. Myocardial lactate production, indicating myocardial ischemia, has been observed in response to dopamine in patients with acute myocardial infarction and pump failure, despite improved systemic hemodynamics.[239] In these patients, left ventricular

function may deteriorate during continued dopamine therapy. Thus, in patients with acute myocardial infarction and shock, a prolonged infusion of dopamine alone should be avoided and other measures, such as the concomitant use of vasodilators or intra-aortic balloon counterpulsation, or both, should be considered.

In addition to an increase in myocardial oxygen consumption and excessive vasoconstriction, dopamine may induce arrhythmias. Prolonged infusion has been reported to precipitate angina, nausea, vomiting, and peripheral gangrene. The duration of action of dopamine is brief, and its half-life of elimination is short. It is metabolized by monoamine oxidase.[229]

DOBUTAMINE

The synthetic sympathomimetic amine dobutamine is a potent β_1-receptor agonist. However, it also possesses β_2- and α-receptor agonist properties.[240] It does not cause neuronal norepinephrine release. Dobutamine is a racemic mixture of L-isomers and D-isomers. The L-isomer is an α_1-receptor agonist and a relatively weak β-receptor agonist. The D-isomer has pronounced effects on β-receptors and little effect on α-receptors. β_2-Receptor-mediated peripheral vasodilation is partly counteracted by the concomitant activation of vascular β_1-receptors. The positive inotropic effect of β_1-receptors is potentiated by simultaneous activation of the myocardial α-receptors. Unlike dopamine, the positive inotropic effect of dobutamine is not related to norepinephrine stores. The usual net hemodynamic effects are a substantial increase in cardiac output, with little or no change in arterial pressure and little or no increase in heart rate.[241] Systemic vascular and pulmonary vascular resistances decrease along with a modest decrease in pulmonary capillary wedge pressure.

In experimental animals with acute ischemia, blood flow in the normal zones and in the moderately ischemic zones increased in response to dobutamine and the blood flow to the severely ischemic zones remained unchanged. However, if significant tachycardia developed, decreased blood flow and endocardial/epicardial blood flow ratio to the ischemic zone along with deterioration in regional myocardial mechanical function were observed.[236] In other experimental studies, in animals with acute or chronic myocardial ischemia, increased blood flow to all myocardial zones in response to dobutamine has been reported.[242] Intact autonomic nervous system activities may prevent tachycardia, and therefore the deleterious effects of dobutamine on myocardial ischemia may be avoided. In anesthetized open-chest dogs with acute myocardial infarction, the magnitude of ST segment elevation may increase, indicating an increase in infarct size probably related to excessive tachycardia frequently observed in these preparations.[242] Marked tachycardia-related increase in oxygen demand and concurrent impairment of myocardial perfusion due to shorter diastole might have contributed to the deleterious effects on the ischemic injury in the presence of myocardial infarction.

In patients with acute myocardial infarction, dobutamine infusion does not appear to increase infarct size, the frequency of reinfarction, or the extension of infarction.[243] In patients with chronic, nonischemic congestive heart failure, improved coronary hemodynamics and myocardial energetics have been observed.[244] With lower (5 µg/kg/min) and higher (10 µg/kg/min) doses of dobutamine, myocardial oxygen consumption and coronary blood flow increased along with improvement in hemodynamics. However, myocardial oxygen/supply ratio remained unchanged and there was no clinical or biochemical evidence for myocardial ischemia. Comparative effects of dobutamine and dopamine on systemic and coronary hemodynamics have been evaluated in patients following cardiac surgery.[245] With similar increases in cardiac output and left ventricular dP/dt, myocardial oxygen consumption increased with both agents. With dobutamine, however, the increase in oxygen uptake was accompanied by a significantly greater increase in coronary blood flow, suggesting that dobutamine does not limit the increase in coronary blood flow associated with increased oxygen demand. In patients with chronic ischemic heart failure, dobutamine increases coronary blood flow and myocardial oxygen consumption (Fig. 3.14).[246] With increasing doses of dobutamine (5, 7.5, and 10 µg/kg/min) there was a progressively significant increase in coronary blood flow. Changes in myocardial oxygen consumption paralleled changes in coronary blood flow, and there was no change in myocardial oxygen extraction. An increase in coronary blood flow may result from decreased coronary vascular resistance secondary to increased metabolic demand. The direct coronary vasodilatory effect of dobutamine, mediated by activation of β_2-adrenergic receptors, may also contribute to decreased coronary vascular resistance and increased coronary blood flow.[247] However, increased myocardial oxygen demands appear to be the important contributing factor for the increase in coronary blood flow in patients with ischemic heart failure. Larger doses of dobutamine (10 µg/kg/min) may cause a greater increase in myocardial oxygen demand than in coronary blood flow, thus enhancing the potential to induce myocardial ischemia.[248] A marked increase in heart rate contributes to an excessive increase in myocardial oxygen requirements. Changes in coronary hemodynamics in response to dobutamine may be influenced by the presence or absence of obstructive coronary artery disease. The increase in coronary blood flow may be substantially greater in patients without coronary artery disease than in patients with coronary artery disease, although changes in systemic hemodynamics and contractility were similar in both groups.[249] Differences in myocardial metabolic function between patients with and without coronary artery disease have been observed following infusion of dobutamine, despite similar improvement in systemic hemodynamics and cardiac performance.[250] In patients with primary dilated cardiomyopathy, myocardial lactate extraction remained unchanged. However, in 11% of patients with coronary artery disease there was myocardial lactate production suggesting myocardial ischemia. About 17% of patients with coronary artery disease also develop angina. As larger doses of dobutamine infusion can induce myocardial ischemia in patients with obstructive coronary artery disease, dobutamine stress echocardiography is evolving as a method of evaluation of coronary artery disease by detecting reversible regional myocardial wall motion abnormalities.[251] With therapeutic doses of dobutamine, however, myocardial ischemia is unlikely to develop, even in patients with obstructive coronary artery disease, provided excessive tachycardia does not occur. This is probably related to the maintenance of myocardial oxygen supply and demand balance.

Figure 3.14 Changes in coronary sinus flow and myocardial oxygen consumption in response to dobutamine infusion in patients with ischemic heart failure. Both coronary sinus flow and myocardial oxygen consumption increased during the higher infusion rate. (Modified from Bendersky R, Chatterjee K, Parmley WW et al: Dobutamine in chronic ischemic heart failure: Alterations in left ventricular function and coronary hemodynamics. Am J Cardiol 48:554, 1981)

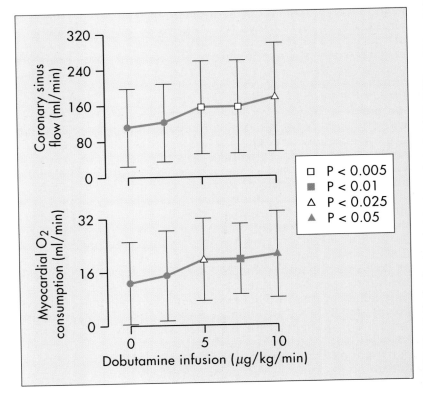

Dobutamine, unlike dopamine, does not stimulate renal dopamine receptors and thus does not selectively increase renal blood flow. However, renal blood flow, urine volume, and sodium excretion may increase along with an increased cardiac output in patients with heart failure.

The hemodynamic effects of dobutamine have been compared with those of other catecholamines and vasodilators. The magnitudes of increase in cardiac output with dobutamine and isoproterenol were similar. Changes in mean arterial pressure, systemic vascular resistance, and mean pulmonary artery and pulmonary capillary wedge pressure were also similar.[252] The increase in heart rate, however, was considerably greater with isoproterenol than with dobutamine. The propensity to induce ventricular arrhythmias is also higher with isoproterenol.

The comparative hemodynamic effects of dobutamine and dopamine were determined in patients with chronic heart failure, cardiogenic shock, and following cardiac surgery.[253,254] Although both dobutamine and dopamine increase cardiac output, pulmonary capillary wedge pressure tends to increase with dopamine, whereas it decreases with dobutamine. Pulmonary artery pressure and pulmonary vascular resistance may also increase with dopamine. Although systemic vascular resistance may decrease with both agents, arterial pressure tends to increase with dopamine, but not with dobutamine, suggesting that for the same magnitude of increase in cardiac output the relative reduction in systemic vascular resistance is less with dopamine than with dobutamine. Increase in cardiac output in response to dopamine is frequently due to an increase in heart rate, whereas dobutamine increases stroke volume consistently.[255]

Compared with nitroprusside, dobutamine causes less reduction in pulmonary capillary wedge pressure for a similar increase in cardiac output.[256] Myocardial oxygen consumption tends to decrease with nitroprusside while it increases with dobutamine. The magnitude of reduction in mean and diastolic arterial pressure is, however, greater with nitroprusside than with dobutamine. Thus, in the presence of myocardial ischemia, nitroprusside has more potential to decrease coronary blood flow by reducing coronary artery perfusion pressure.

The systemic hemodynamic effects of dobutamine infusion and intravenous digoxin were evaluated in patients with mild to moderate heart failure complicating acute myocardial infarction.[89] Although dobutamine consistently increased cardiac output and decreased pulmonary capillary wedge pressure, hemodynamic changes following digoxin were variable and no improvement in left ventricular function was observed. Systemic vascular resistance fell with dobutamine but remained unchanged with digoxin.

Dobutamine is effective in the management of both acute and chronic heart failure. In patients with pump failure and low cardiac output, if inotropic support seems necessary, dobutamine is preferable to dopamine, particularly when the pulmonary capillary wedge pressure is elevated and the arterial pressure is adequate. When severe hypotension (mean arterial pressure < 60 mm Hg) accompanies low cardiac output, dobutamine should not be used initially and a

vasopressor agent, such as dopamine, should be started to increase arterial pressure to the adequate range. For a further increase in cardiac output, dobutamine can then be added.[233] A combination of dopamine and dobutamine has also been shown to reduce the adverse hemodynamic effects of each. Dopamine in low doses may be added for its renal effects when urine output remains low, despite an increase in cardiac output with dobutamine. Dobutamine and nitroprusside can also be used concurrently because the combination may result in a higher cardiac output and lower pulmonary capillary wedge pressure than with either drug alone. In the presence of hypotension, however, this combination should be avoided, since further hypotension may ensue.

Dobutamine is effective in increasing cardiac output in patients with predominant right ventricular infarction. Right and left ventricular ejection fractions improve with little or no change in systemic and pulmonary venous pressure. The hemodynamic effects of dobutamine and nitroprusside have been compared in right ventricular infarction, and a greater increase in cardiac output with dobutamine has been observed.[257] Dobutamine is also effective in improving cardiac function in patients following cardiac surgery; the indications for its use in these patients are similar to those for patients with acute myocardial infarction or chronic heart failure.

Dobutamine is frequently used for treating exacerbation of chronic heart failure. Chronic intermittent infusion of dobutamine has been found effective in maintaining clinical improvement.[258–260] Once-per-week dobutamine infusion for 24 weeks improved exercise tolerance and left ventricular function of patients with moderate to severe congestive heart failure.[258] A similar phenomenon was observed after a single 3-day infusion of dobutamine.[261] A double-blind placebo-controlled study has confirmed sustained improvement in exercise tolerance and left ventricular ejection fraction at 4 weeks after a single 3-day infusion of dobutamine in patients with severe chronic congestive heart failure.[260] The effects of intermittent administration of dobutamine to ambulatory patients, using a portable infusion pump, has been assessed for the long-term management of patients with severe chronic heart failure.[262–264] Although there was a tendency to clinical improvement in many patients, there was a strong tendency for a higher mortality rate in the dobutamine-treated patients. Many of the patients who died, died suddenly. Thus, dobutamine infusion is not recommended without supervision and monitoring for arrhythmias. The mechanism for improvement in left ventricular function and clinical improvement with intermittent dobutamine infusion remains unclear. Chronic dobutamine infusion into sedentary dogs has been reported to produce a "conditioning effect."[265] A similar conditioning effect has been proposed in patients with chronic heart failure receiving intermittent dobutamine infusions.[247] Myocardial biopsy of patients with chronic heart failure, before and after 3 days of infusion of dobutamine, demonstrated a decrease in mitochondrial size in the responders.[266] The significance of such findings, however, remains unclear.

Adverse effects are less frequent with dobutamine

than with other catecholamines. Excessive tachycardia and ventricular tachyarrhythmias are less common, unless a very large dose is used, which may also induce hypotension. Increased myocardial oxygen consumption and the possibility of worsening myocardial ischemia remain potential disadvantages. The elimination half-life is short, only 2 to 3 minutes. The usual dose of dobutamine is 2.5 to 10 μg/kg/min. An excess of 10 μg/kg/min of dobutamine infusion is likely to induce undesirable tachycardia. The dose, however, should be titrated, starting with a lower infusion rate to obtain an adequate hemodynamic response.

EPHEDRINE[229]

Although some beneficial effects have been reported in patients with chronic heart failure, the use of ephedrine has not gained any popularity because of its unpredictable and inconsistent hemodynamic effects and because of the availability of more effective sympathomimetic amines that can also be administered orally. Similarly, its use has been abandoned for treatment of the Stokes-Adams syndrome since artificial pacemaker therapy has been available.

MEPHENTERMINE, METARAMINOL, AND PHENYLEPHRINE

The sympathomimetic amines with predominantly α-receptor stimulating properties are seldom used today, except occasionally to terminate supraventricular tachycardia. Intravenous verapamil and adenosine have almost totally replaced the vasopressor sympathomimetic amines in pharmacologic termination of supraventricular tachycardia. In experimental animals, reduction of infarct size has been reported to be significantly greater with the combined use of methoxamine or phenylephrine and nitroglycerin.[267] Such a beneficial response to phenylephrine in attenuating the adverse effects of nitroglycerin (reflex tachycardia) on infarct size has not been proven in patients with evolving myocardial infarction.

SALBUTAMOL AND PIRBUTEROL

Improvement in left ventricular function with these agents results primarily from a decrease in systemic vascular resistance due to activation of the β_2-receptors, although a modest increase in contractility may also be contributory. The systemic hemodynamic effects consist of an increase in cardiac output, a modest increase in heart rate, and a decrease in pulmonary capillary wedge pressure, along with a significant decrease in systemic vascular resistance.

Salbutamol has been used to treat left ventricular failure complicating acute myocardial infarction with some success.[268] However, the experience is limited and the incidence of adverse effects has not been determined. Salbutamol has also been used in the treatment of chronic heart failure, and some clinical benefit has been observed; the addition of isosorbide dinitrate to salbutamol was found to be more effective.[269–271] Without prospective, controlled studies, the potential benefit in the long-term management of chronic heart failure remains uncertain. The recommended oral dose of salbutamol is 4 to 8 mg three to four times daily.

The mechanism of action and hemodynamic effects of pirbuterol are similar to those of salbutamol. In experimental animals, left ventricular dP/dt increases in response to pirbuterol; however, whether the increased dP/dt results from increased contractility or from changes in ventricular loading conditions and heart rate has not been clarified.[272] Intravenous administration of pirbuterol to healthy volunteers has been associated with increased heart rate and stroke volume and decreased systemic vascular resistance.[273] In patients with chronic heart failure, however, the chronotropic effect is usually absent and a significant increase in cardiac output, along with a reduction in pulmonary capillary wedge pressure, may occur.[274,275] Myocardial oxygen and lactate extraction remain unchanged, suggesting that improved cardiac performance is not associated with increased metabolic cost.

Conflicting results have been reported regarding the efficacy of pirbuterol in the long-term management of patients with chronic heart failure. In some studies, improvement in treadmill exercise time following 6 weeks of chronic therapy has been observed.[275] A sustained increase in left ventricular ejection fraction also resulted from chronic maintenance therapy. However, in other studies there was no significant improvement in exercise tolerance or maximal oxygen consumption following chronic pirbuterol therapy.[276] A decline in ejection fraction after an initial increase has also been observed in some patients with chronic heart failure following maintenance therapy with pirbuterol.[277] This attenuation of the hemodynamic and clinical responses has been attributed to a down-regulation of β-receptor density in the myocardium and vascular beds following long-term treatment with pirbuterol.[277] The changes in β-receptor density were estimated in peripheral blood lymphocytes (β_2-receptors), which may not necessarily reflect changes in myocardial β_1-receptors.

Adverse effects such as ventricular tachyarrhythmias and fluid retention, nervousness, headache, tremors, dry mouth, palpitations, nausea, dizziness, fatigue, malaise, and insomnia have been observed during clinical trials. Because of these potential adverse effects and the uncertainty of clinical efficacy, the use of pirbuterol is usually not recommended for the long-term management of patients with chronic heart failure. After oral administration of pirbuterol, maximal plasma concentrations occur within 30 minutes to 4 hours, and the estimated half-life is 1 to 2 hours. It is readily metabolized following oral or intravenous administration, and in humans, biotransformation to the sulfate conjugate occurs extensively. Pirbuterol and its metabolites are primarily excreted via the kidney. In most clinical trials, a dose of 0.4 mg/kg or 10 mg three times daily has been used.

PARTIAL β_1-RECEPTOR AGONISTS

Prenalterol is a partial β_1-receptor agonist with minimal β_2-receptor stimulating effects. It has a more pronounced positive inotropic effect than chronotropic effect. In experimental animals, prenalterol increased left ventricular dP/dt through its positive inotropic effect.[278] Contractile force also increased in the nonischemic zones in myocardial infarction in experimental animals.[279] In normal volunteers, in patients with acute myocardial infarction, and in patients with chronic congestive heart failure, intravenous prenalterol increased cardiac output and decreased pulmonary capillary wedge pressure and systemic vascular resistance with little or no change in arterial pressure.[280,281] In normal volunteers, a considerable increase in heart rate may occur[281]; however, in patients with heart failure, there was usually little or no increase in heart rate.[282]

Systemic hemodynamic effects of both intravenous and oral prenalterol have been compared in patients with chronic congestive heart failure.[282] The magnitude of increase in cardiac index and the decrease in systemic vascular resistance were similar after intravenous and oral administration of prenalterol. The changes in heart rate, mean arterial pressure, stroke volume, stroke work, and pulmonary capillary wedge pressure were also similar.

Prenalterol, whether given orally or intravenously, tends to increase coronary blood flow and myocardial oxygen consumption.[282] Increased oxygen consumption occurs in the absence of any significant increase in the rate–pressure product, suggesting that the increased inotropic effect enhances myocardial oxygen consumption.

Although acute intravenous or oral prenalterol therapy is associated with hemodynamic improvement, clinical improvement during chronic therapy has not been established. In a double-blind, randomized trial, oral prenalterol therapy for 2 weeks did not improve exercise tolerance or maximal exercise after maintenance therapy.[283] The heart rate response during exercise was also attenuated. In some patients, relative bradycardia and evidence of low cardiac output may develop during chronic oral prenalterol therapy. The mechanisms of these adverse effects remain unclear. In animal experiments, prenalterol was found to possess 70% of the sympathomimetic activity of isoproterenol and was classified as a partial agonist with some β-antagonistic effect. During acute prenalterol therapy, β-antagonist effects, such as reduction in heart rate, may not be observed. During long-term therapy, it is possible that down-regulation of β-receptors occurs and the responsiveness to β_1-receptor activation declines. In these circumstances, the β-antagonist effect may be manifest. Since evidence for a long-term clinical benefit is lacking and the adverse effects may be considerable, long-term prenalterol therapy cannot be recommended in patients with chronic heart failure.

Xamoterol is another selective β_1-agonist that has been evaluated for the treatment of heart failure. In patients with mild to moderate heart failure, a positive inotropic effect with improved hemodynamics has been observed.[270,284] An increase in cardiac index and stroke volume index, and decreased systemic vascular resistance without any change in arterial pressure, pulmonary capillary wedge pressure, or ejection fraction have been reported in response to intravenous xamoterol.[285] In patients with more severe heart failure, such beneficial hemodynamic effects may not be seen.[286]

The safety and efficacy of oral xamoterol in patients with moderate to severe heart failure despite treatment with diuretics and angiotensin-converting enzyme inhibitors were evaluated in a randomized double-blind trial.[287] The three-month survival probability was significantly less for xamoterol-treated

patients than for placebo-treated patients. Progression of heart failure occurred in 4.8% of xamoterol-treated patients and 1.2% of controls, and sudden death occurred in 3.7% of xamoterol-treated patients and 1.8% of controls. The overall mortality within 100 days of randomization was 9.2% in xamoterol-treated patients and 3.7% in the controls. Lack of a beneficial response has also been observed in patients with acute myocardial infarction complicated by heart failure.[288] Xamoterol, however, has been shown to improve exercise tolerance and cardiac function, compared with digoxin, in patients with mild heart failure. The mechanism of such benefit is not fully understood but is probably not solely due to its β-agonist activity; it may also depend on the β-antagonist effect and improvement in ventricular diastolic function.[126]

The differences in hemodynamic response to xamoterol in patients with mild and severe heart failure remain unexplained. Xamoterol is a partial agonist with approximately 43% of the inotropic/chronotropic response attainable with isoprterenol.[289] With this relatively modest β-agonist activity, significant inotropic stimulation would not be anticipated, particularly when the β-receptor density and myocardial responsiveness to catecholamines are diminished, as observed in patients with severe chronic heart failure. In these patients, a full agonist, such as dobutamine, is more likely to be effective. Xamoterol might still exert positive inotropic effects in patients with mild heart failure if myocardial responsiveness to β-receptor activation is relatively maintained.

It is apparent that partial β-agonists are unlikely to be effective inotropic agents for the management of patients with more severe heart failure. This may be because sympathetic tone is already markedly activated in severe heart failure, with an associated decrease in myocardial β-adrenoreceptor density. In mild or moderate heart failure there is a net stimulant (agonist) effect when sympathetic tone is low and a net blocking (antagonist) effect when the sympathetic tone is high. Consequently, xamoterol is believed to modulate the range over which sympathetic nervous activity can modulate cardiac function.

OTHER β-RECEPTOR AGONISTS

A number of new sympathomimetic agents with varying degrees of β-receptor agonist properties have been developed. Most of these agents are undergoing clinical trials and their relative effectiveness, potential adverse effects, and clinical usefulness have not been delineated.

TA-064, (—)-(R)-L-(P-hydroxyphenyl)-2-(93,4-dimethoxyphenyl 6)-amino ethanol, appears to have selective β_1-receptor agonist properties, and its positive inotropic effect is greater than its chronotropic effect. In a limited number of patients with congestive heart failure, left ventricular dP/dt and cardiac output increased, and this enhanced contractility was dose-dependent.[290] TA-064 also causes dilatation of isolated vascular segments, especially the coronary arteries, but also the renal, mesenteric, and large intestinal arteries.[291] Peripheral vascular vasodilation is thought to be mediated by β-receptor stimulation. TA-064 can be administered both intravenously and orally.

Butopamine, a synthetic sympathomimetic amine, is similar to dobutamine except that its molecules are resistant to *O*-methylation because of structural changes, and thus it can be administered orally.[292] In normal volunteers and in some patients with congestive heart failure, acute administration in doses of 0.08 to 1 µg/kg/min was associated with positive inotropic effects; however, it appeared to produce undesirable chronotropic effects that may limit its clinical usefulness.[293]

L-DOPA AND OTHER DOPAMINERGIC RECEPTOR AGONISTS

L-Dopa is a dopamine pro-drug that is converted to dopamine by the enzymatic aromatic amino acid decarboxylase in the liver and other tissues. After its oral administration, the peak blood levels of L-dopa and dopamine are attained in 1 to 3 hours. Previous studies in patients with Parkinson's disease have suggested that the cardiac effects of 1 to 1.5 g of L-dopa are similar to those of 2 to 4 µg/kg/min infusion of dopamine.[294] Based on this experience, the hemodynamic and clinical effects of 1 to 2 g of L-dopa given orally every 6 to 8 hours have been evaluated in patients with severe chronic congestive heart failure.[295,296] In the majority of patients, cardiac output increases without any significant change in arterial pressure or heart rate and pulmonary capillary wedge pressure also remains unchanged. In patients with an elevated pulmonary capillary wedge pressure, agents with the potential to decrease pulmonary capillary wedge pressure are preferable. A combination of L-dopa and captopril, an angiotensin-converting enzyme inhibitor, appears to produce a more advantageous hemodynamic effect than L-dopa alone.[297] This combination therapy maintained the augmented cardiac output by the L-dopa, and the pulmonary capillary wedge pressure decreased with the addition of captopril.

Despite the potential inotropic effect of L-dopa, myocardial oxygen consumption remained unchanged, presumably due to the concomitant reduction in systemic vascular resistance. With combined L-dopa and captopril, there was no significant change in coronary blood flow or myocardial oxygen consumption.[297] Following oral administration there was a significant increase in the level of arterial dopamine; however, there was no correlation between the magnitude of increase in dopamine concentration and the hemodynamic response. Although without controlled studies the efficacy of long-term therapy cannot be established, uncontrolled studies suggest that in some patients clinical and hemodynamic improvement is maintained after chronic therapy with L-dopa.[295]

Intolerable side effects, particularly nausea, vomiting, lack of appetite, hallucinations, dyskinetic movement, nervousness, anxiety, and insomnia, limit the use of L-dopa in many patients. These symptoms are partly reduced if the dose is gradually increased from 250 mg four times daily to 1.5 to 2.0 g four times daily over 5 to 7 days. The concomitant daily administration of 50 mg of pyridoxine, which is required for the decarboxylation of L-dopa, has also been recommended.[295]

Approximately 95% of absorbed L-dopa is decarboxylated to dopamine by the aromatic L-amino acid decarboxylase in the peripheral tissues. A small amount is methylated to 3-*O*-methyldopa. Rapid biotransformation of dopamine occurs to its principal metabolites, 3,4-dihydroxyphenylacetic acid (DOPAC) and 3-methoxy-4-hydroxyphenylacetic acid (homovanillic acid [HVA]), and these metabolites are rapidly excreted in the urine.[229]

IBOPAMINE

Ibopamine is an analogue of dopamine, and it undergoes hydrolysis to epinine (*N*-methyl dopamine), the active metabolite, which activates vascular α_1-adrenoreceptors, β-adrenoreceptors, and dopamine receptors.[298] In laboratory animals left ventricular dP/dt increases along with an increase in aortic blood flow, stroke volume, and arterial pressure.[298] In experimental studies in animals, with adequate doses of both dopamine and epinine, the systemic hemodynamics may improve; however, although renal blood flow increases consistently with dopamine, it may not increase with epinine because of the more potent α-adrenoreceptor activity of epinine.[299] In patients with heart failure, ibopamine increases cardiac index, stroke volume index, and stroke work index; heart rate, mean arterial pressure, and systemic and pulmonary venous pressures usually remain unchanged.[300] In some patients, a transient increase in right atrial and pulmonary capillary wedge pressures and total pulmonary resistance has been observed.[301] A few controlled studies have demonstrated hemodynamic and clinical improvement and increased exercise tolerance in ibopamine-treated patients compared with patients treated either with placebo or conventionally.[302] Improved left ventricular ejection fraction has also been observed, but the number of patients studied was small and the duration of therapy was short. Furthermore, after an initial improvement an attenuation of the hemodynamic response and maximal oxygen uptake during exercise has also been observed.[303] Ibopamine potentially may improve renal function, presumably due to activation of renal dopamine receptors. Urine output, urinary sodium and potassium clearance, renal blood flow, and creatinine clearance may also increase in some patients with heart failure associated with renal failure. Ibopamine may also reduce plasma norepinephrine concentrations either as a direct effect of DA_2- receptor stimulation or secondary to improved cardiac function. The recommended oral dose of ibopamine in congestive heart failure is 100 to 200 mg three times daily. Gastric paresis, increased frequency of premature ventricular beats, ventricular tachycardia, increased angina, and insomnia are the potential adverse effects of ibopamine.

Dopexamine hydrochloride is a short-acting dopamine analogue, with predominantly β_2-receptor and DA_1-receptor agonist activity. It has minimal or no β_1-agonist or α-agonist activity.[304] Dopexamine has also been shown to inhibit directly uptake of norepinephrine.[305] It can only be administered intravenously, and following an adequate dose there is usually a significant reduction in right atrial and pulmonary capillary wedge pressures and systemic vascular resistance. Mean arterial pressure and pulmonary artery pressure tend to decrease, and heart rate may increase slightly along with a significant increase in cardiac index and stroke volume index.[306]

The improvement in left ventricular function by dopexamine is likely to be caused, at least in part, by the reduction of left ventricular outflow resistance, as systemic vascular resistance falls consistently. Enhanced contractility mediated by activation of myocardial β_2-receptors may also contribute. Increased contractility may partly be mediated through enhanced sympathoadrenergic activity as a result of norepinephrine uptake inhibition by dopexamine.[305]

Although dopexamine tends to increase heart rate and possibly contractility, the overall myocardial oxygen consumption remains unchanged. Concomitant reduction of left ventricular afterload, which decreases myocardial oxygen demand, probably offsets the increased oxygen requirements owing to increased heart rate and contractility. Lack of increase in myocardial oxygen consumption may be an advantage of dopexamine over other catecholamines with positive inotropic effect. Dopexamine potentially can increase renal plasma flow and renal function in patients with congestive heart failure.

Propylbutyl dopamine is another parenteral dopaminergic receptor agonist with both DA_1- and DA_2- receptor activity.[307] In patients with severe congestive heart failure, a significant increase in cardiac output, along with a reduction in pulmonary capillary wedge pressure, was observed. There was no change in heart rate, but mean arterial pressure declined. The beneficial hemodynamic effects of propylbutyl dopamine result primarily from reduction of systemic vascular resistance, presumably due to activation of the DA_1 and DA_2 receptors.

Bromocriptine, an ergot derivative and a dopamine agonist, has been used in patients with severe congestive heart failure.[308] It has been shown to possess DA_2 agonist activity in peripheral nerves, but it also decreases sympathetic activity via a central nervous system mechanism. After its oral administration (2.5 mg), stroke volume increased, together with a reduction of heart rate and mean arterial, right atrial, and left ventricular end-diastolic pressures. Plasma norepinephrine concentrations decreased, suggesting that the withdrawal of sympathetic activity contributed to its beneficial hemodynamic effects.

Fenoldopam is a selective DA_1 agonist; after its oral administration (200 mg), the cardiac index increases along with a decrease in pulmonary capillary wedge pressure and systemic vascular resistance.[309] Increased renal blood flow and sodium excretion have been observed in hypertensive patients and normal volunteers. In patients with congestive heart failure, however, renal function may not improve despite increase in cardiac output and improved left ventricular function if arterial pressure falls concomitantly, which reduces renal perfusion pressure. The orally active dopamine pro-drug TA-870 produced in experimental animals a dose-dependent increase in contractile force, renal blood flow, urine flow, and urinary sodium excretion, and decrease in renal vascular resistance. Oral administration for 2 weeks in these animals did not produce attenuation of systemic and renal hemodynamic effects.[310,311]

It is apparent that a number of new dopamine agonists are being developed and have the potential to improve cardiac function and hemodynamics in patients with heart failure; however, the safety and efficacy of these agents during long-term therapy remain to be determined. Further studies will be required to establish their clinical usefulness.

GLUCAGON

Glucagon is a pancreatic polypeptide; it exerts its positive inotropic effects by stimulating myocardial glucagon receptors and activating the adenylate cyclase system. It is a relatively weak inotropic agent, and its clinical use is limited because of its high incidence of gastrointestinal side effects (nausea, vomiting) and rapid attenuation of its inotropic effect.[312] It is sometimes used to correct the low cardiac output resulting from β-blocker overdose. Glucagon is usually administered intravenously in a dose of 1 mg.

HISTAMINE

Stimulation of histamine-2 receptors in myocardial tissue by histamine is associated with positive inotropic effects.[313] Specific histamine-2 agonists, impromidine or dimaprit, exert a marked positive inotropic effect[314]; however, appropriate clinical studies will be required to determine their effectiveness in the management of heart failure. Furthermore, systemic administration of histamine is associated with severe adverse effects, and thus it is unlikely to be clinically useful.

FORSKOLIN

Forskolin, a diterpene compound, is derived from the extracts of an Indian coleus plant, and it exerts potent positive inotropic and vasodilating effects when given intravenously and orally.[315] In patients with congestive heart failure, a substantial increase in cardiac output and reduction in systemic vascular resistance have been reported. Marked tachycardia has been observed with high intravenous doses.

The mechanism of action of forskolin appears to be due to direct activation of the catalytic unit of the adenylate cyclase with a marked increase in cardiac cyclic AMP production.[316] Since its site of action is distal to the β-adrenergic receptor, attenuation of the positive inotropic effects due to desensitization, as occurs with β-adrenergic agonists, is not expected with forskolin. Further clinical studies are warranted to establish its value in the management of heart failure.

DIBUTYRYL-CYCLIC AMP

Dibutyryl-cyclic AMP is a phosphodiesterase-resistant cyclic nucleotide analogue, and it produces a prolonged positive inotropic effect in isolated papillary muscles. Exogenous cyclic AMP is rapidly metabolized and therefore cannot be used clinically, but its analogue, dibutyryl-cyclic AMP, is resistant to degradation by phosphodiesterase. Intravenous administration of dibutyryl-cyclic AMP in patients with chronic congestive heart failure has produced a significant increase in cardiac output and a decrease in systemic vascular resistance.[317] A modest decrease in left ventricular filling pressure was also noted. These hemodynamic effects, however, can result either from enhanced contractility or from cyclic AMP-mediated peripheral vasodilatation.

PHOSPHODIESTERASE INHIBITORS

The existence of several isozymes of cyclic nucleotide phosphodiesterase has been recognized in mammalian cells.[318] Although in cardiac muscle three distinct forms of phosphodiesterase isozymes, designated as peak I, II, or III, have been identified, peak III phosphodiesterase is the predominant form. A number of relatively specific peak III phosphodiesterase inhibitors have been developed that are undergoing clinical trials for short-term and long-term treatment of congestive heart failure. Inhibition of peak III phosphodiesterase results in increased intracellular cyclic AMP in cardiac muscle and subsequent phosphorylation of cellular proteins by cyclic AMP-dependent protein kinase. Increased cyclic AMP in cardiac muscle leads to increased contractility and to enhanced rate of myocardial relaxation.

In contrast to cardiac muscle, both cyclic AMP and cyclic GMP have been identified as second messengers for relaxation of vascular smooth muscle.[319] However, peak III phosphodiesterase in vascular smooth muscle is pharmacologically similar to peak III phosphodiesterase in cardiac muscle.[320] Thus, peak III phosphodiesterase inhibitors not only enhance cardiac contractility but also promote vascular smooth muscle relaxation (Fig. 3.15).[318]

Theophylline and methylxanthine are nonspecific phosphodiesterase inhibitors, and their positive inotropic effects are partly related to inhibition of phosphodiesterase.[320] However, other mechanisms such as direct antagonism of the effects of adenosine, an endogenous nucleotide with negative inotropic actions, inhibition of calcium reuptake by the sarcoplasmic reticulum, and enhanced synthesis and release of endogenous catecholamines have also been believed to be contributory. Although theophylline and methylxanthine have been shown to exert positive inotropic effects in in vitro studies as well as in humans, these agents are seldom used as inotropic agents for the treatment of heart failure. Their inotropic potency is relatively weak, and undesirable gastrointestinal and central nervous sys-

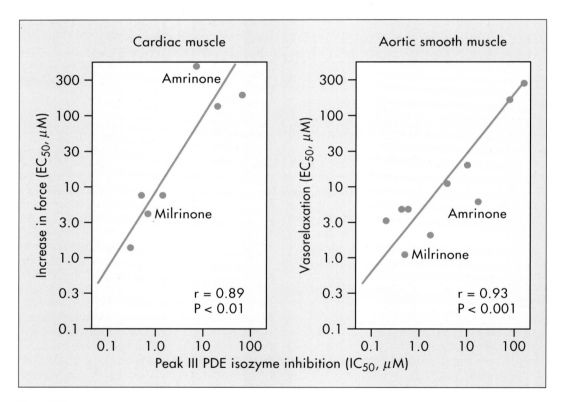

Figure 3.15 Enhanced inotropy (left panel) and vasorelaxation (right panel) as a function of peak III phosphodiesterase (PDE) inhibition in guinea pig (GP) cardiac and aortic smooth muscle. The potency (IC_{50}, μM) for isozyme inhibition and the potency (EC_{50}, μM) for increasing developed force in paced guinea pig papillary muscle or relaxation of phenylephrine-contracted aortic smooth muscle were determined for several PDE III inhibitors. (Modified from Silver PJ: Biochemical aspects of inhibition of cardiovascular low (Km) cyclic adenosine monophosphate phosphodiesterase. Am J Cardiol 63:2A, 1989)

tem side effects are considerable. These agents are also prone to induce excessive tachycardia and arrhythmias. A number of other pharmacologic agents, including papaverine, isobutyl-methylxanthine, the piperidine derivatives buquineran and carbazeran, and the coronary vasodilator trapidil, have been shown to exert positive inotropic effects by phosphodiesterase inhibition.[321–324] A number of other, newer phosphodiesterase inhibitors are undergoing extensive clinical evaluation. These agents are structurally dissimilar to one another and to the methylxanthines but share similar pharmacophysiologic properties. These drugs, in general, do not inhibit Na^+,K^+-ATPase, and their actions are not blocked by histamine-2 antagonists or agents that block synthesis of prostaglandins. The principal mechanism of action of these agents is inhibition of peak III phosphodiesterase, which increases intracellular cyclic AMP concentrations.

The magnitude of response to a peak III phosphodiesterase inhibitor is likely to be partly determined by the levels of cyclic AMP present in the tissue. The contractile response of failing myocardium to the peak III phosphodiesterase inhibitors has been shown to be reduced compared with that of normal tissues,[325] presumably because of lower levels of cyclic AMP in the failing myocardium due to dysfunction of the β_1-adrenergic system. In vitro studies have demonstrated that pre-exposure of failing myocardium to low-dose dobutamine enhances myocardial contractile response to milrinone, a peak III phosphodiesterase inhibitor.[325] The cyclic AMP levels presumably increase in response to dobutamine, providing increased substrate for the peak III phosphodiesterase inhibitors. This provides the rationale for combination of a β_1-adrenoreceptor agonist and a peak III phosphodiesterase inhibitor for inotropic therapy of severe heart failure.

Amrinone, milrinone, and enoximone are three phosphodiesterase inhibitors that have been studied extensively for treatment of heart failure. Several other agents are also undergoing clinical trials. The relative efficacy of these various drugs and, in many instances, their long-term effects in the management of heart failure still need to be determined.

Amrinone

Amrinone is a bipyridine derivative shown to have positive inotropic effects in in vitro studies. It increases peak development tension, maximal rate of tension development, and maximal rate of relaxation.[326] After acute administration of amrinone, either intravenously or orally, substantial improvement in hemodynamics, cardiac performance, and clinical status can occur, even in patients with severe refractory heart failure.[325,327–331] Cardiac output and stroke vol-

ume increase significantly, along with a reduction in right and left ventricular filling pressures. Pulmonary artery pressure and pulmonary vascular resistance also tend to decrease. A slight reduction in mean arterial pressure and a modest increase in heart rate may also be observed. Systemic vascular resistance decreases significantly. With larger doses, significant and undesirable hypotension and tachycardia may occur.

Although in in vitro studies, direct positive inotropic effects and primary peripheral vasodilation have been documented, the relative contributions of these two mechanisms in improving left ventricular function in patients with heart failure remain uncertain. In some studies, there was an increase in left ventricular dP/dt, despite no change in heart rate and a decrease in left ventricular filling pressure, indicating augmented contractility. There was also a significant reduction in systemic vascular resistance; thus, both positive inotropic and vasodilatory effects were evident.[328] In other studies, there were no changes in indices of contractility, such as dP/dt, contractile element velocity, and the end-systolic pressure–volume relation, although there was a significant reduction in systemic vascular resistance.[330] In some studies, intracoronary injections of amrinone were not associated with any evidence of enhanced myocardial contractility.[330] It appears, therefore, that the vasodilatory effect may be more pronounced than the inotropic effect in patients with chronic heart failure. Amrinone has been shown to produce direct smooth muscle relaxation in the coronary artery.[332,333] Changes in coronary hemodynamics and myocardial energetics have been assessed in a small number of patients with heart failure, and no significant changes in rate–pressure product, coronary blood flow, or myocardial oxygen consumption were observed.[334] In occasional patients, however, myocardial lactate production occurred, suggesting myocardial ischemia.

Intravenous administration of amrinone, followed by short-term oral therapy, is associated with both hemodynamic and clinical improvement in patients with severe refractory heart failure. In patients with acute myocardial infarction and pump failure, amrinone increases cardiac output and decreases systemic vascular resistance and pulmonary capillary wedge pressure, with little or no change in heart rate and blood pressure, when a low dose (200 µg/kg/hr) is infused.[335,336] With larger doses, although there is a greater decrease in pulmonary capillary wedge pressure, tachycardia and hypotension develop, which might be deleterious.

Intravenous amrinone has been found effective in the management of postoperative heart failure. Compared with dobutamine, amrinone appears to cause a greater reduction of systemic and pulmonary venous pressures.[337,338] In patients with severe postoperative pump failure or cardiogenic shock refractory to catecholamines and intra-aortic balloon pump therapy, amrinone may cause a substantial increase in cardiac output and stroke volume, reduction of pulmonary capillary wedge pressure and systemic vascular resistance, and improved tissue perfusion (Fig. 3.16).[339,340] In postoperative cardiac surgical patients both low-dose (0.75 mg/kg loading dose and 10 μg/kg/min infusion) and high-dose (2.25 mg/kg loading dose and 20 μg/k/min infusion) amrinone increased heart rate and cardiac output and decreased mean arterial pressure and mean pulmonary arterial, right atrial, and pulmonary capillary wedge pressures. Arterial oxygen saturation decreased significantly after both low-dose and high-dose amrinone. Pulmonary shunt increased slightly following the low dose but markedly after the high dose of amrinone.[341] Thus, high-dose amrinone should be avoided. The major indications for the use of intravenous amrinone in patients with postoperative pump failure are elevated left ventricular filling pressure, low cardiac output, and poor peripheral perfusion, particularly when these hemodynamic abnormalities persist despite conventional therapy. The major undesirable effect in patients with acute heart failure is hypotension, which can be corrected by concomitant adminstration of norepinephrine.[340]

The efficacy of long-term oral amrinone therapy in the management of patients with chronic heart failure remains uncertain. In uncontrolled studies, amrinone has been shown to improve exercise tolerance both during short-term and long-term oral therapy.[342–344] An improvement in left ventricular pump function and maximal oxygen consumption during exercise has been noted after short-term and long-term therapy. Controlled studies, however, have failed to demonstrate any benefit during long-term therapy.[345,346] Compared with placebo, there was no improvement in clinical status or exercise tolerance during maintenance amrinone therapy. Furthermore,

some adverse effects were more frequently seen in the amrinone treated group. Thus, presently, amrinone therapy should be considered only for short-term therapy in patients with heart failure.

Gastrointestinal adverse effects, such as nausea, anorexia, abdominal pain, vomiting, and diarrhea occurred in 27% of patients receiving amrinone. Central nervous system complications, such as dizziness, headache, lightheadedness, and paresthesia, were also more frequent. Unexplained fever, abnormal liver function, and rash with pruritus may also occur. Thrombocytopenia is frequently seen with amrinone therapy, but clinically relevant (platelet counts < 50,000/mm³) thrombocytopenia is uncommon. Thrombocytopenia appears to be dose-related and is usually reversed by lowering the dose to 275 mg/d.[346]

Amrinone appears to increase the maximal velocity, overshoot, and duration of the slow response action potential, due to its effects on the slow inward calcium current. Amrinone also shortens the atrio-His interval, AV nodal effective refractory period, and maximal corrected sinus node recovery time. It does not appear to have any significant effect on ventricular arrhythmogenesis.[347,348]

However, clinical experience suggests that ventricular arrhythmias occur in up to 3% of patients receiving intravenous amrinone. Intravenous amrinone therapy is initiated with a 0.75 mg/kg bolus slowly over 2 to 3 minutes, and the infusion is then continued at a rate between 5 and 10 μg/kg/min. The total daily dose should not exceed 10 mg/kg. The oral dose should be less than 300 mg/day to avoid adverse effects, particularly thrombocytopenia.

Sudden withdrawal of amrinone therapy may be associated with rapid hemodynamic deterioration and thus should be avoided.[349,350] Deterioration of hemodynamics has been observed following withdrawal of amrinone after 2 to 10 weeks of oral therapy. The mechanisms for such deterioration after withdrawal of therapy remain unclear and speculative.

Figure 3.16 Improvement in left ventricular function in a patient with severe postoperative heart failure following the addition of a peak III phosphodiesterase inhibitor, amrinone, to initial combination therapy with dopamine, dobutamine, and nitroglycerin (NTG). (Modified from Goener M et al: Heart failure after open heart surgery. In Perret C, Vincent JL (eds): Update in Intensive Care and Emergency Medicine, p 146. Berlin, Springer-Verlag, 1988)

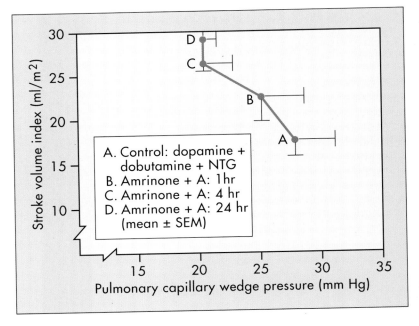

A. Control: dopamine +
   dobutamine + NTG
B. Amrinone + A: 1 hr
C. Amrinone + A: 4 hr
D. Amrinone + A: 24 hr
   (mean ± SEM)

Milrinone

Milrinone is also a bipyridine derivative and is closely related to amrinone; however, it is approximately 15 times more potent than amrinone.[351-353] Its positive inotropic effects have been well documented in papillary muscles, as evident from the increase in developed tension and the rate of tension development.[354,355] Intracoronary infusion of doses of milrinone that did not have any significant effects on arterial pressure and systemic vascular resistance was associated with an increase in left ventricular dP/dt, along with an increased stroke volume and decreased left ventricular end-diastolic pressure (Fig. 13.17).[356]

A substantial dose-dependent increase in left ventricular dP/dt along with an increase in stroke work index has been observed in response to intravenous milrinone.[357,358] In normal subjects, a dose-dependent increase in load-independent end-systolic indices of contractility in response to milrinone has been observed.[359] Milrinone administered orally also increased dP/dt, $dP/dt/P$, V_{max}, and left ventricular end-systolic pressure–volume ratio.[360,361] The direct vasodilatory effect of milrinone has also been demonstrated in isolated limb preparations. Intra-arterial injection of smaller doses of milrinone, which did not produce any significant change in systemic hemodynamics, decreased forearm vascular resistance and increased forearm blood flow.[362] Forearm venous capacitance increases substantially following intravenous administration of milrinone, and this venodilation appears to be due to both direct effect on the veins and an indirect effect due to withdrawal of vasoconstrictor tone.[363]

Milrinone may also improve left ventricular relaxation and diastolic distensibility.[364] A downward and rightward shift of the left ventricular diastolic pressure–volume curve has been observed. An increase in left ventricular negative dP/dt, the time constant for left ventricular relaxation, and the peak rate of diastolic filling also occurred. Increased left ventricular compliance is associated with a left and upward shift of the left ventricular function curve. The relative contributions of the positive inotropic effect, peripheral vasodilation, and improved left ventricular compliance to improved left ventricular function are difficult to determine.

Milrinone, like amrinone, does not appear to increase myocardial oxygen consumption.[365] Coronary sinus blood flow, however, tends to increase, together with a decrease in myocardial oxygen extraction. Since the heart rate–blood pressure product also remains unchanged, increased coronary blood flow appears to result from the primary decrease in coronary vascular resistance.

Such primary coronary arteriolar dilatation can result in redistribution of myocardial blood flow and may not contribute to improvement of myocardial ischemia. Comparative effects of milrinone, nitroprusside, and dobutamine on coronary hemodynamics and myocardial energetics have been evaluated.[366,367] Nitroprusside, a pure vasodilator, tends to decrease myocardial oxygen consumption more than milrinone; while with dobutamine myocardial oxygen consumption increases consistently.

Oral milrinone therapy does not appear to increase renal blood flow or glomerular filtration rate despite

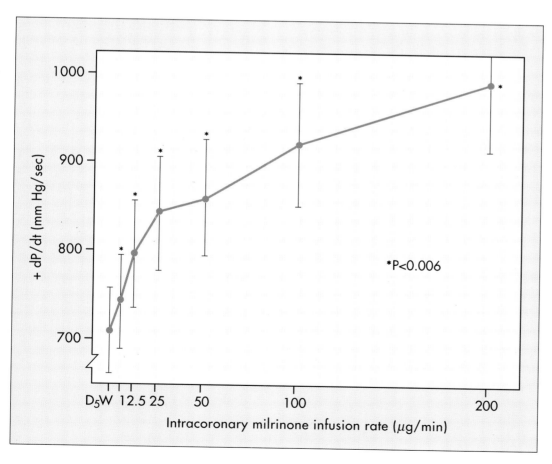

Figure 3.17 Dose-related increase in left ventricular positive dP/dt caused by intracoronary infusion of milrinone. (Modified from Ludmer PL, Wright RF, Arnold MO et al: Separation of the directed myocardial and vasodilator actions of milrinone administered by an intracoronary infusion technique. Circulation 73:130, 1986)

a substantial increase in cardiac output. However, forearm blood flow increases proportionately with cardiac output, suggesting that milrinone preferentially increases skeletal muscle blood flow. Lack of increase in renal blood flow with milrinone may result from shunting of blood flow from the kidney or alternatively from activation of renal cellular mechanisms that might offset the anticipated favorable response from increased cardiac output.

Comparative effects of milrinone and captopril on renal and skeletal muscle blood flow have been evaluated in patients with chronic congestive heart failure after their acute administration.[369] Relative to the increase in cardiac output, the increase in renal blood flow with captopril was greater and there was no change in skeletal muscle blood flow, suggesting a direct effect of captopril on renovascular resistance. With milrinone, skeletal muscle flow increased but the increase in renal blood flow was relatively less (relative to the increase in cardiac output), indicating that milrinone probably does not exert a direct effect on renovascular resistance.

Electrophysiologic studies have demonstrated that milrinone improves conduction and reduces postrepolarization refractoriness in ischemic gap preparations. These findings suggest that milrinone may exert antiarrhythmic or arrhythmogenic effects by restoring or improving conduction in areas of depressed conductivity.[348] Although milrinone mildly improves AV nodal conduction, it does not change atrial AV nodal, or ventricular refractoriness. Potential proarrhythmic effects of milrinone have not been substantiated during prospective Holter monitoring or electrophysiologic studies.[349]

Systemic hemodynamic effects of milrinone are similar to those of other phosphodiesterase inhibitors with combined inotropic and vasodilating properties.

There is usually a significant increase in cardiac index, stroke volume, and stroke work index, along with a decrease in pulmonary capillary wedge and right atrial pressures (Fig. 3.18).[370] A significant decrease in mean arterial pressure and an increase in heart rate may also occur. Reduction in arterial pressure and systemic vascular resistance appears to be dose-dependent; a marked reduction in systemic vascular resistance with hypotension may be observed with larger doses.[371]

Short-term therapy with milrinone in uncontrolled studies has been reported to improve exercise tolerance and maximal oxygen consumption in patients with chronic heart failure.[372] However, some controlled studies have failed to demonstrate a sustained improvement in exercise tolerance during long-term oral therapy.[373]

In a large multicenter, double-blind, randomized, controlled study, changes in exercise tolerance of patients with chronic congestive heart failure were assessed during 3 months of therapy with milrinone alone, digoxin alone, milrinone and digoxin, or placebo. All three treatment groups experienced better exercise performance than the placebo group, significantly so in the groups treated with milrinone alone and digoxin alone. Milrinone-treated patients also experienced better quality of life.[133] In another study, 155 patients with congestive heart failure, whose condition was stable on digitalis and diuretics, were randomized for 3 months to milrinone, milrinone and digoxin, or digoxin alone[374] and the hemodynamic studies did not show any evidence for tolerance to milrinone. Although the quality of life was favorably influenced by milrinone therapy, clinical class was not affected.

Milrinone is usually well tolerated. Diarrhea or other gastrointestinal symptoms are uncommon.

Figure 3.18 Acute and chronic hemodynamic effects of oral milrinone in 25 patients with severe congestive heart failure. Hemodynamic effects are expressed as percentage change from baseline (control). Chronic hemodynamic effects were determined after an average of 37 days (range 19 to 89 days) of therapy. (P values are compared with baseline.) There was no significant difference between acute and chronic responses. (Modified from Simonton CA, Chatterjee K, Cody RJ et al: Milrinone in congestive heart failure: Acute and chronic hemodynamic and clinical evaluation. J Am Coll Cardiol 6:453, 1985)

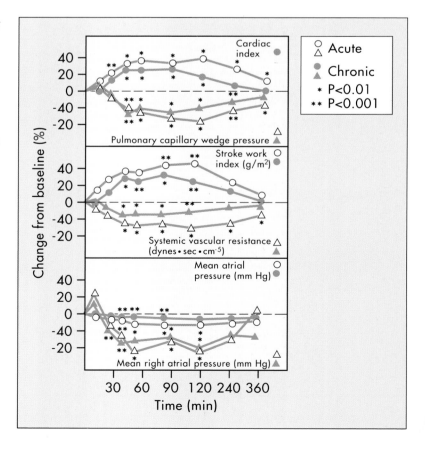

Rash, thrombocytopenia, and fever have not been observed. Fluid retention occurs in over 80% of patients, requiring increased diuretics during maintenance therapy.[371] Milrinone therapy did not improve survival in patients with severe heart failure. In one uncontrolled study, survival at 6 months was only 34%,[370] and in another similar study, 1-year survival was 39%.[375]

In the multicenter placebo-controlled milrinone-digoxin trial of 230 patients with chronic heart failure, during 3 months of therapy, 10 of 119 patients assigned to treatment with milrinone died, compared with only 6 of 111 patients assigned to the control group. These findings suggested an adverse influence of milrinone therapy on survival of patients with severe chronic congestive heart failure.[133] The Prospective Randomized Milrinone Survival Evaluation (PROMISE) study reported a 34% increase in cardiovascular mortality in patients treated with milrinone during a relatively short follow-up.[376] Milrinone or placebo was added to diuretics and, in most patients, digoxin and angiotensin-converting enzyme in-j42 hibitors. The increased mortality with the addition of milrinone was most prominent with the patients with severe heart failure (NYHA class IV). Thus, long-term milrinone therapy should be avoided in patients with severe heart failure.

Enoximone[377, 378]

Enoximone, an imidazole derivative, is also a peak III phosphodiesterase inhibitor and has been extensively evaluated for the management of patients with acute and chronic heart failure. Enoximone increases intracellular concentrations of cyclic AMP but not that of cyclic GMP. In experimental animals, it increases myocardial contractile force and the slope of the peak isovolumetric pressure-volume relation, which has been shown to represent the maximal elastance (E_{max}) of the ventricle for a given contractile state.[379,380] In patients with severe chronic heart failure, calculated E_{max} also tends to increase in response to intravenous enoximone.[380] In patients with impaired left ventricular function, peak dP/dt increases despite a decrease in left ventricular filling pressure and in the absence of any significant change in heart rate or blood pressure.[381] These findings suggest that enoximone exerts direct positive inotropic effect. Enoximone is also a potent vasodilator. In isolated canine hind limb preparation, enoximone produces direct relaxation of vascular smooth muscle.[378] A decrease in calculated systemic vascular resistance has also been observed in patients with chronic heart failure.[382] There is also evidence that enoximone increases left ventricular distensibility.[382] In some patients, left ventricular end-diastolic volume increases despite a marked decrease in pulmonary capillary wedge pressure, which suggests a down and rightward shift of the left ventricular diastolic pressure–volume curve (Fig. 3.19). Such a shift is associated with left and upward shift of the ventricular function curve. However, increased left ventricular distensibility in response to enoximone is not a uniform finding.[383] In only approximately 30% of patients, a downward shift of the left ventricular pressure–volume curve occurred in response to enoximone. Furthermore, when the relationship between changes in transmural pressure (estimated by subtracting right atrial pressure from left ventricular diastolic pressure) and changes in left ventricular diastolic volume was determined, no shift in the left ventricular pressure–volume relationship was found.[383]

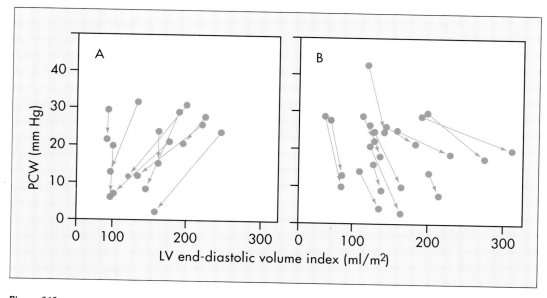

Figure 3.19 Relationship between changes in pulmonary capillary wedge pressure (PCW) and radioangiographically calculated left ventricular end-diastolic volume index in response to intravenous enoximone. In patients in **B**, a marked decrease in PCW was associated with an increase in EDVI. (Modified from Kereiakes DJ, Viquerat C, Lanzer P et al: Mechanisms of improved left ventricular function following intravenous MDL 17043 in patients with severe heart failure. Am Heart J 108:1278, 1984)

Both intravenous and oral enoximone produce a marked increase in cardiac index stroke volume and stroke work index and a significant decrease in pulmonary capillary, right atrial, and pulmonary artery pressures (Fig. 3.20). A slight increase in heart rate and a modest decrease in mean arterial pressure are frequently observed.[384,385]

In experimental animals, improved cardiovascular effects were not accompanied by any significant alterations in myocardial oxygen consumption.[378] Clinical studies on the effects of enoximone on myocardial energetics have suggested that there may be no change or modest increase in coronary blood flow with no change or decrease in myocardial oxygen consumption.[386,387] In one study, in which much larger doses of enoximone were used, a substantial increase in coronary blood flow and myocardial oxygen consumption was observed.[388] Coronary sinus venous oxygen content tends to increase and myocardial oxygen extraction tends to decrease, suggesting primary coronary vasodilatation by enoximone. Primary coronary vasodilatation may, however, be associated with shunting of blood to less metabolically active areas of the myocardium, which may induce myocardial ischemia.[387] Myocardial efficacy is usually estimated by computing the ratio of left ventricular stroke work to myocardial oxygen consumption. Following enoximone, myocardial efficiency usually increases, even when there is some increase in myocardial oxygen requirements.[386–388] Enoximone has also been shown to improve global ejection fraction and regional wall motion in patients after infarction.[389] There was marked improvement of regional wall motion of the noninfarcted segments, myocardial segments that were hypokinetic at control be-

came normokinetic, and the extent of akinesis decreased by 40%.[389]

Enoximone does not appear to change significantly the flow or resistance of renal or hepatic-splanchnic flow, although limb blood flow increases.[390] In normal volunteers, however, improved renal function has been observed with enoximone.[391] Electrophysiologic effects of enoximone have not been adequately evaluated. Like other phosphodiesterase inhibitors, it has little effect on His-Purkinje conduction but tends to shorten the atrio-His interval and ventricular refractoriness.[392]

Clinical improvement is observed during short-term therapy even in patients with severe refractory heart failure.[388] In patients with acute myocardial infarction complicated by left ventricular failure, improved clinical status and hemodynamics have been observed during short-term intravenous enoximone treatment.[393] In some patients with cardiogenic shock refractory to dobutamine, intravenous enoximone treatment improved hemodynamics with resolution of signs of circulatory shock.[394] Intravenous enoximone therapy has also been found to be effective in the management of refractory low output state following cardiac surgery.[395] Rapid and sustained hemodynamic and clinical improvements have been observed in these patients.

Efficacy of long-term maintenance therapy on hemodynamics, exercise tolerance, and clinical status has been assessed mostly in uncontrolled studies. In some studies, no sustained improvement in hemodynamics or exercise tolerance was noted.[396,397] On the other hand, a number of other studies have reported sustained hemodynamic improvement and improvement in clinical status, exercise tolerance, and maxi-

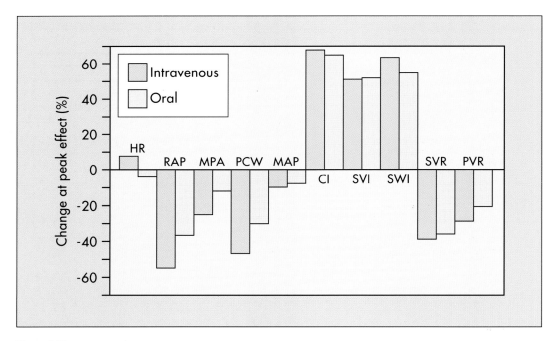

Figure 3.20 Comparative magnitude of the effect of intravenous and oral enoximone (MDL 17043) in 38 patients with congestive heart failure. The percentage change from baseline at peak drug effect of each hemodynamic variable is similar after either route of administration. Cardiac index (CI), stroke volume index (SVI), and stroke work index (SWI) increased markedly along with decreased systemic vascular resistance (SVR), pulmonary vascular resistance (PVR), pulmonary capillary wedge pressure (PCW), mean pulmonary artery pressure (MPA), and right atrial pressure (RAP). There was only a slight change in heart rate (HR) and mean arterial pressure (MAP).

mal oxygen consumption in many patients with chronic heart failure during long-term maintenance therapy.[398-401]

A few controlled studies have indicated that during 12 weeks of enoximone therapy, a sustained improvement in exercise tolerance can be observed in patients with moderately severe chronic heart failure.[402-404] Some studies have noted a similar increase in exercise duration with captopril and enoximone.[400,404] These findings suggest that during relatively shorter periods of treatment with enoximone, sustained clinical improvement is to be expected in patients with moderately severe congestive heart failure.

No large-scale controlled long-term studies have been performed to assess survival rate in patients treated with enoximone. Results of an uncontrolled study suggest that the mortality of patients with severe chronic heart failure, particularly in patients refractory to vasodilators and angiotensin-converting enzyme inhibitors, remains very high. The overall mortality at 6 months, in such patients, in one study was 55%.[388] In another study, mortality rates at 6 and 12 months were 50% and 58%, respectively. In patients who are dependent on intravenous inotropic drugs, the mortality was higher: 64% at 6 months and 73% at 1 year.[405] In a multicenter, prospective, randomized trial, the efficacy of oral enoximone was compared to placebo in patients wth moderate to moderately severe congestive heart failure who were treated with digoxin and diuretics but not with vasodilators or angiotensin-converting enzyme inhibitors. There was no significant improvement in exercise tolerance or anaerobic threshold in the enoximone-treated patients. Furthermore, there was a higher mortality in the enoximone-treated group.[406] Another phosphodiesterase inhibitor, imazodan, has been reported to be associated with increased mortality in a multicenter trial.[407] It is apparent that with the cardiospecific phosphodiesterase inhibitors that have been evaluated, mortality of patients with chronic heart failure increases; thus they should not be considered for long-term management. These agents can be of use for short-term therapy of severe refractory heart failure. Enoximone has also been used for stabilizing patients awaiting cardiac transplant (pharmacologic bridge to cardiac transplant).[408,409]

The major side effects of enoximone are gastrointestinal: nausea, anorexia, vomiting, diarrhea, and abdominal bloating. Thrombocytopenia, rash, and altered taste sensation occur infrequently. Fluid retention and need for increased diuretics are common. An increased incidence of ventricular arrhythmias, particularly during acute intravenous therapy, has also been suspected. Hypotension, insomnia, somnolence, agitation anxiety, and headache have been reported.[410]

PIROXIMONE

Piroximone is also an imidazole derivative that has been demonstrated in vitro and in experimental animals to have direct positive inotropic and vasodilator actions.[411] After acute intravenous and oral administration in patients with chronic congestive heart failure, cardiac output stroke volume and stroke work

increase, while pulmonary capillary wedge and right atrial pressures decrease.[412,413] Heart rate and blood pressure usually do not change, but systemic vascular resistance declines. Left ventricular *dP/dt* increases due to the drug's inotropic effects. Piroximone also tends to increase left ventricular distensibility in some patients.[413] Following acute intravenous therapy, a reduction in plasma norepinephrine levels and a tendency to increased plasma renin activity have been reported.[412]

Piroximone is effective when administered orally, and its inotropic potency appears to be five to ten times that of enoximone.[414] After an oral dose, the peak hemodynamic effects occur in about 30 minutes, and the hemodynamic effects may last for 10 hours or longer. The effects of piroximone on regional blood flow have not been evaluated in patients with congestive heart failure. In experimental animals with heart failure, it does not appear to increase renal blood flow.[415] Clinical experience with piroximone is too limited to determine its long-term efficacy and side effect profile.

POSICOR (RO 13-6438)

Posicor is an imidazoquinazolinone derivative, which is also a peak III phosphodiesterase inhibitor. Its inotropic potency in vitro appears to be less than that of amrinone. Its inotropic effects are partially attenuated by pretreatment with reserpine and, like those of amrinone or milrinone, can be almost totally reversed by carbachol.[416]

Like other phosphodiesterase inhibitors, posicor increases cardiac output, stroke volume, and stroke work, while reducing right atrial and pulmonary capillary wedge pressure.[417] There is usually a slight increase in heart rate and a modest decrease in mean arterial pressure. Its vasodilatory action is evident from the marked reduction in systemic vascular resistance. The peak hemodynamic effects tend to occur within 1 hour, and the effects last for approximately 8 hours after a single oral dose.[417]

Posicor appears to produce primary coronary vasodilation as it decreases myocardial oxygen extraction and increases coronary sinus venous oxygen content.[417] Myocardial oxygen consumption does not increase, and the ratio of minute work/myocardial oxygen consumption, an index of left ventricular efficiency, tends to improve. Information regarding its clinical efficacy and side effects is not available to determine its role in the long-term management of patients with chronic heart failure.

SULMAZOLE (ARL 115BS)

Sulmazole is a phenylimidazopyridine derivative and also a phosphodiesterase inhibitor. It has been suggested that its positive inotropic effect may result, in part, from the release of endogenous catecholamines. It apparently also increases the sensitivity of myofibrils to calcium.[418,419] Its hemodynamic effects are similar to those of other phosphodiesterase inhibitors, and improvement in left ventricular function has been demonstrated in patients with severe congestive heart failure with sulmazole.[420,421] The long-term efficacy of this drug, however, has not been established. Serious gastrointestinal side effects, visual disturbances, and thrombocytopenia have been observed, even during short-term therapy. Hepatic neoplasms have developed in sulmazole-treated rodents.

CALCIUM-SENSITIZING AND OTHER INOTROPIC AGENTS[422–428]

Enhanced contractility (positive inotropism) is caused by or associated with alterations in calcium exchange in heart muscles. Some inotropic agents can increase the sensitivity of the myofilaments to calcium. In papillary muscle preparations, calcium-sensitizing inotropic agents cause an upward and leftward shift of the calcium–force relation.[425–427] This calcium-sensitizing property appears to be related to an increased binding of calcium to troponin.[425,426] However, calcium-sensitizing inotropic agents may impair myocardial relaxation in myopathic hearts, resulting in a reduced contractile reserve and diminished active force production.[428] Pimobendan, sulmazol, and DPI 201-106 are examples of calcium-sensitizing inotropic agents. CI-914 is an imidazolphyenyl pyridazinone that possesses phosphodiesterase-inhibiting properties. The benzimidazole derivatives UD-CG 212 and UD-CG 115 (pimobendan), a quinolone derivative OPC 8212, and other phosphodiesterase inhibitors have been shown to have positive inotropic properties. CI-914, like other phosphodiesterase inhibitors, improves hemodynamics in patients with chronic heart failure; however, mortality in patients treated with CI-914 appears to be higher than among those treated with placebo.[429] The benzimidazol analogue BM14.478, a phosphodiesterase inhibitor, also produces beneficial hemodynamic effects with a substantial increase in cardiac index and stroke volume index and a decrease in systemic and pulmonary venous pressure and systemic and pulmonary vascular resistance.[430] There were, however, no significant favorable neuroendocrine changes. The long-term clinical effects also remain unknown. OPC-8212 is an inotropic and vasodilator agent that increases contractility by an effect on ion channels and by increasing action potential duration. A randomized, double-blind, placebo-controlled trial in patients with congestive heart failure indicated that patients treated with OPC-8212 have decreased morbidity and mortality.[431] The hemodynamic effects of OPC-8212 are similar to those of other inotropic agents.

Pimobendan (UD-CG115), which has phosphodiesterase-inhibiting, vasodilatory, and calcium-sensitizing properties, has also been shown to improve cardiac performance and exercise tolerance of patients with severe chronic congestive heart failure refractory

FIGURE 3.21 RELATIVE CHANGES (COMPARED WITH CONTROL) IN SYSTEMIC HEMODYNAMICS AND OBSERVED SIDE EFFECTS DURING THERAPY WITH NEWER PHOSPHODIESTERASE INHIBITORS IN CHRONIC CONGESTIVE HEART FAILURE— EXPERIENCE AT THE UNIVERSITY OF CALIFORNIA, SAN FRANCISCO

Drug	Change in Systemic Hemodynamics (%)						Adverse Effects
	CI	PCWP	RAP	HR	MAP	SVR	
Milrinone (n = 37)	+49	−31	−39	+0	−13	−30	Fluid retention Ventricular arrhythmias Occasional gastrointestinal symptoms
Amrinone (n = 10)	+67	−36	−42	+3	−17	−48	Nausea Anorexia Loose bowel motions Fever Hepatic dysfunction Rash Ventricular arrhythmias Thrombocytopenia Fluid retention
Enoximone (n = 38)	+75	−42	−50	+9	−10	−42	Diarrhea Nausea Anorexia Fluid retention Hepatic dysfunction Ventricular arrhythmias Rarely thrombocytopenia
Piroximone (n = 15)	+53	−18	−43	+2	−3	−26	Nausea Anorexia Fluid retention Arrhythmia
Posicor	+58	−38	−45	+4	−10	−37	Fluid retention Arrhythmia Visual disturbances Nausea Anorexia

(CI = Cardiac index; PCWP = Pulmonary capillary wedge pressure; RAP = Right atrial pressure; HR = Heart rate; MAP = Mean arterial pressure; SVR = Systemic vascular resistance)

to digitalis, diuretics, and angiotensin-converting enzyme inhibitors.[432] A multicenter, prospective, randomized double-blind trial reported that pimobendan, (5 mg/d) significantly increased exercise duration, peak maximal oxygen consumption (peak VO$_2$), and quality of life. There were no significant changes in ejection fraction or mortality during 12 weeks follow-up.[433] The efficacy and safety of pimobendan have been compared to enalapril in patients with moderate congestive heart failure.[434] Both pimobendan and enalapril improved exercise tolerance by a similar magnitude. However, it is uncertain whether combination therapy is better. Furthermore, the effect of pimobendan on survival of patients with chronic heart failure needs to be determined.

Preliminary studies indicate that berberine, a plant alkaloid, and D13625, both orally active drugs, produce beneficial hemodynamic effects in patients with severe heart failure. Their mechanisms of action have not been clarified. The slow calcium channel agonist Bay K 8644 has been shown to exert positive inotropic effects by promoting calcium influx.[435] These agents also produce peripheral vasoconstriction and raise arterial pressure and coronary vascular tone. The co-enzyme Q$_{10}$ is a mitochondrial respiratory chain redox component and reports suggest that it produces beneficial hemodynamic effects in patients with heart failure, after intravenous as well as oral administration. Co-enzyme Q$_{10}$ plays an important role in myocardial energy metabolism and improvement in myocardial metabolic function has been believed to be the mechanism for hemodynamic improvement.[436] In a double-blind crossover placebo-controlled study, CoQ$_{10}$ was reported to exert a beneficial effect on exercise capacity, quality of life, and ejection fraction in patients with moderate to severe congestive heart failure.[437] Intravenous administration of inosine and adenosine has been reported to improve left ventricular contractile function and to produce beneficial hemodynamic effects. It has been postulated that these agents facilitate myocardial adenine nucleotide repletion and augment myocardial metabolic and contractile function.[438] However, appropriate studies are lacking to demonstrate the clinical efficacy of these agents in the treatment of heart failure.

CLINICAL USE OF INOTROPIC AGENTS
Acute Heart Failure

It is apparent that a number of potent inotropic agents are now available that can be used clinically for the management of heart failure. The systemic hemodynamic effects of adrenergic agents are qualitatively similar, irrespective of their primary mechanisms of action. The acute hemodynamic effects of different phosphodiesterase inhibitors are also very similar, and the choice of a given agent should depend on its side effects and patient tolerance (Fig. 3.21). The systemic hemodynamic effects of most vasodilators are also qualitatively similar to those of the inotropic agents. However, adrenergic inotropic agents, in general, increase myocardial oxygen consumption, and with phosphodiesterase inhibitors, it may remain unchanged. In contrast, myocardial oxygen consumption tends to decrease in response to most vasodilators. Vasodilators can produce hypotension, which may preclude their use in relatively hypotensive patients. For the effective management of acutely decompensated patients and for appropriate selection of inotropic or vasodilator agents, hemodynamic monitoring is preferable, which also allows a change of therapy if response to a given agent is inadequate. The general guidelines for the use of inotropic agents in the management of acutely decompensated heart failure patients are summarized in Figure 3.22.

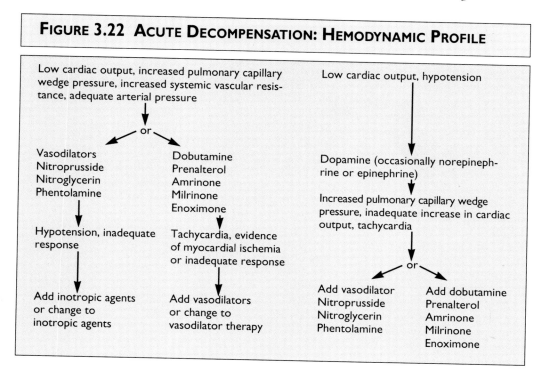

FIGURE 3.22 ACUTE DECOMPENSATION: HEMODYNAMIC PROFILE

Low cardiac output, increased pulmonary capillary wedge pressure, increased systemic vascular resistance, adequate arterial pressure

→ or →

Vasodilators
Nitroprusside
Nitroglycerin
Phentolamine

Dobutamine
Prenalterol
Amrinone
Milrinone
Enoximone

Hypotension, inadequate response

Tachycardia, evidence of myocardial ischemia or inadequate response

Add inotropic agents or change to inotropic agents

Add vasodilators or change to vasodilator therapy

Low cardiac output, hypotension

Dopamine (occasionally norepinephrine or epinephrine)

Increased pulmonary capillary wedge pressure, inadequate increase in cardiac output, tachycardia

→ or →

Add vasodilator
Nitroprusside
Nitroglycerin
Phentolamine

Add dobutamine
Prenalterol
Amrinone
Milrinone
Enoximone

Septic Shock

In patients with septic shock, hypotension is caused by marked peripheral vasodilatation and abnormally low systemic vascular resistance. Cardiac output may remain in the normal range or may be elevated. Right and left ventricular filling pressures may be normal, low, or elevated, depending on the degree of right and left ventricular dysfunction. Clinically, resuscitation from septic shock is usually initiated with repletion of a presumed volume deficit. Frequently, however, intravenous fluid therapy proves inadequate to correct hypotension and vasopressor agents must be used in addition. To increase systemic vascular resistance, the dose of dopamine that is likely to cause vasoconstriction due to activation of peripheral vascular α-receptors is frequently used. In some patients with severe hypotension, even large doses of dopamine may be ineffective in increasing systemic vascular resistance. It has been shown that the peripheral vasculature in patients with severe septic shock is relatively unresponsive to vasoconstricting effects of dopamine.[439] Norepinephrine, in these circumstances, may be effective in maintaining arterial pressure and cardiac performance, and anticipated norepinephrine-induced renal insufficiency may not occur.[440] Improved renal function may occur due to decreased proximal tubular reabsorption with increased renal perfusion pressure with norepinephrine. Increased arterial pressure with norepinephrine may also improve right ventricular myocardial perfusion, which is dependent on the gradient from mean arterial pressure to right ventricular end-diastolic pressure.[441] Right ventricular dysfunction and pulmonary hypertension may complicate septic shock and adversely influence the prognosis.[442-444] Relative effects of norepinephrine and dopamine on hemodynamics and right ventricular performance in septic shock have been evaluated.[445] Dopamine infusion increased cardiac index, systemic oxygen delivery, and systemic oxygen consumption without any change in systemic and pulmonary vascular resistance and right ventricular volume and right ventricular ejection fraction. With norepinephrine, there was also no change in right ventricular volume and ejection fraction and cardiac index. Both systemic and pulmonary vascular resistance increased with norepinephrine. Thus, although norepinephrine may improve the right ventricular oxygen supply–demand ratio, this potentially beneficial effect may be offset by a concomitant increase in right and left ventricular afterload that may prevent an increase in right and left ventricular stroke output. To increase cardiac output, dobutamine or a phosphodiesterase inhibitor can be added to norepinephrine.

In septic shock, increasing oxygen delivery by increasing cardiac output with the use of inotropic drugs has been found to be useful in some patients and has been reported to decrease mortality and morbidity in critically ill patients.[446,447] Critically ill patients suffering from sepsis syndrome, trauma, or acute respiratory failure or undergoing extended surgery have high oxygen requirements and need higher cardiac output to maintain adequate oxygen delivery and tissue perfusion. Frequently, blood lactate levels are measured to assess adequacy of cardiac output and tissue perfusion,[448] although measurements of lactate levels have limitations since concentration of lactate depends on its production as well as its elimination, which also can be altered in shock state.[449]

Inotropic drugs, particularly dobutamine, have been used for maximizing oxygen delivery in patients with septic shock, even in the presence of normal or high cardiac output.[450] Dobutamine infusion increased cardiac output, oxygen delivery, and oxygen consumption without any significant change in ventricular filling pressures.[451] Furthermore, hypotension did not result with the dose of dobutamine (5 µg/kg/min) used. It should be noted, however, that although dobutamine improves oxygen delivery, the impact of such therapy on the mortality and morbidity of septic shock remains to be established. Nevertheless, dobutamine therapy in addition to other supportive measures deserves consideration in the presence of evidence for inadequate oxygen delivery. Phosphodiesterase inhibitors are also potentially useful in increasing cardiac output and oxygen delivery in these patients.

Chronic Heart Failure

In patients with overt chronic congestive heart failure, resulting from depressed left ventricular function, vasodilators, particularly angiotensin-converting enzyme inhibitors, should be added to "digitalis and diuretic" therapy since these agents not only relieve symptoms and improve exercise tolerance and cardiac performance but also improve survival.[452-455] Long-term inotropic therapy with digoxin is indicated except in patients with significant renal failure or in those who are prone to develop digitalis toxicity. In asymptomatic patients with left ventricular dysfunction, digitalis is ineffective compared to angiotensin-converting enzyme inhibitors in preventing ventricular enlargement and remodeling.[456] Thus, digitalis therapy is not indicated in asymptomatic postinfarction patients with left ventricular systolic dysfunction. Patients who become refractory to vasodilators or angiotensin-converting enzyme inhibitors and patients who cannot tolerate vasodilators or angiotensin-converting enzyme inhibitors are presently considered for long-term treatment with newer inotropic agents. Patients with severe pump failure with low cardiac output and hypotension, particularly during exacerbation of chronic heart failure, are frequently treated with intermittent dobutamine and/or dopamine infusion or with intermittent parenteral phosphodiesterase inhibitors. Nonparenteral phosphodiesterase inhibitors are also effective in some patients. Such therapy is also frequently employed as a pharmacologic bridge to cardiac transplantation. Intermittent dobutamine infused through a surgically implanted venous access (Hickman or Cormed Mediport catheters) and via an ambulatory infusion pump has been used in out-patients with end-stage heart failure.[457] Dobutamine infusion for 4 days may attenuate the hemodynamic effects; thus, usually 48 hours of infusion (2.5 to 10 µg/kg/min) are used. A substantial improvement in clinical status and decreased frequency of hospitalization have been reported.[458] However, there is no evidence that such therapy prolongs life.

Intermittent amrinone infusion, titrated to augment cardiac output by more than 30% (mean dose, 1.0 mg/kg bolus and 15 μg/kg/min), has also been used for out-patient or home treatment of end-stage heart failure.[457,459] Amrinone infusions can be used once or twice weekly. Uncontrolled studies indicated that up to 65% of patients derived clinical symptomatic benefit. However, presently available data do not suggest that such therapy improves survival of patients with severe heart failure.

REFERENCES

1. Fabiato A, Fabiato F: Calcium and cardiac excitation-contraction coupling. Annu Rev Physiol 41:473, 1979
2. Wohlfart B, Noble MIM: The cardiac excitation-contraction coupling. Pharmacol Ther 16:1, 1982
3. Chapman RA: Control of cardiac contractility at the cellular level. Am J Physiol 245:H535, 1983
4. Katz AM: Discussion section. Article by Endoh M, Yanagisawa T, Taira N, Blinks JR: Effects of new inotropic agents on cyclic nucleotide metabolism and calcium transients in canine ventricular muscle. Circulation 73(Suppl III):III-117, 1986
5. Katz AM: Cyclic adenosine monophosphate effects on the myocardium: A man who blows hot and cold with one breath. J Am Coll Cardiol 2:143, 1983
6. Sperelakis N: Cyclic AMP and phosphorylation in regulation of Ca^{++} influx into myocardial cells and blockade by calcium antagonist drugs. Am Heart J 107:347, 1984
7. Kranias EG, Solaro J: Coordination of cardiac sarcoplasmic reticulum and myofibrillar function by protein phosphorylation. Fed Proc 42:33, 1983
8. Ikemoto N: Structure and function of the calcium pump protein of sarcoplasmic reticulum. Annu Rev Physiol 44:297, 1982
9. Strada SJ, Thompson WJ: Cyclic nucleotide phosphodiesterase. Adv Cyclic Nucleotide Protein Phosphorylation Res 16:1, 1984
10. Tada M, Kirchberger MA, Li H-C: Phosphoprotein phosphatase-catalyzed dephosphorylation of 22,000 dalton phosphoprotein of cardiac sarcoplasmic reticulum. J Cyclic Nucleotide Res 1:329, 1975
11. Withering W: An account of the foxglove and some of its medical uses with practical remarks on dropsy and other diseases. In Willius FA, Keys TE (eds): Classics of Cardiology, p 231. New York, Henry Schuman, 1941
12. McKenzie J: Digitalis. Heart 2:273, 1911
13. Katzung BG, Parmley WW: Cardiac glycosides and other drugs used in the treatment of congestive heart failure. In Katzung BG (ed): Basic and Clinical Pharmacology, p 143. Los Altos, Lange, 1984
14. Greenberger NJ, Caldwell JH: Studies on the intestinal absorption of ^{3}H-digitalis glycosides in experimental animals and man. In Marks BH, Weissler A (eds): Basic and Clinical Pharmacology of Digitalis, p 15. Springfield, IL, Charles C Thomas, 1972
15. Caldwell JH, Martin JF, Dutta S, Greenberger NJ: Intestinal absorption of digoxin ^{3}H in the rat. Am J Physiol 217:1747, 1969
16. Greenberger NJ et al: Intestinal absorption of six tritium-labeled digitalis glycosides in rats and guinea pigs. J Pharmacol Exp Ther 167:265, 1969
17. Oliver GCH, Taxman R, Frederickson R: Influence of congestive heart failure on digoxin blood levels. In Stor-Stein O (ed): Digitalis Symposium, p 336. Oslo, Gyldenal Norsk Forlag, 1973
18. Ohnhaus EE, Vozel S, Nuesch E: Absorption of digoxin in severe right heart failure. Eur J Clin Pharmacol 15:115, 1979
19. Lindenbaum J, Mellow MH, Blackstone MO, Butler VP: Variation in biological availability of digoxin from four preparations. N Engl J Med 285:1344, 1971
20. Greenblatt DJ, Duhme DW, Koch-Weser J, Smith TW: Equivalent bioavailability from digoxin elixir, and rapid dissolution tablets. JAMA 29:1774, 1974
21. Lindenbaum J: Greater bioavailability of digoxin solution in capsules. Clin Pharmacol Ther 21:278, 1977
22. Gold H, Catell M, Greiner T et al: Clinical pharmacology of digoxin. J Pharmacol Exp Ther 109:45, 1953
23. Marcus FI, Quinn EJ, Horton H et al: The effects of jejunoileal bypass on the pharmacokinetics of digoxin in man. Circulation 55(3):537, 1977
24. White RJ, Chamberlain DA, Howard M, Smith TW: Plasma concentrations of digoxin after oral administration in the fasting and postprandial state. Br Med J 1:380, 1971
25. Greenblatt DJ, Duhme DW, Koch-Weser J, Smith TW: Bioavailability of digoxin tablets and elixir in the fasting and postprandial states. Clin Pharmacol Ther 16:444, 1974
26. Moe GK, Farah AE: Digitalis and allied cardiac glycosides. In Goodman LS, Gilman A (eds): The Pharmacologic Basis of Therapeutics, p 653. New York, Macmillan, 1975
27. Keys W: Digoxin. In Evans WE, Schentag JJ, Jusko WJ (eds): Applied Pharmacokinetics: Principles of Therapeutic Drug Monitoring, p 319. San Francisco, Applied Therapeutics, 1980
28. Doherty JE, deSoyza N, Kane JJ et al: Clinical pharmacokinetics of digitalis glycosides. Prog Cardiovasc Dis 21:141, 1978
29. Smith TW, Antman EM, Friedman PL et al: Digitalis glycosides: Mechanisms and manifestations of toxicity. Prog Cardiovasc Dis 26:413, 1984

30. Smith TW, Antman EM, Friedman PL et al: Digitalis glycosides: Mechanisms and manifestations of toxicity (Part III). Prog Cardiovasc Dis 27:21, 1984

31. Warner NJ, Barnard T, Bigger T: Tissue digoxin concentrations and digoxin effect during the quinidine-digoxin interaction. J Am Coll Cardiol 5:680, 1985

32. Steiner E: Renal tubular secretion of digoxin. Circulation 50:103, 1974

33. Beard OW, Perkins WH: Titrated digoxin XTL: Enterohepatic circulation absorption and excretion studies in human volunteers. Circulation 42:867, 1970

34. Lukas DS, DeMartino AG: Binding of digitoxin and some related cardenolides to human plasma proteins. J Clin Invest 48:1041, 1969

35. Solomon HM, Abrams WB: Interactions between digitoxin and other drugs in man. Am Heart J 83:277, 1972

36. Bigger JT, Strauss HC: Digitalis toxicity: Drug interactions promoting toxicity and the management of toxicity. Semin Drug Treat 2:147, 1972

37. Allen DG, Blinks JR: Calcium transients in aquorin-injected frog cardiac muscle. Nature 273:509, 1978

38. Lullman H, Peters T: Action of cardiac glycosides on the excitation-contraction coupling in heart muscle. Prog Pharmacol 2:5, 1979

39. Ghysel-Barton J, Godfraind T: Stimulation and inhibition of the sodium pump by cardioactive steroids in relation to their binding sites and their inotropic effect on guinea-pig isolated atria. Br J Pharmacol 66:175, 1979

40. Cohen I, Daut J, Noble D: An analysis of the actions of low concentrations of ouabain on membrane currents in Purkinje fibers. J Physiol 260:75, 1976

41. Sharma VK, Banerjee SP: Regeneration of [^{3}H] ouabain binding to (Na$^+$-K$^+$)-ATPase in chemically sympathectomized cat peripheral organs. Mol Pharmacol 15:35, 1979

42. Sharma VK, Banerjee SP: Ouabain stimulation of adrenalin transport in guinea pig heart. Nature 286:817, 1980

43. Wier WG, Hess P: Excitation-contraction coupling in cardiac Purkinje fibers: Effects of cardiotonic steroids on the intracellular [Ca^{2+}] transient, membrane potential and contraction. J Gen Physiol 83:395, 1984

44. Sheu S-S, Fozzard HA: Transmembrane Na$^+$ and Ca^{2+} electrochemical gradients in cardiac muscle and their relationship to force development. J Gen Physiol 80:325, 1982

45. Lee CO, Dagostine M: Effects of strophanthidin on intracellular Na ion activity and twitch tension of constantly driven canine cardiac Purkinje fibers. Biophys J 40:185, 1982

46. Sheu S-S, Sharma VK, Banerjee SP: Measurement of cytosolic free calcium concentration in isolated rat ventricular myocytes with Quin 2. Circ Res 55:830, 1984

47. Weingart R, Kass RS, Tgien RW: Is digitalis inotropy associated with enhanced slow inward calcium current? Nature 273:389, 1978

48. Marban E, Tgien RW: Enhancement of calcium current during digitalis inotropy in mammalian heart; positive feedback regulation by intracellular calcium? J Physiol (Lond) 329:589, 1982

49. Gillis RA, Quest JA: The role of the nervous system in the cardiovascular effects of digitalis. Pharmacol Rev 31:19, 1980

50. Ellis D: The effects of external cations and ouabain on the intracellular sodium activity of sheep heart Purkinje fibers. J Physiol (Lond) 273:211, 1977

51. Warserstrom JA, Schwartz DJ, Fozzard HA: Relation between intracellular sodium and twitch tension in sheep cardiac Purkinje strands exposed to cardiac glycosides. Circ Res 52:697, 1983

52. Katz AM: Effects of digitalis on cell biochemistry: Sodium pump inhibition. J Am Coll Cardiol 5:16A, 1985

53. Hoffman BF: Effects of digitalis on electrical activity of cardiac membranes. In Marks BH, Weissler AM (eds): Basic and Clinical Pharmacology of Digitalis, p 118. Springfield, IL, Charles C Thomas, 1972

54. Rosen MR, Wit AL, Hoffman BF: Electrophysiology and pharmacology of cardiac arrhythmias: Cardiac antiarrhythmic and toxic effects of digitalis. Am Heart J 89:391, 1975

55. Rosen MR: Cellular electrophysiology of digitalis toxicity. J Am Coll Cardiol 5:22A, 1985

56. Watanabe AM: Digitalis and the autonomic nervous system. J Am Coll Cardiol 5:35A, 1985

57. Dhingra RC, Amat-y-Leon F, Wyndham C et al: The electrophysiologic effects of ouabain on sinus node and atrium in man. J Clin Invest 56:555, 1975

58. Goodman DJ, Rossen RM, Cannon DS et al: Effect of digoxin on atrioventricular conduction. Studies in patients with and without cardiac autonomic innervation. Circulation 51:251, 1975

59. Sleight P, Kaal A, Muens M: Reflex cardiovascular effects of epicardial stimulation by acetylstophanthidin in dogs. Circ Res 25:705, 1969

60. Thames MD, Waickman LA, Abboud FM: Sensitization of cardiac receptors (vagal afferents) by intracoronary acetylstrophanthidin. Am J Physiol 239:H628, 1980

61. Nakamura M: Digitalis induced augmentation of cardiopulmonary baroreflex control of forearm vascular resistance. Circulation 71:11, 1985

62. Kent FM, Epstein SE, Cooper T, Jacobowitz DM: Cholinergic innervation of the canine and human ventricular conducting system: Anatomic and electrophysiologic correlations. Circulation 23:1197, 1974

63. Schmid PG, Greif B, Lund DD, Roskoski T: Regional choline acetyl transferase activity in the guinea pig heart. Circ Res 42:657, 1976

64. Brown OM: Cat heart acetylcholine structural proof and distribution. Am J Physiol 231:781, 1976

65. Vatner SF, Rutherford JD, Ochs HR: Baroreflux and vagal mechanisms modulating left ventricular contractile response to sympathetic amines in conscious dogs. Circ Res 44:195, 1979

66. Levy MN, Blattberg B: Effect of vagal stimulation on the outflow of norepinephrine into the coronary sinus during cardiac sympathetic nerve stimulation in the dog. Circ Res 38:81, 1976

67. Braunwald E: Effects of digitalis on the normal and failing heart. J Am Coll Cardiol 5:51A, 1985

68. Sonnenblick EH, Williams JF Jr, Glick G et al: Studies on digitalis XV: Effects of cardiac glycosides on myocardial force-velocity relations in the now failing human heart. Circulation 34:532, 1966

69. Spann JF Jr, Buccino RA, Sonnenblick EH, Braunwald E: Contractile state of cardiac muscle obtained from cats with experimentally produced ventricular hypertrophy at heart failure. Circ Res 21:341, 1967

70. Mahler F, Karliner JS, O'Rourke RA: Effects of chronic digoxin administration on left ventricular performance in the normal conscious dog. Circulation 50:720, 1974

71. Crawford MH, Karliner JS, O'Rourke RA, Amon KW: Effects of chronic digoxin administration on left ventricular performance in normal subjects. Echocardiographic study. Am J Cardiol 38:843, 1976

72. Mason DT, Braunwald E: Studies on digitalis X: Effects of ouabain on forearm vascular resistance and venous tone in normal subjects and in all patients in heart failure. J Clin Invest 43:532, 1964

73. Shanbour LL, Jacobson ED: Digitalis and the mesenteric circulation. Am J Dig Dis 17:826, 1972

74. Ross J Jr, Braunwald E, Waldhausen JA: Studies of digitalis. II: Extracardiac effects on venous return and on the capacity of peripheral vascular bed. J Clin Invest 39:936, 1960

75. Sugar KB, Hanson EC, Powell WJ: Neurogenic vasoconstrictor effects during acute global ischemia in dogs. J Clin Invest 60:1248, 1977

76. DeMots H, Rahimtoola SH, McAnulty JH, Porter GA: Effects of ouabain on coronary and systemic vascular resistance and myocardial oxygen consumption in patients without heart failure. Am J Cardiol 41:88, 1978

77. Garan H, Smith TW, Powell WJ Jr: The central nervous system as a site of action for the coronary vasoconstrictor effect of digoxin. J Clin Invest 54:1365, 1974

78. Arnold SB, Byrd RC, Meister W et al: Long-term digitalis therapy improves left ventricular function in heart failure. N Engl J Med 303:1443, 1980

79. Ferguson DW, Berg WJ, Sanders JS et al: Sympathoinhibitory responses to digitalis glycosides in heart failure patients: Direct evidence from sympathetic neural recordings. Circulation 80:65, 1989

80. Ferguson DW, Abboud FM, Mark AL: Selective impairment of baroreflex-mediated vasoconstrictor responses in patients with ventricular dysfunction. Circulation 69:451, 1984

81. Torretti J, Hendler E, Weinstein E: Functional significance of Na-K-ATPase in the kidney: Effects of ouabain inhibition. Am J Physiol 222:1398, 1972

82. Covit AB, Schaer GL, Sealy JE et al: Suppression of the renin-angiotensin by intravenous digoxin in chronic congestive heart failure. Am J Med 75:445, 1983

83. Banka VS, Schadda KD, Bodenheimer MM et al: Digitalis in experimental acute myocardial infarction. Am J Cardiol 35:801, 1975

84. Hood WB Jr, McCarthy B, Lown B: Myocardial infarction following coronary ligation in dogs. Hemodynamic effects of isoproterenol and acetyl strophanthidin. Circ Res 21:191, 1967

85. Rahimtoola SH, Sinno MZ, Chuquimia R et al: Effects of ouabain on impaired left ventricular function in acute myocardial infarction. N Engl J Med 287:527, 1972

86. Forrester J, Bezdek W, Chatterjee K et al: Hemodynamic effects of digitalis in acute myocardial infarction. Ann Intern Med 76:863, 1972

87. Cohn JN, Tristani FE, Khatri IM: Cardiac and peripheral vascular effects of digitalis in clinical cardiogenic shock. Am Heart J 78:318, 1969

88. Lipp H, Denes P, Gametta M et al: Hemodynamic response to acute intravenous digoxin in patients with recent myocardial infarction and coronary insufficiency with and without heart failure. Chest 63:862, 1972

89. Goldstein RA, Passamani ER, Roberts R: A comparison of digoxin and dobutamine in patients with acute infarction and cardiac failure. N Engl J Med 303:846, 1980

90. Forrester JS, Chatterjee K: Preservation of ischemic myocardium. In Vogel JHK (ed): Advances in Cardiology, p 158. Basel, S Karger, 1974

91. Gunner RM, Loeb HS, Pietras RJT: Hemodynamic measurements in the coronary care unit. Prog Cardiovasc Dis 11:29, 1968

92. Gander MP, Kazamias TM, Henry P et al: Serial determinations of cardiac output and response to digitalis in patients with acute myocardial infarction. Circulation 42(Suppl 3):155, 1970

93. DeMots H, Rahimtoola SH, Kremkau EL et al: Effects of ouabaïn on myocardial oxygen supply and demand in patients with chronic coronary artery disease: A hemodynamic, volumetric and metabolic study in patients without heart failure. J Clin Invest 58:312, 1976

94. Kotter V, Schurer K, Schroder R: Effect of digoxin on coronary blood flow and myocardial oxygen consumption in patients with coronary artery disease. Am J Cardiol 42:563, 1978

95. Watanabe T, Covell JW, Maroko PR et al: Effects of increased arterial pressure and positive inotropic agents on the severity of myocardial ischemia in the acutely depressed heart. Am J Cardiol 30:371, 1972

96. Varomkov Y, Shell WE, Smirnov V et al: Augmentation of serum CPK activity in digitalis in patients with acute myocardial infarction. Circulation 55:719, 1977

97. Morrison J, Pizzarello R, Reduto L, Gulotta S: Effects of digitalis on predicted myocardial infarct size in man (abstr). Clin Res 23:198, 1975

98. Moss AJ, Davis HT, Conard DL et al: Digitalis associated cardiac mortality after myocardial infarction. Circulation 64:1150, 1981

99. Bigger JT, Fleiss JL, Rolnitsky LAM et al: Effect of digitalis treatment on survival after acute myocardial infarction. Am J Cardiol 55:629, 1985

100. Iesaka Y, Aonuma K, Gosselin AJ et al: Susceptibility of infarcted canine hearts to digitalis-toxic ventricular tachycardia. J Am Coll Cardiol 2:45, 1983

101. Goldstein S, Friedman L, Hutchinson R et al: Timing, mechanism and clinical setting of witnessed deaths in post-myocardial infarction patients. J Am Coll Cardiol 3:1111, 1984

102. Mukherji J, Rude RE, Poole WK et al: Risk factors for sudden death after acute myocardial infarction: Two-year follow-up. Am J Cardiol 54:31, 1984

103. The Multicenter Post-Infarction Trial Research Group: Risk stratification and survival after myocardial infarction. N Engl J Med 309:331, 1983

104. The Multicenter Diltiazem Post-Infarction Trial Research Group: The effect of diltiazem on mortality and reinfarction after myocardial infarction. N Engl J Med 319:335, 1988

105. Ruberman W, Weinblatt E, Goldberg JD et al: Ventricular premature complexes and sudden death after myocardial infarction. Circulation 64:297, 1981

106. The Miami Trial Research Group: Metoprolol in acute myocardial infarction (MIAMI): A randomized placebo-controlled international trial. Eur Heart J 6:199, 1985

107. Capone RJ, Pawitan Y, El-Sherif N et al: Events in the cardiac arrhythmia suppression trial: Baseline predictors of mortality in placebo-treated patients. J Am Coll Cardiol 18:1434, 1991

108. Chatterjee K, Parmley WW: Therapy of acute myocardial infarction. In Cohn PF (ed): Diagnosis and Therapy of Coronary Artery Disease, p 357. The Hague, Martinus Nijhoff Publishers, 1985

109. Ryan TJ, Baily KR, McCabe CH et al: The effects of digitalis treatment on survival after acute myocardial infarction. Circulation 67:735, 1983

110. Davidson C, Gibson D: Clinical significance of positive inotroplc action of digoxin in patients with left ventricular disease. Br Heart J 35:970, 1973

111. Goldman RH: Left ventricular dynamics during long term digoxin treatment in patients with stable coronary artery disease. Am J Cardiol 41:937, 1978

112. Carliner NH, Gilbert CA, Puritt AW, Goldberg LI: Effects of maintenance digoxin therapy on systolic time intervals and serum digoxin concentrations. Circulation 50:94, 1974

113. Hoeschen RJ, Cuddy TE: Dose-response relation between therapeutic levels of serum digoxin and systolic time intervals. Am J Cardiol 35:469, 1975

114. Selzer A, Malmborg RO: Hemodynamic effects of digoxin in latent cardiac failure. Circulation 25:695, 1962

115. Vogel R, Frischknecht J, Stelle P: Short and long term effects of digitalis on resting and post-handgrip hemodynamics in patients with coronary heart disease. Am J Cardiol 40:171, 1977

116. Cohn K, Selzer A, Kersh ES et al: Variability of hemodynamic responses to acute digitalization in chronic cardiac failure due to cardiomyopathy and coronary artery disease. Am J Cardiol 35:461, 1975

117. Murray RG, Tweddel AC, Martin W et al: Evaluation of digitalis in cardiac failure. Lancet 1:1526, 1982

118. Murlow CD, Feussner JR, Velez R: Re-evaluation of digitalis efficacy. New light on old leaf. Ann Intern Med 101:113, 1984

119. Rader BR, Smith WW, Berger AR, Eichna LW: Comparison of the hemodynamic effects of mercurial diuretics and digitalis in congestive heart failure. Circulation 29:328, 1964

120. McHaffie D, Purcell H, Mitchell-Heggs P, Guz A: The clinical value of digoxin in patients with heart failure and sinus rhythm. Q J Med 47:401, 1978

121. Hutcheon D, Nemeth E, Quinland D: The role of furosemide alone and in combination with digoxin in the relief of symptoms of congestive heart failure. J Clin Pharmacol 20:59, 1980

122. Dobbs SM, Kenyon WI, Dobbs RJ: Maintenance digoxin after an episode of heart failure: Placebo-controlled trial in outpatients. Br Med J 1:749, 1977

123. Lee DC, Johnson RA, Bingham JB: Heart failure in outpatients: A randomized trial of digoxin versus placebo. N Engl J Med 306:699, 1982

124. Fleg JL, Gottlieb SH, Lakatia EG: Is digoxin really important in treatment of compensated heart failure: A placebo-controlled crossover study in patients with sinus rhythm. Am J Med 73:244, 1983

125. Gheorghiade M, Beller GA: Effects of discontinuing maintenance digoxin therapy in patients with ischemic heart disease and congestive heart failure in sinus rhythm. Am J Cardiol 51:1243, 1983

126. German and Austrian Xamoterol Study Group: Double-blind placebo-controlled comparison of digoxin and xamoterol in chronic heart lailure. Lancet 1:489, 1988

127. The Captopril-Digoxin Multicenter Research Group: Comparative effects of therapy with captopril and digoxin in patients with mild to moderate heart failure. JAMA 259:539, 1988

128. Beaune J, for the Enalapril Versus Digoxin French Multicenter Study Group: Comparison of enalapril versus digoxin for congestive heart failure. Am J Cardiol 63:22D, 1989

129. Davies RF, Beanlands DS, Nadeau C et al: Enalapril versus digoxin in patients with congestive heart failure: A multicenter study. J Am Coll Cardiol 18:1602, 1991

130. Young JB, Uretsky F, Shahidi E et al: Multicenter, double-blind, placebo-controlled randomized withdrawal trial of the efficacy and safety of digoxin in patients with mild to moderate chronic heart failure not treated with converting enzyme inhibitors (abstr). J Am Coll Cardiol 19:259A, 1992

131. Packer M, Gheorghiade M, Young JB, et al: Randomized, double-blind, placebo-controlled withdrawal study of digoxin in patients with chronic heart failure treated with converting enzyme

inhibitors (abstr). J Am Coll Cardiol 19:260A, 1992

132. Guyatt GH, Sullivan MJJ, Fallen EL et al: A controlled trial of digoxin in congestive heart failure. Am J Cardiol 62:372, 1988

133. DiBianco R, Shabetai R, Kostruk W et al for the Milrinone Multicenter Trial Group: A comparison of oral milrinone, digoxin, and their combination in the treatment of patients with chronic heart failure. N Engl J Med 320:677, 1989

134. Cohn JN, Archibald DG, Ziesche S et al: Effect of vasodilator therapy on mortality in chronic congestive heart failure: Results of a Veterans Administration Cooperative Study. N Engl J Med 314:1547, 1988

135. CONSENSUS Trial Study Group: Effects of enalapril on mortality in severe congestive heart failure: Results of the Cooperative North Scandinavian Enalapril Survival Study (CONSENSUS). N Engl J Med 316:1429, 1987

136. Gheorghiade M, Hall V, Lakier JB, Goldstein S: Comparative hemodynamic and neurohormonal effects of intravenous captopril and digoxin and their combinations in patients with severe heart failure. J Am Coll Cardiol 13:134, 1989

137. DiCarlo L, Chatterjee K, Parmley WW et al: Enalapril: A new angiotensin-converting enzyme inhibitor in chronic heart failure: Acute and chronic hemodynamic evaluations. J Am Coll Cardiol 2:865, 1983

138. Mettauer B, Rouleau JL, Bichet D et al: Differential long-term intrarenal and neurohumoral effects of captopril and prazosin in chronic heart failure: Importance of initial plasma renin activity. Circulation 73:492, 1986

139. Crawford MH, LeWinter MM, O'Rourke RA et al: Combined propranolol and digoxin therapy in angina pectoris. Ann Intern Med 83:449, 1975

140. Harding PR, Aronow WS, Eisenman J: Digitalis as an antianginal agent. Chest 64:439, 1973

141. Nederberger M, Bruce RA, Frederick R et al: Reproduction of maximal exercise performance in patients with angina pectoris despite ouabain treatment. Circulation 49:309, 1974

142. Vatner SF, Braunwald E: Effects of chronic heart failure on the inotropic response of the right ventricle of the conscious dog to a cardiac glycoside and to tachycardia. Circulation 50:728, 1974

143. Berglund E, Widimsky J, Malmberg R: Lack of effect of digitalis in patients with pulmonary disease with and without heart failure. Am J Cardiol 11:477, 1963

144. Ferrer MI, Harvey RM, Cathcart RT et al: Some effects of digoxin upon the heart and circulation in man: Digoxin in chronic cor pulmonale. Circulation 1:161, 1950

145. Baum GL, Dick MM, Schotz S, Gumpel RC: Digitalis toxicity in chronic cor pulmonale. South Med J 49:1037, 1956

146. Williams JF Jr, Boyd DC, Border JF: Effects of acute hypoxia and hypercapnic acidosis on the development of acetyl strophanthidin induced arrhythmias. J Clin Invest 47:1885, 1968

147. Goldman RH, Harrison DC: The effect of hypoxemia and hypercapnia on myocardial catecholamines. J Pharmacol Exp Ther 307:174, 1970

148. Johnson LW, Dickstein RA, Fruehass CT et al: Prophylactic digitalization for coronary artery bypass surgery. Circulation 53:819, 1976

149. Tyras DH, Stothert JC Jr, Kaiser GC et al: Supraventricular tachyarrhythmias after myocardial revascularization: A randomized trial of prophylactic digitalization. J Thorac Cardiovasc Surg 77:310, 1979

150. Aronson JK: Digitalis intoxication. Clin Sci 64: 253, 1983

151. Ogilvie RJ, Ruedy J: Adverse drug reactions during hospitalization. Can Med Assoc J 97:1450, 1967

152. Hurwitz N, Wade OL: Intensive hospital monitoring of adverse reaction to drugs. Br Med J 1: 531, 1969

153. Beller CA, Smith TW, Abelmann WH et al: Digitalis intoxication: Prospective clinical study with serum level correlations. N Engl J Med 284:989, 1971

154. Carter BL, Small RE, Garnett WR: Monitoring digoxin therapy in two long-term facilities. J Am Geriatr Soc 29:263, 1981

155. Lely AH, VanEnter CHJ: Noncardiac symptoms of digitalis intoxication. Am Heart J 83:149, 1972

156. Gazes P, Holmes CR, Mosely V, Pratt-Thomas HR: Acute hemorrhage and necrosis of the intestine associated with digitalization. Circulation 23:358, 1961

157. Longhurst JC, Ross J: Extracardiac and coronary vascular effects of digitalis. J Am Coll Cardiol 5:99A, 1985

158. Fisch C, Knoebel SB: Digitalis cardiotoxicity. J Am Coll Cardiol 5:91A, 1985

159. Wellens HJJ: The electrocardiogram in digitalis intoxication. In Yu PN, Goodwin JF (eds): Progress in Cardiology, vol 5, chap 10, p 271. Philadelphia, Lea & Febiger, 1976

160. Surawicz B: Factors affecting tolerance to digitalis. J Am Coll Cardiol 5:69A, 1985

161. Marcus FI: Current status of therapy with digoxin. In Proctor HW (ed): Current Problems in Cardiology, vol III, no 5, p 1. Chicago, Year Book Medical Publishers, 1978

162. Madsen EB, Oilpin E, Henning H et al: Prognostic importance of digitalis after acute myocardial infarction. J Am Coll Cardiol 3:681, 1984

163. Surawicz B: Use of the chelating agent EDTA in digitalis intoxication and cardiac arrhythmias. Prog Cardiovasc Dis 2:432, 1960

164. Goldman RH, Kleiger RE, Schweizer E, Harrison DC: The effect on myocardial 3-H digoxin of magnesium deficiency. Proc Exp Biol Med 136: 747, 1971

165. Tackett RL, Holl JE: Increased automaticity and decreased inotropism of ouabain in dogs with furosemide-induced hypomagnesemia. J Cardiovasc Pharmacol 3:1269, 1981

166. Storstein O, Hansteen V, Hatle L et al: Studies on digitalis: XIV. Is there any correlation between hypomagnesemia and digitalis intoxication? Acta Med Scand 202:445, 1977

167. Cohen L, Kitrzes R: Magnesium sulfate and digitalis-toxic arrhythmias. JAMA 249:2808, 1973

168. Brater DC, Morelli HF: Systemic alkalosis and digitalis-related arrhythmias. Acta Med Scand (Suppl) 647:79, 1981

169. Doherty JE, Perkins WH: Digoxin metabolism in hypo- and hyperthyroidism: Studies with titrated digoxin in thyroid disease. Ann Intern Med 64:489, 1966

170. Ebert PA, Morerow AG, Austen WG: Clinical studies of the effect of extracorporeal circulation on myocardial digoxin concentration. Am J Cardiol 11:201, 1963

171. Ditchey RV, Curtis GP: Effects of apparently nontoxic doses of digoxin on ventricular ectopy after direct-current electrical shocks in dogs. J Pharmacol Exp Ther 218:212, 1981

172. Doherty JE: Conventional drug therapy in the management of heart failure. In Cohn JN (ed): Drug Treatment of Heart Failure, p 91. New York, Yorke Medical Books, 1983

173. Marcus FI: Pharmacokinetic interactions between digoxin and other drugs. J Am Coll Cardiol 5:82A, 1985

174. Bigger JT, Leahey EB: Quinidine and digoxin—an important interaction. Drugs 24:229, 1982

175. Warner NJ, Barnard JT, Bigger JT: Tissue digoxin concentrations and digoxin effect during the quinidine-digoxin interactions. J Am Coll Cardiol 5:680, 1985

176. Graves SW, Brown B, Valdes R: An endogenous digoxin like substance in patients with renal impairment. Ann Intern Med 99:604, 1983

177. Eraker SA, Sasse L: The serum digoxin test and digoxin toxicity: A Bayesian approach to decision making. Circulation 2:409, 1981

178. Wotman S, Bigger JT Jr, Mandel ID et al: Salivary electrolytes in the detection of digitalis toxicity. N Engl J Med 285:871, 1971

179. Aronson JK, Grahame-Smith DG, Hallis KF et al: Monitoring digoxin therapy: I. Plasma concentrations and in vitro assay of tissue response. Br J Clin Pharmacol 4:213, 1977

180. Klein MD, Lown B, Barr I et al: Comparison of serum digoxin level measurement with acetyl strophanthidin tolerance testing. Circulation 49:1053, 1974

181. Caldwell JH, Bush CA, Greenberger NJ: Interruption of the enterohepatic circulation of digitoxin by cholystyramine: II. Effect on metabolic disposition of tritium-labeled digitoxin and cardiac systolic intervals in man. J Clin Invest 50:2638, 1971

182. Bazzano G, Bazzano GS: Digitalis intoxication: Treatment with new steroid binding resin. JAMA 220:828, 1972

183. Garan H, Ruskin JN, Powell WJ: Centrally mediated effect of phenytoin on digoxin induced ventricular arrhythmias. Am J Physiol 241:H67, 1981

184. Castellanos A, Ferreiro J, Pefkaros K et al: Effects of lidocaine on bidirectional tachycardia and on digitalis induced atrial tachycardia with block. Br Heart J 48:27, 1982

185. Davis LD, Temte JV: Effects of propranolol on the transmembrane potentials of ventricular muscle on Purkinje fibers of the dog. Circ Res 22:261, 1968

186. Gillis RA, Clancy MM, Anderson RJ: Deleterious effects of bretylium in cats with digitalis induced ventricular tachycardia 57:974, 1973

187. Cohen L, Kitzes R: Magnesium sulfate and digitalis toxic arrhythmias. JAMA 249:2808, 1983

188. Lown B, Levine SA: The carotid sinus. Circulation 23:766, 1961

189. Lown B, Kleiger R, Williams J: Cardioversion and digitalis drugs: Changes in threshold to electric shock in digitalized animals. Circ Res 57:519, 1965

190. Ditchey RV, Karliner JS: Safety of electrical cardioversion in patients without digitalis toxicity. Ann Intern Med 95:676, 1981

191. Gilfrich HJ, Kasper W, Meinertz T et al: Treatment of massive digitoxin overdose by charcoal hemoperfusion. Lancet 1:505, 1978

192. Buller VP, Chen JP: Digoxin specific antibodies. Proc Natl Acad Sci USA 57:71, 1967

193. Curd J, Smith TW, Jaton J, Haber E: The isolation of digoxin specific antibody and its use in reversing the effects of digoxin. Proc Natl Acad Sci USA 68:2401, 1971

194. Haber E: Antibodies and digitalis: The modern revolution in the use of an ancient drug. J Am Coll Cardiol 5:111A, 1985

195. Mandel WJ, Bigger JT Jr, Butler VP Jr: The electrophysiologic effects of low and high digoxin concentrations on isolated mammalian cardiac tissue reversal by digoxin-specific antibody. J Clin Invest 51:1378, 1972

196. Lloyd BL, Smith TW: Contrasting rates of reversal of digoxin toxicity by digoxin-specific IgC and Fab fragments. Circulation 58:280, 1978

197. Ochs HR, Vatner SF, Smith TW: Reversal of inotropic effects of digoxin by specific antibodies and their Fab fragments in the conscious dog. J Pharmacol Exp Ther 207:64, 1978

198. Clarke W, Ramoska EA: Acute digoxin overdose: Use of digoxin-specific antibody fragments. Am J Emerg Med 6:465, 1988

199. Erdmann E, Mair W, Knedel M, Schaumann W: Digitalis intoxication and treatment with digoxin antibody fragments in renal failure. Klin Wochenschr 67:16, 1989

200. Schaumann W, Kaufmann B, Neubert P, Smolarz A: Kinetics of the Fab fragments of digoxin antibodies and of bound digoxin in patients with severe digoxin intoxication. Eur J Clin Pharmacol 30:527, 1986

201. Smith TW, Butler VP Jr, Haber E et al: Treatment of life threatening digitalis intoxication with digoxin-specific Fab antibody fragments: Experience in 26 cases. N Engl J Med 307:1357, 1982

202. Wenger TL, Butler VP, Haber E, Smith TW: Treatment of 63 severely digitalis-toxic patients with digoxin-specific antibody fragments. J Am Coll Cardiol 5:118A, 1985

203. Bismuth C, Gautlier M, Corso F, Efehymiou ML: Hyperkalemia in acute digitalis poisoning: Prognostic and therapeutic implications. Clin Toxicol 6:153, 1973

204. Ekins BR, Watanabe AS: Acute digoxin poisoning: Review of therapy. Am J Hosp Pharm 35:268, 1978

205. Ahlquist RP: A study of adrenotropic receptors. Am J Physiol 153:586, 1948

206. Watanabe AM: Recent advances in knowledge

about beta-adrenergic receptors: Application to clinical cardiology. J Am Coll Cardiol 1:82, 1983

207. Langer SZ: Presynaptic regulation of catecholamine release. Biochem Pharmacol 23:1793, 1974

208. Goldberg M, Robertson D: Evidence for the existence of vascular alpha adrenoreceptors in humans. Hypertension 6:551, 1984

209. Colucci WS: Alpha-adrenergic receptors in cardiovascular medicine. In Karliner JS, Haft JI (eds): Receptor Science in Cardiology, p 43. Mt Kisco, NY, Futura Publications, 1984

210. Lefkowitz RJ, Stadel JM, Caron MG: Adenylate cyclase-coupled beta adrenergic receptors: Structure and mechanisms of activation and desensitization. Annu Rev Biochem 52:159, 1983

211. Viquerat CE, Daly P, Swedberg K et al: Endogenous catecholamines in chronic heart failure: Relation to the severity of hemodynamic abnormalities. Am J Med 78:455, 1985

212. Hasking GJ, Esler MD, Jennings GL et al: Norepinephrine spillover to plasma in patients with congestive heart failure: Evidence of increased overall and cardiorenal sympathetic nervous activity. Circulation 73:615, 1986

213. Swedberg K, Viquerat C, Rouleau J-L et al: Comparison of myocardial catecholamine balance in chronic congestive heart failure and in angina pectoris without failure. Am J Cardiol 54:783, 1984

214. Chidsey CA, Braunwald EB, Morrow AG, Mason DT: Myocardial norepinephrine concentration in man: Effects of reserpine and of congestive heart failure. N Engl J Med 269:653, 1963

215. Pierpont GL, Francis GS, DeMaster EG et al: Elevated left ventricular myocardial dopamine in preterminal idiopathic dilated cardiomyopathy. Am J Cardiol 52:1033, 1983

216. Sole MJ, Helke CJ, Jascobowitz DM: Increased dopamine in the failing hamster heart: Transvesicular transport of dopamine limits the rate of norepinephrine synthesis. Am J Cardiol 49:1682, 1982

217. Bristow MR: Myocardial beta-adrenergic receptor down regulation in heart failure. Int J Cardiol 5:648, 1984

218. Bristow MR, Ginsburg R, Minobe W et al: Decreased catecholamine sensitivity and beta-adrenergic receptor density in failing human hearts. N Engl J Med 307:205, 1982

219. Bristow MR, Port JD, Sandoval AB et al: β-Adrenergic receptor pathways in the failing human heart. Heart Failure 5:77, 1989

220. Karliner JS: Myocardial adrenergic function in heart failure. In Chatterjee K (ed): Dobutamine: A Ten Year Review, pp 5–31. New York, NCM Publishers, 1989

221. Lee HR: α_1-Adrenergic receptors in heart failure. Heart Failure 5:62, 1989

222. Scholz H: Effects of beta- and alpha-adrenoreceptor activators and adrenergic transmitter releasing agents on the mechanical activity of the heart. In Szekeres L (ed): Handbook of Experimental Pharmacology, Part 1, Adrenergic Activators and Inhibitors, vol 54, pp 651–733. Berlin, Springer-Verlag, 1980

223. Reuter H: Localization of beta adrenergic receptors and effects of noradrenaline and cyclic nucleotides on action potentials, ionic currents and tension in mammalian cardiac muscle. J Physiol (London) 242:429, 1974

224. Reiter M: Drugs and heart muscle. Annu Rev Pharmacol 12:111, 1972

225. Berridge MJ, Irvine RF: Inositol triphosphate, a novel second messenger in cellular signal transduction. Nature 312:315, 1984

226. Kikkawa U, Nishizuka Y: The role of protein kinase in transmembrane signaling. Annu Rev Cell Biol 2:149, 1986

227. Aronson RS, Celles JM: Electrophysiologic effects of dopamine on sheep cardiac Purkinje fibers. J Pharmacol Exp Ther 188:595, 1974

228. Abrams E, Forrester JS, Chatterjee K et al: Variability in response to norepinephrine in acute myocardial infarction. Am J Cardiol 32:919, 1973

229. Innes IR, Nickerson M: Norepinephrine, epinephrine and the sympathomimetic amines. In Goodman LS, Gilman A (eds): Pharmacological Basis of Therapeutics, 5th ed, p 477. New York, Macmillan, 1975

230. Goldberg LI, Rafzer SI: Dopamine receptors. Applications in clinical cardiology. Circulation 72:245, 1985

231. Goldberg LI: Cardiovascular and renal actions of dopamine. Potential applications. Pharmacol Rev 24:1, 1972

232. Goldberg LI, Hsieh YY, Resnekov L: Newer catecholamines for treatment of heart failure and shock: An update on dopamine and a first look at dobutamine. Prog Cardiovasc Dis 4:327, 1977

233. Richard C, Ricome JL, Rimailho A et al: Combined hemodynamic effects of dopamine and dobutamine in cardiogenic shock. Circulation 67:620, 1983

234. Miller RR, Awan NA, Joye JA et al: Combined dopamine and nitroprusside therapy in congestive heart failure: Greater augmentation of cardiac performance by addition of inotropic stimulation to afterload reduction. Circulation 55:881, 1977

235. Loeb HS, Ostrenga JP, Gaul W et al: Beneficial effects of dopamine combined with intravenous nitroglycerin on hemodynamics in patients with severe left ventricular failure. Circulation 68:813, 1983

236. Vatner SF, Baig H: Importance of heart rate in determining the effects of sympathomimetic amines on regional myocardial function and blood flow in conscious dogs with acute myocardial ischemia. Circ Res 45:793, 1979

237. Ramanathan KB, Bodenheimer MM, Banka VS et al: Contrasting effects of dopamine and isoproterenol in experimental myocardial infarction. Am J Cardiol 39:413, 1977

238. McClenathan JH, Guyton RA, Breyer RH et al: The effects of isoproterenol and dopamine on regional myocardial blood flow after stenosis of circumflex coronary artery. J Thorac Cardiovasc Surg 73:431, 1977

239. Mueller HS, Evans R, Ayers SM: Effect of do-

pamine on hemodynamics and myocardial metabolism in shock following acute myocardial infarction in man. Circulation 57:361, 1978

240. Ruffolo RR Jr, Spradlin TA, Pollock GD et al: Alpha and beta adrenergic effects of the stereoisomers of dobutamine. J Pharmacol Exp Ther 219:447, 1981

241. Chatterjee J, Bendersky R, Parmley WW: Dobutamine in heart failure. Eur Heart J 3:107, 1982

242. Willerson JT, Hutton I, Watson JT et al: Influence of dobutamine on regional myocardial blood flow and ventricular performance during acute and chronic myocardial ischemia in dogs. Circulation 53:828, 1976

243. Gillespie TA, Ambos HD, Sobel BE et al: Effects of dobutamine in patients with acute myocardial infarction. Am J Cardiol 39:588, 1977

244. Magotrien RD, Unverferth DV, Brown GP et al: Dobutamine and hydralazine: Comparative influences of positive inotropy and vasodilation on coronary blood flow and myocardial energetics in nonischemic congestive heart failure. J Am Coll Cardiol 1:499, 1983

245. Fowler MB, Alderman EL, Oesterle SN et al: Dobutamine and dopamine after cardiac surgery: Greater augmentation of myocardial blood flow with dobutamine. Circulation 70(Suppl 1):1103, 1984

246. Bendersky R, Chatterjee K, Parmley WW et al: Dobutamine in chronic ischemic heart failure: Alterations in left ventricular function and coronary hemodynamics. Am J Cardiol 48:554, 1981

247. Hamilton FN, Feigl ED: Coronary vascular sympathetic β-receptor innervation. Am J Physiol 230:1569, 1976

248. Kupper W, Waller D, Hanrath P et al: Hemodynamic and cardiac metabolic effects of inotropic stimulation with dobutamine in patients with coronary artery disease. Eur Heart J 3:29, 1982

249. Meyer SL, Curry GC, Donsky MS et al: Influence of dobutamine on hemodynamics and coronary blood flow in patients with and without coronary artery disease. Am J Cardiol 38:103, 1976

250. Pozen RC, DiBianco R, Katz RJ et al: Myocardial metabolic and hemodynamic effects of dobutamine in heart failure complicating coronary artery disease. Circulation 63:1279, 1981

251. Sawada SG, Segar DS, Brown SE et al: Dobutamine stress echocardiography for evaluation of coronary disease (abstr). Circulation 80:II-66, 1989

252. Loeb HS, Khan M, Saudeye A, Gunnar RM: Acute hemodynamic effects of dobutamine and isoproterenol in patients with low output heart failure. Circ Shock 3:55, 1976

253. Leier CV, Heban PT, Huss P et al: Comparative systemic and regional hemodynamic effects of dopamine and dobutamine in patients with cardiomyopathic heart failure. Circulation 58:466, 1978

254. Loeb HS, Bvedakis J, Gunnar RM: Superiority of dobutamine over dopamine in patients with low output cardiac failure. Circulation 55:375, 1977

255. Stoner JD III, Bolen JL, Harrison DC: Comparison of dobutamine and dopamine in treatment of severe heart failure. Br Heart J 39:536, 1977

256. Berkowitz C, McKeever L, Croke RP et al: Comparative responses to dobutamine and nitrprusside in patients with chronic low output cardiac failure. Circulation 56:918, 1977

257. Dell'Italia LJ, Starling MR, Blumhardt R et al: Comparative effects of volume loading, dobutamine and nitroprusside in patients with predominant right ventricular infarction. Circulation 72:1327, 1985

258. Unverferth DV, Magorien RD, Lewis RP, Leier CV: Long-term benefit of dobutamine in patients with congestive cardiomyopathy. Am Heart J 100:622, 1980

259. Unverferth DV, Magorien RD, Altschuld R et al: The hemodynamic and metabolic advantages gained by a three-day infusion of dobutamine in patients with congestive cardiomyopathy. Am Heart J 106:29, 1983

260. Liang C, Sherman LG, Doherty JU et al: Sustained improvement of cardiac function in patients with congestive heart failure after short-term infusion of dobutamine. Circulation 69:113, 1984

261. Leier CV, Huss P, Lewos RP, Unverferth DV: Drug-induced conditioning in congestive heart failure. Circulation 65:1382, 1981

262. Applefeld MM, Newman KA, Grove WR et al: Intermittent continuous outpatient dobutamine infusion in the management of congestive heart failure. Am J Cardiol 51:455, 1983

263. Krell MJ, Kline EM, Bates ER et al: Intermittent ambulatory dobutamine infusions in patients with severe congestive heart failure. Am Heart J 112:787, 1986

264. Dies F: Intermittent dobutamine in ambulatory patients with chronic cardiac failure. Br J Clin Pract 45:37, 1986

265. Liang C, Tuttle RR, Hood WB Jr, Gavras H: Conditioning effects of chronic infusions of dobutamine: Comparison with exercise training. J Clin Invest 64:613, 1979

266. Unverferth DV, Leier CV, Magorien RD et al: Improvement of human myocardial mitochondria after dobutamine: A quantitative ultrastructural study. J Pharmacol Exp Ther 215:527, 1980

267. Hirshfeld JW Jr, Borer JS, Goldstein RE et al: Reduction in severity and extent of myocardial infarction when nitroglycerin and methoxamine are administered during coronary occlusion. Circulation 49:291, 1974

268. Timmis AD, Strak SK, Chamberlin PA: Hemodynamic effects of salbutamol in patients with acute myocardial infarction and severe left ventricular dysfunction. Br Med J 2:1101, 1979

269. Sharma B, Goodwin JF: Beneficial effect of salbutamol on cardiac function in severe congestive cardiomyopathy: Effect on systolic and diastolic function of the left ventricle. Circulation 58:449, 1978

270. Bourdillon PDV, Dawson JR, Foale RA et al: Salbutamol in the treatment of heart failure. Br Heart J 43:206, 1980

271. Mifune J, Kuramoto K, Ueda K et al: Hemodynamic effects of salbutamol, an oral long-acting beta stimulant, in patients with congestive heart failure. Am Heart J 104:1011, 1982

272. Gold FL, Horwitz LD: Hemodynamic effects of pirbuterol in conscious dogs. Am Heart J 102:591, 1981

273. Leier CV, Nelson S, Huss P et al: Intravenous pirbuterol. Clin Pharmacol Ther 31:89, 1982

274. Rude RE, Turi Z, Brown EJ et al: Acute effects of oral pirbuterol on congestive heart failure. Circulation 64:139, 1981

275. Awan NA, Needham K, Evenson MK et al: Therapeutic efficacy of oral pirbuterol in severe chronic congestive heart failure: Acute hemodynamic and long-term ambulatory evaluation. Am Heart J 102:555, 1981

276. Weber KT, Andrews V, Janicki JS: Pirbuterol in the long-term treatment of congestive heart failure. Circulation 65(Suppl 4):307, 1981

277. Colucci WS, Alexander RW, Williams GH et al: Decreased lymphocyte beta-adrenergic-receptor density in patients with heart failure and tolerance to the beta-adrenergic agonist pirbuterol. N Engl J Med 305:185, 1981

278. Manders WT, Watner SF, Braunwald E: Cardioselective beta adrenergic stimulation with prenalterol in the conscious dog. J Pharmacol Exp Ther 215:266, 1980

279. Kirlin PC, Pitt B, Lucchesi BR: Comparative effects of prenalterol and dobutamine in a canine model of acute ischemic heart failure. J Cardiovasc Pharmacol 3:896, 1981

280. Kirlin PC, Pitt B: Hemodynamic effects of intravenous prenalterol in severe heart failure. Am J Cardiol 47:670, 1981

281. Wahr D, Swedberg K, Rabbino M et al: Intravenous and oral prenalterol in congestive heart failure. Effects on systemic and coronary hemodynamics and myocardial catecholamine balance. Am J Med 76:999, 1984

282. Svendsen TL, Harling OJ, Tap-Jensen J: Immediate haemodynamic effects of prenalterol, a new adrenergic beta-1 receptor agonist, in healthy volunteers. Eur J Clin Pharmacol 18:219, 1980

283. Roubin GS, Choong CVP, Devenish-Meares S et al: β-Adrenergic stimulation of the failing ventricle: A double-blind, randomized trial of sustained oral therapy with prenalterol. Circulation 69:955, 1984

284. Simonsen S: Hemodynamic effects of ICI 118,587 in cardiomyopathy. Br Heart J 51:654, 1984

285. Virk SJS, Anfilogoff NH, Lawson N et al: The acute effects of intravenous xamoterol (Corwin, I.C.I. 118,587) on resting and exercise hemodynamics in patients with mild to moderate heart failure. Eur Heart J 10:227, 1989

286. Bhatia JSS, Swedberg K, Chatterjee K: Acute hemodynamic and metabolic effects of ICI 118,587 (Corwin), a selective partial beta agonist, in patients with dilated cardiomyopathy. Am Heart J 111:692, 1986

287. The Xamoterol in Severe Heart Failure Study Group: Xamoterol in severe heart failure. Lancet 336:1, 1990

288. Svensson G, Rehnqvist N, Sjogren A, Erhardt L: Hemodynamic effects of ICI 118,587 (Corwin) in patients with mild cardiac failure after myocardial infarction. J Cardiovasc Pharmacol 7:97, 1985

289. Nuttal A, Snow HM: The cardiovascular effects of ICI 118,587: A beta-1 adrenoreceptor partial agonist. Br J Pharmacol 77:381, 1982

290. Kino M, Hirota Y, Yamamoto S et al: Cardiovascular effects of a newly synthesized cardiotonic agent (TA-064) on normal and diseased hearts. Am J Cardiol 51:802, 1983

291. Ozaki N, Bito K, Kinoshita M, Kawakita S: Effects of a cardiotonic agent, TA-064, on isolated canine cerebral, coronary, femoral, mesenteric and renal arteries. J Cardiovasc Pharmacol 5:818, 1983

292. Thompson MJ, Huss P, Unverferth DV et al: Hemodynamic effects of intravenous butopamine in congestive heart failure. Clin Pharmacol Ther 28:324, 1980

293. Nelson S, Leier CV: Butopamine in normal human subjects. Curr Ther Res 30:405, 1981

294. Goldberg LI: Cardiovascular and renal actions of dopamine: Potential clinical applications. Pharmacol Rev 24:1, 1972

295. Rajfer SI, Anton AH, Rossen J, Goldberg LI: Beneficial hemodynamic effects of oral levodopa in heart failure: Relationship to the generation of dopamine. N Engl J Med 310:1357, 1984

296. Chatterjee K, De Marco T: Central and peripheral adrenergic receptor agonists in heart failure. Eur Heart J 10(Suppl B):55, 1989

297. Daly PA, Curran D, Chatterjee K: Effects of L-dopa and captopril on resting neurodynamics and coronary blood flow (abstr). Circulation 72(Suppl III):406, 1985

298. Harvey CA, Owen DAA: Hemodynamic responses to ibopamine, an orally active dopamine analogue, in anesthetized cats. Br J Pharmacol 78:127P, 1983

299. Itoh H, Kohli JD, Rajfer SL et al: Comparison of the cardiovascular actions of dopamine and epinine in the dog. J Pharmacol Exp Ther 283:87, 1985

300. Dei Cas L, Manca C, Bermardini B et al: Noninvasive evaluation of the effects of oral ibopamine (SB 7505) on cardiac and renal function in patients with congestive heart failure. J Cardiovasc Pharmacol 4:436, 1982

301. Leier CV, Ren JH, Huss P et al: The hemodynamic effects of ibopamine, a dopamine congener in patients with congestive heart failure. Pharmacotherapy 6:35, 1986

302. Cantelli I, Lolli C, Bomba E et al: Sustained oral treatment with ibopamine in patients with chronic heart failure. Curr Ther Res 39:900, 1986

303. Rajter SI, Rossen JD, Douglas FL et al: Effects of long-term therapy with oral ibopamine on resting hemodynamics and exercise capacity in patients with heart failure: Relationship to the generation of N-methyldopamine and to plasma norepinephrine levels. Circulation 73:740, 1986

304. Brown RA, Dixon J, Farmer JB et al: Dopexamine: A novel agonist at peripheral dopamine receptors and beta$_2$ adrenoreceptors. Br J Pharmacol 85:599, 1985

305. Bass AS, Kohli JD, Lubbers NL et al: Potentiation of cardiovascular effects of norepinephrine by dopexamine. Fed Proc 46:205, 1987

306. De Marco T, Kwasman M, Lau D et al: Dopex-amine hydrochloride improved cardiac performance without increased metabolic cost. Am J Cardiol 62:57C, 1988

307. Fennell WH, Taylor AA, Young JB et al: Propyl-butyldopamine: Hemodynamic effects in conscious dogs, normal human volunteers and patients with heart failure. Circulation 67:829, 1983

308. Francis GS, Parks R, Cohn JN: The effects of bromocriptine in patients with congestive heart failure. Am Heart J 106:100, 1983

309. Leon CA, Suarez JM, Aranoff RD et al: Fen-oldopam: Efficacy of a new orally active dopamine analog in heart failure. Circulation 70 (Suppl II):II-307, 1984

310. Nishiyama S, Yamaguchi I: A novel orally active dopamine prodrug TA-870: V. Natriuretic and positive inotropic effects in rats: An assessment after chronic administration. J Cardiovasc Pharmacol 17:768, 1991

311. Nishiyama S, Yoshikawa M, Yamaguchi I: A novel orally active dopamine (DA) prodrug TA-870: IV. renal vasodilatory and negative chronotropic effects in anesthetized dogs: Influence of DA_1 and DA_2 dopamine receptor selective antagonists. J Cardiovasc Pharmacol 17:560, 1991

312. Goldstein RE, Skelton CL, Levey GS et al: Effects of chronic heart failure on the capacity of glucagon to enhance contractility and adenyl cyclase activity of human papillary muscles. Circulation 44:638, 1971

313. Bristow MR, Cubicciotti R, Ginsburg R et al: Histamine-mediated adenylate cyclase stimulation in human myocardium. Mol Pharmacol 21:671, 1982

314. Baumann G, Felix SB, Riess G et al: Effective stimulation of cardiac contractility and myocardial metabolism by impromidine and dimaprit—two new H_2-agonist compounds—in the surviving catecholamine-insensitive myocardium after coronary occlusion. J Cardiovasc Pharmacol 4:542, 1982

315. Linderer T, Biamino G, Bruggeman T et al: Hemodynamic effects of forskolin, a new drug with combined positive inotropic and vasodilating properties (abstr). J Am Coll Cardiol 3:562, 1984

316. Daly JW: Forskolin, adenylate cyclase, and cell physiology: An overview. Adv Cyclic Nucleotide Protein Phosphorylation Res 17:81, 1984

317. Matsue S, Murakami E, Takekoshi N et al: Hemodynamic effects of dibutyryl cyclic AMP in congestive heart failure. Am J Cardiol 51:1364, 1983

318. Silver PJ, Harris AL: Phosphodiesterase isozyme inhibitors and vascular smooth muscle. In Halpern W, Pegram B, Brayden J et al (eds): Proceedings of the Second International Symposium on Resistance Arteries, pp 284–291. Ithaca, Perinatology Press, 1988

319. Silver PJ, Hamel LT, Perrone MH et al: Differential pharmacologic sensitivity of cyclic nucleotide phosphodiesterase isozymes isolated from cardiac muscle, arterial and airway smooth muscle. Eur J Pharmacol 150:85, 1988

320. Stirt JA, Sullivan SF: Aminophylline. Anesth Analg 60:587, 1981

321. Chasin M, Harris D: Inhibitors and activators of cyclic nucleotide phosphodiesterase. Adv Cyclic Nucleotide Res 7:225, 1976

322. Endoh M, Sato K, Yamashita S: Inhibition of cyclic AMP phosphodiesterase activity and myocardial contractility: Effects of cilostamide, a novel PDE inhibitor, and methylisobutylxanthine on rabbit and canine ventricular muscle. Eur J Pharmacol 66:43, 1980

323. Hutton I, Hillis WS, Langhan CE et al: Cardiovascular effects of a new inotropic agent, UK 14275, in patients with coronary heart disease. Br J Clin Pharmacol 4:513, 1977

324. Azuma J, Harada H, Sawamura A et al: Concentration-dependent effect of trapidil on slow action potentials in cardiac muscle. J Mol Cell Cardiol 15:43, 1983

325. Mancini D, LeJemtel T, Sonnenblick E: Intravenous use of amrinone for the treatment of the failing heart. Am J Cardiol 56:8B, 1985

326. Endoh M, Yamashita S, Taira N: Positive inotropic effect of amrinone in relation to cyclic nucleotide metabolism in the canine ventricular muscle. J Pharmacol Exp Ther 221:775, 1982

327. Likoff M, Weber KT, Andrews V et al: Amrinone in the treatment of chronic heart failure. J Am Coll Cardiol 3:1281, 1984

328. Benotti JR, Crossman W, Braunwald E et al: Hemodynamic assessment of amrinone: A new inotropic agent. N Engl J Med 299:1373, 1978

329. LeJemtel TH, Keung E, Sonnenblick EH et al: Amrinone: A new non-glycosidic, non-adrenergic cardiotonic agent effective in the treatment of intractable myocardial failure in man. Circulation 59:1098, 1979

330. Wilmshurst PT, Thompson DS, Juul SM et al: Comparison of the effects of amrinone and sodium nitroprusside on haemodynamics, contractility, and myocardial metabolism in patients with cardiac failure due to coronary artery disease and dilated cardiomyopathy. Br Heart J 52:38, 1984

331. Firth B, Ratner AV, Grassman ED et al: Assessment of the inotropic and vasodilator effects of amrinone versus isoproterenol. Am J Cardiol 54:1331, 1984

332. Millard RW, Dube G, Grupp G et al: Direct vasodilator and positive inotropic actions of amrinone. J Mol Cell Cardiol 12:647, 1980

333. Toda N, Nakajima M, Nishimura K, Miyazaki M: Responses of isolated dog arteries to amrinone. Cardiovasc Res 18:174, 1984

334. Benotti JR, Grossman W, Braunwald E, Carabello BA: Effects of amrinone on myocardial energy metabolism and hemodynamics in patients with severe congestive heart failure due to coronary artery disease. Circulation 62:28, 1980

335. Baim DS: Effects of amrinone on myocardial energetics in severe congestive heart failure. Am J Cardiol 56:16B, 1985

336. Taylor SH, Verma SP, Hussain M et al: Intravenous amrinone in left ventricular failure complicated by acute myocardial infarction. Am J Cardiol 56:29B, 1985

337. Klein M, Siskind S, Frishman W et al: Hemodynamic comparison of intravenous amrinone and dobutamine in patients with chronic congestive heart failure. Am J Cardiol 48:160, 1981

338. Goener M, Pedemonte O, Baele P et al: Amrinone in the management of low cardiac output after open heart surgery. Am J Cardiol 56:33B, 1985

339. Goener M: Severe perioperative cardiogenic shock in open heart surgery: Benefits of combined therapy. In Unger F (ed): Coronary Artery Surgery in the Nineties. Berlin, Springer-Verlag, 1987

340. Robinson RJJ, Tehervenkov C: Treatment of low cardiac output after aorto-coronary bypass surgery using a combination of norepinephrine and amrinone. J Cardiothorac Anesth 1:229, 1987

341. Prielipp RC, Butterworth JF, Zaloga GP: Effects of amrinone on cardiac index, venous oxygen saturation and venous admixture in patients recovering from cardiac surgery. Chest 99:820, 1991

342. Weber KT, Andrews V, Janicki JS et al: Amrinone and exercise performance in patients with chronic heart failure. Am J Cardiol 48:164, 1981

343. Siegel LA, LeJemtel TH, Strom J et al: Improvement in exercise capacity despite cardiac deterioration: Noninvasive assessment of long-term therapy with amrinone in severe heart failure. Am Heart J 106:1042, 1983

344. Leier CV, Dalpiaz K, Huss P et al: Amrinone therapy for congestive heart failure in outpatients with idiopathic dilated cardiomyopathy. Am J Cardiol 52:304, 1983

345. DiBianco R, Shabetai R, Silverman BD et al (with the Amrinone Multicenter Study Investigators): Oral amrinone for the treatment of chronic congestive heart failure: Results of a multicenter randomized double-blind and placebo-controlled withdrawal study. J Am Coll Cardiol 4:855, 1984

346. Massie B, Bourassa M, DiBianco R et al: Long-term oral administration of amrinone for congestive heart failure: Lack of efficacy in a multicenter controlled trial. Circulation 71:963, 1985

347. Naccarelli GV, Gray EL, Dougherty AH et al: Amrinone: Acute electrophysiologic and hemodynamic effects in patients with congestive heart failure. Am J Cardiol 54:600, 1984

348. Naccarelli GV, Goldstein RA: Electrophysiology of phosphodiesterase inhibitors. Am J Cardiol 63:35A, 1989

349. Maskin CS, Forman R, Klein NA et al: Long-term amrinone therapy in patients with severe heart failure: Drug-dependent hemodynamic benefits despite progression of disease. Am J Med 72:113, 1982

350. Packer M, Medina N, Yushak M: Hemodynamic and clinical limitations of long-term therapy with amrinone in patients with severe chronic heart failure. Circulation 70:1038, 1984

351. Alousi AA, Canter JM, Montenaro MJ et al: Cardiotonic activity of milrinone, a new and potent cardiac bipyridine on the normal and failing heart of experimental animals. J Cardiovasc Pharmacol 5:792, 1983

352. Alousi AA, Canter JM, Cicero F et al: Pharmacology of milrinone. In Braunwald E, Sonnenblick EH, Chakrin LW, Schwartz RP Jr (eds): Milrinone: Investigation of New Inotropic Therapy for Congestive Heart Failure, p 21. New York, Raven Press, 1984

353. Alousi AA, Stankus GP, Stuart JC, Walton LH: Characterization of the cardiotonic effects of milrinone, a new and potent cardiac bipyridine, on isolated tissues from several animal species. J Cardiovasc Pharmacol 5:804, 1983

354. Alousi AA, Iwan T, Edelson J, Biddlecome C: Correlation of the hemodynamic and pharmacokinetic profile of intravenous milrinone in anesthetized dog. Arch Int Pharmacodyn Ther 267:59, 1984

355. Harris AL, Wassey ML, Grant AM, Alousi AA: Direct vasodilating effect of milrinone and sodium nitrite in the canine coronary artery (abstr). Fed Proc 43:938, 1984

356. Ludmer PL, Wright RF, Arnold MO et al: Separation of the direct myocardial and vasodilator actions of milrinone administered by an intracoronary infusion technique. Circulation 73:130, 1986

357. Baim DS, McDowell AV, Chernileo J et al: Evaluation of a new bipyridine inotropic agent—milrinone—in patients with severe congestive heart failure. N Engl J Med 309:748, 1983

358. Jaski BE, Fifer MA, Wright RF et al: Positive inotropic and vasodilator actions of milrinone in patients with severe congestive heart failure. J Clin Invest 75:643, 1985

359. Borow KM, Come PC, Neumann et al: Physiologic assessment of the inotropic, vasodilator and afterload reducing effects of milrinone in subjects without cardiac disease. Am J Cardiol 55:1204, 1985

360. Timmis AD, Smyth P, Monaghan M et al: Milrinone in heart failure. Acute effects on left ventricular systolic function and myocardial metabolism. Br Heart J 54:36, 1985

361. Piscione F, Serruys PW, Hugenholtz PG: Left ventricular function after oral milrinone in patients with congestive heart failure: A hemodynamic and angiographic study. In Erdmann E, Greef K, Skou JC (eds): Cardiac Glycosides 1785–1985, pp 237–244. New York, Springer-Verlag, 1986

362. Cody RJ, Muller FB, Kubo SH et al: Identification of the direct vasodilator effect of milrinone with an isolated limb preparation in patients with chronic congestive heart failure. Circulation 73:124, 1986

363. Arnold JM, Ludmar PL, Wright RF et al: Role of reflex sympathetic withdrawal in the hemodynamic response to an increased inotropic state in patients with severe heart failure. J Am Coll Cardiol 8:413, 1986

364. Monrad ES, McKay RG, Baim DS et al: Improvement in index of diastolic performance in patients with congestive heart failure treated with milrinone. Circulation 70:1030, 1984

365. Monrad ES, Baim DS, Smith HS et al: Effects of milrinone on coronary hemodynamics and myocardial energetics in patients with congestive heart failure. Circulation 71:972, 1985

366. Grose R, Strain J, Greenberg M et al: Systemic and coronary effects of intravenous milrinone

and dobutamine in congestive heart failure. J Am Coll Cardiol 7:1107, 1986

367. Monrad ES, Baim DS, Smith HS et al: Milrinone, dobutamine and nitroprusside: Comparative effects on hemodynamics and myocardial energetics in patients with severe congestive heart failure. Circulation 73(Suppl III):III-168, 1986

368. Cody RJ: Renal and hormonal effects of phosphodiesterase III inhibition in congestive heart failure. Am J Cardiol 63:31A, 1989

369. LeJemtel TH, Maskin CS, Mancini D et al: Systemic and regional effects of captopril and milrinone administration alone and concomitantly in patients with heart failure. Circulation 72:364, 1985

370. Simonton CA, Chatterjee K, Cody RJ et al: Milrinone in congestive heart failure: Acute and chronic hemodynamic and clinical evaluation. J Am Coll Cardiol 6:453, 1985

371. Kubo SH, Cody RJ, Chatterjee K et al: Acute dose-range study of milrinone in congestive heart failure. Am J Cardiol 55:726, 1985

372. White HD, Ribeiro JP, Hartley LH, Colucci WS: Immediate effects of milrinone on metabolic and sympathetic response to exercise in severe congestive heart failure. Am J Cardiol 56:93, 1985

373. Schoeller R, Bruggemann T, Vohringer H et al: Long-term oral administration of milrinone for dilated cardiomyopathy (abstr). J Am Coll Cardiol 7:180A, 1986

374. Chesbro JH, Browne KF, Fenster PE et al: The hemodynamic effects of oral milrinone therapy: A multicenter controlled trial (abstr). J Am Coll Cardiol 11:144A, 1988

375. Baim DS, Colucci WS, Monrad SE et al: Survival of patients with severe congestive heart failure treated with oral milrinone. J Am Coll Cardiol 7:661, 1986

376. Packer M, Carver MD, Rodaheffer RJ et al: Effect of oral milrinone on mortality in severe chronic heart failure. N Engl J Med 325:1468, 1991

377. Kariya T, Wille LJ, Dage RC: Biochemical studies on the mechanism of cardiotonic activity of MDL 17043. J Cardiovasc Pharmacol 4:509, 1982

378. Roebel LE, Dage RC, Cheng HC, Woodward JK: Characterization of the cardiovascular activities of a new cardiotonic agent, MDL 17043 (1,3-dihydro-4-methyl-5,4-(methylthio)-benzoyl)-2H-imidazole-2-one). J Cardiovasc Pharmacol 4:721, 1982

379. Dage RE, Kariya T, Hsieh CP et al: Pharmacology of enoximone. Am J Cardiol 60:10C, 1987

380. Janicki JS, Shnoff SG, Weber KT: Physiologic response to the inotropic and vasodilator properties of enoximone. Am J Cardiol 60:15C, 1987

381. Crawford MH, Richards KL, Sodums MT, Kennedy GT: Positive inotropic and vasodilator effects of MDL 17043 in patients with reduced left ventricular performance. Am J Cardiol 53:1051, 1984

382. Kereiakes DJ, Viquerat C, Lanzer P et al: Mechanisms of improved left ventricular function following intravenous MDL 17043 in patients with severe chronic heart failure. Am Heart J 108:1278, 1984

383. Herman HC, Ruddy TD, Dee GW et al: Diastolic function in patients with severe heart failure: Comparison of the effects of enoximone and nitroprusside. Circulation 75:1214, 1987

384. Kereiakes D, Chatterjee K, Parmley WW et al: Intravenous and oral MDL 17043 (a new inotrope-vasodilator agent) in congestive heart failure: Hemodynamic and clinical evaluation in 38 patients. J Am Coll Cardiol 4:884, 1984

385. Uretsky BF, Generalovich T, Reddy PS et al: Acute hemodynamic effect of oral MDL 17043: A new inotropic vasodilator agent in patients with severe heart failure. J Am Coll Cardiol 5:326, 1985

386. Amin DK, Shah PK, Hulse S et al: Myocardial metabolic and hemodynamic effects of intravenous MDL-17043, a new cardiotonic drug in patients with chronic severe heart failure. Am Heart J 108:1285, 1984

387. Martin JL, Likoff MJ, Janicki JS et al: Myocardial energetics and clinical response to the cardiotonic agent MDL 17043 in advanced heart failure. J Am Coll Cardiol 4:875, 1984

388. Viquerat CE, Kereiakes D, Morris DL et al: Alterations in left ventricular function, coronary hemodynamics, and myocardial catecholamine balance with MDL 17043: A new inotropic vasodilator agent in patients with severe heart failure. J Am Coll Cardiol 5:326, 1985

389. Rigaud M, Benit E, Castadot M et al: Comparative effects of enoximone and nitroglycerin on left ventricular performance and regional wall motion in ischemic cardiomyopathy. Br J Clin Pract 42(Suppl 64):26, 1988

390. Leier CV, Meiler SEL, Mathews S et al: A preliminary report of the effects of orally administered enoximone on regional hemodynamics in congestive heart failure. Am J Cardiol 60:27C, 1987

391. Clifton GG, Macmahon FG, Ryan FR et al: Effects of enoximone on renal function and plasma volume in normal volunteers. Curr Ther Res 39:436, 1986

392. Miles WM, Heger JJ, Minardo JD et al: Electrophysiologic and hemodynamic effects of intravenous enoximone (abstr). Circulation 74 (Suppl II):II-38, 1986

393. Renard M, Dereppe H, Henuzet C et al: Effects of enoximone in patients with cardiac failure after myocardial infarction. Br J Clin Pract 42 (Suppl 64):37, 1988

394. Vincent JL, Carlier E, Berre J et al: Administration of enoximone in cardiogenic shock. Am J Cardiol 62:419, 1988

395. Gonzales M, Desager JP, Jacquemart JL et al: Efficacy of enoximone in the management of refractory low output states following cardiac surgery. J Clin Pract 42(Suppl 64):53, 1988

396. Shah PK, Amin DK, Hulse S et al: Inotropic therapy for refractory congestive heart failure with oral enoximone (MDL-17,043): Poor long-term results despite early hemodynamic and clinical improvement. Circulation 71:326, 1985

397. Rubin SA, Tabak L: MDL 17,043: Short and long-term cardiopulmonary and clinical effects in patients with heart failure. J Am Coll Cardiol 5:1422, 1985

398. Weber KT, Janicki JS, Jain MC: Enoximone (MDL 17,043) for stable chronic heart failure secondary to ischemic or idiopathic cardiomyopathy. Am J Cardiol 58:589, 1986

399. Maskin CS, Weber KT, Janicki JS: Long-term oral enoximone therapy in chronic cardiac failure. Am J Cardiol 60:63C, 1987

400. Schriven AJI, Lipkin DP, Anand IS et al: A comparison of hemodynamic effects of one-month oral captopril and enoximone treatment for severe congestive heart failure. Am J Cardiol 60:68C, 1987

401. Triese N, Erbel R, Pilcher J et al: Long-term treatment with oral enoximone for chronic congestive heart failure: The European experience. Am J Cardiol 60:85C, 1987

402. Khalife K, Zannad F, Brunotte F et al: Placebo-controlled study of oral enoximone in congestive heart failure with initial and final intravenous hemodynamic evaluation. Am J Cardiol 60:75C, 1987

403. Narahara K and Western Enoximone Study Group: Enoximone versus placebo: A double-blind trial in chronic congestive heart failure (abstr). Circulation 80(Suppl II):II-175, 1989

404. Crawford MH, Deedwania P, Massie B et al: Comparative efficacy of enoximone versus captopril in moderate heart failure. Circulation 80(Suppl II):II-175, 1989

405. Jessup M, Ulrich S, Samaha J et al: Effects of low dose enoximone for chronic congestive heart failure. Am J Cardiol 60:80C, 1987

406. Uretsky BF, Jessup M, Konstam MA et al: Multicenter trial of oral enoximone in patients with moderate to moderately severe congestive heart failure. Circulation 82:774, 1990

407. Goldberg AD, Goldstein S, Nicklas J: Multicenter trial of imazodan in patients with chronic congestive heart failure (abstr). Circulation 82(Suppl III):III-673, 1990

408. Dubois-Rande JL, Loisance D, Duval AM et al: Enoximone: A pharmacological bridge to transplantation. Br J Clin Pract 42(Suppl 64):73, 1988

409. Bristow MR, Lee HE, Gilbert EM et al: Use of enoximone in patients awaiting cardiac transplant. Br J Clin Pract 42(Suppl 64):69, 1988

410. Crawford MH: Intravenous use of enoximone. Am J Cardiol 60:42C, 1987

411. Okerholm RA, Keeley FJ, Weiner DL, Spangenberg RB: The pharmacokinetics of a new cardiotonic agent, MDL 19205, 4-ethyl-1,3-dihydro-5-(4-pyridinyl)-2H-imidazol-2-one (abstr). Fed Proc 42:1131, 1983

412. Petein M, Levine B, Cohn JN: Hemodynamic effects of a new inotropic agent, piroximone (MDL 19,205) in patients with chronic heart failure. J Am Coll Cardiol 4:364, 1984

413. Axelrod RJ, De Marco T, Dae M et al: Hemodynamic and clinical evaluation of piroximone, a new inotrope-vasodilator agent in severe congestive heart failure. J Am Coll Cardiol 9:1124, 1987

414. Dage RC, Roebel LE, Hsieh CP, Woodward JK: Cardiovascular properties of a new cardiotonic agent, MDL 19,205. J Cardiovasc Pharmacol 6:35, 1984

415. Petein M, Pierpont GL, Heppner B et al: Hemodynamic and regional blood flow response to MDL-19205 in dogs: A comparison with dobutamine (abstr). Circulation 68(Suppl III):III-128, 1983

416. Holck M, Thorens S, Muggli R, Eigenmann R: Studies on the mechanism of positive inotropic activity: RO13-6438, a structurally novel cardiotonic agent with vasodilating properties. J Cardiovasc Pharmacol 6:520, 1984

417. Daly PA, Chatterjee K, Viquerat CE et al: RO13-6438, a new inotrope-vasodilator: Systemic and coronary hemodynamic effects in congestive heart failure. Am J Cardiol 55:1539, 1985

418. Pouleur H, Marechal G, Balasim H et al: Effects of dobutamine and sulmazol (AR-L 115BS) on myocardial metabolism and coronary, femoral, and renal blood flows: A comparative study in normal dogs and in dogs with chronic volume overload. J Cardiovasc Pharmacol 5:861, 1983

419. Pouleur H, Rousseau MF, VanMechelen H et al: Cardiovascular effects of AR-L 115BS in conscious dogs with and without chronic congestive heart failure. J Cardiovasc Pharmacol 4:409, 1982

420. Renard M, Jacobs P, Dechamps P et al. Hemodynamic and clinical response to three-day infusion of sulmazol (AR-L 115BS) in severe congestive heart failure. Chest 84:408, 1983

421. Thormann J, Schlepper M, Kramer W et al: Effects of AR-L 115BS (sulmazol), a new cardiotonic agent in coronary artery disease: Improved ventricular wall motion, increased pump function and abolition of pacing induced ischemia. J Am Coll Cardiol 2:332, 1983

422. Evans DB, Potoczak RE, Newton RS et al: Preclinical cardiovascular pharmacology of CI-914, a novel pyridiazinone cardiotonic (abstr). Circulation 70(Suppl II):II-307, 1984

423. Mancini D, Sonnenblick EH, Latts JR et al: Hemodynamic and clinical benefits of CI-914, a new cardiotonic agent. Circulation 70(Suppl II):II-307, 1984

424. Colucci WS, Wright RF, Braunwald E: New positive inotropic agents in the treatment of congestive heart failure. N Engl J Med 314:349, 1986

425. Fujino K, Sperelakis N, Solaro RJ: Sensitization of dog and guinea pig heart myofilaments to calcium activation and the inotropic effect of pimobendan: Comparison with milrinone. Circ Res 63:911, 1988

426. Solaro RJ, Fujuro K, Sparelakis N: The positive inotropic effect of pimobendan involves stereospecific increases in the calcium sensitivity of cardiac filaments. J Cardiovasc Pharmacol 14 (Suppl 2):57, 1989

427. Endoh M, Shibasaki T, Satoh H et al: Different mechanisms involved in the positive inotropic effects of benzimidazole derivative UD-CG115BS (pimobendan) and its demethylated metabolite UD-CG212C1 in canine ventricular myocardium. J Cardiovasc Pharmacol 17:365, 1991

428. Hajjar RJ, Gwathmey JK: Calcium-sensitizing inotropic agents in the treatment of heart failure: A critical view. Cardiovasc Drug Ther 5:961, 1991

429. Packer M: Effects of phosphodiesterase inhibitors on survival of patients with chronic congestive heart failure. Am J Cardiol 63:41A, 1989

430. Rauch B, Zimmerman R, Kapp M et al: Hemodynamic and neuroendocrine responses to acute adminstration of the phosphodiesterase inhibitor. BM14,478 in patients with congestive heart failure. Clin Cardiol 14:386, 1991

431. Feldman AM, Baughman KL, Lee WK et al: Randomized double-blind placebo trial of OPC-8212 in patients with heart failure: Morbidity/mortality in 80 patients (abstr). Circulation 80(Suppl II):II-176, 1989

432. Katz SD, Kubo SH, Jessup M et al: Pimobendan improves exercise capacity in digitalized patients with severe congestive heart failure (abstr). Circulation 80(Suppl II):II-176, 1989

433. Kubo SH, Gollub S, Bourge R et al: Beneficial effects of pimobendan on exercise tolerance and quality of life in patients with heart failure. Results of a multicenter trial. Circulation 85:942, 1992

434. Remme W, Krayenbuhl H, Baumann G: Efficacy and safety of pimobendan in moderate CHF: a double-blind parallel 6 month comparison with enalapril (abstr). J Am Coll Cardiol 19:261A, 1992

435. Gross R, Schramm M, Thomas G, Toward R: Bay K8644, a positive inotropic dihydropyridine with Ca^{++} agonist properties. J Mol Cell Cardiol 15(Suppl 4):29, 1983

436. Judy WV, Hall JH, Toth PD, Fokers K: Influence of coenzyme Q10 on cardiac function in congestive heart failure (abstr). Fed Proc 43:358, 1984

437. Hoffman-Bang C, Rehnquist N, Swedberg K et al: Coenzyme Q10 as an adjunctive in treatment of congestive heart failure. J Am Coll Cardiol 19:216A, 1992

438. Smiseth OA: Inosine infusion in dogs with acute ischemic left ventricular failure: Favorable effects on myocardial performance and metabolism. Cardiovasc Res 17:192, 1983

439. Chernow B, Roth BL: Pharmacologic manipulation of the peripheral vasculature in shock: Clinical and experimental approaches. Circ Shock 18:141, 1986

440. Deojars P, Pinaud M, Potel G et al: Reappraisal of norepinephrine therapy in human septic shock. Crit Care Med 15:134, 1987

441. Vlahakes GJ, Turley K, Hoffman JIE: The pathophysiology of failure in right ventricular hypertension: Hemodynamic and biochemical correlations. Circulation 63:87, 1981

442. Hoffman MJ, Greenfield LJ, Sugarman HJ et al: Unsuspected right ventricular dysfunction in shock and sepsis. Ann Surg 198:307, 1983

443. Kimchi A, Ellrodt AG, Berman DS et al: Right ventricular performance in septic shock: A combined radionuclide and hemodynamic study. J Am Coll Cardiol 4:945, 1984

444. Sibbald WJ, Driedger M: Right ventricular function in acute disease states: Pathophysiologic considerations. Crit Care Med 11:339, 1983

445. Schreuder WO, Schneider AJ, Groeneveld ABJ et al: Effect of dopamine vs. norepinephrine on hemodynamics in septic shock: Emphasis on right ventricular performance. Chest 95:1282, 1989

446. Shoemaker WC, Appel PL: Pathophysiology of adult respiratory distress syndrome after sepsis and surgical operations. Crit Care Med 13:166, 1985

447. Shoemaker WC: A new approach to physiology, monitoring and therapy of shock states. World J Surg 11:113, 1987

448. Gilbert EM, Haupt MT, Mandanas RY et al: The effect of fluid loading, blood transfusion and catecholamine infusion on oxygen delivery and consumption in patients with sepsis. Am Rev Respir Dis 134:873, 1986

449. Vincent JL, Dufaye P, Berre J et al: Serial lactate determinations during circulatory shock. Crit Care Med 11:449, 1983

450. Shoemaker WC, Appel PL, Kramm HB: Hemodynamic and oxygen transport effects of dobutamine in critically ill general surgical patients. Crit Care Med 14:1032, 1986

451. Vincent JL, Roman A: Dobutamine infusion in septic shock: Effects on arterial pressure (abstr). Chest 94(Suppl):75, 1988

452. Cohn JN, Archibald DG, Ziesche S et al: Effect of vasodilator therapy on mortality in chronic congestive heart failure: Results of Veterans Administration Cooperative Study. N Engl J Med 134:1547, 1986

453. Chatterjee K, Parmley WW, Cohn JN et al: A cooperative multicenter study of captopril in congestive heart failure: Hemodynamic effects and long-term response. Am Heart J 110:439, 1985

454. Consensus Trial Study Group: Effects of enalapril on mortality in severe congestive heart failure: Results of the Cooperative North Scandinavian Enalapril Survival Study (CONSENSUS). N Engl J Med 316:1429, 1987

455. Newman TJ, Maskin CS, Dennick LG et al: Effects of captopril on survival in patients with heart failure. Am J Med 84(Suppl 3A):140, 1988

456. Bonaduce D, Petretta M, Arrichiello P et al: Effects of captopril treatment on left ventricular remodelling and function after anterior myocardial infarction: Comparison with digitalis. J Am Coll Cardiol 19:858, 1992

457. Maskin CS: Intermittent parenteral inotropic therapy in patients with chronic congestive heart failure: Concept and clinical results. Heart Failure 2:117, 1986

458. Miller LW, Merkle EJ, Herrmann V: Out-patient dobutamine for end-stage congestive heart failure. Crit Care Med 18:530, 1990

459. Baptista RJ, Mitrano FP, Perri-LaFrancesca: Home intermittent amrinone infusions in terminal congestive heart failure. Ann Pharmacother 23:59, 1989

Nitrates

4

Jonathan Abrams

The use of nitroglycerin (NTG) and other organic nitrate esters in cardiovascular medicine has increased substantially during the past decade. These drugs, once used only for the treatment of angina pectoris, are playing an increasing role in the management of patients with unstable angina and acute myocardial infarction, as well as in vasodilator therapy for acute and chronic congestive heart failure. Nitrates represent one of the oldest cardiac therapies; an oral solution of NTG was first employed in the treatment of angina over 100 years ago.

Vasodilatation of arteries and veins is the major physiologic characteristic of organic nitrates. These drugs are classified as direct-acting vasodilators; they act on vascular smooth muscle to induce vasodilatation throughout the body. Nitrates have potent venodilating activity, a unique feature compared with most vasodilators; their effect on veins is more prominent than on arteries and arterioles. Nitrates have no direct action on cardiac contractility or electrophysiologic properties of the heart.

NTG and other nitrates may induce reflex sympathetic nervous system discharge. Resultant vasoconstriction in the various regional circulations may counteract the vasodilating actions of nitrates. Vascular beds that have dense sympathetic innervation are particularly likely to respond to nitrate-induced hypotension with arterial and venous vasoconstriction. Reflex tachycardia is commonly seen when central aortic pressure falls following nitrate administration. Activation of baroreceptor reflexes is prominent in individuals with normal cardiac function. However, when nitrates are given to patients with impaired left ventricular contractility or overt congestive heart failure, the vasodilating actions of these drugs are not usually accompanied by reflex sympathetic discharge. It is important to keep in mind the differences in the hemodynamic effects of nitrates in the normal and failing circulations.

The mechanisms of action and clinical pharmacology of nitrates are reviewed in this chapter, and the efficacy of nitrate therapy in the various ischemic syndromes as well as in vasodilator therapy of congestive heart failure will be discussed.

MECHANISMS OF ACTION OF NITROGLYCERIN AND ORGANIC NITRATES

Nitrates produce vascular smooth muscle relaxation through a direct action on blood vessels. Their vasodilating effects are not modulated through neurohu-

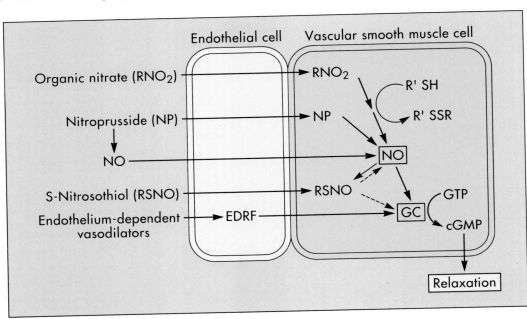

Figure 4.1 Current hypothesis of intracellular events leading to vascular smooth muscle relaxation after nitrate or nitroprusside (NP) administration (see text). Both compounds are metabolized near the cell membrane. The organic nitrates are converted to nitric oxide (NO) and require reduced sulfhydryl groups (R' SH) for the dinitration process. Nitroprusside is more directly converted to NO and does not require thiols for its metabolic activation. Note that endothelium-dependent relaxing factor (EDRF) is produced by endothelial cells and diffuses into smooth muscle cells of arteries and veins. EDRF is believed to be NO or a closely related molecular species. NO activates guanylate cyclase (GC), leading to smooth muscle relaxation. The likeliest cause of nitrate tolerance occurs during the dinitration process of the organic nitrate (RNO$_2$) to NO, with a relative unavailability of adequate numbers of reduced sulfhydryl groups. Recent work suggests that organic nitrates may be converted directly to NO, and they also can react with exogenously administered sulfhydryl groups outside of vascular smooth muscle to form extravascular S-nitrosothiols (RSNO). It is controversial whether RSNO is obligatory in the intracellular dinitration of organic nitrates. (Modified from Kowaluk E, Fung H-L: Pharmacology and pharmacokinetics of nitrates. In Abrams J, Pepine CJ, Thadani U (eds): Medical Therapy of Ischemic Heart Disease, Nitrates, Beta Blockers, and Calcium Antagonists, p. 155. Boston, Little, Brown & Co, 1992)

moral mechanisms as are those of the angiotensin-converting enzyme inhibitors (captopril, enalapril) or sympatholytic agents (prazosin, trimazosin). The precise cellular mode of action of nitrates remains controversial. Some years ago Needleman proposed that nitrates induce vascular relaxation by interacting with a sulfhydryl group on a putative "nitrate receptor" on the surface of vascular smooth muscle cells.[1]

Recent evidence indicates that organic nitrates are converted or dinitrated to nitric oxide (NO) within the smooth muscle cell (Fig. 4.1). The dinitration process requires sulfhydryl (SH) groups that are present as cysteine moieties located near the plasma membrane. Nitric oxide activates the enzyme guanylate cyclase, which in turn increases intracellular cyclic guanosine monophosphate (cGMP). This results in protein kinase phosphorylation, decreased intracellular calcium, and smooth muscle relaxation.[2] Thus veins and arteries dilate through a mechanism involving NO production. The guanylate cyclase–cyclic GMP pathway is activated by NO or a close molecular species. Other nitrovasodilators, such as molsidomine and nitroprusside, release NO directly and produce smooth muscle relaxation through the same final pathway (see Fig. 4.1). However, these compounds do not require a sulfhydryl group for the dinitration process; significant nitrate tolerance has not been observed with either nitrovasodilator.

It remains controversial whether the NO molecule must first combine with an additional thiol group to form an S-nitrosothiol compound in order to activate guanylate cyclase. The nitrosothiols are also capable of directly releasing NO and stimulating guanylate cyclase. Nitrates may also form S-nitrosothiol groups outside the vascular smooth muscle cell which can enter the cell and produce vascular relaxation.[3]

Sodium nitroprusside also induces vascular relaxation by conversion to S-nitrosothiols with subsequent stimulation of the enzyme guanylate cyclase. Thus, it appears that cyclic GMP is the final common pathway for these two vasodilators, although intracellular metabolism of these two drugs is different.[2] Figure 4.1 represents a current hypothesis regarding the cellular mechanism of action of the organic nitrates and nitroprusside.

It has been suggested that NTG and other nitrates may act by stimulation of prostaglandins.[4] NTG induces prostacyclin production by smooth muscle endothelial cells; at high nitrate concentrations thromboxane A$_2$ production is inhibited. However, recent work suggests that the prostaglandin system is not an important modulator of nitrate effects.[5]

Of great importance has been the discovery that nitric oxide is one of the main endothelium-dependent relaxant factors (EDRF), if not EDRF itself. Nitroglycerin and the organic nitrates act on vascular tissue independently of intact endothelial function, and along with molsidomine and nitroprusside, are known as nitrovasodilators. These compounds are all endothelium-independent relaxers of vascular smooth muscle. Thus, the nitrates are capable of dilating the coronary arteries when endothelial function is impaired, as is often the case in coronary atherosclerosis.

Although an antiaggregatory action of the organic nitrates has been previously documented in vitro, this phenomenon has not been felt to be clinically relevant because such platelet effects were only demonstrable at very high (i.e., pharmacologic) concentrations. Recent work from a number of centers has suggested that nitrates, particularly intravenous NTG, may have significant antiplatelet activity in humans at readily obtainable plasma nitrate concentrations.[6–8] If the nitrates do have significant antiplatelet and antithrombotic actions, these drugs would have a potentially important additional role in the treatment of acute ischemic syndromes, such as unstable angina and acute myocardial infarction. Antiplatelet and antithrombotic effects would help explain the demonstrated efficacy of these drugs in these major ischemic conditions.

Nitrate Tolerance

The clinical aspects of this important subject are discussed later in the chapter. It is presently believed that intracellular events involved in nitrate metabolism are critical to the development of tolerance. Specifically, the relative unavailability of reduced sulfhydryl (–SH) moieties within vascular smooth muscle cells limits organic nitrate conversion to nitric oxide (see Fig. 4.1) and subsequent vasodilatation. The sulfhydryl groups are "depleted" during the conversion of the organic nitrate to nitric oxide. The classic hypothesis is still unproven; recent evidence does not support true –SH depletion.

HEMODYNAMIC EFFECTS OF NITRATES

Nitrates induce vasodilatation of veins, arteries, and arterioles. Responsiveness to nitrates varies according to the type of vascular tissue. Differing vascular nitrate metabolism and kinetics may account for the differences in response of various vascular beds to NTG. For instance, following systemic NTG administration veins have a higher concentration of NTG per weight than arteries.[9]

Venodilation

Nitrates induce venodilation at very low doses. The venous dose–response curve is relatively flat; as NTG plasma concentration increases there is little additional venous vasodilation, which is near maximal at

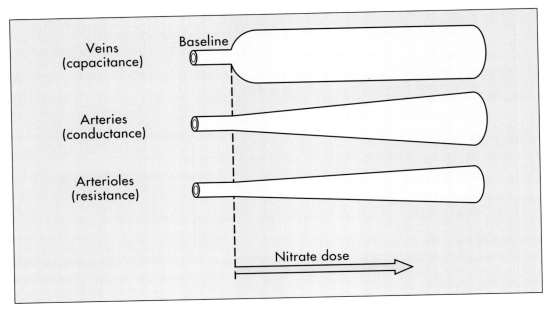

Figure 4.2 Actions of organic nitrates on the major vascular beds and relationship of vasodilatation to the size of the administered dose. The venous or capacitance system dilates maximally with very low doses of organic nitrates. Increasing the amount of drug does not cause appreciable additional venodilatation. Arterial dilation and enhanced arterial conductance begin at low doses of nitrates with further vasodilation appearing as the dosage is increased. With high plasma concentrations of nitrates the arteriolar or resistance vessels dilate, resulting in a decrease in systemic and regional vascular resistance (see text). (Modified from Abrams J: Hemodynamic effects of nitroglycerin and long-acting nitrates. Am Heart J 110(Part 2):216, 1985)

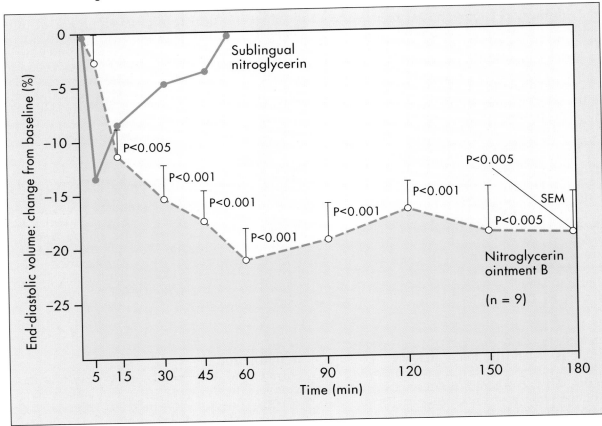

Figure 4.3 Reduction in left ventricular end-diastolic volume following administration of sublingual nitroglycerin or 2% nitroglycerin ointment in normal subjects. The data represent calculations derived from measurements of left ventricular diameter obtained by M-mode echocardiography in nine normal subjects. Similar reductions in left ventricular end-systolic diameter and volume were observed. (Modified from Abrams J: Pharmacology of nitroglycerin and long-acting nitrates and their usefulness in the treatment of congestive heart failure. In Gould L, Reddy CVR (eds): Vasodilator Therapy for Cardiac Disorders, pp 129–167. Mt. Kisco, NY, Futura Publishing, 1979)

low plasma concentrations (Fig. 4.2). Both regional and systemic venous beds dilate following nitrate administration.

In the normal subject, venodilation results in pooling or sequestration of blood in the venous or capacitance circulation. Seventy to 75% of the circulating blood volume is stored in the veins. Nitrates shift the distribution of blood into the central venous circulation at a reduced venous pressure; this results in decreased return of blood to the right side of the heart. Intracardiac pressures and volumes decrease and are accompanied by a fall in stroke volume and cardiac output. Reflex tachycardia, if marked, may limit or even prevent a decrease in cardiac output.

Some experts believe that the pronounced systemic venodilation is responsible for much of the beneficial effect of nitrates in ischemic heart disease. These potent venodilating actions result in a decrease in myocardial oxygen requirements owing to a reduction in cardiac preload accompanying the decrease in ventricular volumes and intracardiac filling pressures. Nitrate venodilation is extremely important in producing beneficial effects in patients with congestive heart failure and contributes to the decrease in signs and symptoms of pulmonary congestion. In normal subjects nitrates substantially reduce left ventricular chamber size (Fig. 4.3), although this effect is not consistently observed in patients with congestive heart failure.

Arterial Vasodilatation

At low doses nitrates have an effect on large arteries,[10] manifested by an increase in arterial conductance and distensibility and an augmented rate of rise of the arterial pulse upstroke. These effects are seen even when systemic blood pressure is not altered. In larger doses nitrates induce more pronounced arterial vasodilatation (see Fig. 4.2). It is not known if minor changes in arterial compliance in the absence of a significant fall in systemic vascular resistance or systolic blood pressure have any positive clinical effect, although it is likely that arterial vasodilatation of various regional circulations, particularly the limbs, may

reduce left ventricular afterload in the absence of a change in arterial pressure.[10]

A recent observation suggests that brachial artery or routine arm cuff measurements of blood pressure may *underestimate* the actual effect of administered nitrate on lowering central aortic pressure.[11] Thus, standard blood pressure determinations may not accurately reflect the maximal effect of nitrates on the arterial system.

Arteriolar Vasodilatation

Large doses of nitrates that produce high plasma and tissue nitrate concentrations induce arteriolar or resistance vessel dilatation (see Fig. 4.2). Systemic vascular resistance falls. Nitrates also decrease resistance in the regional circulations, such as the coronary, splanchnic, and renal beds.

The combination of vasodilatation of the systemic arterioles and generalized venodilatation resulting in decreased return of blood to the central circulation can reduce central aortic pressure, often excessively. Tachycardia is common after nitrate administration. Increased sympathetic tone may attenuate or even prevent nitrate-induced decreases in systolic blood pressure; such reflex adrenergic responses occasionally produce untoward reactions to nitrate administration, such as palpitations and rare episodes of angina pectoris.

Nitrate-induced arteriolar vasodilatation appears to be an important component of the beneficial response of the failing circulation to nitrate administration. A decrease in regional bed and systemic vascular resistance improves the efficiency of left ventricular emptying in congestive heart failure.

Modulators of Nitrate Action (Figure 4.4)
SYMPATHETIC NERVOUS SYSTEM
It has already been stressed that sympathetic activation following nitrate administration plays an important role in modulating the effects of NTG and other nitrates on the systemic and regional circulations.

FIGURE 4.4 IMPORTANT MODULATORS OF NITRATE ACTIVITY

Reflex sympathetic nervous system discharge

Status of left ventricular function

Normal left ventricle

Congestive heart failure and/or dilated ventricle

Presence or absence of nitrate tolerance

Size of administered dose

Reflex tachycardia and vasoconstriction may counteract the desired effects of nitrates in patients with ischemic heart disease. These responses may also prevent or limit adverse sequelae relating to marked nitrate hypotension.

Status of Left Ventricular Function

Nitrates produce a different hemodynamic profile depending on whether cardiac function is normal or abnormal. The classic circulatory response to nitrates in an individual with normal ventricular function consists of a pronounced fall in systolic blood pressure, a reduction in cardiac output, and an increase in heart rate. On the other hand, in the presence of congestive heart failure or significant left ventricular dysfunction, nitrates do not usually decrease cardiac output. In fact, if arteriolar vasodilatation occurs, cardiac performance may actually be enhanced, with an increase in stroke volume and cardiac output, usually in the absence of reflex tachycardia. In addition, blood pressure responses to nitrates in patients with congestive heart failure are much less prominent than in patients with normal left ventricular function. Because cardiac output is maintained or even augmented in congestive heart failure after nitrate administration, reflex sympathetic vasoconstriction is uncommon. In addition, the biphasic response of various regional circulations to nitrates (initial vasodilation followed by reflex vasoconstriction) is less likely to occur.

Presence or Absence of Nitrate Tolerance

There is no longer any doubt that inappropriate dosing with organic nitrates will induce attenuation or tolerance to the hemodynamic and clinical actions of nitrates in many individuals (see below). If a state of partial or complete vascular tolerance exists, the expected response to nitrates will be diminished or absent.

Size of Dose

Small doses of nitrates will induce systemic venodilatation with relatively little arteriolar effect. Large doses will produce a greater fall in arterial pressure and a decrease in systemic vascular resistance. Regional circulatory responses probably share the systemic vascular dose–response relationship to nitrate administration, with regional bed venous capacitance changes occurring at lower nitrate concentrations than will induce vasodilatation of the arteriolar resistance vessels.

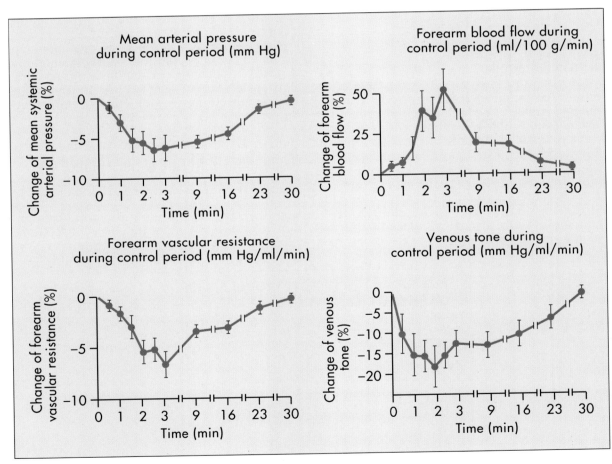

Figure 4.5 Nitroglycerin-induced changes in arterial pressure, forearm blood flow and resistance, and venous tone in normal subjects. Values are expressed as percent changes from control. Eight normal subjects were given 0.6 mg to 0.9 mg of sublingual nitroglycerin. (Modified from Mason DT, Braunwald E: The effects of nitroglycerin and amyl nitrite on arteriolar and venous tone in the human forearm. Circulation 32:755, 1965)

circumstances. It has been demonstrated that exertion can induce coronary vasoconstriction or spasm in some patients; this observation lends credence to the hypothesis that changes in vasomotor tone may play a role in precipitating angina at rest as well as during physical activity.

If coronary vasoconstriction does play a role in precipitating myocardial ischemia in patients with coronary atherosclerosis, nitrate-induced coronary vasodilatation is another potential mechanism to account for the beneficial effects of these drugs.

Of great potential importance has been the observation from a number of laboratories that coronary atherosclerotic lesions are capable of changing diameter in response to various endogenous and exogenous stimuli.[19,22,23] Such responses are often paradoxic in that coronary arterial vasodilatation is the normal consequence of the particular stimulus, whereas constriction may occur in diseased vessel segments. If there is sufficient residual smooth muscle in the coronary arterial media at the site of a stenosis, the stenotic segment may be able to enlarge or constrict (see Fig. 4.7). Transient total obstruction may even occur; this is reversible with nitroglycerin.[23] The phenomenon of stenosis constriction offers new insights into the pathophysiology of coronary artery disease. Nitrates have been shown to reverse this constriction, whether it be during exercise or acetylcholine administration or cold-pressor induced. Enlargement of the atherosclerotic stenosis itself (see Fig. 4.7) may play an important part in the relief of acute myocardial ischemia with nitrates in some patients. It is of interest that both mild and severe coronary stenoses are capable of paradoxic constriction, lending further evidence that the coronary circulation is dynamic even in the setting of advanced atherosclerosis. NTG, an endothelium-independent coronary vasodilator, should be of particular benefit in such circumstances.

CLINICAL INDICATIONS FOR NITRATE USE
Ischemic Heart Disease

NTG and nitrates remain a mainstay for the treatment for coronary heart disease. Many consider these drugs to be the first-line agents for use in patients with stable or unstable angina pectoris. There is a considerable amount of evidence that nitrates may reduce infarct size in acute myocardial infarction. Recent data suggest that nitrates may have a "protective" action in the postmyocardial infarction patient.[24] It has been demonstrated that infusion of intravenous NTG for 48 hours beginning early in the acute infarct period may protect the left ventricle from the deleterious effects of infarct expansion, wall thinning, and left ventricular cavity dilatation in the weeks to months following transmural myocardial infarction.[25]

STABLE ANGINA PECTORIS

Sublingual NTG remains the primary therapy for acute episodes of angina pectoris. Long-acting nitrate formulations are extremely effective in the treatment of chronic effort-induced angina pectoris. In my opinion, nitrates should be the initial therapy for most patients with untreated angina pectoris.[21,26] There is an extensive worldwide experience with long-acting nitrates in patients with angina pectoris.[21]

The use of long-acting nitrates in ischemic heart disease has had a checkered history; during the 1960s and early 1970s most physicians believed that these drugs were of little benefit in the treatment of angina pectoris. It was widely thought that orally administered nitrates could not be effective because of extensive hepatic nitrate metabolism. This hypothesis, promulgated by Needleman and others, was extremely influential in convincing clinicians

FIGURE 4.8 POTENTIAL MECHANISMS OF NITRATE EFFICACY IN ANGINA PECTORIS

Decreased left ventricular preload
    Systemic venous dilatation
    Pulmonary venous dilatation
    Decrease in left ventricular diastolic compressive forces
    Decreased left venterical volume and filling pressure
Decreased left ventricular afterload
    Decreased aortic impedance
    Decreased systolic arterial pressure
    Decreased systemic vascular resistance
    Decreased left ventricular end-diastolic volume
Coronary circulation
    Coronary artery dilatation
    Spasm reversal or prevention
    Stenosis dilatation
    Increased collateral flow
    Prevention or reversal of collateral or distal coronary artery vasoconstriction supplying an occluded vessel
Improvement in disordered endothelial function

that these drugs were of no value in clinical practice.[27] In addition, the quality of many of the early published investigations using nitrates in angina pectoris was uneven, lending considerable uncertainty as to the efficacy of these agents. By the mid to late 1970s, however, the use of nitrate formulations in angina pectoris became increasingly widespread as much new favorable clinical evidence convinced physicians that these drugs have major benefits.

Many well-designed double-blind randomized trials using a variety of nitrate compounds have shown unequivocally positive effects.[21,26,27] Decreased angina attacks and reduced NTG consumption rates have been reported. More importantly, objective assessment of myocardial ischemia during placebo-controlled treadmill or bicycle exercise testing has repeatedly documented that nitrates improve exercise duration to the onset of angina.

Although the other two major classes of antianginal agents, the β-blockers and calcium channel antagonists, are also effective in angina pectoris, it seems reasonable to initiate therapy with a long-acting nitrate in any patient with angina pectoris shown to be responsive to sublingual NTG.[26] Classic improvement of chest pain, that is, relief of discomfort within 3 to 10 minutes after sublingual NTG, should prompt a trial of nitrate therapy in patients who require chronic antianginal prophylaxis. Some patients cannot tolerate nitrates because of adverse side effects, and in such instances excellent alternative therapy is available. Reflex increase in sympathetic activity resulting in excessive tachycardia and contractility may blunt the efficacy of nitrates. Concomitant administration of β-adrenergic blocking agents prevents these undesirable effects and produces beneficial synergetic effects for the treatment of angina.

Nitrates are particularly indicated in patients with angina who have impaired left ventricular function or in those in whom it is believed that an element of coronary vasoconstriction or spasm plays a role in the ischemic syndrome. In several double-blind studies nitrates have been shown to be equally effective as calcium channel blockers for patients with variant or Prinzmetal's angina.[28] There are no available data to indicate which class of drugs is more effective in "mixed angina," and in fact there is no evidence demonstrating that nitrates are less effective than β-blockers or calcium channel blocking agents in any anginal syndrome.

Figure 4.9 lists angina patient subsets who should be preferentially considered for nitrate therapy.

UNSTABLE ANGINA PECTORIS

Nitrates are appropriate first-line therapy in patients with unstable angina. This syndrome, while variably defined, consists of accelerating angina and/or the onset of episodes of rest pain with objective evidence for myocardial ischemia. Such patients should be promptly hospitalized, usually in an intensive care unit. In this setting, the administration of NTG in intravenous or ointment form is usually beneficial.[29] Many of these patients may require an additional class of antianginal medication.

A variety of clinical investigations have demonstrated the benefits of nitrates when used aggressively in hospitalized patients with unstable angina.[30,31] It is possible that the antiplatelet actions of these compounds (see above) provide additional benefit in this syndrome. Most experts agree that an intravenous NTG infusion is a mainstay of therapy in severe unstable angina.

ACUTE MYOCARDIAL INFARCTION

The use of NTG and long-acting nitrates in the setting of acute myocardial necrosis has been the subject of numerous animal and human investigations. A variety of earlier studies indicated that nitrate adminis-

FIGURE 4.9 GUIDELINES FOR SELECTION OF ANGINA PATIENTS FOR LONG-ACTING NITRATE THERAPY

Demonstrated responsiveness to sublingual or oral NTG spray
Any normotensive subject with typical angina pectoris
Symptoms suggestive of intermittent increases in coronary vasomotor tone:
    Variable angina threshold
    Common occurrence of episodes of pain at rest or during slight physical activity
    Early morning angina
    Cold-induced angina
    Emotion-induced angina
Overt vasospastic anginal attacks
History or evidence of congestive heart failure
Depressed LV ejection fraction (<0.40) and/or major cardiomegaly
Presence of mitral regurgitation
Postinfarction angina
Relative or absolute contraindications of β-adrenergic blockers and/or calcium
    channel antagonists

tered early during acute myocardial infarction may reduce infarct size and decrease complications of acute myocardial infarction.[32] Nevertheless, until recently nitrate therapy in acute infarction has been limited to those patients with continuing or recurrent ischemic pain, acute heart failure, or hypertension. New data, however, suggest a more expanded role for nitrate therapy in acute infarction.[25,33]

A recent meta-analysis of a number of clinical trials employing intravenous nitroglycerin suggested a substantial mortality benefit over placebo-treated subjects when the drug was administered within the first 48 hours after admission.[34] More recently, an important trial from Canada demonstrated a major reduction of both early and late (1 year) mortality in patients with anterior wall myocardial infarction given intravenous NTG for 48 hours or more (Fig. 4.10).[25,33] Not only was mortality reduced, but many serious complications of acute infarction were decreased in the NTG-treated cohort; in addition, late postinfarction remodeling was prevented in the nitrate-treated patients.

Thus, it can now be suggested that routine (albeit careful) administration of nitroglycerin for 24 to 48 hours in the early hours of the postinfarction period may be appropriate in Q wave infarcts, particularly anterior. Such a recommendation may be premature, but the available data are most encouraging.[25,32–34] It had been previously suggested that patients who have had a myocardial infarction and who continue to take nitrates may have a better long-term prognosis than individuals who do not use nitrates.[24]

Nitrates are indicated in certain clinical situations following acute myocardial infarction. Recurrent episodes of chest pain may be effectively treated with intravenous or topical NTG. Patients with persistent hypertension represent another indication for nitrate therapy. In such cases intravenous NTG should be carefully administered to lower systolic blood pressure. Persistent hypertension may also be treated with sodium nitroprusside. The use of sodium nitroprusside in acute myocardial infarction may be deleterious in some patients,[32] particularly in those who are normotensive and do not show evidence of congestive heart failure.[35] For this reason some advocate that administration of intravenous NTG for complications of acute myocardial infarction may be a better initial choice than nitroprusside, although this remains controversial.

Patients with pump failure are definite candidates for nitrate administration. The beneficial effects of these drugs in individuals with depressed left ventricular function, particularly when ischemic, is often striking. NTG usually results in an improvement in left ventricular regional wall motion and global ejection fraction as well as a decrease in cardiac dimensions and left ventricular filling pressure. Nitrates may normalize ventricular dyssynergy.

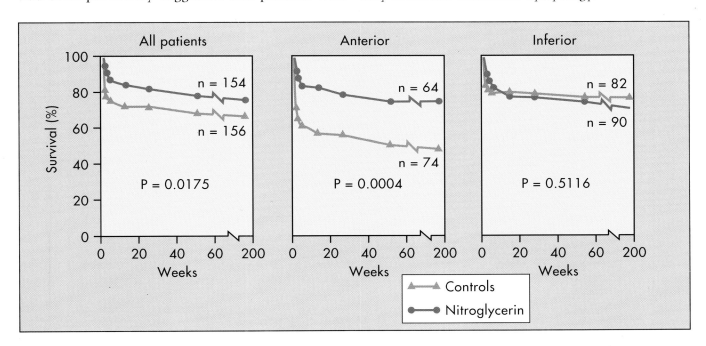

Figure 4.10 Improved mortality with the use of a 48-hour infusion of intravenous nitroglycerin in acute myocardial infarction. In this protocol, 310 patients, immediately after hospitalization, were randomized to begin an infusion of low-dose intravenous NTG or placebo. Mortality, both early and late, was decreased in the NTG group due to a marked reduction in early deaths in the anterior wall myocardial infarction cohort. There was a 46% reduction in hospital deaths up to 38 days from admission in the NTG patients, with the benefit mainly seen in the anterior Q wave infarction group. Note that the curves remain parallel for 43 months of follow-up. In addition, Kilip score, infarct expansion and extension, left ventricular thrombus, and cardiogenic shock were all considerably reduced in the NTG group. (Modified from Jugdutt BI, Warnica JW: Intravenous nitroglyerin therapy to limit myocardial infarct size, expansion, and complicaations. Effect of timing, dosage, and infarct location. Circulation 78:706, 1988)

The clinical indications for nitrate therapy in acute myocardial infarction are listed in Figure 4.11. It is important to ensure that the systolic arterial pressure and left ventricular filling pressure are adequate before using intravenous NTG. Invasive monitoring is essential in patients with complicated infarction.

Coronary Vasospasm

Organic nitrates are effective in reversing coronary vasospasm. This has been shown repeatedly in the cardiac catheterization laboratory. Sublingual NTG remains the drug of choice for acute episodes of chest pain in patients who have documented variant angina. In addition, long-acting nitrate therapy has been shown to be beneficial in this syndrome. Some experts believe that patients with documented coronary spasm should preferentially receive a calcium channel blocker, either alone or in combination with a long-acting nitrate. Nevertheless, available data at this time do not clearly indicate that calcium channel blockers are more effective than nitrates.

Congestive Heart Failure

Nitrates are one of the major classes of drugs that have been successfully employed for vasodilator treatment of congestive heart failure.[17,36,37] These agents have been repeatedly shown to be effective in Class III–IV patients with heart failure. Several well-designed double-blind studies indicate that nitrates have sustained beneficial actions over a period of months.[37,38]

The concept of vasodilator therapy is reviewed elsewhere. This therapeutic approach is based on the beneficial hemodynamic response of the failing or impaired left ventricle to afterload reduction. Afterload, defined as ventricular wall stress in early systole, is increased in patients with congestive heart failure. Left ventricular dilatation, an abnormal cavity–wall thickness ratio, and systemic arterial vasoconstriction all contribute to an increase in left ventricular wall stress. A reduction of afterload produced by an arteriolar vasodilator will result in improved left ventricular emptying with an augmented ejection fraction.[36]

Nitrates have a modest effect in increasing cardiac output in congestive heart failure compared with more potent arterial vasodilators, such as hydralazine. However, the action of nitrates in reducing left ventricular preload by systemic and regional bed venodilatation gives these drugs a unique advantage over relatively pure arterial vasodilators. Nitrates reduce pulmonary capillary wedge pressure and right heart filling pressures owing to a redistribution of circulating blood volume and increase in systemic venous pooling. At the same time the arteriolar vasodilating action of these drugs helps in "unloading" the left ventricle and results in enhanced systolic performance; left ventricular function improves and stroke volume usually rises. In patients with heart failure, nitrate-induced arteriolar vasodilatation results in enhanced left ventricular performance, and this prevents the decrease in cardiac output that typically accompanies the reduction in left ventricular preload occurring in normal subjects after nitrate administration.

It is difficult to demonstrate that nitrates significantly reduce left ventricular cavity size in patients with severe heart failure. Nitrates may decrease left ventricular compliance by reducing intrapericardial pressure. In patients with ischemic heart disease nitrates may have an additional beneficial effect if nutrient myocardial blood flow is increased. Nitrates usually improve mitral regurgitation, a common accompaniment of severe left ventricular decompensation.

ACUTE CONGESTIVE HEART FAILURE

Nitrates, particularly the rapid-acting formulations such as intravenous sublingual, oral spray, or buccal NTG, are very effective in decreasing the elevated left ventricular filling pressure of acute pulmonary edema. At the same time, the arteriolar vasodilating effects of nitrates reduce left ventricular work and improve forward cardiac output. Although there are limited published data on nitrate therapy in pulmonary edema or acute congestive heart failure, clinical experience indicates that these drugs are very useful adjunctive agents in reducing the signs and symptoms of severe pulmonary congestion.

CHRONIC CONGESTIVE HEART FAILURE

Numerous studies have shown that long-acting nitrates are beneficial for patients with chronic congestive heart failure.[36] Pulmonary capillary wedge and pulmonary artery pressure are reduced at rest and during exercise; stroke volume may increase modestly or remain unchanged but rarely falls after nitrate administration. Systemic and pulmonary vascular resistance decrease.

Several long-term trials indicate that nitrates maintain their effectiveness in reducing pulmonary capillary wedge pressure during chronic therapy.[37,38]

FIGURE 4.11 INDICATIONS FOR NITRATES IN ACUTE MYOCARDIAL INFARCTION

Persistent or recurrent chest pain
Sustained hypertension (BP >140/90 mm Hg)
Major left ventricular dysfunction: acute pulmonary edema or congestive heart failure
Diastolic dysfunction with high left ventricular filling pressure
Papillary muscle dysfunction with mitral regurgitation
Potential role for careful routine administration of intravenous NTG during the first 24–48 hours of acute
    Q wave infarction (see text)

Exercise performance in patients with congestive heart failure treated with isosorbide dinitrate (ISDN) increases over time when compared with placebo treatment.[38] Present evidence indicates that ISDN and angiotension converting enzyme inhibitors are the only vasodilator drugs that have consistently been shown to produce beneficial effects in patients with chronic congestive heart failure over a period of months.[37,38]

In summary, nitrates are an excellent choice for patients with symptoms of pulmonary venous congestion, such as orthopnea, paroxysmal nocturnal dyspnea, and dyspnea on exertion. Evidence of pulmonary congestion on radiography, the presence of rales on physical examination, and an elevated jugular venous pressure are all clues that nitrate administration will be beneficial. Patients with congestive heart failure typically require larger doses of nitrates than those with normal ventricles.

Of major importance have been the results of the Veterans Administration Cooperative Trials of Congestive Heart Failure that have demonstrated a significant long-term reduction in mortality in patients with heart failure treated with the combination of isosor-

bide dinitrate and hydralazine for several years (Fig. 4.12).[39,40] The initial trial, V-HEFT 1, provided the first evidence that any pharmacologic intervention in congestive heart failure can exert a positive benefit on mortality.[39] Although it is not known for certain which drug (or both) provided the protective benefit, it is likely that isosorbide dinitrate played an important role. This suggests but does not prove that long-term administration of nitrates in subjects with heart failure may be truly cardioprotective.

In V-HEFT 2, the same combination of hydralazine and isosorbide dinitrate was compared to enalapril in a comparable patient population.[40] In this trial, enalapril produced a greater survival benefit than the original drug combination. No placebo group was included. Because the baseline characteristics of the subjects appeared to be identical in the two V-HEFT trials, the investigators concluded that in V-HEFT 2 there was a protective effect from the ISDN–hydralazine combination, identical to V-HEFT 1, but this combination was not as potent as enalapril in reducing death from congestive heart failure.[40] Most experts believe that nitrates are more adjunctial as agents in heart failure when compared to ACE inhibitors.

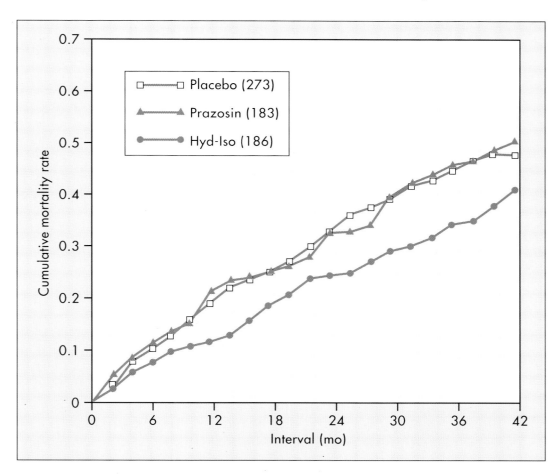

Figure 4.12 Improvement in mortality in the VA Cooperative Trial of Congestive Heart Failure. In this multicenter trial of patients with class II–III heart failure, individuals were treated with placebo, prazosin, or the combination of hydralazine, 75 mg qid, and isosorbide dinitrate, 40 mg qid (Hyd-Iso). There was a reduction of mortality seen at 1, 2, and 3 years after onset of the study; the major benefits were derived in the first year. This study was the first to document that medical therapy for congestive heart failure can impart an improvement in longevity. Subsequent analysis demonstrated that only persons with an increase in ejection fraction enjoyed a mortality benefit. (Modified from Cohn JN et al, 1986)

Additional Uses for Nitroglycerin and Long-Acting Nitrates

PULMONARY HYPERTENSION

Nitrates are effective pulmonary vasodilators. They reduce pulmonary vascular resistance and pulmonary artery pressure in a variety of conditions. Several studies indicate that intravenous NTG is quite effective in lowering pulmonary artery pressure after open heart surgery. Long-acting nitrates have been used successfully in occasional patients with chronic severe pulmonary hypertension. Recent studies show nitric oxide-induced vasodilation in pulmonary hypertension.

HYPERTENSION

During the 1940s and 1950s the organic nitrates were used for the treatment of hypertension. Although it is true that acute nitrate administration decreases systolic blood pressure, particularly in the upright position, tolerance to the hypotensive effects of these drugs rapidly occurs; after 1 or more weeks of therapy a given dose of nitrate no longer has the same effect on systemic arterial pressure as it did initially. Thus, these drugs are not appropriate choices for the outpatient treatment of hypertension. Nevertheless, a recent report suggests that oral ISDN has a favorable effect on systolic hypertension in the elderly.[41]

Acute administration of intravenous NTG, on the other hand, is a safe and effective mode of therapy for lowering blood pressure in the intensive care unit setting. Intravenous NTG infusion usually results in a gradual decline in blood pressure. The hypotensive effects are directly related to the infusion rate. With moderate to high concentrations of NTG, arteriolar vasodilatation occurs and the drug achieves a hypotensive potency comparable to sodium nitroprusside. Intravenous NTG does not lower blood pressure as rapidly as nitroprusside, diazoxide, or sublingual nifedipine. The magnitude and response time of blood pressure lowering may be greater with these other vasodilators, but this has not been subjected to rigorous clinical testing.

MITRAL REGURGITATION

Nitrates reduce the degree of the mitral regurgitation; the height of the left atrial *v* wave and mean atrial pressure fall after nitrate administration.[42] Stroke volume is often augmented. Nitrates are probably not as effective as are pure arterial vasodilators (such as hydralazine) in reducing the regurgitant fraction in mitral or aortic regurgitation. These drugs are particularly useful if there is underlying left ventricular dysfunction or in subjects with ischemic heart disease with papillary muscle dysfunction.

ESOPHAGEAL SPASM

Nitrates have potent relaxant effects on smooth muscle throughout the body, including the esophagus, gallbladder, and uterus. These actions have been used to prevent or reverse esophageal spasm in patients who have motility disorders of the esophagus.[43] In addition, efforts have been made to use nitrates to lower portal venous pressure in individuals with cirrhosis of the liver.

CONTROLLED ARTERIAL PRESSURE DURING SURGICAL PROCEDURES

Intravenous NTG has been effectively used to control blood pressure in a variety of surgical procedures. It has been used successfully to treat intraoperative and postoperative hypertension associated with coronary bypass grafting and has been employed to induce deliberate hypotension during neurosurgery, hip surgery, and abdominal aneurysm repair.[44,45]

INTERVENTIONAL CARDIOLOGY

The use of intravenous NTG has been increasing in patients undergoing percutaneous coronary angioplasty. This drug appears to be useful in preventing early spasm or reclosure of the target artery.[46] One study suggested a benefit in ventricular function when NTG was given in addition to intracoronary streptokinase in acute myocardial infarction.[47] It is likely that intravenous NTG given concomitantly with fibrinolytic therapy would have beneficial effects, although no major trials have been reported to date.

PHARMACOLOGY OF NITROGLYCERIN AND LONG-ACTING NITRATRES

A wide variety of organic nitrate esters are available to clinicians. Some agents, such as erythrityl tetranitrate and mannitol hexanitrate, have fallen into disuse. The most widely used compounds are NTG and

FIGURE 4.13 METABOLISM OF NITROGLYCERIN, ISOSORBIDE DINITRATE, AND 5-ISOSORBIDE MONONITRATE

Parent Compound/ Metabolites	Hemodynami- cally Active	Elimination Half-life
Nitroglycerin	Yes	1.5–4.5 min
1,2-glyceryl dinitrate	No	
1,3-glyceryl dinitrate	No	
Isosorbide dinitrate	Yes	1.2 hr
2-isosorbide mononitrate	Possible	1.8 hr
5-isosorbide mononitrate	Yes	4–4.5 hr

ISDN. The majority of published clinical investigative studies in patients with angina and congestive heart failure have been carried out with these two agents. Pentaerythritol tetranitrate and 5-isosorbide mononitrate (5-ISMN) are currently available. The former is not widely used, and clinical data supporting its efficacy are limited. On the other hand, 5-ISMN enjoys considerable popularity in Europe and has recently been approved in the United States for use in angina pectoris. This interesting compound is one of the two major metabolites of ISDN and has a much longer duration of action than ISDN (Figs. 4.13 and 4.14).[48,49]

Metabolism of Nitroglycerin, Isosorbide Dinitrate, and 5-Isosorbide Mononitrate (see Figure 4.13)

NITROGLYCERIN

The half-life of NTG is very short (less than 5 minutes). NTG is rapidly converted into two inactive metabolites, the 1,2- and 1,3-glyceryl dinitrates. Both metabolites are found in the urine after oral administration. These compounds have little hemodynamic activity. Because of the large amounts of the enzyme glutathione organic nitrate reductase in the liver, it has been assumed that hepatic metabolism is solely responsible for NTG degradation. This led to the hypothesis that orally administered nitrates could not produce clinically useful effects because of potent hepatic first-pass metabolism. It is now recognized that the blood vessels of the body directly metabolize nitrates and appear to be responsible for considerable degradation of these compounds,[9,49] particularly after systemic (nonoral) administration. After intravenous administration of NTG there is a large systemic arteriovenous NTG gradient with higher arterial than venous NTG concentrations.[50] This observation is consistent with substantial vascular uptake of NTG.

NTG is available in the United States in sublingual, intravenous, oral spray, buccal, oral, ointment, and transdermal disc or patch formulations.

ISOSORBIDE DINITRATE AND 5-ISOSORBIDE MONONITRATE

ISDN and 5-ISMN have theoretic advantages over NTG because of their much longer half-lives as well as higher plasma nitrate concentations. ISDN is converted to two active metabolites, 2- and 5-isosorbide mononitrate. While both metabolites have vasodilatory activity, 5-ISMN is more potent than 2-ISMN and achieves higher blood levels. 5-ISMN has been shown to be an effective drug for the treatment of angina and congestive heart failure, and has been approved in the United States for use in angina. The metabolism and clearance of the parent compound ISDN is more rapid than that of the metabolites; after dosing, plasma concentrations of ISDN are considerably lower than those of 5-ISMN and 2-ISMN.[48,49,51] Plasma levels of 5-ISMN remain elevated for hours (Fig. 4.14). The half-life of 5-ISMN is approximately 4 1/2 hours, considerably longer than that of ISDN.

Only 20% to 25% of an oral dose of ISDN is bioavailable because of active hepatic nitrate metabolism.[51] The metabolites of ISDN appear unchanged in the urine. 5-ISMN, however, does not undergo hepatic metabolism and is therefore virtually completely bioavailable. This compound appears to have

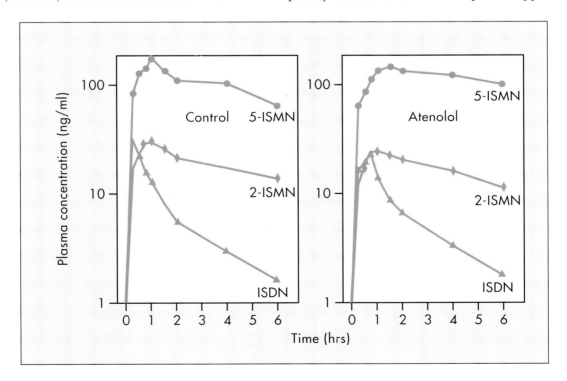

Figure 4.14 Plasma concentrations of isosorbide dinitrate (ISDN), isosorbide 2-mononitrate (2-ISMN), and isosorbide 5-mononitrate (5-SMN) following administration of 10 mg of oral ISDN before and after treatment with 100 mg of atenolol. Note that the plasma concentration of 5-ISMN is substantially higher than that of the parent compound ISDN and that 5-ISMN persists in the plasma at a constant level for several hours longer than ISDN. β-Blocker administration did not alter ISDN pharmacokinetics. (Modified from Bogaert MG, Rosseel MT: Fate of orally given isosorbide dinitrate in man: Factors of variability. Z Kardiol 72(Suppl 3):11, 1983)

a vasodilating potency at least equal to ISDN; some believe that 5-ISMN is responsible for the majority of nitrate effect following oral administration of ISDN. Approximately 60% of a dose of ISDN is converted to 5-ISMN. It is estimated that 40 mg of oral ISDN is approximately equivalent to 20 mg of 5-ISMN.

ISDN is currently available in sublingual, chewable, and oral formulations. Intravenous ISDN and topical ISDN cream have been clinically tested and are used in other countries. An oral ISDN spray is available in West Germany, and a new translucent plastic wrap impregnated with ISDN may undergo clinical trials in the future.

5-ISMN is now available in a standard oral formulation in the United States. In Europe and Scandinavia, sustained release 5-ISMN is widely used, and this formulation has recently been approved for use in the United States.

NITRATE PLASMA CONCENTRATIONS

There is considerable uncertainty and controversy regarding the value of nitrate blood levels. It is not easy to obtain accurate and reliable measurements of NTG, ISDN, and 5-ISMN, although the latter two are more readily assayed because their higher plasma concentrations and longer half-lives. Gas chromatographic techniques for nitrate measurement have become available in recent years, but these assays are performed in only a very few laboratories because of technical difficulties in obtaining reliable and reproducible data.

In acute dosing studies, NTG plasma nitrate concentrations bear a proportional relationship to the hemodynamic effects of the administered drug. However, with chronic dosing, plasma nitrate concentrations no longer are predictive of the hemodynamic effects (Fig. 4.15).[52] It has been observed that plasma nitrate concentrations tend to increase with chronic dosing (see Fig. 4.15).[52,53] This appears to result from a decreased clearance of the parent nitrate compound apparently due to a reduction of vascular nitrate metabolism.[9,49] Alterations in nitrate vascular kinetics with chronic dosing may be related to the development of nitrate tolerance.[49] Uptake and metabolism of organic nitrate by veins and arteries is diminished in the presence of nitrate tolerance; tolerance is associated with higher plasma nitrate levels (see Fig. 4.15) and decreased clearance of the drug from the systemic circulation.[9]

Factors Influencing Nitrate Pharmacokinetics

Data have become available evaluating potential alterations of nitrate metabolism during varying physiologic states. It is difficult to demonstrate any significant impact on nitrate metabolism during differing clinical conditions. Plasma ISDN and 5-ISMN levels are not affected by whether the dose is taken before or after a meal; cigarette smoking does not alter ISDN pharmacokinetics.[54] Nitrate levels do not appear to be affected by the presence of reduced renal function.[55] Limited data do suggest that in cirrhotic patients plasma ISDN concentrations may be higher after oral dosing.[55] Congestive heart failure does not appear to affect nitrate kinetics.[54] β-Blockers and cimetidine, drugs that are known to alter hepatic enymatic function and thus potentially alter the metabolism of other drugs, do not influence nitrate metabolism (see Fig. 4.14).[55]

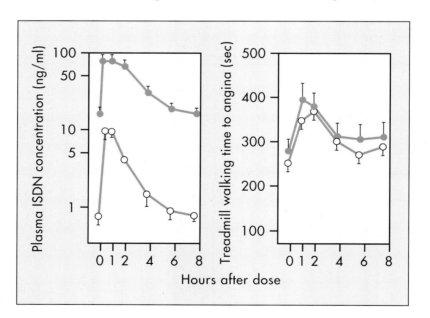

Figure 4.15 Relationship of plasma isosorbide dinitrate (ISDN) concentration to improvement in treadmill walking time in a double-blind, placebo-controlled study of patients with angina. These data from the study of Thadani and co-workers[52] compare plasma ISDN concentrations and treadmill walking time in patients who took 15 mg of ISDN four times daily for 1 week (open circles) and 120 mg of ISDN four times daily for 1 week (closed circles). In the acute dosing study (not illustrated) there was a dose–response relationship between the amount of administered ISDN and improvement in treadmill walking time. However, after chronic short-term therapy the small dose of 15 mg produced the same improvement as the large dose of 120 mg; both resulted in marked attenuation of exercise improvement at 4, 6, and 8 hours, a finding indicative of nitrate tolerance. During the acute dosing study, exercise performance was improved over a placebo from 4 to 8 hours (not shown). Plasma ISDN concentrations were higher after chronic therapy than with acute dosing. (Modified from Fung H-L: Pharmacokinetic determinants of nitrate action. Am J Med 76:22, 1984)

Nitrate Delivery Systems

A wide variety of nitrate formulations are presently available.[56] Nitrates are well absorbed across the skin and mucosal surfaces, and the diverse dosing forms take advantage of this characteristic. When a sufficient amount of oral nitrate is given, hepatic metabolism is readily bypassed and "therapeutic" concentrations of nitroglycerin and ISDN appear in the blood.

The currently available nitrate delivery systems, dose recommendations, the time to peak effect, and the total duration of activity of each compound are listed in Figure 4.16. Nitrate pharmacokinetics in a given patient are not predictable; the pharmacokinetic information listed in Figure 4.16 represents averages of many studies.

Rapid-Onset Formulations

SUBLINGUAL NITRATES

The gold standard of therapy for angina attacks is sublingual NTG, an extremely effective formulation. Sublingual or chewable ISDN tablets are also useful for acute therapy, but their onset of action is somewhat slower than that of sublingual NTG. Sublingual ISDN has a longer duration of activity than sublingual NTG and may be desirable for patients who need sustained protection after an episode of angina. Neither of these formulations represent practical therapy for long-term angina prophylaxis in individuals who have frequent attacks of chest pain.

It is important for patients with angina to be instructed to use sublingual NTG or ISDN prophylactically *prior to* activities or situations that are likely to induce chest pain. If this is done, potential angina attacks can be prevented and patients may be able to conduct normal activities without interruption. Oral NTG and ISDN sprays have been evaluated that appear to be effective in aborting episodes of angina. An oral NTG spray has recently become available in the United States. It acts comparably to sublingual NTG.

BUCCAL OR TRANSMUCOSAL NITROGLYCERIN

A buccal tablet of NTG has been available for several years, consisting of NTG dispersed in a special cellulose matrix.[56,57] The unique property of buccal NTG is its extremely rapid onset of action combined with sustained hemodynamic and clinical effects. The medication is placed in the buccal pouch between the upper lip and teeth. A gel or seal rapidly forms and the tablet subsequently adheres to the mucosa. Most patients find that they can eat, drink, and talk without difficulty once the medication is in place. NTG is released immediately across the mucosal membranes into the rich capillary bed of the mouth; the onset of NTG effect is as rapid as with sublingual NTG.[57] Thus, this drug can be used for acute prophylaxis of anginal attacks instead of sublingual NTG or ISDN. NTG is absorbed at a constant rate while the buccal tablet remains intact in the mouth. Studies have indicated that the average duration of availability of the tablet ranges between 3 and 6 hours. NTG plasma concentrations are well in the therapeutic range after buccal NTG administration.[57]

Long-Acting Nitrates

ORAL NITRATES

Both NTG and ISDN have been available for many years. These drugs are manufactured in standard formulation and as sustained-action tablets or capsules.

Oral nitrates produce prolonged hemodynamic effects that last from 3 to 8 hours with acute dosing. Therapeutic plasma concentrations are sustained for many hours. Unfortunately, gastrointestinal absorption of oral nitrates is variable and unpredictable from one patient to the next. Thus, a fixed oral dose of NTG or ISDN should not be employed; rather, patients should be given oral nitrates in increasing amounts until the clinical syndrome is well controlled and/or side-effects occur.

Numerous studies attest to the efficacy of ISDN in both angina pectoris and congestive heart fail-

---

FIGURE 4.16 SUBLINGUAL AND LONG-ACTING NITROGLYCERIN, ISOSORBIDE DINITRATE AND ISOSORBIDE 5-MONONITRATE: PHARMACOKINETICS AND RECOMMENDED DOSAGE

Medication	Recommended Dosage (mg)*	Onset of Action (minutes)	Peak Action (minutes)	Duration
Sublingual NTG	0.3–0.8	2–5	4–8	10–30 minutes
Sublingual ISDN	2.5–10	5–20	15–60	45–120 minutes†
Oral NTG spray	0.4	2–5	4–8	10–30 minutes
Buccal NTG	1–3	2–5	4–10	30–300 minutes
Oral ISDN	10–60	15–45	45–120	2–6 hours
Oral 5-ISMN‡	20	30–90	90–180	2–8 hours
Oral NTG	6.5–19.5	20–45	45–120	2–6 hours
NTG ointment (2%)	1/2–2 inches	15–60	30–120	3–8 hours
NTG discs (transdermal)	10–20 mg	30–60	60–180	Up to 24 hours§

* Higher doses may be needed, especially in congestive heart failure.
† Up to 3 to 4 hours in some studies.
‡ Give 2 doses daily, 7 hours apart.
§ Clinical effects may not persist for 24 hours.
NTG = Nitroglycerin; ISDN = Isosorbide dinitrate

ure.[21,26-28,36,38,52] This compound has been investigated more thoroughly than any other nitrate. Data on oral NTG are more limited. It is probable that when sufficient oral NTG is given its effects are similar to those of ISDN, although direct comparative studies are few. Many experts believe that oral ISDN is a more effective formulation than oral NTG.

Oral 5-ISMN, now available in the United States, is approved to be given twice daily in an asymmetric dosing regimen, with 7 hours between doses. This unusual recommendation is based on the pharmacokinetics of this compound, which has the longest half-life of any organic nitrate used in clinical medicine. Studies have shown antianginal protection after the first and second doses, when 20 mg of 5-ISMN is given at 8 AM and 2 PM.[58] There are very few comparative studies of ISDN and 5-ISMN. It is likely that these compounds are equally effective; the dose of oral ISDN is approximately twice that of 5-ISMN to achieve a comparable effect.

Patients too often receive smaller doses of oral nitrates than are optimal. Although high-dose nitrate therapy may be more likely to induce nitrate tolerance, it is important that a dose be established that is clinically effective. Physicians should follow patients closely when nitrate therapy is instituted. In those with angina pectoris, angina attack rates should be markedly decreased with an effective dosing regimen. In congestive heart failure, it is best to carefully assess clinical parameters, such as the signs and symptoms of pulmonary congestion, as a rough guide to dose adequacy.

It is important to begin nitrate therapy with low doses and then to increase the dosage to reach an effective dosing regimen. At the same time, one should always attempt to use as little nitrate as possible because of the possibility that higher doses will more readily induce nitrate tolerance. The physician must strike a balance in prescribing a nitrate dosing regimen that ensures nitrate efficacy while minimizing the likelihood of tolerance.

NITROGLYCERIN OINTMENT

A 2% NTG ointment formulation has been available for many years. In 1974 Reichek and co-workers published the results of a double-blind, placebo-controlled study that demonstrated a prolonged (3-hour) protective action of 2% NTG ointment in patients with angina.[59] Numerous other investigations in patients with angina and heart failure have demonstrated the effectiveness of NTG ointment. The effects of this compound last 4 to 6 hours or longer in acute dosing trials.

As with oral nitrates the effective dosage of NTG ointment is variable and unpredictable. There is some argument about the size of the skin area over which the ointment should be spread; some believe that a 6 x 6-inch area is necessary, while others believe that a smaller surface area is satisfactory. It is best to spread the NTG ointment on the chest or arms. This formulation is relatively messy and readily soils clothes. It is particularly useful for patients in intensive care units who require the long-acting nitrates. A recently developed adhesive unit that prevents leakage of the ointment from the bandage has made NTG ointment more practical for active patients.

NTG ointment should also be considered in patients who have nocturnal symptoms of chest pain or those with congestive heart failure who have orthopnea and paroxysmal nocturnal dyspnea.

TRANSDERMAL NITROGLYCERIN PATCHES

The NTG disc or patch units were introduced in 1982 and have received an enthusiastic welcome by patients and physicians. The NTG discs consist of NTG impregnated into a silicone gel or matrix. The discs provide a constant NTG delivery across the skin barrier for 24 to 48 hours, at a release rate of approximately 0.5 mg NTG per square centimeter of disc area. New FDA guidelines require manufacturers to list the actual NTG release rate per hour for each size of dosing unit.

A number of investigations indicate that lower doses of the disc (0.2 to 0.4 mg/h) are not very effective in many patients with angina.[60,61] One should begin with a minimum of 0.4 mg/h and increase the NTG dose to 0.8 to 1.6 mg/h in patients who continue to have the symptoms of angina or heart failure. In the latter situation, particularly large doses are usually necessary.

The NTG patches have stimulated a considerable amount of controversy since their introduction. Early studies suggested less than optimal efficacy in "standard" doses (e.g., 5 to 10 mg per 24 hours). It is not clear that a predictable and classic nitrate effect can be obtained with higher doses; in general, a minimum of 10 to 15 mg per 24 hours (0.4 to 0.6 mg/h) is necessary, and often more, especially in heart failure patients.

The more important aspect of the patch controversy was stimulated by early observations that classic nitrate effects appeared in many studies to wane by 24 hours in angina and congestive heart failure.[60-63] A subsequent major investigation has confirmed this phenomenon in a large number of patients.[64] Although not every subject will become tolerant to continuous patch administration, this is likely to occur in the majority of individuals. Many clinical investigations of tolerance have confirmed that dosing regimens designed to provide sustained nitrate exposure to the vasculature will readily induce some degree of attenuation of nitrate activity. The NTG patches have been a pharmacologic innovation that has elucidated much information about tolerance.

It is now well established that an intermittent or on-off dosing strategy can maintain responsiveness to NTG patches (Fig. 4.17).[65-67] Thus, removing the unit nightly for 10 to 12 hours is a reasonable strategy that will provide continued nitrate efficacy during the patch-on period.

Intravenous Nitroglycerin

Intravenous NTG has been commercially available in the United States since the early 1980s. This formulation has achieved widespread popularity in intensive care units. It is an excellent drug for patients with acute myocardial infarction complicated by hypertension, recurrent chest pain, or pump failure. Intravenous NTG is also useful in acute pulmonary edema or severe congestive heart failure.

Intravenous NTG has a rapid onset of action; similarly, its effects quickly disappear when the infusion is discontinued. At low NTG concentrations venodilatation is dominant, but as the infusion rate increases arterial and arteriolar vasodilatation occur and systemic vascular resistance decreases (see Fig. 4.2).

It is not necessary to use specialized polyethylene tubing and infusion sets when administering intravenous NTG. This has been suggested because NTG is readily absorbed onto conventional polyvinyl chloride (PVC) tubing. In one study it was demonstrated that the benefits of using polyethylene tubing instead of PVC tubing were insignificant.[68]

Intravenous NTG infusion should begin at a rate 5 to 20 μg/min and be increased by 5 to 10 μg/min every 5 to 10 minutes until the desired clinical or hemodynamic effect is achieved. Hypotension, tachycardia, nausea, and headache are potential complications. Particular care should be used in hypovolemic patients.

PROBLEMS WITH NITRATE THERAPY

The two major areas of difficulty resulting from nitrate administration are the acute side effects and the potential for induction of nitrate tolerance.

Adverse Effects

Classic nitrate side effects include headache and dizziness. Headaches are the most debilitating feature relating to nitrate administration and preclude continuation of long-acting nitrates in approximately 20% of patients. The headache may be mild or intense; it may consist of a throbbing sensation or a severe generalized headache. Nitrate headaches frequently attenuate or completely disappear after several days to 2 weeks of daily therapy. If patients take mild analgesics concomitantly with nitrates for several days they will often be able to tolerate nitrates on a long-term basis when the headaches disappear. Some subjects, however, refuse to use sublingual NTG or other nitrates because of an unhappy experience with initial doses. It is important for the physician to inform patients in advance that headache is to be expected and to encourage the short-term use of analgesics.

Nausea and vomiting occasionally result from nitrate therapy, but these symptoms are not usually serious or persistent. Acute hypotensive reactions to sublingual NTG or other nitrates may cause dizziness and even syncope. These reactions tend not to persist, since the blood pressure and heart rate responses following nitrate administration rapidly become attenuated with chronic dosing.

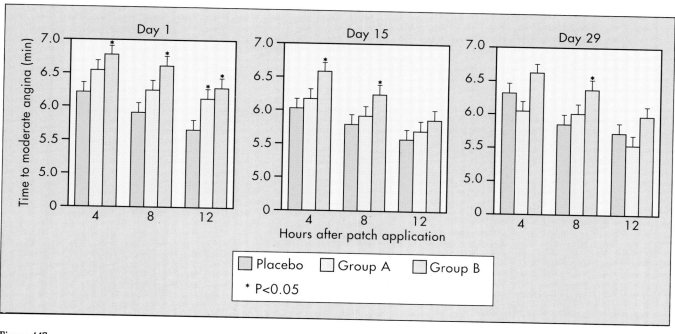

Figure 4.17 Efficacy of intermittent nitroglycerin patch administration to avoid tolerance in angina pectoris. The results are from a multicenter placebo-controlled trial involving 215 randomized patients. The groups included placebo, low-dose transdermal NTG (10–20 cm², group A) and high-dose transdermal NTG (30–40 cm², group B). Patients wore a placebo or active patch for 12 hours each day for a total of 29 days. Treadmill time to angina of moderate intensity is shown in the vertical column for each group at 4, 8, and 12 hours on the three testing days: days 1, 15, and 29. An antianginal response was seen in the high-dose group on day 1 and day 15 (except at 12 hours); after 1 month, exercise duration was longer than placebo at all testing intervals but reached statistical significance only at hour 8 on day 29. There was a reduction in anginal attacks and sublingual NTG consumption per week in both groups, although the frequency of angina was low in this study. A retrospective analysis of the 20-cm² group indicated that there was a similar trend toward improvement of angina, compared with placebo, at this dosage strength. Attenuation or tolerance seemed to be more of a problem after 4 weeks of long-term therapy compared with day 15 in both dosing groups. (Modified from DeMots H, Glasser SP. Intermittent transdermal nitroglycerin therapy in the treatment of chronic stable angina. J Am Coll Cardiol 13:786, 1989)

Topical nitrates may cause skin irritation and dermatitis. The adhesive or metallic components of the NTG discs may result in erythema and occasional skin reactions.

Paradoxic bradycardia and hypotension may follow sublingual or intravenous nitrate administration (Fig. 4.18).[69] Such reactions usually occur when sublingual NTG is given to a patient with acute myocardial infarction or ischemia. This paradoxic response to nitroglycerin appears to result from reflex activation of afferent cardiac mechanoreceptors (Bezold-Jarisch reflex) and can be promptly reversed by administration of atropine.

NTG has been shown to reduce systemic oxygen saturation in patients with chronic obstructive lung disease. In patients with right ventricular dysfunction related to pulmonary hypertension, NTG may decrease right ventricular stroke work as well as right ventricular diastolic dimensions. Thus, in patients with significant chronic lung disease the use of nitrates might be deleterious, although the clinical significance of these observations remains to be elucidated. In patients with right ventricular infarction, cardiac output and blood pressure may decrease markedly following administration of NTG and nitrates and therefore these drugs should be avoided.

Several investigators have measured elevated methemoglobin levels in patients receiving large amounts of nitrates.[70] The clinical significance of this problem is minimal. It is not necessary to monitor methemoglobin levels in patients on chronic nitrate therapy, although this might be a consideration in a subject receiving enormous doses of NTG who develops unexplained cyanosis.[45]

Nitrate Tolerance

Tolerance to NTG and long-acting nitrates is a controversial problem that has been argued for many years.[4,71–74] The development of nitrate vascular tolerance occurs rapidly in experimental animals given frequent doses of NTG. It has long been known that the blood pressure reduction following acute nitrate administration rapidly becomes attenuated. Decreased blood pressure and heart rate responses as well as the loss of headaches during chronic therapy certainly represent manifestations of nitrate tolerance. Until recently, however, it had not been demonstrated unequivocally that the desired clinical actions of these drugs become less effective during chronic therapy.

Many studies, particularly from Europe and Canada, indicate that clinically relevant tolerance to nitrates is a real phenomenon and is more common than previously thought.[2,52,73,74] In one early investigation in patients with angina pectoris it was demonstrated that the duration of effect of ISDN shortened considerably and the dose–response relationship between the amount of administered ISDN and the resultant beneficial effects on treadmill walking time disappeared after several weeks of ISDN therapy.[52] As discussed previously, many additional reports have documented the development of partial or complete nitrate tolerance in angina pectoris and congestive heart failure with various dosing regimens and nitrate compounds.

Parker and colleagues have shown that chronic therapy with NTG discs or a long-acting ISDN cream resulted in complete attenuation of nitrate

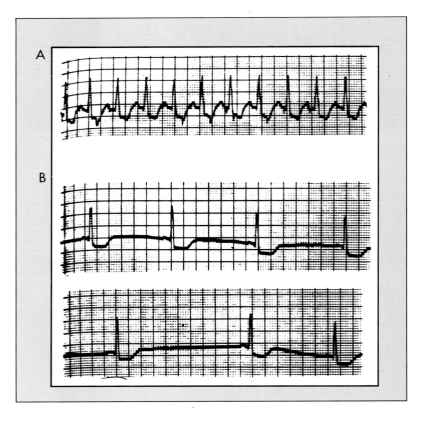

Figure 4.18 Profound sinus bradycardia and arterial hypotension developing in a patient with an acute anteroseptal myocardial infarction and congestive heart failure given an intravenous infusion of nitroglycerin. The fall in the heart rate was associated with a marked decline in mean arterial pressure from 84 mm Hg to 36 mm Hg, as well as a substantial drop in the pulmonary artery diastolic pressure, which fell from 23 mm Hg to 7 mm Hg. All hemodynamic parameters returned to baseline after administration of intravenous atropine and discontinuation of intravenous nitroglycerin. Reinfusion of nitroglycerin at a lower rate than before produced similar but less marked changes 30 minutes later. **A** Before NTG. **B** After NTG. (Come PC, Pitt B: Nitroglycerin-induced severe hypotension and bradycardia in patients with acute myocardial infarction. Circulation 54:624, 1976)

effect at all testing intervals in patients with angina.[53,63] These data suggest that any nitrate formulation providing 12 or more hours of sustained nitrate availability may induce a more complete form of tolerance than intermittent nitrate dosing regimens.

Tolerance is not related to a specific formulation. Large doses, frequent dosing schedules, and sustained-acting formulations are all pro-tolerant; conversely, small doses, less frequent dosing, and shorter-acting compounds may avoid the induction of tolerance. Of great importance is the presence or absence of a *nitrate-free interval* each day. Thus, a designated period of no nitrate exposure each day for at least 10 to 12 hours should be part of each patient's dosing program. Fewer doses, e.g., two to three times daily for oral nitrates, have been associated with less tolerance.[75,76] Twelve to 14 hours of NTG patch application, with removal on a daily basis, are also recommended.[65-67] It is important for the vasculature to be exposed to declining nitrate plasma levels for a protracted period each day; the longer the better.

Guidelines for Nitrate Therapy

Current recommendations for nitrate therapy should take into account the newer data regarding nitrate tolerance (Fig. 4.19). Nitrates are best administered using the smallest effective dose and the least number of doses that control the clinical syndrome. Sustained-action formulations, transdermal NTG discs,

and large or frequent nitrate doses may quickly induce a hyperreactive state in blood vessels. Intermittent nitrate therapy employing a nitrate-free interval of at least 8 to 10 hours may avoid or delay the development of nitrate tolerance. Many patients treated with nitrates do not need "around the clock" protection; clinicians should give serious consideration to having patients take the last daily dose of nitrates in the late afternoon or early evening, including the NTG patches.

ISDN should be administered two to three times daily, but not four times per day. Oral 5-ISMN can also induce tolerance. The standard formulations of 5-ISMN have been shown to produce attenuation of effect when given every 12 hours in some studies, but not all. Sustained release 5-ISMN, soon to be available in America, readily induces tolerance when given twice a day. The current dosing recommendation for regular-acting 5-ISMN is twice daily with a 7 hour interval between the first and second doses (e.g., 7–8 AM, 2–3 PM). Figure 4.20 indicates current recommendations for long-acting nitrate compounds.

CLINICAL IMPLICATIONS

Nitrate therapy represents one of the oldest forms of treatment for cardiovascular diseases. Physicians have had extensive experience with these agents,

FIGURE 4.19 CURRENT GUIDELINES FOR INITIATION OF NITRATE THERAPY

1. Begin with small dose.
2. Establish a dose threshold that achieves the desired clinical effect.
3. Use the least amount of nitrate that provides continued symptomatic benefit.
4. Use caution with sustained-action formulations; these preparations may more readily induce nitrate tolerance.
5. Establish a dosing regimen that provides a nitrate-free interval of at least 10–12 hours each day.

FIGURE 4.20 SPECIFIC DOSING RECOMMENDATIONS FOR LONG-ACTING NITRATES

Nitroglycerin	
Buccal	1–3 mg bid–tid
Patch	0.4–0.8 mg/hr for 12–14 hrs; remove 10–12 hr
Isosorbide dinitrate	
Regular	20–60 mg bid–tid
Sustained release	80–120 mg once daily
5-Isosorbide mononitrate	
Regular	20 mg bid, 7 hours apart (e.g., taken 7–8 AM, 2–3 PM)
Sustained release	40–60 mg once daily

which are relatively safe and well tolerated. Side effects are circumscribed and predictable. These drugs are not costly, although the NTG disc systems are expensive.

Nitrates have important actions in patients with ischemic heart disease. These compounds lower the preload and afterload of the heart and result in a reduction in myocardial energy requirements and an increased efficiency of left ventricular ejection. Nitrates have direct effects on the coronary circulation, such as increasing coronary collateral flow, stenosis dilatation, and enhancement of nutrient subendocardial perfusion during myocardial ischemia. These actions may be important in relieving chest pain in a variety of anginal syndromes. Nitrates are beneficial in acute myocardial infarction complicated by hypertension, recurrent chest pain, or congestive heart failure. Routine administration of these compounds in acute myocardial infarction is not indicated. There are suggestive data that long-term nitrate administration in patients who have chronic coronary heart disease may improve longevity. Nitrates in the post-MI subject may limit remodelling.

Nitrates are useful in congestive heart failure. These drugs lower intracardiac filling pressures and improve exercise capacity when taken for several weeks or months. They are particularly indicated in patients who have signs and symptoms of an elevated pulmonary capillary wedge pressure, or pulmonary hypertension, or associated right ventricular failure.

Nitrate side effects of headache and transient hypotension are common with initial therapy but usually attenuate over time. Some patients cannot be maintained on long-term nitrate administration because of adverse effects. Nitrate tolerance remains a problem, but its clinical implications are still unclear. It is prudent to use the least amount of nitrate that controls the clinical syndrome.

Patients with angina, acute myocardial infarction, and congestive heart failure can derive important clinical benefits from the proper use of nitrate therapy. When used intelligently these drugs provide consistent and effective cardiovascular therapy at low cost and with rare serious side effects.

REFERENCES

1. Needleman P, Johnson EM: The pharmacological and biochemical interaction of organic nitrates with sulfhydryls: Possible correlations with the mechanism for tolerance development, vasodilation and mitochondrial and enzyme reactions. In Needleman P (ed): Organic Nitrates. Handbook of Experimental Pharmacology, vol 40, pp 97–114. New York, Springer-Verlag, 1975

2. Armstrong PW, Moffat JA: Tolerance to organic nitrates: Clinical and experimental perspectives. Am J Med 74(Suppl):73, 1983

3. Kowaluk E, Fung HL: Pharmacology and pharmacokinetics of organic nitrates. In Abrams J, Pepine C, Thadani V (eds): Medical Therapy of Ischemic Heart Disease, pp 151–176. Boston, Little, Brown & Co, 1992

4. Levin RI, Jaffe EA, Weksler BB et al: Nitroglycerin stimulates synthesis of prostaglandin by cultured human endothelial cells. J Clin Invest 67:762, 1981

5. Rehr RB, Jackson JA, Winniford MD et al: Mechanism of nitroglycerin-induced coronary dilatation: Lack of relations to intracoronary thromboxane concentrations. Am J Cardiol 54:971, 1984

6. Lam JYT, Chesebro JH, Fuster V: Platelets, vasoconstriction and nitroglycerin during arterial wall injury. Circulation 78:712, 1988

7. Diodati J, Theroux P, Latour J-G et al: Nitroglycerin at therapeutic doses inhibits platelet aggregation in man. J Am Coll Cardiol 11:54A, 1988

8. Johnstone M, Lam JYT, Waters D: The antithrombotic action of nitroglycerin: Cyclic GMP as a potential mediator. J Am Coll Cardiol 13:231A, 1989

9. Fung H-L, Sutton SC, Kamiya A: Blood vessel uptake and metabolism of organic nitrates in the rat. J Pharmacol Exp Ther 228:334, 1984

10. McGregor M: Pathogenesis of angina pectoris and role of nitrates in relief of myocardial ischemia. Am J Med 74(Suppl):21, 1983

11. Kelly R, Gibbs R, Morgan J, et al: Nitroglycerin has more favorable effects on left ventricular afterload than apparent from measurements of pressure in peripheral artery. Eur Heart J 11: 138–144, 1990

12. Mason DT, Braunwald E: The effects of nitroglycerin and amyl nitrite on arteriolar and venous tone in the human forearm. Circulation 32:755, 1965

13. Vatner SF, Pagani M, Rutherford JD et al: Effects of nitroglycerin on cardiac performance and regional blood flow distribution in conscious dogs. Am J Physiol 234(3):H244, 1978

14. Ferrer MI, Bradley SE, Wheeler HO et al: Some effects of nitroglycerin upon the splanchnic, pulmonary and systemic circulations. Circulation 33:357, 1966

15. Manyari DE, Smith ER, Spragg J: Isosorbide dinitrate and glyceryl trinitrate: Demonstration of cross tolerance in the capacitance vessels. Am J Cardiol 55:927, 1985

16. Abrams J: Hemodynamic effects of nitroglycerin and long-acting nitrates. Am Heart J 110(Part 2):216, 1985

17. Leier CV, Magorien RD, Desch CE et al: Hydralazine and isosorbide dinitrate: Comparative central and regional hemodynamic effects when administered alone or in combination. Circulation 63:102, 1981

18. Ganz W, Marcus HS: Failure of intracoronary nitroglycerin to alleviate pacing-induced angina. Circulation 46:880, 1972

19. Brown G, Bolson E, Petersen RB et al: The mechanisms of nitroglycerin action: Stenosis vasodilatation as a major component of drug response. Circulation 64:1089, 1981

20. Conti CR, Feldman RL, Pepine CJ et al: Effect of glyceryl trinitrate on coronary and systemic hemodynamics in man. Am J Med 74(Suppl):28, 1984

21. Abrams J: The role of nitroglycerin and long-acting nitrates in the treatment of angina. In Weiner

DA, Frishman W (eds): Therapy of Angina, pp 53–81. New York, Marcel Dekker, 1986

22. Gage JE, Hess OM, Murakami T et al: Vasoconstriction of stenotic coronary arteries during dynamic exercise in patients with classic angina pectoris: reversibility by nitroglycerin. Circulation 73:865, 1986

23. Ludmer PL, Selwyn AP, Shook TL et al: Paradoxical vasoconstriction induced by acetylcholine in atherosclerotic coronary arteries. N Engl J Med 315:1046, 1986

24. Rapaport E, Remedios P: The high risk patient after recovery from myocardial infarction: Recognition and management. J Am Coll Cardiol 1: 391, 1983

25. Jugdutt BI, Warnica JW: Intravenous nitroglycerin therapy to limit myocardial infarct size, expansion, and complications. Effect of timing, dosage, and infarct location. Circulation 78:706, 1988

26. Hoekenga D, Abrams J: Rational medical therapy for stable angina pectoris. Am J Med 76:309, 1984

27. Abrams J: Usefulness of long-acting nitrates in cardiovascular disease. Am J Med 64:183, 1978

28. Hill JA, Feldman RL, Pepine CJ et al: Randomized double-blind comparison of nifedipine and isosorbide dinitrate in patients with coronary arterial spasm. Am J Cardiol 49:431, 1982

29. Curfman GD, Heinsimer JA, Lozner EC et al: Intravenous nitroglycerin in the treatment of spontaneous angina pectoris: A prospective randomized trial. Circulation 67:276, 1983

30. Conti CR: Use of nitrates in unstable angina pectoris. Am J Cardiol 60:31H, 1987

31. Horowitz JD, Henry CA, Syranen ML, et al: Combined use of nitroglycerin and N-acetylcysteine in the management of unstable angina pectoris. Circulation 77:787, 1988

32. Flaherty JT: Comparison of intravenous nitroglycerin and sodium nitroprusside in acute myocardial infarction. Am J Med 74(Suppl):53, 1983

33. Jugdutt BI: Nitroglycerin in acute myocardial infarction. Can J Cardiol 5:110, 1989

34. Yusuf S, Collins R, MacMahon S, Peto R: Effect of intravenous nitrates on mortality in acute myocardial infarction: An overview of the randomized trials. Lancet 1:1088–1092, 1988

35. Cohn JN, Franciosa JA, Francis GA: Effect of short-term infusion of sodium nitroprusside on mortality rate in acute myocardial infarction complicated by left ventricular failure. N Engl J Med 306:1129, 1982

36. Abrams J: Pharmacology of nitroglycerin and long-acting nitrates and their usefulness in the treatment of congestive heart failure. In Gould L, Reddy CVR (eds): Vasodilator Therapy for Cardiac Disorders, pp 129–167. Mt Kisco, NY, Futura Publishing, 1979

37. Packer M: New perspectives on therapeutic application of nitrates as vasodilator agents for severe chronic heart failure. Am J Med 74(Suppl):61, 1983

38. Leier CV, Huss P, Magorien RP et al: Improved exercise capacity and differing arterial and venous tolerance during chronic isosorbide dinitrate therapy for congestive heart failure. Circulation 67:817, 1983

39. Cohn JN et al: Effect of vasodilator therapy on mortality in chronic congestive heart failure. Results of a Veterans Administration cooperative study. N Engl J Med 374:1547, 1986

40. Cohn JN, Johnson G, Ziesche S et al: A comparison of enalapril with hydralazine–isosorbide dinitrate in the treatment of chronic congestive heart failure. N Engl J Med 325:303, 1991

41. Duchier J, Iannoscoli F, Safar M: Antihypertensive effect of sustained-release isosorbide dinitrate for isolated systolic systemic hypertension in the elderly. Am J Cardiol 60:99, 1987

42. Chatterjee K, Parmley WW, Swan HJC et al: Beneficial effects of vasodilator therapy in severe mitral regurgitation due to dysfunction of subvalvular apparatus. Circulation 48:684, 1973

43. Swamy N: Esophageal spasm: Clinical and manometric response to nitroglycerine and long-acting nitrates. Gastroenterology 72:23, 1977

44. Hill NS, Antman EM, Green LH et al: Intravenous nitroglycerin: A review of pharmacology, indications, therapeutic effects and complications. Chest 79:69, 1981

45. Herling IM: Intravenous nitroglycerin: Clinical pharmacology and therapeutic considerations. Am Heart J 108:141, 1984

46. Margolis JR, Chen C: Coronary artery spasm complicating PTCA: role of intracoronary nitroglycerin. Z Kardiol 78(Suppl 2):41, 1989

47. Rentrop KP, Feit F, Sherman W et al: Late thrombolytic therapy preserves left ventricular function in patients with collateralized total coronary occlusion: Primary and point findings of the Second Mount Sinai–New York University Reperfusion Trial. J Am Coll Cardiol 14:58, 1989

48. Abrams J: Pharmacology of nitroglycerin and long-acting nitrates. Am J Cardiol 56:12A, 1985

49. Fung H-L: Pharmacokinetic determinants of nitrate action. Am J Med 76(6A):22, 1984

50. Armstrong PW, Moffat JA, Marks GS: Arterial-venous nitroglycerin gradient during intravenous infusion in man. Circulation 66:1273, 1982

51. Chasseaud LF: Newer aspects of the pharmacokinetics of organic nitrates. Z Kardiol 72(Suppl 3): 20, 1983

52. Thadani U, Fung H-L, Darke AC et al: Oral isosorbide dinitrate in angina pectoris: Comparison of duration of action and dose response relationship during acute and sustained therapy. Am J Cardiol 49:411, 1982

53. Parker JO, Van Koughnett KA, Fung H-L: Transdermal isosorbide dinitrate in angina pectoris: Effect of acute and sustained therapy. Am J Cardiol 54:8, 1984

54. Fung H-L, Ruggirello D, Stone JA et al: Effects of disease, route of administration, cigarette smoking, food intake on the pharmacokinetics and circulatory effects of isosorbide dinitrate. Z Kardiol 72(Suppl 3):5, 1983

55. Bogaert MG, Rosseel MT: Fate of orally given isosorbide dinitrate in man: Factors of variability. Z Kardiol 72(Suppl 3):11, 1983

56. Abrams J: Nitrate delivery systems in perspective: A decade of progress. Am J Med 76:38, 1984

57. Abrams J: New nitrate delivery systems: Buccal nitroglycerin. Am Heart J 105:848, 1983

58. Thadani U: Isosorbide-5-mononitrate (5-ISMN) in angina pectoris: Efficacy of AM and PM doses,

lack of tolerance and zero hour effect during eccentric BID therapy. Circulation 84(Suppl II):II-730, 1991

59. Reichek N, Goldstein RE, Redwood DR et al: Sustained effects of nitroglycerin ointment in patient with angina pectoris. Circulation 50:348, 1974

60. Abrams J: The brief saga of transdermal nitroglycerin discs: Paradise lost? Am J Cardiol 54:220, 1984

61. Abrams J: Transcutaneous nitroglycerin: Ointment or disc? Am Heart J 108:1597, 1984

62. Reichek N, Priest C, Zimrin D et al: Limited antianginal effects of nitroglycerin patches. Am J Cardiol 54:1, 1984

63. Parker JO, Fung H-L: Transdermal nitroglycerin in angina pectoris. Am J Cardiol 54:471, 1984

64. Multicenter Transdermal Nitroglycerin Trial (in press)

65. Schaer DH, Buff LA, Katz RJ: Sustained antianginal efficacy of transdermal nitroglycerin patches using an overnight 10-hour nitrate-free interval. Am J Cardiol 61:46, 1988

66. Sharpe N, Coxon R, Webster M, Luke R: Hemodynamic effects of intermittent transdermal nitroglycerin in chronic congestive heart failure. Am J Cardiol 59:895, 1987

67. DeMots H, Glasser SP: Intermittent transdermal nitroglycerin therapy in the treatment of chronic stable angina. J Am Coll Cardiol 13:786, 1989

68. Young JB, Pratt CM, Farmer JA et al: Specialized delivery systems for intravenous nitroglycerin: Are they necessary? Am J Med 76:27, 1984

69. Come PC, Pitt B: Nitroglycerin-induced severe hypotension and bradycardia in patients with acute myocardial infarction. Circulation 54:624, 1976

70. Arsura E, Lichstein E, Guadagnino V et al: Methemoglobin levels produced by organic nitrates in patients with coronary artery disease. J Clin Pharmacol 24:160, 1984

71. Abrams J: Nitrate tolerance and dependence. Am Heart J 99:113, 1980

72. Abrams J: Nitrate tolerance in angina pectoris. In Cohn J, Rittinghausen R (eds): Mononitrates, pp 154–170. Berlin, Springer-Verlag, 1985

73. Blasini R, Froer KL, Blume I et al: Wirkungsverlust von Isosorbiddinitrat bei Langzeitbetrandlung der chronischen Herzinsuffizienz. Herz 7:250, 1982

74. Armstrong PW, Moffat JA: Tolerance to organic nitrates: Clinical and experimental perspectives. Am J Med 74(Suppl):73, 1983

75. Parker JO: Intermittent transdermal nitroglycerin therapy in the treatment of chronic stable angina. J Am Coll Cardiol 13:794, 1989

76. Elkayam U, Jamison M, Roth A et al: Oral isosorbide dinitrate in chronic heart failure: Tolerance development to QID vs TID regimen. J Am Coll Cardiol 13:178A, 1989

The α- and β-Adrenergic Blocking Drugs

William H. Frishman
Shlomo Charlap

Catecholamines are neurohumoral substances that mediate a variety of physiologic and metabolic responses in humans. The effects of the catecholamines ultimately depend on their physiologic interactions with receptors, which are discrete macromolecular components located on the plasma membrane. Differences in the ability of the various catecholamines to stimulate a number of physiologic processes were the criteria used by Ahlquist in 1948 to separate these receptors into two distinct types: α- and β-adrenergic.[1] Subsequent studies suggested that β-adrenergic receptors exist as two discrete subtypes called β_1 and β_2.[2] It is now also appreciated that there are two subtypes of α-receptors, designated α_1 and α_2.[3] Specific drugs are available that will inhibit or block these receptors. In this chapter we examine the adrenergic receptors and the drugs that can inhibit their function. The rationale for use and clinical experience with α- and β-adrenergic blocking drugs in the treatment of various cardiovascular and noncardiovascular disorders are also discussed.

α-ADRENERGIC BLOCKERS
Clinical Pharmacology

When an adrenergic is nerve stimulated, catecholamines are released from their storage granules in the adrenergic neuron, enter the synaptic cleft, and bind to α-receptors on the effector cell.[4] A feedback loop exists by which the amount of neurotransmitter released can be regulated: accumulation of catecholamines in the synaptic cleft leads to stimulation of α-receptors on the neuronal surface and inhibition of further catecholamine release. Catecholamines from the systemic circulation can also enter the synaptic cleft and bind to presynaptic or postsynaptic receptors.

Initially it was believed that α_1-receptors were limited to postsynaptic sites where they mediated vasoconstriction, whereas the α_2-receptors only existed at the prejunctional nerve terminals and mediated the negative feedback control of norepinephrine release. The availability of compounds with high specificity for either α_1- or α_2-receptors demonstrated that while presynaptic α-receptors are almost exclusively of the α_2-subtype, the postsynaptic receptors are made up of comparable numbers of α_1- and α_2-receptors.[4] Stimulation of the postsynaptic α_2-receptors also causes vasoconstriction. However, a functional difference does exist between the two types of postsynaptic receptors. The α_1-receptors appear to exist primarily within the region of the synapse and respond preferentially to neuronally released catecholamine, whereas α_2-receptors are located extrasynaptically and respond preferentially to circulating catecholamines in the plasma.

Drugs having α-adrenergic blocking properties are of several types (Fig. 5.1).[4–12]

1. Nonselective α-blockers having prominent effects on both the α_1 and α_2-receptors (e.g., the older drugs such as phenoxybenzamine

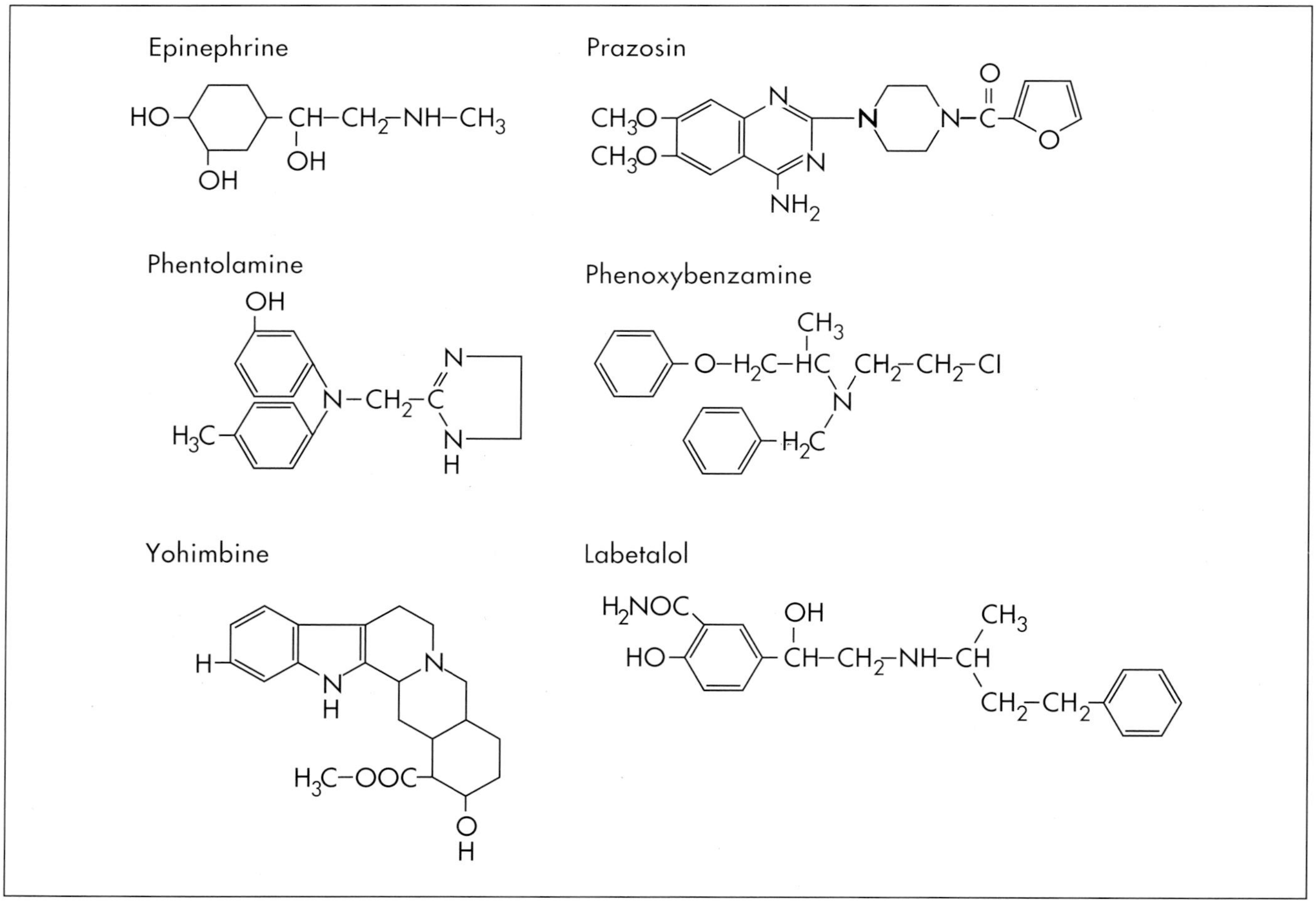

Figure 5.1 Molecular structure of the α-adrenergic agonist epinephrine and some α-blockers.

and phentolamine). Although virtually all of the clinical effects of phenoxybenzamine are explicable in terms of α-blockade, this is not the case with phentolamine, which also possesses several other properties, including a direct vasodilator action and sympathomimetic and parasympathomimetic effects.

2. Selective α_1-blockers having little affinity for α_2-receptors (e.g., prazosin, terazosin, doxazosin, and other quinazoline derivatives). Originally introduced as direct-acting vasodilators, it is now clear that these drugs exert their major effect by reversible blockade of postsynaptic α_1-receptors. Other selective α_1-blockers include indoramin, trimazosin, and urapadil (Fig. 5.2). Urapadil is of interest because of its other actions, which include stimulation of presynaptic α_2-adrenergic receptors and a central effect.

3. Selective α_2-blockers (e.g., yohimbine). The primary use of these drugs has been as tools in experimental pharmacology. Yohimbine is now marketed in the United States as an oral sympatholytic and mydriatic agent. Male patients with impotence from vascular or diabetic origins or from psychogenic origin have been treated successfully with yohimbine.

4. Blockers that inhibit both α- and β-adrenergic receptors (e.g., labetalol). Labetalol, like prazosin and terazosin, is a selective α_1-blocker. Since this agent is more potent as a β-blocker than an α-blocker, it is discussed in greater detail in the section on β-blockers.

5. Agents having α-adrenergic blocking properties but whose major clinical use appears unrelated to these properties (e.g., chlorpromazine, haloperidol, quinidine, bromocriptine, amiodarone, and ketanserin, a selective blocking agent of serotonin-2 receptors). It has been demonstrated that verapamil, a calcium channel blocker, also has α-adrenergic blocking properties. Whether this is a particular property of verapamil and its analogues or is common to all calcium channel blockers is not clear.[13] Also to be clarified is whether verapamil-induced α-blockade occurs at physiologic plasma levels and helps to mediate the vasodilator properties of the drug.

All the α-blockers in clinical use inhibit the postsynaptic α-receptor and result in relaxation of vascular smooth muscle and vasodilation. However, the nonselective α-blockers also antagonize the presynaptic α_2-receptors, allowing for increased release of neuronal norepinephrine. This results in attenuation of the desired postsynaptic blockade and spillover stimulation of the β-receptors and, consequently, in troublesome side effects such as tachycardia and tremulousness and increased renin release. The α_1-selective agents that preserve the α_2-mediated presynaptic feedback loop prevent excessive norepinephrine release and thus avoid these adverse cardiac and systemic effects.

Because of these potent peripheral vasodilatory properties, however, one would anticipate that even the selective α_1-blockers would induce reflex stimulation of the sympathetic and renin-angiotensin system similar to that seen with other vasodilators such as hydralazine and minoxidil. The explanation for the relative lack of tachycardia and renin release observed after prazosin, doxazosin, and terazosin may, in part, be due to the drugs' combined action of reducing vascular tone in both resistance (arteries) and capacitance (veins) beds. Such a dual action may prevent the marked increases in venous return and cardiac output observed with agents that act more selectively to reduce vascular tone only in the resistance vessels. The lack of tachycardia with prazosin, doxazosin, and terazosin use has also been attributed by some investigators to a significant negative chronotropic action of the drug independent of its peripheral vascular effect.[14]

Use in Cardiovascular Disorders

HYPERTENSION

Increased peripheral vascular resistance is present in the majority of patients with long-standing hypertension. Since dilation of constricted arterioles should result in lowering of elevated blood pressure, interest has focused on the use of α-adrenergic blockers in the medical treatment of systemic hypertension. The experience with nonselective α-blockers in the treatment of hypertension was disappointing because of

FIGURE 5.2 PHARMACOKINETICS OF SELECTIVE α_1-ADRENERGIC BLOCKING DRUGS

Selective α_1-Blocker	Daily Dose (mg)	Frequency per Day	Bioavailability (% of Oral Dose)	Plasma Half-life (h)	Urinary Excretion (% of Oral Dose)
Doxazosin	1–16	1	65	10–12	NA
Indoramin*	50–125	2–3	NA	5	11
Prazosin	2–20	2–3	44–69	2.5–4	10
Prazosin GITS†*	2.5–20	1			
Terazosin	1–20	1	90	12	39
Trimazosin*	100–900	2–3	61	2.7	NA

*Investigational drug
†Gastrointestinal therapeutic system
NA = Not available

(Adapted from Luther RR: New perspectives on selective α_1-blockade. Am J Hypertens 2:731, 1989)

accompanying reflex stimulation of the sympathetic and renin-angiotensin system, resulting in frequent side effects and limited long-term antihypertensive efficacy. However, the selective α_1-blockers prazosin, doxazosin, and terazosin have been shown to be effective antihypertensive agents.[4,5,12]

Prazosin, doxazosin, and terazosin decrease blood pressure in both the standing and supine positions, although blood pressure decrement tends to be somewhat greater in the upright position. Because their antihypertensive effect is accompanied by little or no increase in heart rate, plasma renin activity, or circulating catecholamines, prazosin, doxazosin, and terazosin, have been found useful as first-step agents in hypertension. Monotherapy with these agents, however, promotes sodium and water retention in some patients, although it is less pronounced than with other vasodilators. The concomitant use of a diuretic prevents fluid retention and in many cases markedly enhances the antihypertensive effect of the drugs. In clinical practice, prazosin, doxazosin, and terazosin have their widest application as adjuncts to one or more established antihypertensive drugs in treating moderate to severe hypertension. Their effects are additive to those of diuretics, β-blockers, α-methyldopa, and the direct-acting vasodilators. The drugs cause little change in glomerular filtration rate or renal plasma flow and can be used safely in patients with severe renal hypertension. There is no evidence for attenuation of the antihypertensive effect of prazosin, doxazosin, or terazosin during chronic therapy.

Selective α_1-blockers appear to have neutral or even favorable effects on plasma lipids and lipoproteins when administered to hypertensive patients. Investigators have reported mild reductions in levels of total cholesterol, low-density lipoprotein (LDL) and very-low-density lipoprotein (VLDL) cholesterol, and triglycerides and elevations in levels of high-density lipoprotein (HDL) cholesterol with prazosin, doxazosin, and terazosin.[15] With long-term use, selective α_1-blockers also appear to decrease left ventricular mass in patients having both hypertension and left ventricular hypertrophy.[16]

A number of prazosin, doxazosin, and terazosin analogues have been developed (e.g., trimazosin) that in preliminary clinical trials have also shown promise as antihypertensive agents.[9,10] Doxazosin and terazosin have a longer duration of action than prazosin and have been shown to produce sustained blood pressure reductions with single daily administration. Indoramin, also a selective α_1-blocker, has been found to be effective in the treatment of systemic hypertension, but it produces many unwanted effects, such as lethargy and impotence, which may limit its clinical value. In contrast to prazosin, the drug appears to have little dilative effect on the venous circulation. Prazosin, doxazosin, and terazosin are available for clinical use in the United States.

A new formulation of prazosin, prazosin GITS (gastrointestinal therapeutic system) has undergone clinical trials and may soon be released. This is an extended once-daily formulation designed as an osmotic pump. Through this innovative delivery system, prazosin is released at an approximately steady rate over a 16-hour period, allowing once-daily clinical administration in hypertension.[7]

α-Adrenergic blocking drugs appear particularly attractive for use in the treatment of heart failure because they hold the possibility of reproducing balanced reductions in resistance and capacitance beds. In fact, phentolamine was one of the earlier vasodilators to be shown effective in the treatment of heart failure.[17,18] The drug was infused into normotensive patients with persistent left ventricular dysfunction after a myocardial infarction and found to induce a significant fall in systemic vascular resistance accompanied by considerable elevation in cardiac output and a reduction in pulmonary artery pressure.[18] Because of its high cost and the frequent side effects that it produces, especially tachycardia, phentolamine is no longer used in the treatment of heart failure. Oral phenoxybenzamine has also been used as vasodilator therapy in heart failure; like phentolamine, it has been replaced by newer vasodilator agents.

Studies evaluating the acute hemodynamic effects of prazosin in patients with congestive heart failure consistently find significant reductions in systemic and pulmonary vascular resistances and left ventricular filling pressures associated with increases in stroke volume.[14] In most studies, there is no change or a decrease in heart rate. The response pattern seen with prazosin is similar to that observed with nitroprusside with the exception that the heart rate tends to be higher with the use of nitroprusside and, therefore, the observed increases in cardiac output are also higher with the latter agent.

Controversy still exists as to whether the initial clinical and hemodynamic improvements seen with prazosin are sustained during long-term therapy.[19] Whereas some studies have demonstrated continued efficacy of prazosin therapy after chronic use, others have found little hemodynamic difference between prazosin- and placebo-treated patients. Some investigators believe that whatever tolerance to the drug does develop is most likely secondary to activation of counterposing neurohumoral forces; if the dose is raised and the tendency toward sodium and water retention is countered by appropriate increases in diuretic dose, prazosin is likely to remain effective. Others argue that sustained increases in plasma renin activity or plasma catecholamines are not seen during long-term therapy and that tolerance is not prevented or reversed by a diuretic. Some clinical studies suggest that patients with initially high plasma renin activity experience attenuation of beneficial hemodynamic effects more frequently. What appears clear is the need to evaluate patients individually as to the continued efficacy of their prazosin therapy. Whether there are subgroups of patients with heart failure (e.g., those with highly activated sympathetic nervous systems) that are more likely to respond to prazosin or other α-blockers remains to be determined.

A multicenter study from the Veterans Administration Hospitals has shown that prazosin, when compared with placebo therapy, did not reduce mortality with long-term use in patients with advanced forms of congestive heart failure.[20] In the same study, a favorable effect on mortality was seen with an isosorbide dinitrate-hydralazine combination.[20]

There is increasing evidence that α_1-adrenergic receptors, different from those of other tissues, also exist in the myocardium and that an increase in the force of contraction may be produced by stimulation of these sites.[21] The mechanism of α-adrenergic positive inotropic response is unknown. What the biologic significance of α-adrenergic receptors in cardiac muscle is and whether these receptors play a role in the response to α-blocker therapy in congestive heart failure also remain to be determined.

ANGINA PECTORIS

α-Adrenergic receptors help mediate coronary vasoconstriction. It has been suggested that a pathologic alteration of the α-adrenergic system may be the mechanism of coronary spasm in some patients with variant angina.[22] In uncontrolled studies, the administration of α-adrenergic blockers, both acutely and chronically, has been shown effective in reversing and preventing coronary spasm. However, in a long-term randomized, double-blind trial prazosin was found to exert no obvious beneficial effect in patients with variant angina.[23] The demonstration of an important role for the postsynaptic α2-receptors in determining coronary vascular tone may help explain prazosin's lack of efficacy. Further study in this area is anticipated.

ARRHYTHMIAS

It has been postulated that enhanced α-adrenergic responsiveness occurs during myocardial ischemia and that it is a primary mediator of the electrophysiologic derangements and resulting malignant arrhythmias induced by catecholamines during myocardial ischemia and reperfusion.[24] In humans, there have been favorable reports of the use of an α-blocker in the treatment of supraventricular and ventricular ectopy. Whether there is a significant role for α-adrenergic blockers in the treatment of cardiac arrhythmias will be determined through further clinical study.

Use in Other Disorders

PHEOCHROMOCYTOMA

α-Blockers have been used in the treatment of pheochromocytoma to control the peripheral effects of the excess catecholamines.[25] In fact, intravenous phentolamine was used as a test for this disorder but the test is now rarely done because of reported cases of cardiovascular collapse and death in patients who exhibited exaggerated sensitivity to the drug. The drug is still rarely used in cases of pheochromocytoma-related hypertensive crisis. However, for long-term therapy, oral phenoxybenzamine is the preferred agent. β-Blocking agents may also be needed in pheochromocytoma for control of tachycardia and arrhythmias. All β-blockers, but primarily the nonselective agents, should not be initiated prior to adequate α-blockade since severe hypertension may occur as a result of the unopposed α-stimulating activity of the circulating catecholamines.

SHOCK

In shock, hyperactivity of the sympathetic nervous system occurs as a compensatory reflex response to reduced blood pressure. Use of α-blockers in shock has been advocated as a means of lowering peripheral vascular resistance and increasing vascular capacitance while not antagonizing the cardiotonic effects of the sympathomimetic amines. Although investigated for many years for the treatment of shock, α-adrenergic blockers are still not approved for this purpose.[26] A prime concern when using α-blockers for shock is that the rapid drug-induced increase in vascular capacitance may lead to inadequate cardiac filling and profound hypotension, especially in the hypovolemic patient. Adequate amounts of fluid replacement prior to use of an α-blocker can minimize this concern.

LUNG DISEASE
Pulmonary Hypertension

The part played by endogenous circulating catecholamines in the maintenance of pulmonary vascular tone appears to be minimal. Studies evaluating the effects of norepinephrine administration on pulmonary vascular resistance have found the drug to have little or no effect. The beneficial effects on the pulmonary circulation that phentolamine and other α-blockers have demonstrated in some studies is most likely primarily due to their direct vasodilative actions rather than to α-blockade.[27] Like other vasodilators, in patients with pulmonary hypertension due to fixed anatomic changes, α-blockers can produce hemodynamic deterioration secondary to their systemic vasodilative properties.[28]

Bronchospasm

Bronchoconstriction is mediated in part through catecholamine stimulation of α-receptors in the lung. It has been suggested that in patients with allergic asthma, a deficient β-adrenergic system or enhanced α-adrenergic responsiveness could result in α-adrenergic activity being the mean mechanism of bronchoconstriction.[29] Several studies have shown bronchodilation or inhibition of histamine and allergen- or exercise-induced bronchospasm with a variety of α-blockers.[30] Additional studies are needed to define more fully the role of α-blockers for use as bronchodilators.

ARTERIOCONSTRICTION

Oral α-adrenergic blockers can produce subjective and clinical improvement in patients experiencing episodic arterioconstriction (Raynaud's phenomenon). α-Blockers may also be valuable in the treating severe peripheral ischemia caused by an α-agonist (e.g., norepinephrine) or ergotamine overdose. In cases of inadvertent infiltration of a norepinephrine infusion, phentolamine can be given intradermally to avoid tissue sloughing.

BENIGN PROSTATIC OBSTRUCTION

α-Adrenergic receptors have been identified in the bladder neck and prostatic capsule of male patients. In clinical studies, use of α-blockers in patients with benign prostatic obstruction has resulted in increased urinary flow rates and reductions in residual volume and obstructive symptoms.[31] It would appear that α-blockers may have an important role in the medical treatment of patients with benign prostatic obstruction.

Clinical Use and Adverse Effects

Oral phenoxybenzamine has a rapid onset of action, with the maximal effect from a single dose seen in 1 to 2 hours.[32,33] The gastrointestinal absorption is incomplete, and only 20% to 30% of an oral dose reaches the systemic circulation in active form. The half-life of the drug is 24 hours, with the usual dose varying between 20 and 200 mg daily in one or two doses. Intravenous phentolamine is initially started at 0.1 mg/min and is then increased at increments of 0.1 mg/min every 5 to 10 minutes until the desired hemodynamic effect is reached. The drug has a short duration of action of 3 to 10 minutes. Little is known about the pharmacokinetics of long-term oral use of phentolamine. The main side effects of the drug include postural hypotension, tachycardia, gastrointestinal disturbances, and sexual dysfunction. Intravenous infusion of norepinephrine can be used to combat severe hypotensive reactions. Oral phenoxybenzamine is approved for use in pheochromocytoma.

Prazosin is almost completely absorbed following oral administration, with peak plasma levels achieved at 2 to 3 hours. The drug is 90% protein bound. Prazosin is extensively metabolized by the liver. The usual half-life of the drug is 2½ to 4 hours; in patients with heart failure, the half-life increases to the range of 5 to 7 hours.

The major side effect of prazosin is the first-dose phenomenon—severe postural hypotension occasionally associated with syncope seen after the initial dose or after a rapid dose increment.[4,5] The reason for this phenomenon has not been clearly established but may involve the rapid induction of venous and arteriolar dilatation by a drug that elicits little reflex sympathetic stimulation. It is reported more often when the drug is administered as a tablet rather than a capsule, possibly related to the variable bioavailability or rates of absorption of the two formulations.[4] (In the United States, the drug is available in capsule form.) The postural hypotension can be minimized if the initial dose of prazosin is not higher than 1 mg and if it is given at bedtime. In treating hypertension, a dose of 2 to 3 mg/d should be maintained for 1 to 2 weeks, followed by a gradual increase in dosage titrated to achieve the desired reductions in pressures, usually up to 20 to 30 mg/d, given in two or three doses. In treating heart failure, larger doses (2 to 7 mg) may be used to initiate therapy in recumbent patients, but the maintenance dose is also usually not more than 30 mg. Higher doses do not seem to produce additional clinical improvement.

Other side effects of prazosin include dizziness, headache, and drowsiness. The drug produces no deleterious effects on the clinical course of diabetes mellitus, chronic obstructive pulmonary disease, renal failure, or gout. It does not adversely affect the lipid profile. Prazosin is presently approved for use in hypertension. Prazosin GITS may soon become available for once-daily use in systemic hypertension. With this formulation, there are narrower peak-to-trough fluctuations in drug plasma levels, which may be associated with less postural hypotension.[7]

Terazosin, which has been approved for once-daily use in hypertension, may be associated with a lesser incidence of first-dose postural hypotension than prazosin.[12] The usual recommended dose range is 1 to 5 mg administered once a day; some patients may benefit from doses as high as 20 mg daily or from divided doses.

Doxazosin is also approved as a once-daily therapy for systemic hypertension. The initial dosage of doxazosin is 1 mg once daily. Depending on the patient's standing blood pressure response, the dosage may then be increased to 2 mg and, if necessary, to 4 mg, 8 mg, or 16 mg to achieve the desired reduction in blood pressure. Doses beyond 4 mg increase the likelihood of excessive postural effects including syncope, postural dizziness/vertigo, and postural hypotension.

The α₂-blocker yohimbine, 5.4 mg orally, is used three times daily to treat male impotence. Urologists have used yohimbine for the diagnostic classification of certain cases of male erectile impotence. Increases in heart rate and blood pressure, piloerection, and rhinorrhea are the most common adverse reactions. Yohimbine should not be used with antidepressant drugs.

β-ADRENERGIC BLOCKERS
Clinical Pharmacology

The β-adrenergic receptor blocking drugs (Fig. 5.3) differ from one another in respect to several pharmacodynamic and pharmacokinetic properties.[34–36] The properties considered here are potency, membrane

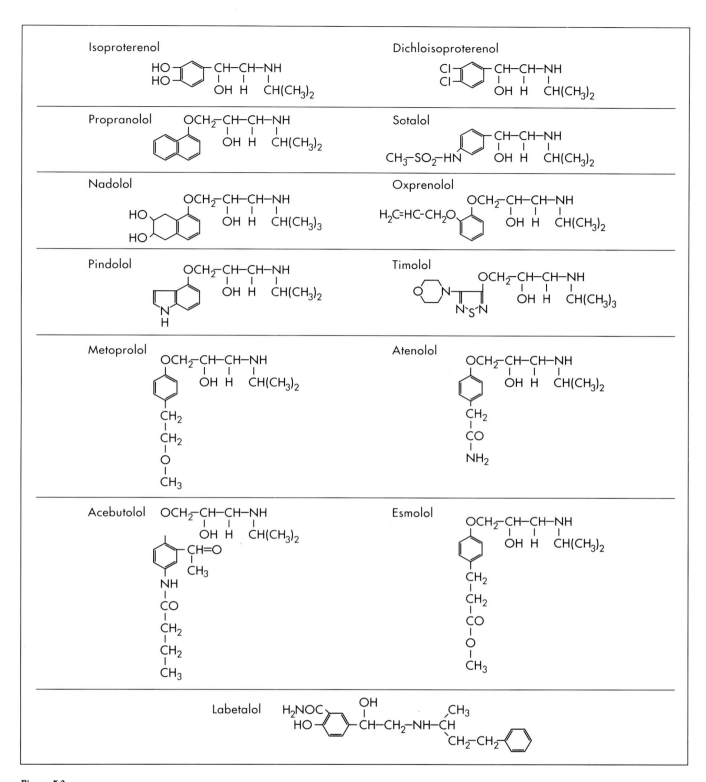

Figure 5.3 Molecular structure of the α-adrenergic agonist isoproterenol and some β-blockers.

stabilizing activity, selectivity, intrinsic sympatho-mimetic activity, and, finally, pharmacokinetic characteristics (Figs. 5.4 and 5.5).

POTENCY

β-Adrenergic receptor blocking drugs are competitive inhibitors of catecholamine binding at β-adrenergic receptor sites. In the presence of a β-blocker, the dose-response curve of the catecholamine is shifted to the right; that is, a higher concentration of the catecholamine is required to provoke the response. The potency of a β-blocker tells us how much of the drug must be administered in order to inhibit the effects of an adrenergic agonist. Potency can be assessed by noting the dose of the drug that is needed to inhibit tachycardia produced by an agonist or by exercise. It has been found that potency differs from drug to drug, with carteolol being the most potent and esmolol the least potent. While differences in potency explain the different dosages needed to achieve effective β-adrenergic blockade, they have no therapeutic relevance, except when switching patients from one drug to another.

MEMBRANE STABILIZING ACTIVITY

At very high concentrations, certain β-blockers have a quinidine or local anesthetic effect on the cardiac action potential. There is no evidence that membrane stabilizing activity is responsible for any direct negative inotropic effect of the β-blockers, since drugs with and without this property equally depress left ventricular function. In therapeutic situations, the concentration of the β-blocker is probably too small to produce the membrane stabilizing activity. Only during massive β-blocker intoxication is the activity manifested.

SELECTIVITY

The β-adrenoceptor blockers can be classified as selective or nonselective, according to their relative abilities to antagonize the actions of sympathomimetic amines in some tissues at lower doses than those required in other tissues.[37] Drugs have been developed with a degree of selectivity for two subgroups of the β-adrenoceptor population receptors, such as those in the heart, and β_2-receptors, such as those in the peripheral circulation and bronchi.

Because selective β_1-blockers have less of an inhibitory effect on β_2-receptors, they offer theoretic advantages. In patients with asthma or obstructive pulmonary disease, in which β_2-receptors must remain available to mediate adrenergic bronchodilatation, relatively low doses of β_1-selective drugs have been shown to cause a lower incidence of side effects than similar doses of a nonselective drug, such as propranolol. It should be noted that even selective β_1-blockers may aggravate bronchospasm in some

FIGURE 5.4 PHARMACODYNAMIC PROPERTIES OF β-ADRENOCEPTOR BLOCKING DRUGS

Drug	β_1 Potency Ratio (Propranolol = 1.0)	Relative β_1 Selectivity	Intrinsic Sympathomimetic Activity	Membrane Stabilizing Activity
Acebutolol	0.3	+	+	+
Atenolol	1.0	++	0	0
Betaxolol	1.0	++	0	+
Bevantolol	0.3	++	0	0
Bisoprotol	10.0	++	0	0
Carteolol	10.0	0	+	0
Carvedilol*	10.0	0	0	++
Celiprolol†	0.4	+	+	0
Dilevalol‡	1.0	0	+	0
Esmolol	0.02	++	0	0
Labetalol§	0.3	0	+	0
Metoprolol	1.0	++	0	0
Nadolol	1.0	0	0	0
Oxprenolol	0.5–1.0	0	+	+
Penbutolol	1.0	0	+	0
Pindolol	6.0	0	++	+
Propranolol	1.0	0	0	++
Sotalol¶	0.3	0	0	0
Timolol	6.0	0	0	0
YM 151‖	1.0	++	0	0
Isomer:				
D-propranolol	—	—	—	++
D-sotalol	—	—	—	—

*Carvedilol has additional α_1-adrenergic blocking activity without peripheral β_2 agonism.
†Celiprolol has peripheral β_2 agonism and may have additional α_2-adrenergic blocking activity at high doses.
‡Dilevalol is an isomer of labetalol with additional peripheral β_2 agonism but no α_1-blocking activity.
§Labetalol has additional α_1-adrenergic blocking activity and direct vasodilatory actions (β_2 agonism).
¶Sotalol has an additional type of antiarrhythmic activity.
‖YM 151 has additional dihydropyridine calcium channel blocker activity.

(Frishman WH: Clinical Pharmacology of the β-Adrenoceptor Blocking Drugs, 2nd ed. Norwalk, CT, Appleton-Century-Crofts, 1984)

patients; therefore, these drugs are not generally recommended for patients with asthma or other bronchospastic disease.

Selective β₁-blockers also have less of an inhibitory effect on the β₂-receptors that mediate dilation of arterioles and are thus less likely to impair peripheral blood flow. In the presence of epinephrine, nonselective β-blockers can cause a vasopressor response by blocking receptor-mediated vasodilation (since α-adrenergic vasoconstriction receptors remain operative). Selective β₁-blockers may not induce this effect. Whether this offers an advantage in treating hypertension is yet to be demonstrated.

INTRINSIC SYMPATHOMIMETIC ACTIVITY

Certain β-adrenoceptor blockers possess partial agonist activity (PAA).[38] These drugs cause a slight to moderate activation of the β-receptor, even as they prevent the access of natural and synthetic catecholamines to the receptor sites. The result is stimulation of the receptor, which is, of course, much weaker than those of the agonists epinephrine and isoproterenol. In laboratory animals, pindolol, for example, may have 50% of the agonist activity of isoproterenol; the activity is probably lower in humans.

The assessment of the PAA of β-blockers in humans is complicated by the need to study the intact subject. However, the significance of PAA can be evaluated in clinical trials in which equivalent pharmacologic doses of β-blockers with and without this property are compared. In such trials, drugs with PAA have been shown to cause less slowing of the resting heart rate than do drugs without PAA. It is important to note, by contrast, that both types of β-blockers similarly reduce the increases in heart rate that occur with exercise or isoproterenol. An explanation for these findings is that the importance of the PAA of pindolol, for example, relative to its β-blocker action, is greatest when sympathetic tone is low, as it is in the resting subject. During exercise, when sympathetic tone is high, the β-blocking effect of pindolol predominates over its PAA. It is for this reason that all β-blockers have been found to be equally effective in reducing the increases in heart rate and blood pressure that occur with exercise.

Whether PAA in a β-blocker offers an overall advantage in cardiac therapy remains a matter of controversy.[38] Some investigators suggest that drugs with this property may reduce peripheral vascular resistance and may depress atrioventricular conduction less than other β-blockers. Other investigators claim that PAA in a β-blocker protects against myocardial depression, bronchial asthma, and peripheral vascular complications in patients receiving therapy. However, these claims have not yet been substantiated by definitive clinical trials.

α-ADRENERGIC ACTIVITY

Labetalol is the first of a group of β-blockers that acts as comparative pharmacologic antagonist at both α- and β-adrenergic receptors.[39] Labetalol is 4 to 16 times more potent at β-adrenergic receptors than at α-adrenergic receptors. In a series of tests, the drug has been shown to be 6 to 10 times less potent than phentolamine at α-adrenergic receptors and 1½ to 4 times less potent than propranolol at α-adrenergic receptors.

FIGURE 5.5 PHARMACOKINETIC PROPERTIES OF VARIOUS β-ADRENOCEPTOR BLOCKING DRUGS

Drug	Extent of Absorption (% of Dose)	Extent of Bioavailability (% of Dose)	Dose-Dependent Bioavailability (Major First-Pass Hepatic Metabolism)	Interpatient Variations in Plasma Levels	β-Blocking Plasma Concentrations	Protein Binding (%)	Lipid Solubility*
Acebutolol	≈70	≈40	No	7-fold	0.2–2.0 μg/ml	25	Moderate
Atenolol	≈50	≈40	No	4-fold	0.2–5.0 μg/ml	<5	Weak
Betaxolol	>90	≈80	No	2-fold	5–20 ng/ml	50	Moderate
Bevantolol	≈90	≈55	No	4-fold	0.13–3.0 μg/ml	95	Moderate
Carteolol	≈90	≈90	No	2-fold	40–160 ng/ml	20–30	Weak
Celiprolol	≈30	≈30	No	3-fold		≈30	Weak
Esmolol†	NA	NA	NA	5-fold	0.15–1.0 μg/ml	55	Weak
Labetalol	>90	≈33	Yes	10-fold	0.7–3.0 μg/ml	≈50	Weak
Metoprolol	>90	≈50	No	7-fold	50–100 ng/ml	12	Moderate
Nadolol	≈30	≈30	No	7-fold	50–100 ng/ml	≈30	Weak
Oxprenolol	≈90	≈40	No	5-fold	80–100 ng/ml	80	Moderate
Penbutolol	>90	≈90	No	4-fold	5–15 ng/ml	98	High
Pindolol	>90	≈90	No	4-fold	50–100 ng/ml	57	Moderate
Propranolol	>90	≈30	Yes	20-fold	50–100 ng/ml	93	High
Long-acting propranolol	>90	≈20	Yes	10- to 20-fold	20–100 ng/ml	93	High
Sotalol	≈70	≈90	No	4-fold	2.4–6.1 μg/ml	0	Weak
Timolol	>90	≈75	No	7-fold	5–10 ng/ml	≈10	

*Determined by the distribution ratio between octanol and water.

†Ultra-short-acting β-blocker available only in intravenous form.

NA = Not applicable.

(Frishman WH: Clinical Pharmacology of the β-Adrenoceptor Blocking Drugs, 2nd ed. Norwalk, CT, Appleton-Century-Crofts, 1984)

Whether concomitant α-adrenergic activity is generally advantageous in a β-blocker is yet to be determined. In the case of labetalol, the additional α-adrenergic blocking action does result in a reduction of peripheral vascular resistance that may be useful in the treatment of hypertensive emergencies, and, unlike other β-blockers, the drug may maintain cardiac output. It has also been suggested that unlike other β-blockers, labetalol may be very effective in the black patient with hypertension. Its overall efficacy in the treatment of arrhythmias, hypertension, and angina pectoris appears to be similar to that of other β-blockers.[35,39]

COMBINED β-ADRENERGIC AND CALCIUM CHANNEL BLOCKADE

An agent, YM 151, has been developed that demonstrates the pharmacologic properties of a β_1-selective adrenergic blocker and a dihydropyridine-like calcium channel blocker (see Fig. 5.4). This unique compound is now undergoing investigation in hypertension and angina pectoris.

PHARMACOKINETIC PROPERTIES

Although the β-adrenergic blocking drugs have similar therapeutic effects, their pharmacokinetic properties differ significantly (see Fig. 5.5),[35,40] that is, in ways that may influence their clinical usefulness in some patients. On the basis of their pharmacokinetic properties, the β-blockers can be classified into two broad categories: those eliminated by the hepatic metabolism and those eliminated unchanged by the kidney. Drugs in the first group, for example, propranolol and metoprolol, are lipid soluble, are almost completely absorbed by the small intestine, and are largely metabolized by the liver. They tend to have highly variable bioavailability and relatively short plasma half-lives. In contrast, drugs in the second category are more water soluble, are incompletely absorbed through the gut, and are eliminated unchanged by the kidney. They show less variable bioavailability and have longer half-lives.

Many of the β-blockers, including those with short plasma half-lives, can be administered as infrequently as once or twice daily. Of course, the longer the half-life, the more useful the drug is likely to be for patients who experience difficulty in complying with β-blocker therapy. An addition to the list of available β-blockers is a long-acting, sustained-release preparation of propranolol that provides β-blockade for 24 hours. Studies have shown that this compound provides a much smoother curve of daily plasma levels than comparable divided doses of conventional propranolol and that it has fewer side effects.

Ultra-short-acting β-blockers, with a half-life of no more than 10 minutes, also offer advantages to the clinician, for example, in patients with questionable congestive heart failure in whom β-blockers may be harmful. Such drugs are now being tested, and one, esmolol, has already been approved for clinical use in patients with supraventricular tachycardias.[41] The short half-life of esmolol relates to the rapid metabolism of the drug by blood tissue and hepatic esterases.

In medical practice, the pharmacokinetic properties of the different β-adrenergic blockers become important. The dose of the drug, for example, depends on its first-pass metabolism; if the first-pass effect is extensive, not much of an orally administered drug will reach the systemic circulation and so dosage will have to be larger than the intravenous dose would be. Knowing if the drug is transformed into active metabolites as opposed to inactive metabolites is important in gauging the total pharmacologic effect. Finally, for some β-blockers, lipid solubility has been associated with the entry of these drugs into the brain resulting in side effects that are probably unrelated to β-blockade, such as lethargy, mental depression, and even hallucinations. Whether drugs that are less lipid soluble cause fewer of these adverse reactions remains to be determined.

Use in Cardiovascular Disorders

HYPERTENSION

It is now well recognized that β-adrenergic blockers are effective in reducing the blood pressure of many patients with systemic hypertension when used as monotherapy or in combination with other antihypertensive agents.[35,42] They are considered to be first-line treatment 5. There is, however, no consensus as to the mechanism(s) by which these drugs lower blood pressure. It is probable that some, or all, of the following proposed mechanisms play a part.

Negative Chronotropic and Inotropic Effects

Slowing of the heart rate and some decrease in myocardial contractility with β-blockers lead to a decrease in cardiac output, which in the short term and long term may lead to a reduction in blood pressure. It might be expected that these factors would be of particular importance in the treatment of hypertension related to high cardiac output and increased sympathetic tone.

Differences in Effects on Plasma Renin

The relation between the hypotensive action of β-blocking drugs and their ability to reduce plasma renin activity remains controversial. There is no doubt that some β-blocking drugs can antagonize sympathetically mediated renin release. However, the important question remains whether there is a clinical correlation between the β-blocker effect on plasma renin activity and the lowering of blood pressure.

Central Nervous System Effect

There is now good clinical and experimental evidence to suggest that β-blockers cross the blood–brain barrier and enter the central nervous system. Although there is little doubt that β-blockers with high lipophilicity enter the central nervous system in high concentrations, a direct antihypertensive effect mediated by their presence has not been well defined.

Venous Tone and Plasma Volume

Decreased plasma volume has been seen with use of β-blockers in hypertension. One would have expected the reduced cardiac output with β-blockade to have caused a reflex increase in plasma volume.

These findings suggest that decreased plasma volume may play a role in the hypotensive action of β-blockers. Further study is anticipated.

Peripheral Resistance

Nonselective β-blockers have no primary action in lowering peripheral resistance and indeed may cause it to rise by leaving the α-stimulatory mechanisms unopposed. The vasodilating effect of catecholamines on skeletal muscle blood vessels is β-mediated, suggesting possible therapeutic advantages in using $β_1$-selective blockers, agents with PAA, and drugs with α-blocking activity when blood pressure control is desired. Since β-selectivity diminishes as the drug dosage is raised, and since hypertensive patients generally have to be given far larger doses than are required simply to block the $β_1$-receptors alone, $β_1$-selectivity offers the clinician little, if any, real specific advantage in antihypertensive treatment.

"Quinidine Effect"

Some early clinical investigations indicated that the antihypertensive effect of propranolol paralleled that of quinidine, suggesting that the "membrane stabilizing" effect in the β-blocker might be important. Subsequent studies refuted these early findings. All β-blockers appear to reduce blood pressure, regardless of "membrane effects."

Resetting of Baroreceptors

In patients with long-standing hypertension, the baroreceptors may react less strongly to a reduction in blood pressure than they would in a normal subject. It may be that β-blockers achieve some of this antihypertensive effect by "resetting" or increasing the sensitivity of the baroreceptor. The clinical significance of this proposed mechanism is unknown.

Effects on Prejunctional Receptors

The stimulation of prejunctional β-receptors is followed by an increase in the quantity of norepinephrine released by the postganglionic sympathetic fibers. Blockade of prejunctional β-receptors should, therefore, diminish the amount of norepinephrine released, leading to a weaker stimulation of postjunctional α-receptors, an effect that would produce less vasoconstriction and lower blood pressure. Opinions differ, however, on the importance of the contribution of presynaptic β-blockade to the antihypertensive effects of β-blocker drugs.

ANGINA PECTORIS

Sympathetic innervation of the heart causes the release of norepinephrine, activating β-adrenergic receptors in myocardial cells. This adrenergic stimulation causes an increment in heart rate, isometric contractile force, and maximal velocity of muscle fiber shortening, all of which lead to an increase in cardiac work and myocardial oxygen consumption. The decrease in intraventricular pressure and volume caused by the sympathetic-mediated enhancement of cardiac contractility tends, on the other hand, to reduce myocardial oxygen consumption by reducing myocardial wall tension (Laplace's law). Although there is a net increase in myocardial oxygen demand, this is normally balanced by an increase in coronary blood flow. Angina pectoris is believed to occur when oxygen demand exceeds supply. Since cardiac sympathetic activity increases myocardial oxygen demand, it might be expected that blockade of cardiac β-adrenergic receptors would relieve the symptoms of the anginal syndrome. It is on this basis that the early clinical studies with β-blocking drugs in angina were initiated.

The reduction in heart rate effected by β-blockade has two favorable consequences: (1) a decrease in cardiac work, thus reducing myocardial oxygen needs, and (2) a longer diastolic filling time associated with a slower heart rate, allowing for increased coronary perfusion.[43,44] β-Blockade also reduces exercise-induced blood pressure increments, the velocity of cardiac contraction, and oxygen consumption at any patient workload. Concomitant with the decrease in myocardial oxygen consumption, β-blockers can cause a reduction in coronary blood flow and a rise in coronary vascular resistance. The reduction in myocardial oxygen demand may be sufficient cause for this decrease in coronary blood flow. Although there is a decrease in total coronary flow, animal studies have demonstrated that β-blocker-induced shunting occurs in the coronary circulation, maintaining blood flow to ischemic areas, especially in the subendocardial region.

Although exercise tolerance and work capacity improve with β-blockade, the rate–pressure product (systolic blood pressure x heart rate) achieved when pain occurs is lower than that reached during a control run. This effect may relate to the action of β-blockers to increase left ventricular size, causing increased left ventricular wall tension and an increase in oxygen consumption at a given blood pressure.

The therapeutic benefit of β-blockers in chronic stable angina is now established beyond question. Many double-blind studies of β-blockers in patients have demonstrated a significant reduction in the frequency of angina attacks. Observed improvement is dose related, and dosage must be titrated for each patient.

Combined Use with Other Antianginal Therapies in Stable Angina

NITRATES Combined therapy with nitrates and β-blockers may be more efficacious for the treatment of angina pectoris than the use of either drug alone. The primary effect of β-blockers is to cause a reduction in both resting heart rate and the response of heart rate to exercise. Nitrates produce a reflex increase in heart rate and contractility, owing to a reduction in arterial pressure, and concomitant β-blocker therapy is extremely effective because it blocks this reflex increment in the heart rate. In patients with a propensity for myocardial failure who may have a slight increase in heart size with the β-blockers, the nitrates will counteract this tendency; the peripheral venodilatory effects of these drugs reduce the left ventricular volume. Similarly, the increase in coronary resistance associated with β-blocker administration can be ameliorated by the administration of nitrates.

CALCIUM CHANNEL BLOCKERS Calcium channel blockers block transmembrane calcium currents in vascular smooth muscle to cause arterial vasodilatation. Some calcium channel blockers also slow the heart rate and reduce atrioventricular conduction. Combined therapy with β-adrenergic and calcium channel blockers can provide clinical benefits for patients with angina pectoris who remain symptomatic with either agent used alone.[44] Because adverse effects can occur (heart block, heart failure), however, patients being considered for such treatment must be carefully selected and observed.

Angina at Rest and Vasospastic Angina

Although β-blockers are effective in the treatment of patients with angina of effort, their use in angina at rest is not so well established. The rationale for therapy with β-blockers was based on the assumption that the pathogenesis of chest pain at rest is similar to that with exertion. However, angina pectoris can be caused by multiple mechanisms, and increased coronary vascular tone may be responsible for ischemia in a significant proportion of patients with angina at rest.[44] Therefore, β-blockers that primarily reduce myocardial oxygen consumption but fail to exert vasodilating effects on coronary vasculature may not be totally effective in patients in whom angina is caused or increased by dynamic alterations in coronary luminal diameter. Despite their theoretic dangers in rest and vasospastic angina, β-blockers have been successfully used alone and in combination with vasodilating agents in many patients.

ARRHYTHMIAS

β-Adrenergic receptor blocking drugs have two main effects on the electrophysiologic properties of specialized cardiac tissue.[35] The first effect results from specific blockade of adrenergic stimulation of cardiac pacemaker potentials. By competitively inhibiting adrenergic stimulation, β-blockers decrease the slope of phase 4 depolarization and the spontaneous firing rate of sinus or ectopic pacemakers and thus decrease automaticity. Arrhythmias occurring in the setting of enhanced automaticity, as seen in myocardial infarction, digitalis toxicity, hyperthyroidism, and pheochromocytoma, would therefore be expected to respond well to β-blockade.[45] The second electrophysiologic effect of β-blockers involves membrane stabilizing activity, also known as "quinidine-like" or "local anesthetic" action. Characteristic of this effect is a reduction in the rate of rise of the intracardiac action potential without an effect on the spike duration of the resting potential. This effect and its attendant changes have been explained by inhibition of the depolarizing inward sodium current.

Sotalol, which has recently become available for treatment of ventricular arrythmias, is unique among the β-blockers in that it possesses class III antiarrhythmic properties, causing prolongation of the action potential period and thus delaying repolarization.[35] Clinical studies have verified the efficacy of sotalol in control of arrhythmias,[46] but additional investigation will be required to determine whether its class III antiarrhythmic properties contribute significantly to its efficacy as an antiarrhythmic agent.

The most important mechanism underlying the antiarrhythmic effect of β-blockers, with the possible exclusion of sotalol, is believed to be β-blockade with resultant inhibition of pacemaker potentials. If this view is accurate, then one would expect all β-blockers to be similarly effective at a comparable level of β-blockade. In fact, this appears to be the case. No superiority of one β-blocking agent over another in the therapy of arrhythmias has been convincingly demonstrated.[35] Differences in overall clinical usefulness are related to their other associated pharmacologic properties.

Supraventricular Arrhythmias

SINUS TACHYCARDIA Sinus tachycardia usually has an obvious cause (e.g., fever, hyperthyroidism, congestive heart failure), and therapy should focus on correcting the underlying condition. If the rapid heart rate itself is compromising the patient, however, causing recurrent angina in a patient with coronary artery disease, for example, then direct intervention with a β-blocker may be effective. Patients with heart failure, however, should not be treated with β-blockers unless they have been placed on diuretic therapy and cardiac glycosides and even then only with extreme caution. Some patients with primary cardiomyopathy with congestive heart failure appear to benefit from prolonged very-low-dose β-blocker therapy; the mechanisms for such beneficial effect, however, remain unclear.

Supraventricular Ectopic Beats

As in sinus tachycardia, specific treatment of these extrasystoles is seldom required and therapy should be directed to the underlying cause. Although supraventricular ectopic beats often are the precursors to atrial fibrillation, there is no evidence that prophylactic administration of β-blockers can prevent the development of atrial fibrillation. Supraventricular ectopic beats due to digitalis toxicity generally respond well to β-blockade.

Paroxysmal Supraventricular Tachycardia

By delaying atrioventricular conduction (e.g., increased atrio-His interval in bundle of His electrocardiograms) and prolonging the refractory period of the reentrant pathways, β-blockers are effective in terminating many cases of paroxysmal supraventricular tachycardia. Vagal maneuvers after β-blockade may effectively terminate an arrhythmia when they previously may have been unsuccessful without β-blockade. Even when β-blockers do not convert an arrhythmia to sinus rhythm, by increasing atrioventricular nodal refractoriness they often will slow the ventricular rate. The use of β-blocking drugs also still allows the option of direct-current countershock cardioversion.

Atrial Flutter

β-Blockade can be used to slow the ventricular rate (by increasing atrioventricular block) and may restore sinus rhythm in a large percentage of patients. This is a situation in which β-blockade may be of diagnostic value; given intravenously, β-blockers slow the ventricular response and permit the differentiation of flutter waves, ectopic P waves, or sinus mechanism.

Atrial Fibrillation

The major action of β-blockers in rapid atrial fibrillation is the reduction in the ventricular response caused by increasing the refractory period of the atrioventricular node. Although β-blocking drugs have been effective in slowing ventricular rates in patients with atrial fibrillation, they are less effective than quinidine or direct-current cardioversion in changing atrial fibrillation to sinus rhythm.

β-Blockers must be used with caution when atrial fibrillation occurs in the setting of a severely diseased heart that depends on high levels of adrenergic tone to avoid myocardial failure. These drugs may be particularly useful in controlling the ventricular rate in situations in which this is difficult to achieve with maximal tolerated doses of digitalis (e.g., thyrotoxicosis, hypertrophic cardiomyopathy, mitral stenosis, and after cardiac surgery).

Ventricular Arryhythmias

The response of ventricular arrhythmias to β-blockade appears to be at least as effective as antiarrhythmic drugs with other therapy.[46] β-Blockers are particularly useful if these arrhythmias are related to excessive catecholamines (e.g., exercise, halothane anesthesia, pheochromocytoma, exogenous catecholamines), myocardial ischemia, or digitalis. Since β-blockers are effective in preventing ischemic episodes, arrhythmias generated by these episodes may be prevented. β-Blockers are also quite effective in controlling the frequency of premature ventricular contractions in hypertrophic cardiomyopathy and in mitral valve prolapse. In controlled studies, β-blockers have been found to be effective in controlling complex life-threatening arrhythmias.[46]

Ventricular Tachycardia

β-Blocking drugs are not the agents of choice in the treatment of acute ventricular tachycardia. Cardioversion or other antiarrhythmic drugs should be the initial mode of therapy. β-Blockers have been shown to be of benefit for prophylaxis against recurrent ventricular tachycardia, particularly if sympathetic stimulation and/or myocardial ischemia appear to be precipitating causes. Several studies have been reported showing the prevention of exercise-induced ventricular tachycardia by β-blockers; in many previous cases there had been a poor response to digitalis or quinidine.[35]

Prevention of Ventricular Fibrillation

β-Blockade agents can attenuate cardiac stimulation by the sympathetic nervous system, and perhaps the potential for reentrant ventricular arrhythmias and sudden death.[47] Experimental studies have shown that β-blockers raise the ventricular fibrillation threshold in the ischemic myocardium.[47] Placebo-controlled clinical trials have shown that β-blockers reduce the number of episodes of ventricular fibrillation and cardiac arrest during the acute phase of myocardial infarction.[43] The long-term β-blocker postmyocardial infarction trials and other clinical studies with β-blockers have demonstrated that there is a significant reduction of complex ventricular arrhythmias.[49]

Use in Survivors of Acute Myocardial Infarction

The results of placebo-controlled long-term treatment trials with some β-adrenergic blocking drugs in survivors of acute myocardial infarction have demonstrated a favorable effect on total mortality, cardiovascular mortality (including sudden and non-sudden cardiac deaths), and the incidence of nonfatal reinfarction.[50,51] These beneficial results with β-blocker therapy can be explained by both the antiarrhythmic and the anti-ischemic effects of these drugs. It has also been proposed that β-blockers could reduce the risk of atherosclerotic placque rupture and subsequent thrombosis.[52] Two nonselective β-blockers, propranolol and timolol, have been approved by the Food and Drug Administration for reducing the risk of mortality in infarct survivors when started 5 to 28 days after an infarction. Metoprolol and atenolol, two β-selective blockers, are approved for the same indication and can be used in both intravenous and oral forms. β-Blockers have also been suggested as a treatment for reducing the extent of myocardial injury and mortality during the hyperacute phase of myocardial infarction with and without thrombolysis, but their exact role in this situation remains unclear.[53]

"Silent" Myocardial Ischemia

In recent years, investigators have observed that not all myocardial ischemic episodes detected by electrocardiography are associated with detectable symptoms.[54] Positron emission imaging techniques have validated the theory that these silent ischemic episodes are indicative of true myocardial ischemia.[55] The prognostic importance of silent myocardial ischemia occurring at rest and/or during exercise has not been determined. β-Blockers are successful in reducing the frequency of silent ischemic episodes detected by ambulatory electrocardiographic monitoring, as in reducing the frequency of painful ischemic events.[54]

Hypertrophic Cardiomyopathy

β-Adrenergic receptor blocking drugs have been proven efficacious in therapy for hypertrophic cardiomyopathy and idiopathic hypertrophic subaortic stenosis (IHSS).[56] These drugs are useful in controlling the dyspnea, angina, and syncope that occur with these disorders. β-Blockers have also been shown to lower the intraventricular pressure gradient both at rest and with exercise.

The outflow pressure gradient is not the only abnormality in hypertrophic cardiomyopathy; more important is the loss of ventricular compliance, which impedes normal left ventricular function. It has been shown that propranolol produces favorable changes in ventricular compliance in some patients with hypertrophic cardiomyopathy. The salutary hemodynamic and symptomatic effects produced by propranolol derive from its inhibition of sympathetic stimulation of the heart. However, there is no evidence that the drug alters the primary cardiomyopathic process; many patients remain in or return to their severely symptomatic state and some die despite its administration.

DILATED CARDIOMYOPATHY

The ability of intravenous sympathomimetic amines to effect an acute increase in myocardial contractility through stimulation of the β-adrenergic receptor has prompted hope that oral analogues may provide long-term benefit for patients with severe heart failure. Recent observations concerning the regulation of the myocardial adrenergic receptor and abnormalities of β-receptor-mediated stimulation in the failing myocardium have caused a critical reappraisal of the scientific validity of sustained β-adrenergic receptor stimulation, however.[57,58] New evidence suggests that β-receptor blockade may, when tolerated, have a favorable effect on the underlying cardiomyopathic process.[59,60]

The excessive catecholamine stimulation of the heart that occurs in chronic congestive heart failure can cause myocardial catecholamine depletion[61,62] a direct toxic effect on the heart,[63–65] and down-regulation of β-adrenergic receptors.[57,58,66] It appears that β-adrenergic blockade can correct these abnormalities and possibly improve left ventricular function.[60]

Preliminary studies with chronic β-blockade have demonstrated improvement in left ventricular function in many patients with advanced cardiomyopathy.[67–70] These studies have included patients who showed dramatic improvement in their hemodynamic situations while awaiting cardiac transplantation.[71] A large, prospective, double-blind multicenter study (Metoprolol in Dilated Cardiomyopathy [MIDICD]) is in progress, evaluating the efficacy of β-blocker therapy in patients with idiopathic cardiomyopathies.

MITRAL VALVE PROLAPSE

Mitral valve prolapse, characterized by a nonejection systolic click, a late systolic murmur, or a midsystolic click followed by a late systolic murmur, has been studied extensively over the past 20 years. Atypical chest pain, malignant arrhythmias, and nonspecific ST and T wave abnormalities have been observed with this condition. By decreasing sympathetic tone, β-adrenergic blockers have been shown to be useful for relieving the chest pains and palpitations that many of these patients experience and for reducing the incidence of life-threatening arrhythmias and other electrocardiographic abnormalities.[72]

DISSECTING ANEURYSMS

β-Adrenergic blockade plays a major role in the treatment of patients with acute aortic dissection.[73] During the hyperacute phase, β-blocking agents reduce the force and velocity of myocardial contraction *(dP/dt)* and hence the progression of the dissecting hematoma. However, such administration must be initiated simultaneously with the institution of other antihypertensive therapy that may cause reflex tachycardia and increases in cardiac output, factors that can aggravate the dissection process. Initially, propranolol is administered intravenously to reduce the heart rate to below 60 beats per minute. Once a patient is stabilized and long-term medical management is contemplated, the patient should be maintained on oral β-blocker therapy to prevent recurrence.

TETRALOGY OF FALLOT

By reducing the effects of increased adrenergic tone on the right ventricular infundibulum in tetralogy of Fallot,[74] β-blockers have been shown to be useful for the treatment of severe hypoxic spells and hypercyanotic attacks. With long-term use, these drugs have also been shown to prevent prolonged hypoxic spells. These drugs should be looked at only as palliative, and definitive surgical repair of this condition is usually required.

QT INTERVAL PROLONGATION SYNDROME

The syndrome of electrocardiographic QT interval prolongation is usually a congenital condition associated with deafness, syncope, and sudden death.[75] Abnormalities in sympathetic nervous system functioning in the heart have been proposed as explanations for the electrophysiologic aberrations seen in these patients. Propranolol appears to be the most effective drug for treatment of this syndrome. It reduces the frequency of syncopal episodes in most patients and may prevent sudden death. This drug will reduce the electrocardiographic QT interval.

EPINEPHRINE-INDUCED HYPOKALEMIA

Experimental studies have established that the infusion of catecholamines decreases serum potassium levels. Recently, it was demonstrated that physiologic concentration of epinephrine, such as that which may be seen with a myocardial infarction, may also induce hypokalemia, primarily through stimulation of β_2-receptors.[76] Subsequent studies have found that only the nonselective β-blockers can completely block the hypokalemic effect of epinephrine.[77] Considering the importance given to avoiding hypokalemia in the patient with an acute myocardial infarction, further study in this area is anticipated.

REGRESSION OF LEFT VENTRICULAR HYPERTROPHY

Left ventricular hypertrophy induced by systemic hypertension is an independent risk factor for cardiovascular mortality and morbidity.[16] Regression of left ventricular hypertrophy with drug therapy is feasible and may improve patient outcome.[16] β-Adrenergic blockers can cause regression of left ventricular hypertrophy, as determined by echocardiography with or without an associated reduction in blood pressure.[16]

Use in Noncardiovascular Disorders

THYROTOXICOSIS

Despite the inability to define precisely the relationship between catecholamines and hyperthyroidism, certain antiadrenergic agents (i.e., reserpine, guanethidine, and β-blockers) are capable of alleviating many of the sympathomimetic manifestations of the thyrotoxic state.[78] Because of their relative freedom from side effects, ease of administration, and rapid onset of action, β-blockers are the agents of choice. The exact mechanism of β-blocker benefit in hyperthyroidism is not fully defined. It is not resolved whether the effects of β-blockade are mediated by adrenergic blockade or by blocking the peripheral conversion of triiodothyronine to thyroxine.

PROPHYLAXIS OF MIGRAINE

The use of β-adrenergic blocking drugs to prevent migraine headache first was suggested in 1966. Clinical trials confirmed the safety and efficacy of propranolol for the prophylaxis of common migraine.[79] Propranolol is approved by the Food and Drug Administration for the treatment of migraine headache.

OPEN ANGLE GLAUCOMA

As early as 1968, topical applications of propranolol were shown to reduce intraocular pressure but its mild local anesthetic properties made investigators reluctant to use it for treatment of glaucoma. Topical application of timolol, a nonselective β-blocker without this local anesthetic property or PAA, also reduced intraocular pressure.[80] The mechanism of its ocular hypotensive effect has not been firmly established, but it may reduce the pressure by decreasing the production of aqueous humor. Of note, aggravation or precipitation of certain cardiovascular and pulmonary disorders has been reported with topical application of the drug and is presumably related to the systemic effects of β-adrenergic receptor blockade. Recently, four new ophthalmic β-blocker solutions were subsequently approved for glaucoma. Betaxolol is a β_1-selective drug that is applied twice daily. Levobunolol and metipranolol are nonselective drugs that can be used once or twice daily. Carteolol is a nonselective drug with partial agonism that can be used once daily. These new drugs do not appear to provide any efficacy or side-effect advantage over timolol.

ESSENTIAL TREMOR

The β-blocker propranolol has been approved for treatment of benign essential tremor.

Adverse Effects

MYOCARDIAL FAILURE

There are two circumstances by which blockade of β-receptors may cause congestive heart failure: (1) in an enlarged heart with impaired myocardial function in which excessive sympathetic drive is essential to maintain the myocardium on a compensated Starling curve and (2) in hearts in which the left ventricular stroke volume is restricted and tachycardia is needed to maintain cardiac output. In patients with impaired myocardial function who require β-blocking agents, digitalis and diuretics can be used, preferably with drugs having intrinsic sympathomimetic activity or β-adrenergic blocking properties.

SINUS NODE DYSFUNCTION AND ATRIOVENTRICULAR CONDUCTION DELAY

Slowing of the resting heart rate is a normal response to treatment with β-blocking drugs with and without PAA. In most cases, this does not present a problem;

healthy persons can sustain a heart rate of 40 to 50 beats per minute without disability unless there is clinical evidence of heart failure. Drugs with PAA do not lower the resting heart rate to the same degree as propranolol.[38] However, all β-blocking drugs are contraindicated (unless an artificial pacemaker is present) in patients with sick sinus syndrome.

β-ADRENERGIC RECEPTOR BLOCKER WITHDRAWAL

Following abrupt cessation of chronic β-blocker therapy, exacerbation of angina pectoris and, in some cases, acute myocardial infarction and death have been reported.[81] The exact mechanism for this reaction is unclear. There is some evidence that the withdrawal phenomenon may be due to the generation of additional β-adrenergic receptors during the period of β-adrenergic receptor blockade (hyperadrenergic state). Other suggested mechanisms for the withdrawal reaction include heightened platelet aggregability, an elevation in thyroid hormone activity, and an increase in circulating catecholamines. However, continuing the same level of activity as during β-blocker therapy appears to be the major contributing mechanism for the exacerbation of angina.

BRONCHOCONSTRICTION

The bronchodilator effects of catecholamines on the bronchial β-receptors (β_2) are inhibited by nonselective β-blockers. Comparative studies have shown that β-blocking compounds with PAA, β_1-selectivity, and α-adrenergic blocking actions are less likely to increase airway resistance in asthmatics than propranolol. β_1-Selectivity, however, is not absolute and may be lost with high therapeutic doses; therefore, all β-blockers should be avoided in patients with bronchospastic disease.

PERIPHERAL VASCULAR EFFECTS (RAYNAUD'S PHENOMENON)

Raynaud's phenomenon is one of the more common side effects of treatment with propranolol. Also, cold extremities and absent pulses have been reported to occur more frequently in patients receiving β-blockers for hypertension than in those receiving methyldopa. This is probably due to the reduction in cardiac output and blockade of β_2-adrenergic receptor-mediated vasodilation, resulting in unopposed α-adrenergic receptor vasoconstriction. β-Blocking drugs with β_1-selectivity or PAA will not affect peripheral vessels to the same degree as propranolol.

MISCELLANEOUS SIDE EFFECTS

Several authors have described severe hypoglycemic reactions during therapy with β-adrenergic blocking drugs. Studies of resting normal volunteers have demonstrated that propranolol produces no alteration in blood glucose values, although the hyperglycemic response to exercise is blunted. The enhancement of insulin-induced hypoglycemia and its hemodynamic consequences may be less with β_1-selective agents and agents with intrinsic sympathomimetic activity. There is also marked diminution in the clinical manifestations of the catecholamine discharge induced by hypo-glycemia (tachycardia).[82] These findings suggest that β-blockers interfere with compensatory responses to hypoglycemia and can mask certain "warning signs" of this condition. Other hypoglycemic reactions, such as diaphoresis, are not affected by β-adrenergic blockade.

Dreams, hallucinations, insomnia, and depression can occur during therapy with β-blockers. These symptoms are evidence of drug entry into the central nervous system and are especially common with the highly lipid-soluble β-blockers.

Diarrhea, nausea, gastric pain, constipation, and flatulence have been noted occasionally with all β-blockers (2% to 11% of patients). Hematologic reactions are rare: purpura and agranulocytosis have been described with propranolol.

A characteristic immune reaction, the oculomuco-cutaneous syndrome, affecting singly or in combination the eyes, mucous and serous membranes, and the skin (often in association with a positive antinu-clear factor), has been reported in patients treated with practolol and has led to the curtailment of this drug in clinical practice. Fears that other β-adrenergic blocker drugs may cause this syndrome have not been substantiated.

Drug Interactions
The wide diversity of diseases for which β-blockers are employed raises the likelihood of their concurrent administration with other drugs. It is imperative,

---

FIGURE 5.6 DRUG INTERACTIONS THAT MAY OCCUR WITH β-ADRENOCEPTOR BLOCKING DRUGS

Drug	Possible Effects	Precautions
Aluminum hydroxide gel	Decreased β-blocker adsorption and therapeutic effect	Avoid β-blocker-aluminum hydroxide combination.
Aminophylline	Mutual inhibition	Observe patient's response.
Amiodarone	May induce cardiac arrest	Combination should be used with extreme caution.
Antidiabetic agents	Enhanced hypoglycemia; hypertension	Monitor for altered diabetic response.
Calcium channel inhibitors (verapamil, diltiazem)	Potentiation of bradycardia, myocardial depression, and hypotension	Avoid use, although few patients show ill effects.
Cimetidine	Prolongs half-life of propranolol	Combination should be used with caution.
Clonidine	Hypertension during clonidine withdrawal	Monitor for hypertensive response; withdraw β-blocker before withdrawing clonidine.
Digitalis glycosides	Potentiation of bradycardia	Observe patient's response; interactions may benefit angina patients with abnormal ventricular function.
Epinephrine	Hypertension; bradycardia	Administer epinephrine cautiously; cardioselective β-blocker may be safer.
Ergot alkaloids	Excessive vasoconstriction	Observe patient's response; few patients show ill effects.
Glucagon	Inhibition of hyperglycemic effect	Monitor for reduced response.
Halofenate	Reduced β-blocking activity; production of propranolol withdrawal rebound syndrome	Observe for impaired respose to β-blockade.
Indomethacin	Inhibition of antihypertensive response to β-blockade	Observe patient's response.
Isoproterenol	Mutual inhibition	Avoid concurrent use or choose cardiac-selective β-blocker.
Levodopa	Antagonism of levodopa's hypotensive and positive inotropic effects	Monitor for altered response; interaction may have favorable results.
Lidocaine	Propranolol pretreatment increases lidocaine blood levels and potential toxicity	Combination should be used with caution; use lower doses of lidocaine.
Methyldopa	Hypertension during stress	Monitor for hypertensive episodes.
Monoamine oxidase inhibitors	Uncertain, theoretical	Manufacturer of propranolol considers concurrent use contraindicated.
Phenothiazines	Additive hypotensive effects	Monitor for altered response, especially with high doses of phenothiazines.
Phenylpropanolamine	Severe hypertensive reaction	Avoid use, especially in hypertension controlled by both methyldopa and β-blockers.
Phenytoin	Additive cardiac depressant effects	Administer IV phenytoin with great caution.
Quinidine	Additive cardiac depressant effects	Observe patient's response; few patients show ill effects.
Reserpine	Excessive sympathetic blockade	Observe patient's response.
Rifampin	Increased metabolism of β-blockers	Observe patient's response.
Smoking	Increased metabolism of β-blockers	Observe etc.
Tricyclic antidepressants	Inhibits negative inotropic and chronotropic effects of β-blockers	Observe patient's response.
Tubocurarine	Enhanced neuromuscular blockade	Observe response in surgical patients, especially after high doses of propranolol.

(Frishman WH: Clinical Pharmacology of the β-Adrenoceptor Blocking Drugs, 2nd ed. Norwalk, CT, Appleton-Century-Crofts, 1984, and Missri JC: How do beta-blockers interact with other commonly used drugs? Cardiovasc Med 8:668, 1983)

therefore, that clinicians become familiar with the interactions of β-blockers with other pharmacologic agents. The list of commonly used drugs with which β-blockers interact is extensive (Fig. 5.6).[35,83] The majority of the reported interactions have been associated with propranolol, the best studied of the β-blockers, and may not apply to other drugs in this class.

Clinical Use

More than 15 β-adrenoceptor blocking drugs are now available world-wide. As of 1993, with the introduction of betaxolol,[84] carteolol, penbutolol,[85] and sotalol, 14 β-blockers are marketed for approved uses in the United States. These are propranolol for angina pectoris, arrhythmia, systemic hypertension, essential tremor, prevention of migraine headache, and reducing the risk of mortality of survivors of acute myocardial infarction; atenolol and nadolol for angina pectoris and hypertension; timolol for hypertension, open angle glaucoma, and reducing the risk of mortality and reinfarction in survivors of acute myocardial in-

farction; metoprolol and atenolol for hypertension, angina pectoris, and reducing the risk of mortality in survivors of acute myocardial infarction; acebutolol for hypertension and ventricular arrhythmias; betaxolol, bisoprolol, carteolol, penbutolol, and pindolol for hypertension; intravenous esmolol for supraventricular tachycardias; sotalol for ventricular arrhythmias; and labetalol for hypertension and hypertensive emergencies. Recently the FDA approved a very low-dose diuretic–blocker combination (6.25 mg hydrochlorothiazide and bisoprolol) as a first line treatment for systemic hypertension. Carvedilol is now being studied actively in clinical trials. Oxprenolol has been approved for use in hypertension but has not yet been marketed in the United States.

The various β-blocking compounds given in adequate dosage appear to have comparable antihypertensive, antiarrhythmic, and antianginal effects. Therefore, the β-blocking drug of choice in an individual patient is determined by the pharmacodynamic and pharmacokinetic differences between the drugs, in conjunction with the patient's other medical conditions (Fig. 5.7).

FIGURE 5.7 CLINICAL SITUATIONS THAT WOULD INFLUENCE THE CHOICE OF A β-BLOCKING DRUG

Condition	Choice of β-Blocker
Asthma, chronic bronchitis with bronchospasm	Avoid all β-blockers if possible; however small doses of β_1-selective blockers (e.g., acebutolol, atenolol, metoprolol) can be used; β_1-selectivity is lost with higher doses; drugs with partial agonist activity (e.g., pindolol, oxprenolol) and labetalol with α-adrenergic blocking properties can also be used.
Congestive heart failure	Drugs with partial agonist activity and labetalol might have an advantage, although β-blockers are usually contraindicated.
Angina	In patients with angina at low heart rates, drugs with partial agonist activity are probably contraindicated; patients with angina at high heart rates but who have resting bradycardia might benefit from a drug with partial agonist activity; in vasospastic angina, labetalol may be useful, but other β-blockers should be used with caution.
Atrioventricular conduction defects	β-Blockers are generally contraindicated by drugs with partial agonist activity and labetalol can be tried with caution.
Bradycardia	β-Blockers with partial agonist activity and labetalol have less pulse-slowing effect and are preferable.
Raynaud's phenomenon, intermittent claudication, cold extremities	β_1-Selective blocking agents, labetalol, and those with partial agonist activity might have an advantage.
Depression	Avoid propranolol; substitute a β-blocker with partial agonist actvity.
Diabetes mellitus	β_1-Selective agents and partial agonist drugs are preferable.
Thyrotoxicosis	All agents will control symptoms, but agents without partial agonist activity are preferred.
Pheochromocytoma	Avoid all β-blockers unless an α-blocker is given; labetalol is the drug of choice.
Renal failure	Use reduced doses of compounds largely eliminated by renal mechanisms (nadolol, acebutolol, sotalol, atenolol) and of those drugs whose bioavailability is increased in uremia (propranolol); also consider possibly accumulation of active metabolites (acebutolol, propranolol)
Insulin and sulfonylurea use	Danger of hypoglycemia; possibly less using drugs with β_1-selectivity
Clonidine	Avoid nonselective β-blockers; severe rebound effects with clonidine withdrawal
Oculomucocutaneous syndrome	Stop drug; substitute any other β-blockers.
Hyperlipidemia	Avoid nonselective β-blockers; use agents with partial agonism, β_1-selectivity, or labetalol.

(Frishman WH: Clinical Pharmacology of the β-Adrenoceptor Blocking Drugs, 2nd ed. Norwalk, CT, Appleton-Century-Crofts, 1984)

REFERENCES

1. Ahlquist RP: Study of the adrenotropic receptors. Am J Physiol 153:486, 1948
2. Lands AM, Luduena FP, Buzzo HJ: Differentiation of receptor systems responsive to isoproterenol. Life Sci 6: 2241, 1967
3. Berthelsen S, Pettinger WA: A functional basis for classification of alpha-adrenergic receptors. Life Sci 21:596, 1977
4. Frishman WH, Charlap S: α-Adrenergic blockers. Med Clin North Am 72:427, 1988
5. Luther RR: New perspectives on selective α_1-blockade. Am J Hypertens 2:729, 1989
6. Taylor SH: Clinical pharmacotherapeutics of doxazosin. Am J Med 87(2A): 2S, 1989
7. Singleton W, Dix RK, Monsen L et al: Efficacy and safety of Minipress XL, a new once-a-day formulation of prazosin. Am J Med 87(2A):45S, 1989
8. Van Zwieten PA: Pharmacology profile of urapadil. Am J Cardiol 64:1D, 1989
9. Elliott HL, Meredith PA, Vincent J et al: Clinical pharmacological studies with doxazosin. Br J Clin Pharmacol 21:27S, 1986
10. Reid JL, Meredith PA, Elliot HL:Pharmacokinetics and pharmacodynamics of trimazosin in man. Am Heart J 106:1222, 1983
11. Archibald JL: Recent developments in the pharmacology and pharmacokinetics of indoramin. J Cardiovasc Pharmacol 8(Suppl 2):516, 1986
12. Frishman WH, Eisen G, Lapsker J: Terazosin: A new long-acting α-adrenergic antagonist for hypertension. Med Clin North Am 72:441, 1988
13. Katz AM, Hager WD, Mesineo FC et al: Cellular actions and pharmacology of the calcium channel blocking drugs. Am J Med 77:2, 1984
14. Ribner HS, Bresnahan D, Hsieh AM: Acute hemodynamic responses to vasodilation therapy in congestive heart failure. Prog Cardiovasc Dis 25: 1, 1982
15. Frishman WH, Johnson BF, Pulos G, et al: The effects of cardiovascular drugs on plasma lipids and lipoproteins. In Frishman WH (ed): Medical Management of Lipid Disorders: Focus on Prevention of Coronary Artery Disease, p 253. New York, Futura Publishing Co, 1992
16. Hachamovitch R, Strom JA, Sonnenblick EH, Frishman WH: Left ventricular hypertrophy in hypertension and the effects of antihypertensive drug therapy. Curr Probl Cardiol 13: 371, 1988
17. Gould L, Reddy CVR: Phentolamine. Am Heart J 92:392, 1976
18. Majid PA, Sharma B, Taylor SH: Phentolamine for vasodilator treatment of severe heart failure. Lancet 2:719, 1971
19. Packer M: Vasodilator and inotropic therapy for severe chronic heart failure: Passion and skepticism. J Am Coll Cardiol 2:841, 1983
20. Cohn JN, Archibald DG, Ziesche S et al: Effect of vasodilator therapy on mortality in chronic congestive heart failure: Results of a Veterans Administration Cooperative Study (V-HEFT). N Engl J Med 314:1547, 1986
21. Scholz H: Inotropic drugs and their mechanism of action. J Am Coll Cardiol 4:389, 1984
22. Orlick AE, Ricci DR, Cipriano PR et al: The contribution of alpha-adrenergic tone to resting coronary vascular resistance in man. J Clin Invest 62:459, 1978
23. Winniford MD, Flipchuk N, Hillis DL: Alpha-adrenergic blockade for variant angina: A long-term double-blind randomized trial. Circulation 67:1185, 1983
24. Corr PB, Shayman JA, Kramer JB et al: Increased α-adrenergic receptors in ischemic cat myocardium: A potential mediator of electrophysiologic derangements. J Clin Invest 67:1232, 1981
25. Manger WM, Gifford RW: Pheochromocytoma. New York, Springer-Verlag, 1977
26. Honston MC, Thompson WL, Robertson D: Shock. Arch Intern Med 144:1433, 1984
27. Fein SA, Frishman WH: The pathophysiology and management of pulmonary hypertension. Cardiol Clin 5:563, 1987
28. Cohen ML, Kronzon I: Adverse hemodynamic effects of phentolamine in primary pulmonary hypertension. Ann Intern Med 95:591, 1981
29. Henderson WR, Shelhamer JH, Reingold DB et al: Alpha-adrenergic hyper-responsiveness in asthma. N Engl J Med 300:642, 1979
30. Barnes PJ, Wilson NM, Vickers H: Prazosin, an alpha α_1-adrenoceptor antagonist, partially inhibits exercise-induced asthma. J Allergy Clin Immunol 68:411, 1981
31. Hedlund H, Andersson KE, Ek A: Effects of prazosin in patients with benign prostatic obstruction. Urol 130:275, 1983
32. Oates JA, Robertson D, Wood AJJ: Alpha and beta-adrenergic agonists and antagonists. In Rosen MR, Hoffman BF (eds): Cardiac Therapy, p 145. Boston, Martinus Nijhoff, 1983
33. Westfall DP: Adrenoceptor antagonists. In Craig CR, Zitzel RE (eds): Modern Pharmacology, p 141. Boston, Little, Brown & Co, 1982
34. Frishman WH: β-Adrenoceptor antagonists. New drugs and new indications. N Engl J Med 305: 500, 1981
35. Frishman WH: Clinical Pharmacology of the β-Adrenoceptor Blocking Drugs, 2nd ed. Norwalk, CT, Appleton-Century-Crofts, 1984
36. Frishman WH β-Adrenergic blockers. Med Clin North Am 72:37, 1988
37. Koch-Weser J: Metoprolol. N Engl J Med 301: 698, 1979
38. Frishman WH: Pindolol: A new β-adrenoceptor antagonist with partial agonist activity. N Engl J Med 308:940, 1983
39. Frishman W, Halprin S: Clinical pharmacology of the new beta-adrenergic blocking drugs VII. New horizons in beta-adrenoceptor blocking therapy: Labetalol. Am Heart J 98:660, 1979
40. Frishman WH, Lazar EJ, Gorodokin G: Pharmacokinetic optimization of therapy with beta-adrenergic blocking agents. Clin Pharmacokin 20:311, 1991
41. Murthy VF, Frishman WH: Controlled beta-receptor blockade with esmolol and flestolol. Pharmacotherapy 8:168, 1988
42. Frishman W, Silverman R: Clinical pharmacology of the new beta-adrenergic blocking drugs: III. Comparative clinical experience and new therapeutic applications. Am Heart J 98:119, 1979
43. Frishman WH: Multifactorial actions of β-adren-

ergic blocking drugs in ischemia heart disease: Current concepts. Circulation 67(Suppl 1):11, 1983

44. Frishman WH: Beta-adrenergic blockade in the treatment of coronary artery disease. In Hurst JW (ed): Clinical Essays on the Heart, vol 2, p 25. New York, McGraw-Hill, 1983

45. Miura D, Frishman WH, Dangman KH: Class II drugs. In Dangman KH, Miura D (eds): Basic and Clinical Electrophysiology and Pharmacology of the Heart, p 665. New York, Marcel Dekker, 1991

46. Anastosioll U, Nana MI, Gilbert EM, Miller RH et al: Usefulness of dil-sotalol for suppression of chronic ventricular arrhythmias. Am J Cardiol 67:511, 1991

47. Pratt C, Lichstein E: Ventricular antiarrhythmic effects of beta-adrenergic blocking drugs: A review of mechanism and clinical studies. J Clin Pharmacol 22:335, 1982

48. Ryden L, Ariniego R, Arnman K et al: A double-blind trial of metoprolol in acute myocardial infarction: Effects on ventricular tachyarrhythmias. N Engl J Med 308:614, 1983

49. Pratt C, Lichstein E: Ventricular anti-arrhythmic effects of beta-adrenergic blocking drugs: A review of mechanism and clinical studies. J Clin Pharmacol 22:335, 1982

50. Frishman WH, Furberg CD, Friedewald WT: β-Adrenergic blockade for survivors of acute myocardial infarction. N Engl J Med 310:830, 1984

51. Frishman WH, Skolnick AE, Lazar EJ: β-Adrenergic blockade and calcium channel blockade in myocardial infarction. Med Clin North Am 73:409, 1989

52. Frishman WH, Lazar EJ: Reduction of mortality, sudden death and non-fatal reinfarction with beta-adrenergic blockers in survivors of acute myocardial infarction: A new hypothesis regarding the cardioprotective action of beta-adrenergic blockade. Am J Cardiol 66:66G, 1990.

53. TIMI Study Group: TIMI II comparison by invasive and conservative strategies after treatment with IV TPA in acute MI: Results of Thrombolysis in MI TIMI phase II trial. N Engl J Med 320(10):618, 1989

54. Frishman WH, Teicher M: Antianginal drug therapy for silent myocardial ischemia. Am Heart J 114:140, 1987

55. Deanfield JE, Shea MJ, Selwyn AP: Clinical evaluation of transient myocardial ischemia during daily life. Am J Med 79(Suppl 3A):18, 1985

56. Swan DA, Bell B, Oakley CM et al: Analysis of symptomatic course and prognosis in treatment of hypertrophic obstructive cardiomyopathy. Br Heart J 33:671, 1971

57. Bristow MR, Ginsberg R, Minobe W et al: Decreased catecholamine sensitivity and β-adrenergic receptor density in failing human hearts. N Engl J Med 307:205, 1982

58. Colucci WS, Alexander RW, Williams GH et al: Decreased lymphocyte beta-adrenergic receptor density in patients with heart failure and tolerance to the beta-adrenergic agonist parbuterol. N Engl J Med 305:185, 1981

59. Bristow MR: The adrenergic nervous system in heart failure. N Engl J Med 311:850, 1984

60. Andersson E, Blomstrom-Lundquist C, Hedner T, Waagstein F: Exercise hemodynamics and myocardial metabolism during long-term beta-adrenergic blockade in severe heart failure. J Am Coll Cardiol 18:1059, 1991

61. Rose CP, Burgess JH, Cousineau D: Reduced aortocoronary sinus extraction of epinephrine in patients with left ventricular failure secondary to long-term pressure or volume overload. Circulation 68:241,1983

62. Sole MJ. Kamble AB, Hussain MN: A possible change in the rate-limiting step for cardiac norepinephrine synthesis in the cardiomyopathic Syrian hamster. Circ Res 41:814, 1977

63. Bloom S, Davis DL: Calcium as mediator of isoproterenol-induced myocardial necrosis. Am J Pathol 69:459,1972

64. Kahn DS, Rona G, Chappel CI: Isoproterenol-induced cardiac necrosis. Ann NY Acad Sci 156:285, 1969

65. Simons M, Downing S: Coronary vasoconstriction and catecholamine cardiomyopathy. Am Heart J 109:297, 1985

66. Heinsimer JA, Lefkowitz RJ: The beta-adrenergic receptor in heart failure. Hosp Pract 18:103, 1983

67. Engelmeier RS, O'Connell JB, Walsh R et al: Improvement in symptoms and exercise tolerance by metoprolol in patients with dilated cardiomyopathy. A double-blind, randomized, placebo-controlled trial. Circulation 72:536, 1985

68. Eichorn EJ, Bedotto JB, Malloy CR et al: Effect of β-adrenergic blockade on myocardial function and energetics in congestive heart failure: Improvements in hemodynamics, contractile, and diastolic performance with bucindolol. Circulation 82:473, 1990

69. Waagstein F, Caidahl K, Wallentin I et al: Long-term β-blockade in dilated cardiomyopathy: Effects of short and long-term metoprolol treatment followed by withdrawal and readministration of metoprolol. Circulation 80:551, 1989

70. Heilbrunn SM, Shah P, Bristow MR et al: Increased β-receptor density and improved hemodynamic response to catecholamine stimulation during long-term metoprolol therapy in heart failure from dilated cardiomypathy. Circulation 79:483, 1989

71. Fowler MB, Bristow MR, Laser JA et al: Beta-blocker therapy in severe heart failure: Improvement related to β-adrenergic receptor regulation? Circulation 70(Suppl 2):112, 1984

72. Winkle RA, Lopes MG, Goodman DS et al: Propranolol for patients with mitral valve prolapse. Am Heart J 93:422, 1970

73. Slater EE, DeSanctis R: Dissection of the aorta. Med Clin North Am 63:141, 1979.

74. Shah PM, Kidd L: Circulatory effects of propranolol in children with Fallot's tetralogy: Observations with isoproterenol infusion, exercise and crying. Am J Cardiol 19:653, 1967

75. Vincent CM, Abildskov JA, Burgess MJ. Q-T interval syndromes. Prog Cardiovasc Dis 16:523, 1974

76. Brown MJ, Brown DC, Murphy MB: Hypokalemia from beta²-receptor stimulation by circulating epinephrine. N Engl J Med 309:1414, 1983

77. Struthers AD, Reid JL, Whitesmith R et al: The effect of cardioselectivity and nonselective beta-adrenoceptor blockade on the hypokalemic and cardiovascular responses to adrenomedullary hormone in man. Clin Sci 65:143, 1983

78. Ingbar SH: The role of antiadrenergic agents in the management of thyrotoxicosis. Cardiovasc Rev Rep 2:683, 1981

79. Caviness VS Jr, O'Brien P: Headache. N Engl J Med 302:446, 1980

80. Heel RC Brogden RN, Speight TM et al: Timolol: A review of its therapeutic efficacy in the topical treatment of glaucoma. Drugs 17:38, 1979

81. Frishman WH: Beta-blocker withdrawal. Am J Cardiol 59:26F, 1987

82. Lloyd-Mostyn RH, Oram S: Modification by propranolol of cardiovascular effects of induced hypoglycemia. Lancet 2:1213, 1975

83. Missri JC: How do beta-blockers interact with other commonly used drugs? Cardiovasc Med 8: 668, 1983

84. Frishman WH, Tepper D, Lazar E, Behrman D: Betaxolol: A new long-acting β-selective adrenergic blocker. J Clin Pharmacol, 30:699, 1990

85. Frishman WH, Covey S: Carteolol and penbutolol, two new β-adrenergic blockers with partial agonist activity. J Clin Pharmacol, 30:412, 1990

Calcium Channel Blockade and Cardiovascular Therapeutics

Bramah N. Singh

It is now more than 30 years since the prototype of calcium channel blockers, verapamil, was first described. Rapid advances in our understanding of the pharmacodynamics of these agents and their clinical applications followed only after the conceptual framework was provided by Fleckenstein in the early 1970s.[1] The pioneering work focused attention on the selectivity of effects of calcium channel blockers on the myocardial slow channel, as the electrophysiologic effects of agents such as verapamil and prenylamine[1] in cardiac muscle were found to be similar to those produced by calcium-free media. The slow channel could be blocked markedly with drug concentrations that had little or no effect on the fast sodium channel. Agents with this selectivity of myocardial action also showed a propensity to block calcium fluxes in vascular smooth muscle; thus, they all are coronary vasodilators and peripheral vasodilators. However, it soon became clear[2-5] that the so-called calcium antagonist compounds (defined primarily as those agents that produced excitation-contraction uncoupling in cardiac muscle by blocking the slow channel) manifest a marked heterogeneity in chemical structure. Some are truly selective for the slow channel in extremely low concentrations (e.g., the dihydropyridines), while others block the slow and fast channels in approximately the same drug concentrations (e.g., perhexiline). Recent approaches have focused attention on the development of agents either with a broad pharmacologic profile or with a particular tissue selectivity.[5] This has led to a plethora of newer calcium channel blocking drugs, many still under investigation, while a number have been introduced into therapeutics.[2-5] Numerous others are under development and are likely to be introduced into therapeutics in the future.

Calcium antagonism has been established as a therapeutic modality in the treatment of various myocardial ischemic syndromes, hypertension, certain cardiac arrhythmias, and hypertrophic cardiomyopathies. Numerous lesser indications are less well established. The effectiveness of calcium channel blockers as a class of agents stems from the pathologic effects of intracellular calcium overload in these disorders.

In this chapter, the pharmacologic basis of the therapeutic actions of calcium channel blockers is discussed, with particular reference to their hemodynamic and electrophysiologic actions. Their expanding role in the management of various cardiocirculatory disorders is delineated in relation to the pharmacodynamic and pharmacokinetic properties of the individual agents. The potential and the expanding roles of the newer agents are emphasized.

ELECTROPHARMACOLOGIC CONSIDERATIONS

The ubiquitous role of calcium in mediating numerous physiologic responses is well recognized. Many physiologic processes, such as excitation-contraction coupling, control of secretion, excitability, and conduction and pacemaker activity, are now known to be mediated through voltage-dependent calcium channels[6,7] The type, density, and function of these channels vary between different type of cells.[7] In relation to the actions of calcium channel blockers, the role of calcium in mediating excitation-contraction coupling in cardiac muscle[6,7] and in vascular smooth muscle[8] is of the greatest significance.

Types and Defining Properties of Calcium Channels

In defining the pharmacologic properties of calcium antagonists, some of the recent knowledge gleaned from patch-clamp and voltage-clamp techniques in isolated myocytes from the mammalian myocardium is useful. Four types of calcium channels have now been described.

In the myocardium, the primary locus of action of these drugs is on the L-type calcium channels; these are 1,4-dihyropyridine-sensitive.[7] The voltage clamp technique has established that the depolarizing current in cardiac muscle is mediated by two discrete components. The first current component ("fast response"), carried by sodium ions, is rapidly activated and inactivated and is blocked selectively by fast-channel blockers, which are essentially local anesthetics. The second component is the slow current ("slow response"), for which the charge carrier is mostly calcium.[7] This current is carried primarily through the L-type calcium channel and it completes the terminal phase of depolarization. It is slowly activated at more positive membrane voltages, and it is much more slowly inactivated than the fast sodium current. Blockade of this channel leads to excitation-contraction uncoupling with little or no change in the gross electrophysiologic parameters of the action potential in fast-channel-dependent fibers. Particularly evident in isolated tissue is the striking reduction in contractility, the overall effect resembling that of calcium-free media.[1] These changes are evident especially in atrial and ventricular myocardium, in which neither conduction nor refractoriness is altered.

An additional calcium channel, the T-type, is activated at still higher membrane potentials than the L-type, but it deactivates much more rapidly.[9] Its physiologic importance remains unknown. It is abundant in sinoatrial cells, in Purkinje fibers, and in the pacemaker cells in the atria and ventricles. The T-channel may play a role in automaticity in these fibers, but its relationship to the so-called pacemaker (I_f) current remains uncertain. The N-type calcium channels have been described in neuronal cells and may play a major role in neurotransmitter release. Finally, high-threshold channels insensitive to 1,4-dihydropyridines but sensitive to certain spider toxins, designated P-type channels, have been described in the Purkinje cells in the mammalian cerebellum. Their precise physiologic significance is currently unknown.

Radioligand Binding of Calcium Channel Blockers

Agents that bind directly to voltage-sensitive calcium channels are called calcium channel ligands, which may function as agonists (e.g., Bay K 4486) or antagonists (e.g., verapamil, diltiazem, nifedipine), respectively increasing or decreasing calcium ion fluxes through the channels. In the case of the best known antagonists, the binding leads to vasodilatation, decreased incidence of certain arrhythmias, or decreased heart rate and contractility, at least in cardiac preparations in vitro.

Thus the effects of myocardial calcium antagonism are minimal in fast-channel-dependent fibers, such as those in atria, ventricles, His–Purkinje system, and atrioventricular bypass tracts, although the effect on the plateau phase of the action potential in the Purkinje fibers and ventricular muscle may be demonstrable. The effects of calcium channel blockers are most pronounced in slow-channel-dependent fibers, namely, in the sinoatrial and atrioventricular nodes. Again, the most consistent depressant effect is seen in isolated preparations devoid of autonomic reflexes. In isolated preparations of smooth muscle cells, slow-channel blockers exert a much more complex effect,

since the process of excitation-contraction coupling is not governed by a single process.[8] Calcium entry across smooth muscle membrane is regulated by a voltage-dependent mechanism and by a receptor-mediated channel. These mechanisms may be affected by different slow-channel blockers, but the net effect is varying degrees of smooth muscle relaxation due to inhibition of calcium influx. The major focus of this chapter is the role of specific blockers of L-type calcium channels, as they constitute an important class of therapeutic agents for major cardiovascular disorders.

A very heterogeneous group of compounds has been shown to block calcium currents through the L-type channels. The structures of the commonly available agents are shown in Figure 6.1. These

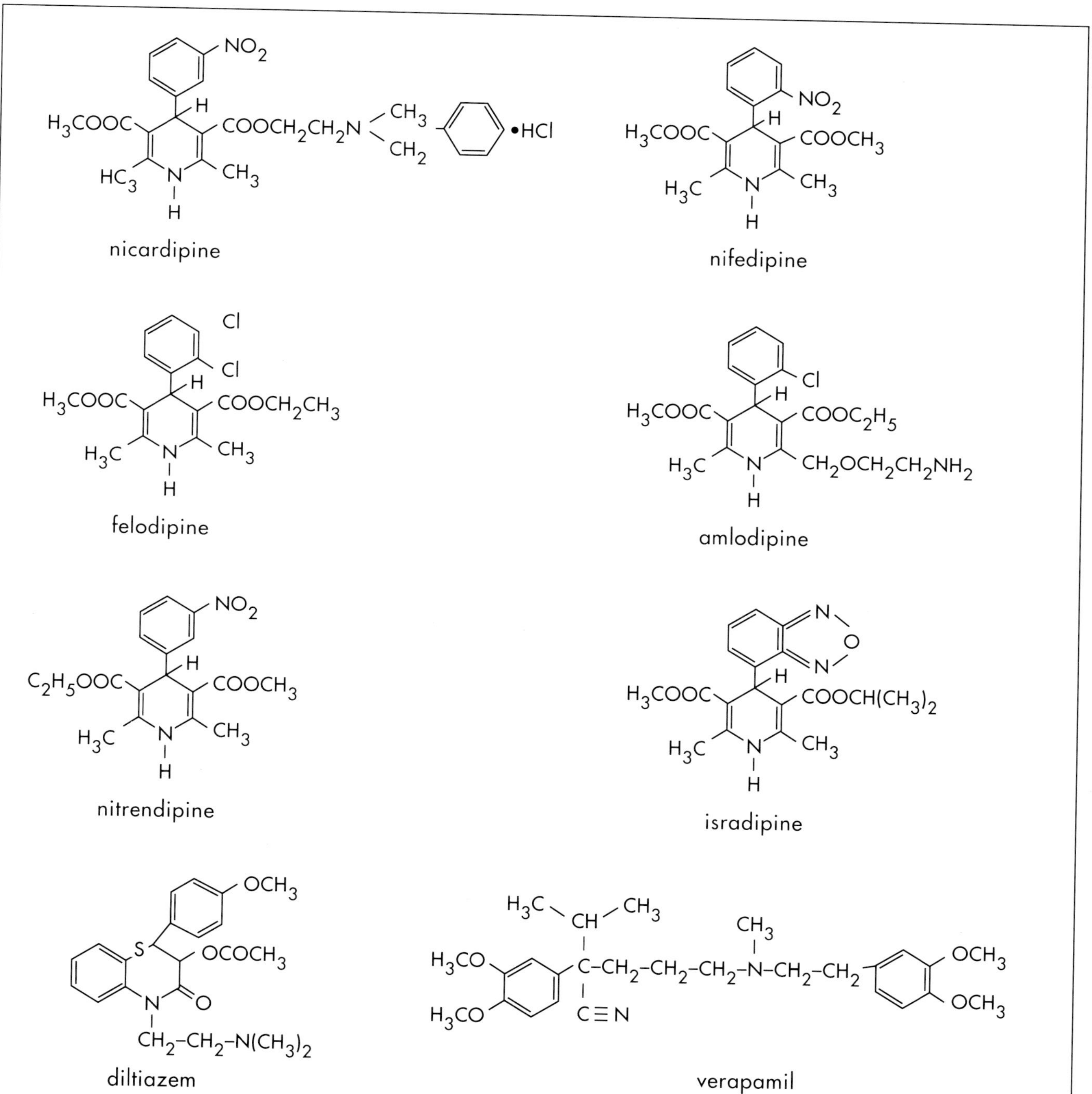

Figure 6.1 The structure of commonly available calcium channel blockers. The structures of verapamil and diltiazem differ from the others, which are all 1,4-dihydropyridines. Over 20 dihydropyridines (e.g., nimodipine, nisoldipine, nilvadipine, niludipine) are under development.

compounds have varying potencies for blocking the myocardial slow channel and for inhibiting calcium fluxes in vascular smooth muscle cells. Furthermore, because of their structural heterogeneity, many of the agents have additional pharmacologic properties. For example, some of the compounds influence the autonomic nervous system by their propensity noncompetitively to inhibit catecholamine α- and β-receptors (e.g., verapamil, diltiazem, bepridil). These properties therefore influence the balance between these compounds' direct myocardial effects on chronotropic, dromotropic, and inotropic properties and the reflex changes caused by the activation of the sympathetic nervous system by peripheral vasodilatation. Some of the agents have additional electrophysiologic actions due to their associated effects on the fast channel and on cardiac repolarization (e.g., bepridil, lidoflazine). It is clear that, unlike β-blockers, the net pharmacologic effects of individual calcium channel blockers may not be predictable solely from their ability to inhibit calcium fluxes competitively in the myocardium or smooth cells. The net effects may differ significantly in vivo from those in vitro; these differences are of clinical significance.

CLASSIFICATION OF CALCIUM ANTAGONISTS

Fleckenstein[1] suggested that calcium antagonists may be classified into two categories. He placed agents such as verapamil, diltiazem, and nifedipine with its

derivatives, which have a marked selectivity for inhibiting the slow channel rather than the fast sodium channel in the heart, into one group (group A), and those such as prenylamine, terodiline, fendiline, and perhexiline, which inhibit the slow channel but also have a broad array of other electrophysiologic actions, into another group (group B). However, the expanding knowledge of the electropharmacology of these and newer agents suggests a need for an alternative classification. The one proposed in Figure 6.2, developed along clinical lines,[5] may also eventually need modification due to the rapidly accumulating clinical and experimental data relating to calcium channel blockers. The ideal classification is likely to be one that not only provides a framework for the conceptual understanding of cellular and subcellular actions of these agents but also provides a correlative link to their clinical and therapeutic effects relative to pathophysiology.

Type I: Calcium Channel Blockers With In Vivo Myocardial and Peripheral Vascular Effects

These agents are moderately potent peripheral vasodilators and are effective in mild to moderate hypertension. Their predominant electrophysiologic actions are to delay conduction and to prolong refractoriness in the AV node, properties that account for many of their known antiarrhythmic effects. The hemodynamic effects in experimental animals and in

---

FIGURE 6.2 CLINICAL CLASSIFICATION OF CALCIUM ANTAGONISTS

Type I	Calcium antagonists with "balanced" in vivo myocardial, electrophysiologic, and vascular effects
	Verapamil Diltiazem
	Gallopamil (D$_{600}$) Tiapamil
	Anipamil
Type II	Calcium antagonists with predominantly vascular effects in vivo
	Nifedipine Niludipine
	Nitrendipine Felodipine
	Nisoldipine Isradipine
	Nimodipine Amlodipine
	Nicardipine
Type III	Calcium antagonists with markedly selective vascular effects
	Cinnarizine
	Flunarizine
Type IV	Calcium antagonists with complex pharmacologic profiles
	Bepridil Perhexiline
	Lidoflazine

(Adapted from Singh BN, Baky S, Nademanee K: Second generation calcium antagonists: Search for greater selectivity and versatility. Am J Cardiol 55:214B, 1985)

patients with varying levels of ventricular function are reasonably well defined for verapamil; there are modest data for diltiazem but very little information for tiapamil, anipamil, and gallopamil (none of the last three is available in the United States). There are preliminary data to indicate that gallopamil might be extremely effective in terminating supraventricular tachycardias and controlling chronic stable angina; further data are needed to determine critically the comparative efficacy of tiapamil, gallopamil, and anipamil on the one hand and verapamil and diltiazem on the other.

Type II: The Dihydropyridines

Over thirty of these compounds have been synthesized. These agents are relatively homogeneous in their overall properties and best demonstrate the scope for the study of structure–activity relationships. The quantitative potencies of individual members of the subclass may differ with respect to the effects on the myocardial slow channel as well as the potencies for inhibiting calcium fluxes in vascular smooth muscle. They also exhibit quantitative differences in their predilection for regional circulations. As a group, the potency of the dihydropyridines is much greater in smooth muscle than in cardiac muscle; these agents in vivo are nearly or completely devoid of clinically significant electrophysiologic properties, their overall hemodynamic effects being dominated by striking peripheral vasodilatation. For agents whose peripheral vasodilator effect far exceeds that in the myocardium, the concept of vasoselectivity has been invoked. Such agents (e.g., nicardipine, felodopine, isradipine, nisoldipine, nitrendipine, nilvadipine, lacidipine, amlodipine) may be essentially devoid of negative inotropic effect in vivo; even in heart failure they may function as potent afterload-reducing agents producing increases in cardiac output and stroke volume and improving contractile indices, including left ventricular ejection fraction. Their role in the treatment of heart failure and in patients with myocardial ischemia in the setting of heart failure is being explored (see below).

From the therapeutic standpoint, the dihydropyridines, though devoid of antiarrhythmic effects, may be of particular value in the control of hypertensive emergencies as well as in the long-term management of essential hypertension, either as single agents or in combination with diuretics, β-adrenergic blocking drugs or other hypotensive agents. Since all of these agents can produce reflex increases in heart rate and contractility, angina may sometimes be aggravated in patients with coronary artery disease if concomitant sympatholytic agents are not used. The cardioprotective effects of these agents appear to be less striking in experimental animals than those of type I agents.

They even have a deleterious effect in the survivors of acute infarction, if not combined with β-blockers.

The first dihydropyridine approved for therapeutic use was nifedipine, but numerous others have more recently been introduced. These include nicardipine, isradipine, felodipine, amlodipine, and nimodipine. The dihydropyridines may exert tissue selectivity.[10] For example, nimodipine was introduced into clinical use for its action in the cerebral vasculature.[10,11]

Type III: The Piperazine Derivatives, Cinnarizine and Flunarizine

The piperazine derivatives of calcium channel blocker drugs, namely cinnarizine and its difluoro derivative, flunarizine, are highly selective for calcium channels in vascular smooth muscle relative to cardiac muscle.[10,12] However, at high concentrations in the myocardium, they affect triggered activity and may therefore be of value for differentiating certain ventricular arrhythmias. The properties and therapeutic uses of flunarizine have been reviewed by Holmes and colleagues.[12] Flunarizine has a much longer plasma elimination half-life than does cinnarizine. The majority of the therapeutic trials with flunarizine have been in the prophylaxis of migraine, occlusive peripheral vascular disease, and vertigo of central and peripheral origin. The preliminary data for the piperazine derivatives appear to offer new and useful pharmacologic approaches to the control of a number of circulatory disorders, but the definition of their precise role in the therapy of such conditions must await results of stringently controlled comparative studies.

Type IV: Calcium Channel Blockers With Complex Pharmacologic Profiles

Another group of pharmacologic agents may be categorized as calcium channel blockers that have a selectivity of action either for vascular tissues (as in the case of lidoflazine)[13] or for both cardiac and smooth muscle (in the case of perhexiline[14] and bepridil[15,16]) while also having the propensity to block the fast sodium channel in the heart to a variable degree. Some of these agents have yet other electrophysiologic properties, such as effects on repolarization (lidoflazine and bepridil). Thus, these agents are not only heterogeneous chemically but, by virtue of their complex overall pharmacologic properties, they may exert a somewhat different spectrum of therapeutic as well as adverse cardiac effects. This pertains particularly to their cardiac electrophysiologic actions.

Bepridil hydrochloride (Fig. 6.3) is the most important compound in this regard. Electrophysiologically, bepridil blocks the slow calcium channel in the heart while inhibiting the fast channel and lengthening the repolarization phase of the cardiac action potential in all myocardial tissues. The compound may produce torsade de pointes in association with prolonged QT interval, especially during electrolyte disturbance. The lengthening of repolarization is related to the drug's inhibition of the delayed rectifier and inward rectifier potassium channels. Bepridil has recently been approved in the United States for refractory angina based on comparative studies with diltiazem[17]; it has been available in some European countries for a number of years. It is an antianginal agent with multiple actions.[15] The drug decreases calcium influx through potential-dependent and receptor-operated sarcoplasmic calcium channels and acts intracellularly as a calmodulin antagonist and calcium sensitizer. In cardiac muscle, it enhances the sensitivity of troponin C to calcium and stimulates myofibrillar ATPase activity. Bepridil also removes calmodulin's inhibitory effects on sarcoplasmic reticulum release and inhibits Na–Ca exchange. These actions are thought to offset the effects of calcium influx blockade on the cardiac contractile force. In vascular smooth muscle, where the calcium–calmodulin complex promotes muscle contraction by activating myosin light-chain kinase phosphorylation of contractile proteins, calmodulin antagonism, coupled with bepridil's inhibition of calcium influx, produces vascular relaxation.[15] It is not known to what extent such a complex pharmacologic profile contributes to bepridil's unusual effectiveness in refractory angina.

Clinical Electrophysiologic Effects

The clinical and experimental electrophysiologic effects of verapamil and its congeners, diltiazem and nifedipine, are consistent with the in vitro and experimental findings.[16] The in vivo electrophysiologic profiles of the newer dihydropyridines (nicardipine, nimodipine, isradipine, felodipine, nisoldipine,

amlodipine) are similar to that of nifedipine. The major effects of verapamil, diltiazem, nifedipine, and bepridil are summarized in Figure 6.4. The effects of tiapamil and gallopamil are qualitatively similar to those of verapamil and diltiazem and differ from those of the dihydropyridines.

The main electrophysiologic effect of conventional calcium channel blockers in therapeutic doses is on the properties of myocardial cells that are dependent on the slow-channel function for depolarization (e.g., sinoatrial and atrioventricular nodes). Thus, the most readily demonstrable effects are on the AV node. Here they increase the intranodal conduction (i.e., prolong AH interval) and prolong the effective and functional refractory periods in the antegrade and retrograde directions (see Fig. 6.4). They also increase the Wenckebach cycle length during right atrial pacing. However, as already indicated, there are differences among various calcium channel blockers in this regard. For example, whereas diltiazem and verapamil (and its congeners) do exert these effects in vitro and in vivo, with the dihydropyridines these effects are either reversed or nullified because of the potent reflex effects generated by their peripheral vasodilator actions. Unlike verapamil and diltiazem, the dihydropyridines do not appear to exert sympatholytic effects. Thus, agents such as nifedipine have actions opposite to those of verapamil and diltiazem on the AV node, reducing rather than prolonging the effective refractory period and shortening the intranodal conduction. A depressant effect on the AV node may become apparent with the dihydropyridines (even the vasoselective ones) if the sympathetic reflexes are blunted, as might occur with substantial β-blockade or pathologically induced autonomic insufficiency. In general, calcium channel blockers have little or no effect on the maximum sinus node recovery time or on sinoatrial conduction in the setting of normal sinus nodal function. However, their depressant effect becomes evident in patients with conduction system disease, but it tends to be less pronounced with the dihydropyridines.

As indicated in Figure 6.4, the net effects of bepridil are broad.[16] Thus, over and above the effect on

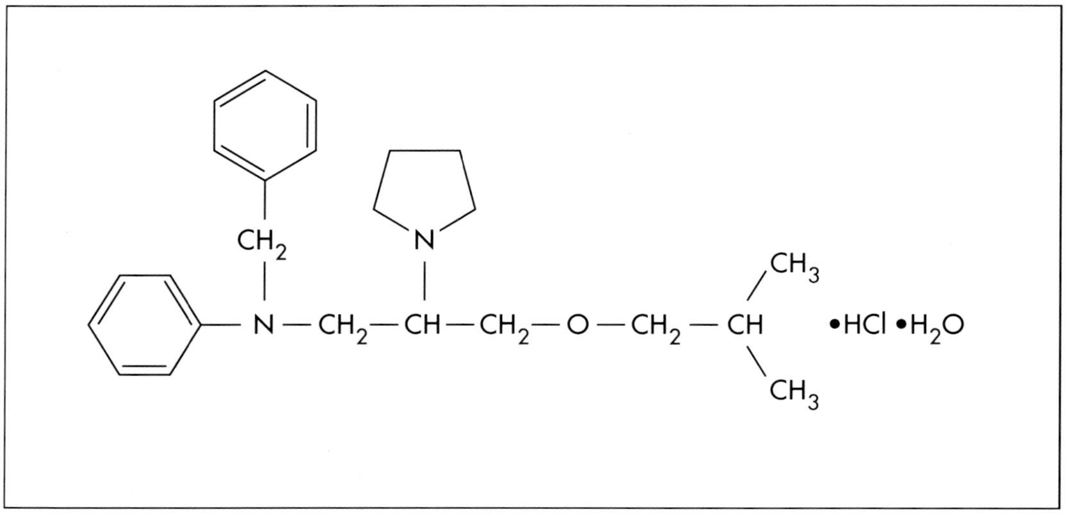

Figure 6.3 The chemical structure of bepridil, a calcium channel blocker with a broad pharmacodynamic profile.

conduction and refractoriness in the AV node, the drug prolongs the effective refractory period of the atria, bypass tracts, ventricles, and His–Purkinje system. It also increases the HV interval. Moreover, the QRS and QTc intervals are lengthened by bepridil and lidoflazine, unlike other calcium channel blockers.

It should also be emphasized that while calcium channel blockers as a class of agents (exclusive of bepridil) exert little effect on the electrophysiologic parameters of normal fast-channel-dependent myocardial fibers, in the setting of ischemia they may increase the effective refractory period and improve conduction. This is not a primary effect. It is likely related to the amelioration of ischemia. It will be evident that an appreciation of the electrophysiologic effects of calcium channel blockers in humans allows choice of an appropriate agent for the elective and prophylactic control of arrhythmias (diltiazem, verapamil). Similarly, the effects of some of these agents (e.g., bepridil and lidoflazine) on ventricular conduction and repolarization may be predictive of the potentially serious pro-arrhythmic reactions (e.g., ventricular tachycardia, fibrillation, torsade de pointes) occurring under certain clinical conditions.

HEMODYNAMIC EFFECTS

The hemodynamic effects of these compounds represent a complex interplay of simultaneous alterations in preload, afterload, contractility, and coronary blood flow.[2,3,18] The net effect is determined by the overall properties of individual calcium channel blockers, the level of baseline ventricular function, the integrity of the autonomic nervous system, and the presence or absence of myocardial ischemia. To these must be added the route and dose of the channel blocker used. In general, the net effect is largely determined by the degree to which the intrinsic negative inotropic effect of the individual agent (determined by its potency as a blocker of the slow calcium channel in the heart) is offset by its peripheral dilator actions in vascular smooth muscle.[2]

Verapamil

In healthy subjects verapamil exerts a trivial degree of negative inotropic effect, which is readily abolished with mild exercise. In patients with cardiac disease who have relatively well preserved ventricular function, intravenous verapamil functions as a moderately potent peripheral vasodilator. It reduces systemic arterial pressure and resistance, with a slight increase in cardiac output and no fall in stroke volume. There is a mild but a significant increase in pulmonary wedge pressure (and other right-sided pressures) accompanied by a decrease in contractility, although the left ventricular ejection fraction as determined by contrast or radionuclide ventriculography is not reduced. In some studies a mild increase has been reported.

In patients with preserved or only moderately impaired ventricular function, hemodynamic variables are not affected adversely by intravenous verapamil, but deterioration may occur in those with severely impaired ventricular performance.[18] For example, in those with left ventricular ejection fraction below 35% and filling pressures exceeding 18 mm Hg, the usual infusion regimen has been shown to induce marked clinical and hemodynamic deterioration, with steep increases in the left ventricular filling pressures.[19] This suggests caution in the intra-

FIGURE 6.4 COMPARATIVE CLINICAL ELECTROPHYSIOLOGIC EFFECTS OF CALCIUM CHANNEL BLOCKERS

Electrophysiologic Parameter	Verapamil	Nifedipine	Diltiazem	Bepridil	Vasoselective Agents**
RR interval	↕	↓	↑	↑	↓
QRS interval	0	0	0	+	0
QTc interval	0	0	0	++	0
PR interval	++	±	++	++	0
AH interval	+++	±	++	+++	0
HV interval	0	0	0	++	0
Atrial ERP	±	0	±	++	0
AV node ERP	++++	±	+++	+++	0
AV node FRP	++++	±	+++	+++	0
Ventricular ERP	0	0	0	++	0
His–Purkinje ERP	0	0	0	++	0
Bypass tract ERP	±	0	±	++	0
Sinus node recovery time	0*	0	0*	+	0
Ventricular automaticity	0	0	0	↓	0

(↓ = decrease; ↑ = increase; ↕ = variable effect; +–++++ = graded increase in intensity of effect;
AV = atrioventricular; ERP = effective refractory period; FRP = functional refractory period)
* Prolonged in sick sinus syndrome
** Felodipine, nicardipine, isradipine, amlodipine (see text) among others

venous use of the drug in patients with severe reduction of left ventricular systolic function, particularly those with a previous history of congestive heart failure and pulmonary edema. However, this does not preclude use of the drug in the setting of myocardial ischemia and cardiac arrhythmias in patients with reduced ejection fraction, because the salutary effects of the drug in ischemia and in arrhythmias may offset the intrinsic depressant effect of the compound. The hemodynamic effects of intravenously administered gallopamil and tiapamil are similar to those of verapamil.

Relatively few data are available on the hemodynamic effects of orally administered verapamil in patients with cardiac disease. Single oral doses of the drug in patients with uncomplicated myocardial infarction have revealed no significant depressant effect.[19] However, chronic therapy at doses of 320 to 480 mg per day in patients with ischemic heart disease or hypertrophic cardiomyopathy has been reported to reduce left ventricular ejection fraction

and to produce heart failure in a small number of cases.[20,21] A more severe depression of ventricular performance may occur in the setting of concomitant β-blockade.

Diltiazem

Diltiazem appears to be a less potent peripheral vasodilator with less negative inotropic effect than verapamil, although a direct comparison between the two agents in humans has not been made. The mean hemodynamic effects of intravenous diltiazem (0.16 to 0.25 mg/kg) in patients with coronary artery disease[22] but a normal or near-normal ejection fraction included a 22% decrease in systemic vascular resistance, 12% decrease in mean arterial pressure, 8% increase in cardiac index, and 10% increase in mean pulmonary wedge pressure (Fig. 6.5). A modest increase in left ventricular ejection fraction was also found. These overall effects are similar to those found

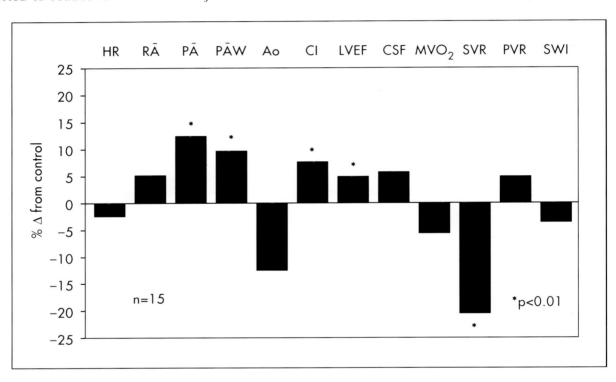

Figure 6.5 The effects of intravenous diltiazem on systemic and coronary hemodynamic features and left ventricular ejection fraction in patients with coronary disease. (HR = heart rate, RA = mean right atrial pressure, PA = mean pulmonary arterial pressure, PAW = mean pulmonary capillary wedge pressure, Ao = mean aortic pressure, CI = cardiac index, LVEF = left ventricular ejection fraction, CSF = coronary sinus flow, MVO_2 = myocardial oxygen consumption, SVR = systemic vascular resistance, PVR = pulmonary vascular resistance, SWI = stroke work index) (Modified from Josephson MA, Hopkins J, Singh BN: Hemodynamic and metabolic effects of diltiazem during coronary sinus pacing with particular reference to left ventricular ejection fraction. Am J Cardiol 55:286, 1985)

with verapamil in a comparable group of patients with cardiac disease. In patients with Class III to IV (New York Heart Association) congestive heart failure and dilated cardiomyopathy who had a mean ejection function of 26% and wedge pressure of 29 mm Hg, studies with intravenous and oral diltiazem (360 mg/d) indicated that the drug does not aggravate heart failure in this subset of patients. In these patients, intravenous diltiazem increased cardiac index by 20%, stroke volume index by 50%, stroke work index by 20%, heart rate by 23%, mean arterial pressure by 18%, and pulmonary wedge pressure by 34% without a change in LV *dP/dt*.[23] Equivalent hemodynamic alterations were produced by short-term oral diltiazem. These findings are in contrast to those reported for verapamil. However, while the short-term studies with diltiazem suggest that the drug can be used with impunity in patients with heart failure, long-term experience is limited and it would not be prudent to advocate the use of the drug as an afterload-reducing agent in preference to conventional vasodilators or cardioselective calcium channel blockers. However, diltiazem has been shown to increase late-onset congestive heart failure in postinfarction patients with early reduction in ejection fraction.[24] These data emphasize the potential negative inotropic effect of the agent.

Bepridil

Because bepridil is a relatively weak peripheral vasodilator, it might be expected to have a significant negative inotropic effect. However, there are major differences in effects when the drug is given intravenously compared to when it is given orally in varying doses. When the drug was given intravenously to patients with preserved or reduced left ventricular ejection fraction, there was a fall in cardiac output and stroke volume, a decrease in LV *dP/dt,* and an increase in the pulmonary capillary wedge pressure. These findings are consistent with a negative inotropic effect and in line with the observation that, unlike the other calcium channel blockers, the drug is not a potent peripheral vasodilator. In contrast, when the drug is given orally in therapeutic doses (200 to 400 mg/d), there is little or no impairment of ventricular function. This is consistent with the knowledge that bepridil rarely induced heart failure when given to a large number of patients with chronic stable angina.[25] Nevertheless caution is warranted in the use of the drug in patients with significantly impaired ventricular function.

Nifedipine and Other Dihydropyridines

Whether administered orally or sublingually or intravenously, the hemodynamic effects of the drug are characterized by a profound fall in arterial pressure and systemic resistance with a corresponding reflex increase in heart rate. This leads to an increase in cardiac index and in many patients a fall in the left ventricular filling pressure with an increase in cardiac contractility. For example, a 20 mg dose of the drug may induce an 18% increase in cardiac index and a 10% increase in the left ventricular ejection fraction. The effects of other dihydropyridines are directionally similar. The intrinsic negative inotropic effect of these calcium channel blockers is nullified or reversed by their reflex effects. However, if the reflex effects are attenuated or abolished by disease or drugs (e.g., β-blockers), a frankly depressant effect may emerge.

The improvement in hemodynamic effects following the use of nifedipine and other dihydropyridines is particularly marked and of clinical utility in the setting of hypertensive crises and pulmonary edema. In this setting the ventricular ejection fraction may increase with a fall in the left ventricular end-diastolic pressure. However, the improved hemodynamic responses after nifedipine in cases of pulmonary edema often are striking only after the initial doses, not being sustained during chronic therapy. Significantly greater enhancement of left ventricular performance has been reported after equihypotensive doses of hydralazine than after nifedipine in patients with congestive heart failure.[26] Hemodynamic deterioration may also occur with nifedipine in a subset of such patients, especially those in whom the drug does not produce increases in heart rate. This is consistent with the recent reports of cardiac failure occurring in patients given nifedipine in combination with β-blockade. In this respect the effects of other dihydropyridines are likely to be similar. However, there are dihydropyridines that exert little or no depressant effect on myocardial function; some improve indices of ventricular function. These so-called vasoselective calcium antagonists, many under investigation, merit further discussion, although it is not uniformly agreed that these so-called second-generation calcium antagonists are free from cardiac depressant effects.[27]

Vasoselective Calcium Antagonists

The best studied of these compounds include nicardipine, felodipine, amlodipine, isradipine, nisoldipine, and nitrendipine. Although the hemodynamic effects of these agents are not identical, as a group they share the common feature of augmenting ventricular performance in patients with congestive heart failure. Their overall effects, however, are dose-dependent. The pattern of responses for four of these agents is presented in Figure 6.6. It is dominated by major decreases in systemic vascular resistance, a fall in systemic and mean arterial pressure, modest increases in heart rate, a fall in pulmonary capillary wedge pressure, and increases in cardiac and stroke volume index and, wherever measured, an increase in the left ventricular ejection fraction and the LV *dP/dt*. The overall pattern is consistent with an improvement in ventricular performance.

The emerging data for these agents indicate that a distinction should be made between the hemody-namic effects of conventional calcium channel blockers and those of vasoselective agents. The conventional agents, such as verapamil, diltiazem, bepridil and, to a lesser extent, nifedipine, are essentially safe in patients without cardiac failure; their use in failure may be attended by unpredictable effects with an aggravation or decompensation in a subset of patients. The experience does not justify their use in preference to the conventional vasodilators as afterload-reducing agents. In contrast, the vasoselective agents function essentially as afterload-reducing agents and may be of value not only in patients with symptomatic ischemia in the setting of heart failure but also in those needing symptomatic relief and improved ventricular performance in other cases of heart failure. However, it must be emphasized that

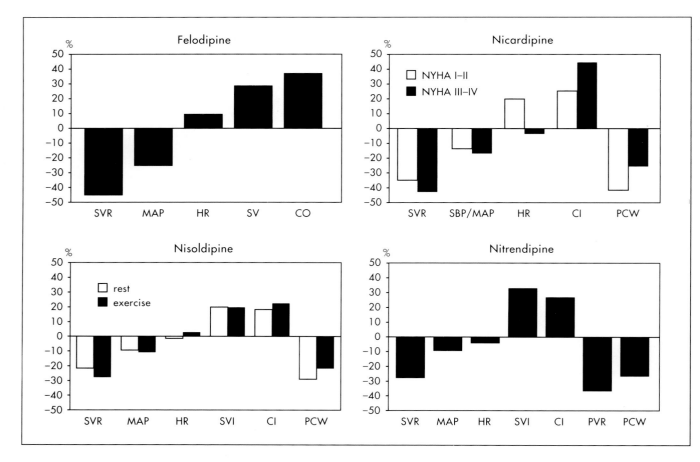

Figure 6.6 Acute hemodynamic effects of various vasoselective calcium antagonists. (SVR = systemic vascular resistance, MAP = mean arterial pressure, HR = heart rate, SV = stroke volume, SVI = stroke volume index, CI = cardiac index, CO = cardiac output, SBP = systolic blood pressure, PVR = pulmonary vascular resis-tance, PCW = pulmonary capillary wedge pressure) (Modified from Hofman-Bang C, Ryden L: Vascular selective calcium-channel antagonists in congestive heart failure. In Singh BN, Dzau V, Vanhoutte P, Woosley R: Textbook of Cardiovascular Pharmacology and Therapeutics. New York, Churchill-Livingstone, 1993 (in press))

the impact of vasoselective calcium channel blockers on prognosis is not known. This issue is under investigation in large multicenter trials involving felodipine and amlodipine.

EFFECTS ON THE CORONARY CIRCULATION

There are major similarities in the pharmacologic actions of these drugs in the coronary circulation with respect to their dilator actions in the resistance and capacitance vessels and in coronary sinus flow as measured by thermodilution in humans.[2,3,29] Although differences in the potency of verapamil, diltiazem, and nifedipine for dilating coronary arteries have been found in experimental models, such differences are difficult to define in humans. Nor do they appear to be of clinical significance if present. When nifedipine, verapamil, and diltiazem are given intravenously, they produce an increase in oxygen tension in the coronary sinus effluent with a small but a significant dilatation of not only normal but also the narrowed segments of the coronary arteries, with a corresponding decrease in the estimated flow resistance as determined by computer-assisted angiographic techniques.[28] Such a vasodilator response is accompanied by a fall in total coronary vascular resistance, with a tendency for the coronary sinus flow to increase, indicating that these agents dilate the resistance as well as capacitance segments of the coronary circulation. However, there is no significant decrease in myocardial oxygen consumption as determined by standard hemodynamic techniques.

Of particular clinical relevance is the finding that these drugs prevent coronary stenosis constriction provoked by α-adrenergic and serotonergic receptor stimulation.[29] For example, handgrip produces a constriction of 20% in the minimal luminal area; such an area may increase by 3% with handgrip during the continuous infusion of diltiazem. Stenosis dilatation is also produced by nitrates but not by such potent coronary arterial dilators as dipyridamole, which does not block handgrip-induced coronary vasoconstriction. It is now believed that stenosis dilatation may be an integral component of the anti-ischemic action of calcium channel blockers.[29] Calcium channel blockers do not appear to produce the "coronary steal syndrome" in humans.

PHARMACOKINETICS

The salient features of the pharmacokinetics of the commonly used conventional calcium channel blockers and bepridil are summarized in Figure 6.7 and those of vasoselective agents in Figure 6.8. The data for the latter agents are not complete.

FIGURE 6.7 CLINICAL PHARMACOKINETIC PARAMETERS OF FOUR CALCIUM ANTAGONISTS

	Verapamil	Nifedipine	Diltiazem	Bepridil
1. Absorption	>79%	>90%	>90%	>90%
Bioavailability	10%–20%	45%–62%	24%–90%	>70%
Onset of action	1–2 hrs (oral)	15 minutes (oral)	15 minutes (oral)	1–2 hours (oral)
	1/2–1 minutes (IV)	2–3 minutes (sublingual)	2–3 minutes (IV)	2–3 minutes (IV)
2. Elimination half-life	3–7 hours* (up to 26 hours in hepatic cirrhosis)	4 hours	4 hours	40 hours
3. Protein binding (approximately)	90%	90%	80%	Low
4. Metabolism	Liver	Liver	Liver	Liver
First pass	85%	20%–30%	50%	<3%
5. Metabolite activity	20%–25% (nor-verapamil)	None	40%–50% (Deacetyldiltiazem and oxidation)	70%–80% Hydroxylation
6. Excretion				
Gastrointestinal	25%	15%	60%	>99%
Renal	75%	85%	40%	0.1%
7. Dose*	IV: 0.075–0.15 mg/kg Oral: 80–120 mg tid or qid	Sublingual: 10–40 mg tid Oral: 10–40 mg tid or qid	IV: 0.15–0.25 mg/kg Oral: 30–90 mg tid or qid	IV: 2–4 mg/kg Oral: 200–400 mg/day
8. Therapeutic plasma level	80–100 ng/ml	25–100 ng/ml	40–200 ng/ml	?
9. Interaction with digoxin	Yes	Minor	No	Minimal

*Long-acting preparations of verapamil, nifedipine, and diltiazem are available.

Nifedipine

Over 90% of orally or buccally administered nifedipine is absorbed, with the drug appearing in the plasma within 3 minutes of buccal and 20 minutes of oral administration. The peak plasma concentrations are reached about 1 to 2 hours after an oral dose. The first-pass effect for nifedipine is low, and systemic bioavailability is over 65%. The drug is metabolized in the liver, but its metabolites are not pharmacologically active. A linear correlation between plasma drug levels and clinical effects for nifedipine has not been demonstrated. Nifedipine does not appear to accumulate after chronic therapy, and its elimination half-life remains stable. Nifedipine is available as short-acting liquid-filled capsules or controlled-release tablets suitable for once-a-day administration; its intravenous formulation is not stable. The dosage regimens are indicated in Figure 6.7.

Diltiazem

This drug is almost completely absorbed following oral administration. It appears in the plasma within 15 minutes of ingestion, with the peak concentration developing after 30 minutes. Diltiazem is subject to extensive hepatic metabolism, the major pathway being deacetylation. Its metabolite deacetyldiltiazem is pharmacologically active, having approximately 40% of the activity of the parent compound. An intravenous formulation for use as an AV nodal blocker has recently become available for the control of supraventricular arrhythmias.

The bioavailability of diltiazem appears to increase with continued drug administration without a change in the elimination half-life, a phenomenon probably due to the saturation of the metabolic pathway of the compound in the liver. The elimination half-life of diltiazem is not altered by renal failure, and there is no known interaction with digoxin, hydrochlorothiazide, warfarin, or propranolol. However, a significant interaction has been demonstrated with cimetidine; during their concomitant administration, dose adjustment of diltiazem is required.

Verapamil

The elimination half-life of verapamil is similar after acute intravenous or oral drug administration; however, during chronic long-term drug administration, there is nonlinear accumulation of the drug with reduced clearance and prolongation of elimination half-life. This indicates that, as in the case of diltiazem, verapamil may be administered twice daily, although sustained-release formulations of both drugs are available. The elimination of verapamil is essentially hepatic metabolism by an enzyme that is inducible by phenobarbitone. Numerous metabolites are formed, but only nor-verapamil is active, having about 25% of the activity of the parent compound. Verapamil exhibits a marked first-pass effect in the liver; thus its serum levels are likely to vary with hepatic disease, especially cirrhosis of the liver. Because of the first-pass effect, the serum concentrations of the drug are likely to vary tenfold or more in different subjects at the same dosage regimens. Verapamil at the protein binding sites in the plasma may be displaced by lidocaine, diazepam, propranolol, and disopyramide, but the clinical significance of this effect is unclear. However, the pharmacokinetic interaction with digoxin is of clinical significance. The steady-state levels of digoxin may be elevated more than 50% by the concomitant administration of verapamil. In part, this may be due to reduced renal clearance, and dose adjustment is usually necessary when the two drugs are given together. It should also be emphasized that the electrophysiologic effects of the two drugs on the AV node may be additive.

Bepridil

After oral administration (300 mg/d chronically), the absorption half-life of bepridil is 1 to 2 hours, with a mean plasma level of 1 μg/ml in healthy volunteers. The hepatic first-pass effect of the drug is less than 3%. In humans, bepridil is extensively metabolized by hydroxylation and oxidation in the liver, but the resulting metabolites are either pharmacologically inactive or considerably weaker than the parent com-

FIGURE 6.8 PHARMACOKINETICS OF NEW DIHYDROPYRIDINE CALCIUM ANTAGONISTS IN HEALTHY SUBJECTS

Drug	Bioavail-ability	Protein-Binding	Elimination Half-Life (Hours)	Metabolism	Excretion	Dose
Nicardipine	10%–30%	>95%	8–9	Liver	60% in urine	20–40 mg tid
Amlodipine	52%–88%	97%	30	Liver		2.5–10 mg qd
Isradipine	15%–20%	97%	9			2.5–10 mg qd
Felodipine	15%–25%	99%	11–17	Liver (Extensive metabolism)	60% – 70% in urine, 10% in feces	5–10 mg qd
Nitrendipine	10%–30%	80%	8–10	Liver		10–20 mg qd or bid
Nimodipine	13%	95%	2–5	Liver	<1%	30–40 mg bid or qid

pound. The renal excretion of the drug does not exceed 0.1%. In patients with chronic stable angina, the elimination half-life of the drug is between 1.6 and 4.5 days; the steady-state plasma levels are thus attained between 5 and 15 days. A more rapid steady-state level may be achieved by giving a higher initial dose on the first day. These data indicate that dose changes should not be made at intervals shorter than a week. There are no significant pharmacokinetic interactions between bepridil and other cardioactive agents, the possible exception being a weak interaction with digoxin.

The Newer Dihydropyridines

The major pharmacokinetic constants and the effective range of oral doses for these agents are shown in Figure 6.8. Of these, amlodipine has the longest elimination half-life (36 hours); it is less lipid-soluble than nifedipine.

Duration of Therapeutic Effects

There now is an increasing appreciation of the need to protect patients from rapid swings of plasma drug concentrations and especially drug responses as a function of time during chronic therapy. This has led to the development of newer calcium channel blockers with long elimination half-lives. For example, of the newer agents, bepridil (see above), amlodipine, and nitrendipine (half-life exceeding 20 hours) can be given once daily for hypertension or angina. However, it must be emphasized that while most of the other agents have relatively short plasma elimination half-lives, many of them are effective in the control of hypertension or angina when given once or twice a day. Nitrendipine doubles the steady-state plasma digoxin levels. There also has been progress in converting the existing compounds with differing delivery systems to prolong their duration of therapeutic action. Several 24-hour acting slow-release verapamil preparations permitting once-daily dosing of the drug has been available for many years; diltiazem slow release (given twice a day) and diltiazem continuous release (given once daily) are also available. While these preparations have longer-lasting therapeutic effects, they do not differ from the ordinary formulation of the drugs. The two preparations of nifedipine, slow-release nifedipine and continuous-release nifedipine (nifedipine GITS) are characterized by a longer elimination half-life than nifedipine capsules and a lower incidence of vasodilator side effects such as flushing, headache, palpitations, and dizziness.[30]

Pharmacodynamic Drug Interactions

Because a large number of cardioactive drugs exert significant hemodynamic or electrophysiologic effects, the scope for pharmacodynamic interactions between calcium channel blockers and other agents is large. For example, the potential negative inotropic effect of certain calcium channel blockers (particularly type I) may be additive with those of β-blockers, disopyramide, and certain class IC agents such as flecainide. Similarly, the electrophysiologic effects may be additive with those of β-blockers and amiodarone or other antiarrhythmic drugs that influence adrenergic and slow-channel functions in the heart. Such interactions are of the greatest importance in patients with overt or covert conduction system disease. In the case of bepridil, there is minimal pharmacokinetic interaction with other cardioactive agents, but the broad electrophysiologic profile of the drug may lead to numerous pharmacodynamic interactions with agents such as β-blockers, class III agents including sotalol, and class I agents.

THERAPEUTIC APPLICATIONS

The major established indications and the newer potential ones are listed in Figure 6.9. The role of calcium antagonists is best established in ischemic myocardial syndromes, especially in Prinzmetal's angina, unstable angina, and chronic stable angina. Their potential role in myocardial protection in the context of cardiac surgery and survivors of acute myocardial infarction remains unclear. Electrophysiologic studies have now established the role of this class of drugs in the control of certain supraventricular tachyarrhythmias, but their place in the treatment of ventricular arrhythmias is less well defined. In the last few years, perhaps the greatest promise that

---

FIGURE 6.9 THERAPEUTIC APPLICATIONS OF CALCIUM ANTAGONISTS

Established Clinical Indications
Ischemic myocardial syndromes
Prinzmetal's angina
Unstable angina
Chronic stable angina
Cardiac arrhythmias
Hypertension and hypertensive emergencies
Hypertrophic cardiomyopathies

Potential Indications
Congestive heart failure
Relieving or preventing spasm during PTCA
Cardioprotection
Pulmonary hypertension
Migraine and cluster headaches
Cerebral insufficiency
Raynaud's phenomenon
Disorders of gastrointestinal motility
Exercise-induced bronchospasm
Prevention of atherosclerosis

these agents have shown is in the control of mild to moderate essential hypertension and in the management of hypertensive emergencies. An additional rare indication for nimodipine is for cerebral protection in subarachnoid hemorrhage.[11]

Myocardial Ischemic Syndromes

Many observations from hemodynamic monitoring, radionuclide perfusion studies, metabolic investigations, and Holter recordings in ambulatory and hospitalized patients have established two important findings about the nature of myocardial ischemia in the setting of coronary artery disease,[31] which have a bearing on the therapeutic effects of calcium channel blockers. First, it is clear that over two thirds of the transient ischemic episodes detected by continuous monitoring in variant angina, unstable angina, and chronic stable angina are not associated with chest pain or equivalents (i.e., they are "silent"). Second, many of the episodes in unstable as well as chronic stable angina are not triggered by increases in heart rate or blood pressure. Thus, episodes of ischemia in coronary artery disease may be due to increases in myocardial work load as well as a primary reduction in myocardial flow as a result of intermittent arterial obstruction produced either by thrombus formation or by coronary vasoconstriction.

These observations have an important bearing on the mechanism of action of various anti-ischemic agents in the several syndromes of myocardial ischemia in patients with coronary artery disease. The human coronary artery is subject to numerous neurohumoral influences that may alter its caliber. If these were to occur in association with eccentrically placed atherosclerotic plaques in juxtaposition to an arc of normal tissue, variations in the caliber of the coronary artery of as little as 10% may lead to a critical reduction in coronary blood flow.[29] Calcium channel blockers are coronary vasodilators and may counteract such a tendency to vasoconstriction in various anginal syndromes. It has also been shown that these drugs reverse or negate the vasoconstrictive effects of ergonovine on the coronary arteries and prevent the sympathetically mediated vasoconstriction induced by handgrip or other physiologic interventions.[29] Thus, unlike the effects of β-blockers, a significant effect of calcium channel blockers in ischemic syndromes may be mediated by their action on coronary vessels rather than on myocardial oxygen consumption. The potential mechanisms that determine the salutary effects of calcium channel blockers in myocardial ischemia are summarized in Figure 6.10.

It must be emphasized that the effects on myocardial oxygen consumption of the various calcium channel blockers may differ significantly. For example, verapamil, diltiazem, and bepridil tend to lower the heart rate, whereas the dihydropyridines induce significant tachycardia, at least during the early stages of therapy. In some patients, the reflex sympathetic activation may lead to an increase in oxygen demand and aggravation of ischemia; rarely, myocardial infarction may be precipitated in the early stages of therapy. Thus, the dihydropyridines are best used in combination with β-blockers in patients with chronic stable angina, although the aggravation of heart rate has not been shown to be of much clinical significance in variant angina or unstable angina, or during long-term therapy with dihydropyridines in chronic stable angina. This suggests that an adaptation in the reflex responses may occur during protracted therapy.

GOALS OF THERAPY

As with any class of anti-ischemic and antianginal agents, the goals and end-points of calcium antagonist therapy should be clearly established for various subsets of patients with coronary artery disease. For the largest majority of patients these are alleviation of angina or angina equivalents, prevention of infarction or reinfarction, regression or progression of existing atherosclerotic lesions, and prolongation of survival. In the case of calcium channel blockers, the greatest success has been in the alleviation of symptoms and the prolongation of exercise capacity. The data on the other end points are limited, equivocal, or at best tentative, and the effects may be agent-specific.

FIGURE 6.10 POTENTIAL MECHANISMS OF ACTION OF CALCIUM ANTAGONISTS IN CHRONIC STABLE ANGINA

Increased Myocardial Oxygen Supply
Increased coronary blood flow (all agents)
Coronary arterial dilatation, including lesion dilatation
Improved subendocardial perfusion
? Decreased platelet aggregability

Decreased Myocardial Oxygen Demand
Decreased peripheral vascular resistance afterload (all agents)
Decreased myocardial contractility (verapamil, bepridil)
Decreased heart rate (verapamil, diltiazem, bepridil)
Decreased intracellular metabolism or change in substrate utilization

*Not all the postulated mechanisms have been verified in patients. They have been extrapolated from findings in experimental models of myocardial ischemia.

It must be emphasized that although various anti-ischemic agents (nitrates, β-blockers, calcium channel blockers) are potent suppressors of myocardial ischemia, there is little to suggest that this effect has any impact on mortality or reinfarction. The impact on mortality in the case of angina appears to be related more to alteration in the coronary anatomy by surgical revascularization in certain subsets of patients. The available data suggest that the number of coronary vessels with stenoses and the severity and the location of such lesions relative to the left ventricular ejection fraction are more powerful discriminants of prognosis than myocardial ischemia, silent or symptomatic. Thus, although silent and symptomatic ischemia may provide important prognostic information, there is currently little evidence to support the use of ischemia as a surrogate end point for determining influence on mortality or morbidity in coronary artery disease. For this reason, unless controlled clinical trials suggest the contrary, the treatment of silent ischemia as a therapeutic end point appears unjustified. Therefore, in the following discussion, attention is drawn only to the alleviation of symptoms, prolongation of exercise duration on treadmill, prevention of reinfarction, and prolongation of life.

VARIANT OR PRINZMETAL'S ANGINA

The advent of calcium channel blockers has been a major advance in the control of variant angina. Verapamil, diltiazem, and nifedipine have been found to reverse coronary artery spasm and reduce the frequency of ischemic episodes as judged by symptoms, nitroglycerin consumption, and reduced ST-segment deviations documented on Holter recordings.[32] The data on bepridil and the newer dihyropyridines are limited. Among the three widely used agents mentioned above, no significant differences in efficacy have been established, and although excellent theoretical reasons may be cited for the use of combination therapy with different calcium channel blockers, at present there is no decisive evidence that combination therapy is superior to the maximal tolerated doses of a single agent. Similarly, it is not certain whether these agents have a greater efficacy compared to nitrates. The available data suggest that the overall efficacy of both classes of compounds may be similar. However, because of their more predictable half-life and easier dosing schedules, with less likelihood of developing tolerance during continuous drug therapy, calcium channel blockers are now used in most cases of Prinzmetal's angina, in conjunction with nitrates.

On pharmacologic grounds, combination therapy of nitrates and calcium channel blockers appears rational and should always be considered in recalcitrant cases. The role of β-blockers in this setting when compared to calcium channel blockers is less well established. In vasotonic angina with normal coronary arteries, β-blockers have been shown to increase the duration of ischemic episodes compared to placebo.[33] On the other hand, a combination of coronary vasodilators and β-blockers in patients with the so-called mixed angina may be helpful, especially in the setting of fixed coronary lesions in patients in

whom myocardial revascularization is thought unnecessary.

The overall clinical impression is that over 80% of patients with Prinzmetal's angina respond to calcium antagonism. However, it remains uncertain whether continuous prophylactic therapy with calcium channel blockers leads to enhanced survival. The drugs are nevertheless effective in relieving symptoms and in preventing recurrent ventricular arrhythmias complicating ischemic episodes, the primary effect being on ischemia rather than on the arrhythmia in this setting. Whether calcium channel blockers exert an effect on mortality, infarction, or sudden death in patients with variant angina is not known. It is not unreasonable to assume, however, that the prognosis in these patients is linked to the underlying severity of coronary artery disease and the level of ventricular ejection fraction.

UNSTABLE ANGINA

At present the exact mechanisms underlying the development of the unstable angina syndrome are unclear.[34] It is known that the rate of progression of the atherosclerotic disease may be accelerated in patients with unstable angina; it is also known that in some there is evidence of coronary vasospasm and in others, especially those who die, the evidence of antemortem clot formation is convincing.[34] Angioscopic studies have now confirmed the role of thrombus formation, a finding of much therapeutic importance.[35] Experimental data (see below) have indicated a beneficial effect of calcium channel blockade in atherosclerosis, and in vitro data involving human platelets have documented significant effects of calcium channel blockers on platelet aggregability (see below). It remains uncertain whether either of these potential mechanisms is related to the salutary effects of calcium channel blockers in unstable angina, although the short-term ability of these drugs to alleviate the symptoms and electrocardiographic abnormalities has been well documented for verapamil, diltiazem, and nifedipine. There is very little experience with bepridil or the newer dihydropyridines.

In contrast to the plethora of data supporting the efficacy of oral calcium channel blockers, there is no systematic experience on the effects of intravenously administered calcium channel blockers in unstable angina. For example, it is not known whether they are as effective as intravenous nitrates. Unlike nitrates, intravenous calcium channel blockers do not appear to exhibit the phenomenon of tachyphylaxis. Whether the combination of intravenous nitrates and calcium channel blockers is superior to the use of the individual agents alone in the control of unstable angina is not known.

Nearly all cases of unstable angina occur in the setting of advanced coronary artery disease and, as indicated above, there may be a significant incidence of abnormal coronary vasomobility in these patients. Therefore, it has been felt that β-blockers might aggravate the development of ischemia in this context. At present, this possibility is no more than theoretical, there being no controlled observations to suggest that β-blockade might exert a deleterious influence on the clinical course of unstable angina. In fact, a recent controlled study comparing the effects of propranolol and diltiazem revealed no differences in morbidity and mortality in unstable angina.[36] Combination therapy with β-blockers and calcium channel blockers has been shown to be more effective than β-blockers alone in unstable angina.[37]

Numerous studies have established the effectiveness of calcium channel blockers in relieving symptoms of unstable angina and reducing the electrocardiographic abnormalities that accompany symptomatic ischemia. Whether these drugs reduce the incidence of silent ischemic episodes in unstable angina and thereby prolong survival has not been established for any antianginal agent, including β-blockers, nitrates, and calcium channel blockers.

CHRONIC STABLE ANGINA

The role of calcium channel blockers in chronic stable angina is now well defined.[3] Numerous studies with verapamil and its congeners, nifedipine and diltiazem, using blind placebo-controlled protocols, have shown that these drugs reduce the frequency of angina and the number of sublingual nitroglycerin tablets consumed, increase the time to development of angina and total exercise duration during the treadmill test, and delay the onset of ischemia as judged by electrocardiographic parameters. These drugs also elevate the anginal threshold and attenuate ischemic manifestations during rapid atrial pacing in patients with coronary artery disease undergoing cardiac catheterization.[38] They also reduce the fall in left ventricular ejection due to ischemia induced either by exercise or by rapid atrial pacing[22,38] and improve radionuclide-documented perfusion deficits induced by exercise.[32]

It is of interest that the product of heart rate and blood pressure, an index of oxygen demand, tends to be lower at any given work load under treatment with calcium channel blockers, although not as low as with β-blockers. However, it is known that the peak heart rate and blood pressure are not significantly different during treadmill exercise whether a patient is on or off calcium channel blockers, although the peak of these variables is delayed when the patient is taking calcium channel blockers.[38]

The data thus suggest that the effects of calcium channel blockers in chronic stable angina differ in mechanism from those of β-blockers, which appear to produce their salutary effects by reducing myocardial oxygen demand, especially by reducing heart rate at rest and during exercise. In the case of calcium channel blockers, the possibility cannot be excluded that these agents act, at least in part, by augmenting regional blood flow through altering coronary vasomobility, even though the precise measurement of

FIGURE 6.11 COMPARISON OF ANTIANGINAL DRUGS

	Nitrate Therapy	β-Blocking Drugs	Calcium Blocking Agents	
Physiologic Effects				
Heart rate	↑	↓	↓(V,D),B	N↑
AV conduction	—	↓	↓	N↑
Systemic resistance	↓	↑(acutely)	↓	N↓
Coronary resistance	↓↓	↑	↓	N↓
Contractility	↑	↓	↓	N±
Therapeutic Effects				
Reduce angina frequency	Yes	Yes	Yes	
Improve exercise tolerance	Yes	Yes	Yes	
Decrease TNG consumption	Yes	Yes	Yes	
Decrease MVO$_2$	Yes	Yes	Yes	
Dilate coronary arteries	Yes	No	Yes	
Reduce silent ischemia	Yes	Yes	Yes	
Favorable and Limiting Factors				
Exertional angina	+	+	+	
Variant angina	+	—	+	
Once-a-day therapy	—	+	+	
Partial tolerance	+	—	—	
Side-effects	+	+	+	
Drug interactions	+	+	+	
May worsen CHF	—	+	+(V>N>D>B)	
May worsen bronchospasm and claudication	—	+ / Yes	— / No	
Bradyarrhythmias	—	+	+(V,D≤B)	
Reduce sudden death and reinfarction	±	+	?	

(AV = atrioventricular; TNG = nitroglycerin; MVO$_2$ = myocardial oxygen consumption; CHF = congestive heart failure; V = verapamil; D = diltiazem; N = nifedipine; B = bepridil).

(Adapted from McCall D, Walsh RA, Frohlich ED et al: Calcium entry blocking drugs: Experiment studies and clinical uses. Curr Probl Cardiol 10:1, 1985)

regional flow in humans is rarely possible. It is also possible that part of the anti-ischemic effect of calcium channel blockers may be mediated through an effect on platelet adhesiveness, since many of these agents exert significant effects on platelet aggregability, an effect that has also been shown for propranolol and other β-blockers. Furthermore, as with other antianginal and anti-ischemic agents, it is not clear whether calcium channel blockers, as a class, influence survival or infarction rate in patients with chronic stable angina.

There are some differences among calcium channel blockers as anti-ischemic agents in terms of subjective as well as objective criteria. For example, bepridil appears to be effective in cases of angina in which other agents produce suboptimal response. In a series of patients who were given diltiazem to maximal tolerated doses, bepridil (300 to 400 mg/d) improved all subjective and objective criteria of ischemia.[25,39]

CALCIUM CHANNEL BLOCKERS AND OTHER ANTI-ISCHEMIC AGENTS

An appreciation of the pharmacodynamic effects of the three classes of antianginal drugs (Fig. 6.11) allows one to predict their overall effects in angina, especially during combination therapy. Since the fundamental mechanisms of action of β-blockers, nitrates, and calcium channel blockers differ somewhat, there exists a rationale for combining these drugs in what has become a "step-care" approach to the therapy of angina pectoris. However, there are a number of limitations to this approach. First, there are multiple objectives in the treatment of angina, and not all three classes of agents are equally effective in this regard. For example, to date only β-blockers have been demonstrated to reduce the incidence of sudden death and reinfarction during chronic prophylactic therapy of the survivors of acute myocardial infarction,[40] although all three classes of agents have been shown to reduce infarct size in laboratory animals and in humans. Second, not all patients can tolerate β-blockers: for example, these agents are contraindicated, relatively or absolutely, in insulin-dependent diabetes, bronchospastic disease, and peripheral vascular disease. These conditions are not influenced adversely by calcium channel blockers. Third, in certain subsets of patients, combination therapy might be deleterious. For instance, in patients with impaired ventricular function, heart failure might be precipitated, and in patients with conduction system disease, serious lapses of conduction might develop if β-blockers and certain calcium channel blockers are combined. The combination of nitrates and large doses of dihydropyridine calcium channel blockers may produce significant hypotension that could lead to potentially serious cardiovascular complications. Thus, in the treatment of chronic stable angina, an individualized approach rather than a simple "step-care" approach is desirable if combination therapy is contemplated. For patients with impaired ventricular performance or conduction system disease, combination of β-blockers with either

verapamil or diltiazem is likely to be more hazardous than with the dihydropyridines (although cases have been reported documenting deleterious effects even with nifedipine in this context). Surprisingly, the combination of β-blockers and bepridil appears to be safe, especially in patients with no history of heart failure or conduction system disease. Emerging data suggest that the newer vasoselective calcium channel blockers (nicardipine, felodipine, amlodipine, isradipine), which are not myocardial depressants, may be of particular value for symptomatic ischemia in patients with markedly impaired ventricular function or manifest heart failure.

CARDIOPROTECTION

There is much evidence that the administration of calcium channel blockers to laboratory animals with coronary artery occlusion leads to smaller infarct size, decreased histologic and ultrastructural damage, increased collateral blood flow to the ischemic areas, and less severe electrocardiographic and enzymatic evidence of ischemic damage.[41] These findings are consistent with the intracellular calcium overload hypothesis of ischemic damage following coronary occlusion. A reduction in myocardial enzyme release has also been demonstrated in humans with acute myocardial infarction when a calcium channel blocker is given in the early stages of acute myocardial infarction.[42] The addition of calcium channel blockers to cardioplegic solutions during cardiopulmonary bypass surgery has been shown to reduce systolic and diastolic abnormalities during protracted total myocardial ischemia; in humans, a decrease in the severity of myocardial ischemic injury as detected by technetium pyrophosphate scintigraphy has also been demonstrated.[43] However, in the controlled experimental setting of an isolated perfused heart, verapamil was shown to be protective only when administered before the onset of ischemia.[44] This requirement for effectiveness may be a reason for the limited clinical success of calcium channel blockers in the treatment of acute myocardial infarction.

Thus, whether the experimental and preliminary observations on cardioprotection will eventually be translated into routine clinical indications remains to be established. The role of focal spasm in mediating coronary obstruction in the setting of infarction now appears to be unlikely in most patients. However, a clear rationale exists for the use of these agents to control persistent or recurrent myocardial ischemia or supraventricular tachyarrhythmias in the early stages of acute myocardial infarction.[3] Oral or intravenous agents may be used for this purpose. However, benefit is not always seen with these agents in acute ischemic syndromes such as unstable angina. For example, in the case of dihydropyridines (especially nifedipine), there appears to be an increase in the incidence of infarction in patients with unstable angina unless a β-blocker is also used.[37] The potential deleterious effect of nifedipine and, by inference, of other dihydropyridines might stem from the reflex tachycardia engendered by potent vasodilatation.

EFFECT OF CALCIUM ANTAGONISM IN SURVIVORS OF ACUTE MYOCARDIAL INFARCTION

The early promise of these agents in this area has not been fulfilled. There is now compelling evidence[41] that β-adrenergic blocking drugs given prophylactically to survivors of acute myocardial infarction reduce the incidence of sudden death and reinfarction.

To date no studies have unequivocally indicated that the prophylactic administration of calcium channel blockers has a salutary effect on mortality or reinfarction rate in survivors of acute myocardial infarction. During the 1980s there were numerous randomized trials of calcium channel blockers given immediately after a myocardial infarction. They have been reviewed and some have been subjected to meta-analysis.[45] The mean data are shown in Figure 6.12. The dihydropyridine calcium channel blockers clearly have a detrimental effect on survival after infarct. The unexpected direction of this result may be explained by the reflex sympathetic activation produced by these compounds. In the setting of non-Q-wave infarction, diltiazem was of no survival benefit but was reported to have a beneficial effect (of borderline statistical significance given the inappro-

priate one-tailed analysis) on reinfarction in the first 2 weeks.[46] About two thirds of the patients in the treatment limb were also on β-blockers. A larger trial of diltiazem after all types of infarcts showed no overall effect on survival.[47] However, breaking the population into two groups, with and without pulmonary congestion at the time of the infarct, revealed a beneficial effect for patients with presumably better left ventricular function and a detrimental effect for those with congestion. The pathophysiologic mechanism for this biphasic result is not clear. Earlier trials with verapamil were smaller and inconclusive; however, a larger more recent trial has had more promising preliminary results.[48] However, unlike β-blockers, there was no benefit in patients with reduced ejection fraction or history of heart failure. In the case of verapamil, a beneficial effect was seen in patients without a history of heart failure, but none in those with impaired ventricular function. Although for many years a very significant number of patients surviving myocardial infarction have been given calcium channel blockers for secondary prevention, the trend is now shifting away from these agents towards β-blockers.[49] It is doubtful whether calcium channel

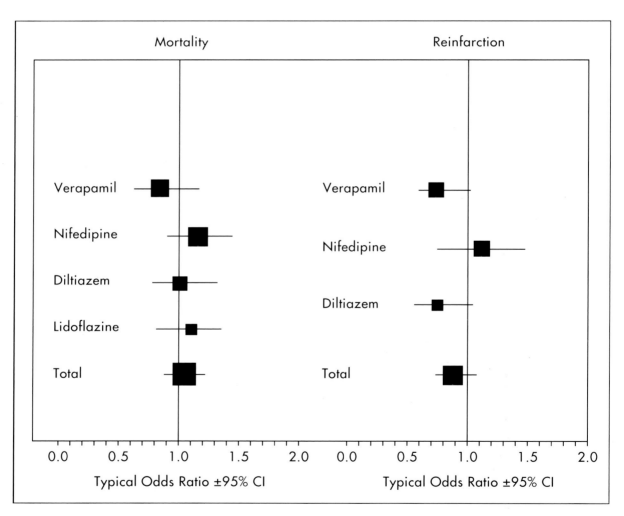

Figure 6.12 Meta-analysis of randomized clinical trials of various calcium channel blockers in unstable angina and in survivors of acute myocardial infarction. (Modified from Held P, Yusuf S: In Singh BN, Wellens HJJ, Hiraoka M (eds): Electropharmacologic Control of Arrhythmias: To Delay Conduction or to Prolong Refractoriness? Mt Kisco, NY, Futura Publishing Company, 1993 (in press))

blockers have a meaningful role in reducing mortality in the survivors of acute myocardial infarction.

REVERSAL OR PREVENTION OF ATHEROSCLEROSIS AND PREVENTION OF RESTENOSIS AFTER PTCA

It has been recognized for a long time that calcium may have a significant role in aggregation of platelets, release of platelet-derived growth factor, smooth muscle cell replication, protein synthesis, and lipid binding to the macromolecules involved in atherogenesis. It might therefore be expected that inhibition of the calcium influx might reduce calcification and atherosclerosis. Fleckenstein[1] and others[35,36] have indeed provided experimental evidence that this might be so. For example, experimental studies have suggested that prophylactic administration of calcium channel blockers delays or reduces the tendency for atherosclerosis to develop in animals fed a high cholesterol diet.[50,51] While these animal studies are of major clinical interest, there are at present no controlled studies in humans to confirm or deny this possibility. Two studies should be mentioned. In the so-called INTACT study,[52] the effects of nifedipine were compared to those of placebo on the rate of progression of atherosclerosis in patients with coronary artery disease and stable angina. Nifedipine did not retard the progression of atherosclerotic lesions but reduced the number of new lesions that developed. Very similar results have been reported with nicardipine.[53] However, to date there is no evidence that calcium channel blockers delay restenosis of lesions after percutaneous transluminal angioplasty.

Cardiac Arrhythmias

The role of calcium channel blockers in the treatment of cardiac arrhythmias is reasonably well defined, especially for supraventricular tachycardias.[54] The spectrum of clinical activity is in line with the electrophysiologic effects (see Fig. 6.4) as summarized in Figure 6.13. The major effects are related to the propensity of these agents predictably to inhibit or completely but transiently to block the anterograde impulses across the AV node and to lengthen its effective and functional refractory periods. Most of the experience relates to the effects of verapamil. Recent data indicate that diltiazem is as effective as verapamil.[55]

PAROXYSMAL SUPRAVENTRICULAR TACHYCARDIAS

When verapamil or diltiazem is given intravenously, paroxysmal supraventricular tachycardia (PSVT) due to AV nodal re-entry is promptly terminated in most cases. However, intravenous adenosine, which has

---

FIGURE 6.13 ANTIARRHYTHMIC EFFECTS OF CALCIUM ANTAGONISTS

Arrhythmia	Response to Parenteral Administration	Response During Long-Term Prophylaxis
1. Sinus tachycardia	Variable	Of little value
2. Paroxysmal supraventricular tachycardia		
a. Atrioventricular (AV) node reentrant	90%–100%	Modest effect in preventing recurrence
b. Circus movement (orthodromic) with bypass tract (overt or concealed)	80%–90%	Modest effect in preventing recurrence
c. Circus movement (antidromic) with bypass tract	No effect	Of little value
d. Sinus node or intra-atrial reentrant	Probably effective	Effect uncertain
e. Ectopic atrial tachycardia	Produced AV block without conversion	Of little value
3. Paroxysmal atrial tachycardia with AV block (with or without digitalis toxicity)	May convert to sinus rhythm (?mechanism)	Effect uncertain
4. Multifocal atrial tachycardia	Variable; often effective in slowing rate	Variable (more data needed)
5. Atrial fibrillation	Slows ventricular response (conversion to sinus rhythm rare)	Control of ventricular response at rest and with exercise excellent
6. Atrial flutter	Slows ventricular response (conversion to sinus rhythm rate)	Control of ventricular response at rest and with exercise good
7. Atrial flutter and fibrillation with Wolff-Parkinson-White syndrome (wide QRS)	May accelerate ventricular response	Contraindicated
8. Ventricular tachyarrhythmias	Generally low rate of conversion except when due to coronary artery spasm	Rarely successful except secondarily by preventing myocardial ischemia and exercise-induced tachycardia
9. Ventricular tachycardia with right bundle and left axis deviation	Effective in producing conversion	Effective in prophylaxis
10. Torsade de pointes	Responses occasionally reported; responses inferior to intravenous magnesium	No significant data available
11. Prevention of sudden death in post-MI survivors	Not available	No effect or possibly deleterious

(Adapted from Singh BN, Ellrodt G, Nademanee K: Calcium antagonists: Cardiocirculatory effects and applications. In Hurst JW (ed): Clinical Essays on the Heart, vol 2, pp 65–98. New York, McGraw-Hill, 1984)

similar electrophysiologic effects but has a much shorter half-life of only seconds, has replaced intravenous verapamil or diltiazem as the agent of choice once the commonly used vagal maneuvers fail in the acute conversion of re-entrant PSVT.[54] Similarly, adenosine is rapidly replacing intravenous verapamil as the agent of choice for distinguishing different forms of narrow WRS tachycardias.[56]

When verapamil is used, the termination is usually prompt (within 2 minutes of a bolus injection); often the conversion is preceded by ventricular ectopic beats, atrial fibrillation, or transient AV dissociation with a junctional escape rhythm. In the case of orthodromic tachycardia complicating the Wolff-Parkinson-White syndrome, cycle length alternation may occur before conversion. Calcium channel blockers may also terminate tachycardia by blocking the retrograde conduction in the AV node. However, the use of calcium channel blockers must be avoided in wide complex tachycardias without known involvement of the AV node. Severe hypotension can occur if verapamil is mistakenly given for ventricular tachycardia. Whether intravenous calcium channel blockers also terminate PSVT involving sinus or intraatrial pre-entry is not certain. Uncertain also is the role of calcium channel blockers in ectopic atrial tachycardia.

While the role of intravenous calcium channel blockers for the treatment of PSVT is well established, the precise role of the oral drugs in the prophylaxis of recurrent arrhythmia is less clear. However, if the intravenous drug is effective in preventing the reinduction of the PSVT in the electrophysiologic laboratory, subsequent oral therapy may be highly effective in preventing recurrences of arrhythmia. At present, there are few studies in which the efficacy of verapamil and other calcium channel blockers versus other agents has been systematically addressed. It should be emphasized that drug therapy for the prophylaxis of PSVT is now being superseded rapidly by radiofrequency catheter ablation, where facilities and resources are available.

Atrial Flutter and Fibrillation

Acute intravenous injections of type I calcium channel blockers predictably reduce the ventricular rate in atrial flutter and fibrillation, with rare cases converting to sinus rhythm, especially if the arrhythmias are of short duration and the heart size is not large. The effect of these agents for conversion might be comparable to that of placebo, although the figures for bepridil might be higher due to the drug's broader spectrum of electrophysiologic effects, but it is unlikely that this drug will be developed for such an indication. In a small number of cases regularization of the ventricular response is seen. Oral verapamil and diltiazem are highly effective in reducing the ventricular response in atrial flutter and fibrillation at rest as well as during exercise, in contrast to the effect of digoxin, which lowers the ventricular response primarily at rest.[54] They are effective alternatives to β-blockers and digoxin in this setting. The longer acting formulations are likely to be of value for 24-hour control of ventricular response in patients with atrial flutter and fibrillation. Neither the electrophysiologic effects nor the clinical experience suggest that these drugs are likely to be effective in preventing relapses of atrial flutter and fibrillation after chemical or electrical conversion of these arrhythmias. Calcium channel blockers are contraindicated in patients with atrial flutter and fibrillation complicating the Wolff-Parkinson-White syndrome, because they aggravate the ventricular response and precipitate ventricular fibrillation.

Multifocal Atrial Tachycardia

It is unclear what the effects are in multifocal atrial tachycardia of calcium channel blockers.[54] They are sometimes of value, especially oral or intravenous verapamil. Their role in ectopic atrial tachycardia is also poorly defined. Anecdotal reports suggest that calcium channel blockers produce transient AV block without terminating the tachycardia.

Ventricular Arrhythmias

As a class of agents, calcium channel blockers have a limited role in the control of ventricular tachyarrhythmias except when the ventricular tachycardia or fibrillation is due to coronary artery spasm. Here, the primary effect is on myocardial ischemia via release of coronary spasm. Calcium channel blockers are weak suppressors of premature ventricular contractions in normal subjects or in those with organic cardiac disease; they rarely suppress ventricular tachycardia that can be induced by programmed electrical stimulation.[57] There is some evidence that calcium channel blockers are effective in controlling ventricular tachycardia induced by exercise in patients with coronary artery disease; they appear also to be effective in young patients without organic heart disease who have ventricular tachycardia with the right bundle branch block morphology associated with left axis deviation. The nature of this arrhythmia is uncertain, but it may result from triggered automaticity responsive to calcium antagonism.[57]

It should also be emphasized that, although heart-rate-lowering calcium channel blockers may produce severe degrees of bradycardia and aggravate the manifestations of the sick sinus syndrome, they do not produce serious proarrhythmic effects. There are two exceptions, however. Bepridil and lidoflazine (not generally available) both exhibit electrophysiologic effects akin to those of quinidine; they both can induce potentially serious proarrhythmic responses—ventricular tachycardia and fibrillation as well as torsade de pointes.

Systemic Hypertension

Although the vasodilator properties of calcium channel blockers have been recognized for many years, it is only in the last 10 to 15 years that numerous reports have suggested a significant role for these drugs in the control of hypertensive emergencies and mild to moderate essential hypertension. Indeed, calcium channel blockers and angiotensin-converting enzyme (ACE) inhibitors have now emerged as two of the most significant classes of agents for lowering high arterial pressure. Interest in these drugs as hypotensive agents has grown pari passu with the concept implicating calcium in the pathogenesis of hypertension.[58,59] It is likely that the overall mechanisms of reduction of high arterial pressure by these agents go beyond their peripheral vasodilator properties, although this may be the principal action. It is a reasonable assumption that these drugs act largely by attenuating the pressor effects of major vasoconstrictor hormones—epinephrine, norepinephrine, and angiotensin II—upon vascular smooth muscle. This would lead to a decrease in the tonic action of the sympathetic and renin systems on the circulation, while reducing the responses to acute stimuli.

Calcium channel blockers improve renal function since their vasodilator effect increases blood flow. Furthermore, their vasodilator effects on the afferent renal arterioles tend to increase the glomerular filtration rate.[60] However, it is not yet clear whether the improvement in blood flow and tubular function in the kidney protects against the long-term structural changes associated with hypertension. It is possible that, in part, the hypotensive effects of calcium channel blockers might stem from their modest natriuretic actions, although not all agents produce a similar effect quantitatively.[60] However, the total amount of sodium depletion produced by this associated property of calcium channel blockers is less than that induced by conventional diuretics. In the case of potent vasodilator calcium channel blockers, the frequently seen pedal edema is not offset by the natriuretic effects of these agents, whereas conventional diuretics are often effective in preventing fluid accumulation. It should be emphasized that calcium channel blockers do not appear to induce long-term changes in the renin–aldosterone axis.

METABOLIC EFFECTS

Calcium channel blockers do not have significant effects on glucose and insulin metabolism nor on uric acid metabolism, nor do they cause metabolic effects relative to changes in overall calcium balance. In this respect, they differ from potassium-losing diuretics. It is known that β-blocking drugs, as a class (with the exception of those which have significant intrinsic sympathomimetic actions), decrease serum lipid levels; α-adrenergic blockers also tend to decrease serum lipids. In this regard, calcium channel blockers are "lipid neutral."

EFFECTIVENESS IN HYPERTENSION

Calcium channel blockers are used in the acute reduction of blood pressure in hypertensive emergencies and for chronic control alone or in combination with other agents.

Hypertensive Emergencies

When calcium channel blockers are given orally or intravenously in patients with hypertension, they reduce systemic vascular resistance, increase cardiac output, and increase the stroke volume index. These properties have been used in the treatment of hypertensive emergencies with or without encephalopathy. Recent experience with intravenous nicardipine indicates that the so-called vasoselective agents are especially effective and do not depress myocardial function.[28] Oral or sublingual nifedipine and nitrendipine have been shown to be quite effective in most patients; the most extensive experience has been with sublingual or oral nifedipine. The usual dose of nifedipine for this purpose is 10 to 20 mg. The hypotensive response is attained rapidly within 30 to 60 minutes and may be maintained with a q 6 h dosage schedule. This modality of therapy may obviate the necessity for the use of parenteral therapy with nitroprusside and other agents in most patients, but further controlled studies are needed to validate this approach.

Chronic Control of Mild to Moderate Hypertension

That calcium channel blockers are effective in controlling mild to moderate essential hypertension is now well established. Numerous studies, many blind as well as placebo-controlled, have indicated that verapamil, nifedipine, and diltiazem are as potent as β-blockers or diuretics in the control of mild to moderate systemic hypertension.[58,59] Most studies have used thrice-daily regimens, but the increasing availability of long-acting formulations of these agents is likely to increase their appeal for control of systemic hypertension. The newest dihydropyridines, felodipine, isradipine, and nicardipine, have all been introduced for the treatment of hypertension based on similar trials.

While this class of agents exhibits a wide diversity of structure and variability of pharmacologic effects, the older and newer agents appear to have comparable efficacy for reducing arterial pressure. Direct comparisons of drugs such as verapamil, diltiazem, nifedipine, and nitrendipine[60] have revealed almost identical efficacy. Newer agents have also shown similar effectiveness. The hypotensive effect of bepridil is not well defined.

As single agents, these drugs are successful in controlling hypertension in 60% to 70% of patients. They tend to be most effective in the patients with the highest pretreatment blood pressures. They can be combined with virtually all other hypotensive agents, especially β-blockers and ACE inhibitors. Less controlled data are available for diuretics, α-adrenergic blockers, and direct-acting vasodilators. However, a combination with diuretics may not be as effective as other combinations. Unlike β-blockers, calcium channel blockers appear to be effective in all races, including black patients, and in young as well as old patients. Baseline renin activity may be a useful predictor of response to treatment. Low-renin patients appear to respond favorably to calcium channel blockers, whereas high-renin patients tend to respond less well. This is the converse of what has been found with β-blockers. The mechanism whereby low-renin patients respond to calcium channel blockers is not known.

β-Blockers and calcium channel blockers are both used widely for the treatment of ischemic myocardial syndromes. Their comparative merits and demerits in patients with hypertension and coronary artery disease should be appreciated. Calcium channel blockers can be given with impunity to patients with diabetes mellitus, bronchospastic disease, and peripheral vascular disease, unlike β-blockers. In the younger patient, β-blockers may seriously interfere with exercise and sexual function; these limitations, as well as central nervous system effects, are considerably less with calcium channel blockers. The major shortcoming of calcium channel blockers in this context is the absence of a favorable effect on mortality. These issues are important in the selection of agents for the treatment of hypertension in patients with ischemic heart disease.

Effects on Left Ventricular Hypertrophy

The development of increased left ventricular mass in hypertensive patients indicates a marked increase in the likelihood of cardiovascular complications, including heart failure, atrial fibrillation, and sudden death. Echocardiography has indicated the development of hypertrophy, dilatation, and changes in systolic and diastolic function. Whether such changes and their attendant complications can be averted by an optimal control of blood pressure is not known. However, it appears that the beneficial effect in terms of regression of hypertrophy may be agent-specific. Along with several other classes of antihypertensives but in contrast to diuretics or pure vasodilators, calcium channel blockers have a beneficial effect on left ventricular hypertrophy in hypertension and diastolic function.[61]

The effects are most striking in the case of ACE inhibitors and calcium channel blockers, less in the case of β-blockers. Further work is needed to define the varying effects of different classes of hypotensive agents in this regard, as well as their impact on the complications of ventricular hypertrophy.

Hypertrophic Cardiomyopathy

Patients with hypertrophic cardiomyopathy are known to have both systolic and diastolic abnormalities of ventricular function.[62] It appears to be a disorder of cellular calcium overload. The degree of dynamic obstruction to left ventricular ejection is directly related to the inotropic state, and for this reason β-blockers have long been used in this condition with a variable degree of success. They increase exercise capacity and decrease the incidence of angina pectoris. Propranolol and other β-blockers may, however, reduce neither the incidence of serious ventricular arrhythmias nor the risk of sudden death. Because of their intrinsic negative inotropic activity, calcium channel blockers might be expected to exert a salutary effect in hypertrophic cardiomyopathy. It has been found that calcium channel blockers prevent the development of hereditary cardiomyopathy in hamsters, a disorder akin to hypertrophic obstructive cardiomyopathy and possibly related to abnormal calcium flux across myocardial cell membranes. These observations have formed the basis for the clinical evaluation of calcium channel blockers in hypertrophic cardiomyopathy.

The most extensive data are available for verapamil. Early studies with the drug (480 mg/d) demonstrated significant improvement in symptoms compared to β-blockers. In uncontrolled clinical stud-

ies involving verapamil therapy, reductions in electrocardiographic signs of left ventricular hypertrophy and heart size (assessed radiographically) were observed. Follow-up catheterization studies have also demonstrated a decline in resting outflow tract obstruction in 50% of patients, with decrease in left ventricular mass in 70% of patients. Extensive studies by Rosing and colleagues[62] have shown a significant improvement in basal and provoked left ventricular outflow gradients in most patients that is dependent on dose. Cardiac output remains unchanged or increases slightly, without a significant increase in left ventricular end-diastolic pressure.

A direct but uncontrolled comparison of verapamil and propranolol at varying doses has shown that both produce an increase in exercise tolerance of about 20% to 25% acutely. However, with long-term therapy, exercise capacity deteriorates more frequently with propranolol and may actually increase with verapamil (120 mg q.i.d.). Patients symptomatically prefer verapamil. Unfortunately, a large number of patients develop significant side effects with long-term verapamil use, including sinoatrial and atrioventricular node dysfunction, and occasionally severe myocardial dysfunction and heart failure. These adverse reactions may be accentuated when propranolol and verapamil are combined, although some refractory cases may respond satisfactorily to the combination therapy. As in the case of β-blockers, calcium channel blockers do not appear to reduce the incidence of life-threatening ventricular arrhythmias and they have no effect on survival. There are preliminary echocardiographic data suggesting that verapamil may reduce the degree of hypertrophy during chronic therapy. Whether other type I calcium channel blockers or the dihydropyridines may also be of value is unclear at present.

The precise mechanism mediating the salutary effects of calcium channel blockers in hypertrophic cardiomyopathy is also uncertain. However, it is known that abnormalities of diastolic function in patients with hypertrophic cardiomyopathy may be improved by calcium channel blockers,[63] an action that correlates with the evidence of objective symptomatic improvement.[63] For example, verapamil has been shown to shorten the abnormally prolonged isovolumic relaxation time in such patients. Nifedipine has also been demonstrated favorably to modify abnormal left ventricular relaxation and diastolic filling rates in hypertrophic cardiomyopathy.[62] This effect does not appear to be related to the depression of left ventricular systolic function. Administration of nifedipine alone could be deleterious due to its potent vasodilator effects with reflex sympathetic discharge. The combined administration of nifedipine and propranolol may be superior to the use of the calcium channel blocker alone. The combination reduces left ventricular peak systolic pressure, total peripheral resistance, and resting left ventricular outflow gradient without altering cardiac index or pulmonary capillary wedge pressure, or inducing conduction defects. In hypertrophic cardiomyopathy, diltiazem exerts effects similar to those of verapamil and attenuates exercise-induced elevation of pulmonary artery diastolic pressure, suggesting an improvement in left ventricular diastolic function.[62]

Thus, calcium channel blockers, alone or in combination with β-blockers, appear to improve both systolic function and diastolic function in hypertrophic cardiomyopathy. Long-term follow-up studies and determination of the comparative efficacy of the various calcium channel blockers and combination regimens may further define the role of these agents. However, there are no definitive data to indicate that these drugs reduce sudden death or the incidence of symptomatic arrhythmias or induce regression of hypertrophy in this form of cardiomyopathy. When used in combination with β-blockers they may, in a proportion of patients, produce sinus arrest, AV block, and cardiac failure.

Pulmonary Hypertension

Although promising from a theoretical and experimental standpoint, the efficacy of calcium channel blockers in the various forms of pulmonary hypertension appears to be limited.[64] Intravenous verapamil (mean dose 9.6 mg), reported[65] in 12 patients with a mean pulmonary artery pressure of 57 mm Hg due to pulmonary fibrosis, congenital heart disease, or primary pulmonary hypertension, produced a slight decrease in mean pulmonary artery pressure and right ventricular performance in several patients, while in others it had a marked negative inotropic effect with an increase in pulmonary arteriolar resistance. Overall, right atrial pressure, right ventricular end-diastolic pressure, pulmonary arteriolar resistance, and cardiac index were unchanged. Perhaps because of nifedipine's lesser inherent negative inotropic properties in humans, preliminary studies have suggested that this drug may be effective in some patients in specific clinical settings. For example, in one case of primary pulmonary hypertension, nifedipine produced a 54% decrease in pulmonary vascular resistance, a 49% decrease in systemic vascular resistance, and a 90% increase in cardiac output.[66] The improvement was maintained over a 3-month period. However, many patients with pulmonary hypertension do not respond so well or may even deteriorate, with severe systemic hypotension, when a calcium channel blocker is given.[64] In another study of patients with acute respiratory failure and chronic airway obstruction, nifedipine dilated pulmonary vessels constricted by hypoxemia but had no further vasodilator effect when hypoxemia was corrected. No adverse effects on arterial oxygenation were noted. Experience with diltiazem and other calcium channel blockers is still limited, but effects similar to those of verapamil and nifedipine are likely.

It is apparent that although available data concerning calcium channel blockers in pulmonary hypertension are encouraging in individual patients, they are preliminary and essentially anecdotal. In addition, adverse effects have been noted, probably due to inherent myocardial depressant properties and possibly also due to differential vasodilatation of the pulmonary and systemic vascular beds. Such adverse effects are most likely in patients whose right ventricular function has been severely impaired by chronic pressure load. In these cases, the marked depressant effect on right ventricular function may outweigh the hemodynamic improvement resulting from a reduction in pulmonary vascular resistance. For this reason it is unlikely that calcium channel blockers will make a major impact on the chronic prophylactic therapy of pulmonary hypertension.

Acute and Chronic Congestive Heart Failure

Although calcium channel blockers are potent vasodilators and may ameliorate heart failure by impedance reduction, it must be emphasized that as a class these compounds are unlikely to be the first-line therapy.[27] Their effects in this setting are unpredictable, variable, and sometimes depressant, even with the dihydropyridines. However, they may be of value in patients who have myocardial ischemia in the setting of cardiac decompensation. Available data suggest that nifedipine and other dihydropyridines may be effective preload- and afterload-reducing agents in the setting of acute pulmonary edema. The administration of 10 mg of nifedipine sublingually may improve congestive heart failure secondary to hypertensive, rheumatic, or primary heart disease.[67] The drug induces a sustained decrease in preload and afterload and appears to enhance contractility. Compared to nitrates, nifedipine has a greater tendency to increase cardiac output, without inducing venous pooling. In patients with advanced chronic congestive heart failure, the acute administration of nifedipine (20 mg sublingual) may increase the cardiac index and stroke work index, while decreasing preload significantly. These changes appear to result from decreased systemic vascular resistance. However, sustained hemodynamic improvement has been noted in less than 50% of patients at 24 hours with continuous therapy, suggesting tolerance or possible sodium retention. Deterioration of ventricular function may also occur in some patients.

As indicated above, the hemodynamic profiles of the newer vasoselective calcium channel blockers (amlodipine, nicardipine, felodipine, isradipine) suggest that they function essentially as afterload-reducing agents with no negative inotropic action. Indeed, they may augment indices of ventricular contractility. They may be of potential value in patients with heart failure, especially in the setting of coronary artery disease. The dihydropyridines may also be of value as afterload-reducing agents in patients with aortic and mitral regurgitation. However, barring the exceptions mentioned above, it is rarely if ever justified to use calcium channel blockers as first-line afterload-reducing agents.

Miscellaneous Cardiovascular and Noncardiovascular Disorders

Numerous studies in a wide variety of cardiovascular and noncardiovascular conditions have suggested that the overall spectrum of therapeutic utility of calcium channel blockers is wide.

MIGRAINE AND CLUSTER HEADACHES

Calcium channel blockers may be effective in the control of migraine and cluster headaches,[68] but their efficacy relative to that of β-blockers or conventional regimens remains unclear.

CEREBROVASCULAR DISORDERS

The rationale for the use of prophylactic calcium channel blocker therapy in evolving cerebral stroke relates to the supposition that the initial event in the development of cerebral arterial spasm is the contraction of smooth muscle cells in the large cerebral arteries. Thus, an agent that inhibits such contractions may prevent spasm as well as the resulting neurologic damage. Experimental data have indicated that certain dihydropyridines may be selective in their action with respect to regional circulatory beds. Thus, they may have the potential to dilate cerebral vessels without producing severe hypotension. This appears to be most striking in the case of nimodipine, which penetrates the blood–brain barrier; it has been released for prevention of cerebral injury in subarachnoid hemorrhage. Preliminary[11] clinical trials have suggested that prophylactic administration also significantly decreases the occurrence of severe neurologic deficits in stroke. However, further vindication of these data is needed before the routine clinical use of calcium channel blockers in this setting can be established.

EXERCISE-INDUCED ASTHMA

Recent studies[69] have emphasized the role of calcium in the control of smooth muscle tone in bronchial tissue. This has provided the basis for clinical trials of calcium channel blockers in bronchial asthma. Although experience is limited, it appears that these agents are weak bronchodilators for symptomatic bronchial asthma, but they may be of therapeutic utility in exercise-induced bronchoconstriction.[70] This has been demonstrated for nifedipine and verapamil. The drugs may be of value as tools to determine the role of calcium in bronchial physiology and in the pathophysiologic mechanism of asthma.

GASTROINTESTINAL DISORDERS

Calcium channel blockers have the potential to alter secretory and motility processes in the gastrointestinal tract.[71] Both in laboratory animals and in humans, diltiazem, verapamil, and nifedipine have been found to decrease contractions in smooth muscle,

decreasing peristalsis and sphincter pressures.[72] Thus, a rational basis exists for the role of this class of drugs in the amelioration of symptoms referable to upper gastrointestinal motility. Their precise role remains to be defined, however.

RAYNAUD'S PHENOMENON

Since calcium channel blockers are often powerful peripheral arterial dilators, they have been used in Raynaud's phenomenon.[73] Their role in this setting remains under clinical evaluation. Agents such as cinnarizine and flunarizine have also been used successfully in the treatment of tissue damage due to vascular obstruction.

SIDE EFFECTS

The major side effects of verapamil, nifedipine, and diltiazem are generally predictable from their inherent vasodilator and relatively negative inotropic and chronotropic properties (see Fig. 6.11). Their side effects may also vary in relation to the route of administration. The nature and incidence of side effects following oral therapy are shown in Figure 6.14. Though the safety of nifedipine and other dihydropyridines has not been thoroughly studied, a review[74] of the records of over 3000 patients treated with the drug provides valuable basic information. In this review of patients with various anginal syndromes, some complicated by congestive heart failure and many studied for longer than 6 months, about 60% of the patients reported no adverse side effects. Dizziness and lightheadedness were reported in 12.1% of the total population but were more frequent in patients with congestive heart failure and in those on long-term therapy. Edema, swelling, and fluid retention occurred in 7.7% of the population and were also more common in patients with congestive heart failure and during long-term therapy. Disturbances of upper gastrointestinal tract function and headaches occurred in about 7% of patients, while flushing or burning or a general or specific feeling of weakness were reported in 7.4% and 5.9% of

---

FIGURE 6.14 ADVERSE EFFECTS OF CALCIUM CHANNEL BLOCKERS

Nifedipine (17%)	Verapamil (9%)*	Diltiazem (4%)*	Bepridil (8%–10%)
Ankle edema	Constipation	Dizziness	Dizziness
Headache	Headache	Headache	Headache
Dizziness	Dizziness	Fatigue	Nausea
Tinnitus	Nausea	Blurred vision	Torsade de pointes
Flushing	Galactorrhea	Flushing	Congestive heart failure
Hypotension	Hepatotoxicity	Atrioventricular	AV block and bradycardia
Aggravation of angina (occasionally)	Atrioventricular block/bradycardia	block/bradycardia	
Nasal congestion	Congestive heart failure		
Palpitations			

*Based on estimated in reported series. The side effect profile of newer dihydropyridines, including vasoselective agents, is similar to that of nifedipine.

cases, respectively. Less common side effects related to cardiovascular function included hypotension, precipitation of angina, preinfarction angina or myocardial infarction, and congestive heart failure, in less than 4% of patients. The total percentage of patients in whom therapy was discontinued due to an adverse experience was 5%, but the overall incidence of side effects has been estimated to be about 17%. The overall side effects of other dihydropyridines are similar, but the problems of rapid peripheral vasodilatation and edema appear to be less with both the newer dihydropyridines and with the controlled-release form of nifedipine.

After administration of intravenous verapamil, the adverse effects reported have been those expected from the drug's known pharmacologic properties. Perhaps the most common is a transient fall in blood pressure. More serious side effects are uncommon, but severe hypotension, bradycardia, and rarely ventricular asystole have all been observed. In general, these latter occurred in patients receiving concomitant β-blocking drugs. Suicidal overdose with verapamil, manifested by unconsciousness, hypotension, anuria, and AV block, has been reported. These severe side effects of verapamil can be successfully treated with intravenous atropine (partially effective), catecholamines (particularly isoproterenol), and intravenous calcium. Occasionally, temporary transvenous ventricular pacing may be necessary. The effects of intravenous diltiazem, gallopamil, tiapamil, and bepridil are likely to be qualitatively similar to those of intravenous verapamil.

Overall, oral verapamil is well tolerated. The most common side effects include constipation, dizzying, nausea, headache, and ankle edema. In general, these symptoms are relatively mild and can be managed symptomatically. Less common side effects include galactorrhea and reversible hepatic toxicity. Prolongation of first-degree AV block occurs in a proportion of patients given chronic oral verapamil therapy, but in the absence of antecedent conduction system disease more advanced grades of heart block are unusual. In patients with normal ventricular function, the precipitation of clinically evident cardiac failure is very uncommon. The overall incidence of side effects following oral verapamil therapy is about 9%.

Experience with diltiazem indicates a spectrum of side effects similar to verapamil, but generally with a lower frequency in data derived from studies of angina. Dizziness, headache, fatigue, blurred vision, flushing, and minor degrees of AV block have been reported when the drug is administered in daily doses of 240 to 360 mg. Overall, however, diltiazem appears to have the lowest incidence of side effects of the calcium channel blockers, with estimates of about 4%.

The side effect profile of bepridil is well described. The major cardiovascular complication is the occurrence of torsade de pointes in the setting of long QT interval and hypokalemia. Proarrhythmic reactions typical of class I agents may also be seen. Minor side effects relate to gastrointestinal or central nervous system reactions.

CHOOSING A CALCIUM ANTAGONIST IN THERAPY

With the increasing number of calcium channel blockers becoming available for use in a wide variety of clinical disorders, a common quandary is which calcium channel blocker to use for which clinical indication. Unlike the β-blockers, which exert the bulk of their therapeutic effects by blocking β-receptors, the overall electrophysiologic and hemodynamic effects of various calcium channel blockers may differ markedly. Thus guidelines can be suggested only on the basis of a thorough knowledge of the pharmacodynamic and pharmacokinetic properties (including the side-effect profile) of the individual agent relative to the pathophysiology of the clinical entity under consideration. For example, it is known that in the case of Prinzmetal's angina, unstable angina, or chronic stable angina all calcium channel blockers are perhaps equally effective if the dosage regimen is appropriate; the choice of one compound over another is likely to depend on the side-effect profile and on the presence of associated features in the patient. Thus, the presence of conduction system disease, bradycardia, or ventricular dysfunction may warrant the use of a dihydropyridine rather than diltiazem, verapamil, or bepridil. On the other hand, it is known that since the dihydropyridines may produce reflex tachycardia, they may aggravate angina or ischemia in a proportion of patients with chronic stable angina; so the efficacy of the dihydropyridines in this setting may be lower. Thus, a rate-lowering calcium channel blocker might be preferred for monotherapy.

Bepridil has been effective in some patients with effort angina refractory to diltiazem. However, its potential for proarrhythmic effects limits it to use as a last resort, and it should be avoided when concomitant use of a diuretic could provoke hypokalemia and in patients whose baseline QT is pathologically increased. In the case of hypertrophic cardiomyopathy, it is likely that a rate-lowering calcium channel blocker that is a less potent vasodilator and exerts a modest negative inotropic effect is preferable. In hypertensive emergencies, dihydropyridines may be preferred because of their rapid onset of action and potent vasodilator effects. On the other hand, in the long-term treatment of mild to moderate hypertension, most calcium channel blockers are effective.

With controlled-release preparations allowing once-a-day dosing now available for verapamil, diltiazem, and nifedipine, an appropriate formulation can be prescribed to maximize patient compliance by taking into account the schedules of other medications used by the patient. Whether striking differences exist in the efficacy of individual agents with respect to other conditions in which these drugs as a class may be effective needs further critical evaluation.

ACKNOWLEDGMENTS

I am indebted to Dr. Malcolm Bersohn, MD, PhD, for comments on this chapter and to Diane Gertschen for help in preparing it.

REFERENCES

1. Fleckenstein A: History of calcium antagonists. Circ Res 52(Suppl II):1, 1983
2. Singh BN, Hecht HS, Nademanee K et al: Electrophysiologic and hemodynamic effects of slow-channel blocking drugs. Prog Cardiovasc Dis 5:103, 1982
3. Singh BN, Ellrodt G, Nademanee K: Calcium antagonists: Cardiocirculatory effects and therapeutic applications. In Hurst JW (ed): Clinical Essays on the Heart, vol 2, pp 65–98. New York, McGraw-Hill, 1984
4. Schwartz A: A view of the latest concept of the voltage-dependent calcium-channel and mechanism of action of calcium-channel modulators. Cardiovasc Drugs Ther 1:439, 1988
5. Singh BN, Baky S, Nademanee K: Second generation calcium antagonists: Search for greater selectivity and versatility. Am J Cardiol 55:214B, 1985
6. Hess P: Calcium channels in vertebrate cells. Annu Rev Neurosci 13:337, 1990
7. Bean BP: Multiple types of calcium channels in heart muscle and neurons. Modulation by drugs and neurotransmitters. Ann NY Acad Sci 560:334, 1989
8. VanBreeman C, Saida K: Cellular mechanisms regulating Ca^{2+} in smooth muscle. Annu Rev Physiol 51:315, 1989
9. Tseng GN, Boyden PA: Multiple types of calcium currents in single canine Purkinje cells. Circ Res 65:1735, 1989
10. Sheridan DJ, Thomas P: Vascular versus myocardial selectivity of calcium antagonists. J Cardiovasc Pharmacol 10(Suppl 1):S165, 1987
11. Allen GS, Ahn HS, Preziosi TJ et al: Cerebral arterial spasm—a controlled trial of nimodipine in patients with subarachnoid hemorrhage. N Engl J Med 308:619, 1983
12. Holmes B, Brogden RN, Heel RG et al: Flunarizine: A review of its pharmacodynamic and pharmacokinetic properties and therapeutic use. Drugs 22:6, 1984
13. Shapiro W, Narahara KA, Park J: The effects of lidoflazine on exercise performance and thallium stress scintigraphy in patients with angina pectoris. Circulation 65(Suppl II):1, 1982
14. Vaughan Williams EM: Antiarrhythmic Action and the Puzzle of Perhexiline, pp 1–143. London, Academic Press, 1980
15. Gill A, Flaim SF, Damiano B et al: Pharmacology of bepridil. Am J Cardiol 69:11D, 1992
16. Singh BN, Nademanee K, Feld G et al: Comparative electrophysiologic profiles of calcium antagonists with particular reference to bepridil. Am J Cardiol 55:14C, 1985
17. Singh BN and the Bepridil Collaborative Group: Comparative efficacy and safety of bepridil and diltiazem in chronic stable angina. Am J Cardiol 68:306, 1991
18. Chew CYC, Hecht HS, Collett JT et al: Influence of the severity of ventricular dysfunction on hemodynamic responses to intravenously administered verapamil in ischemic heart disease. Am J Cardiol 47:917, 1981
19. Theroux P, Waters DD, Debaisieux JC et al: Hemodynamic effects of calcium ion antagonists after acute myocardial infarction. Clin Invest Med 50:689, 1982
20. O'Rourke RA, Walsh RA: Experience with calcium antagonist drugs in congestive heart failure. Am J Cardiol 59:64B, 1987
21. Bonow R: Effects of calcium-channel blocking agents on left ventricular diastolic function in hypertrophic cardiomyopathy and in coronary artery disease. Am J Cardiol 55:172B, 1985
22. Josephson MA, Hopkins J, Singh BN: Hemodynamic and metabolic effects of diltiazem during coronary sinus pacing with particular reference to left ventricular ejection fraction. Am J Cardiol 55:286, 1985
23. Walsh RA, Porter CB, Starling MR et al: Beneficial hemodynamic effects of intravenous and oral diltiazem in severe congestive heart failure. J Am Coll Cardiol 3(4):1044, 1984
24. Goldstein RE, Boccuzzi SJ, Cruess D et al: The Adverse Experience Committee and the Multicenter Diltiazem Post-Infarction Research Group: Diltiazem increases late-onset congestive heart failure in post infarction with early reduction in ejection fraction. Circulation 83:52, 1991
25. Singh BN: Safety profile of bepridil determined from clinical trials in chronic stable angina in the United States. Am J Cardiol 69:68D, 1992
26. Elkayam U, Weber L, McKay CR et al: Differences in hemodynamic response to vasodilatation due to calcium channel antagonism with nifedipine and direct-acting agonism with hydralazine in chronic refractory congestive heart failure. Am J Cardiol 54:126, 1984
27. Packer M: Second generation calcium-channel blockers in the treatment of chronic heart failure: Are they any better than their predecessors? Circulation 14:1339, 1989
28. Hofman-Bang C, Ryden L: Vascular selective calcium-channel antagonists in congestive heart failure. In Singh BN, Dzau V, Vanhoutte P, Woosley R: Textbook of Cardiovascular Pharmacology and Therapeutics. New York, Churchill-Livingstone, 1993 (in press)
29. Brown BG, Bolson EL, Dodge HT: Dynamic mechanisms in human coronary stenosis. Circulation 10:917, 1984
30. Parmley WW, Nesto RW, Singh BN et al: Attenuation of the circadian patterns of myocardial ischemia with nifedipine GITS in patients with chronic stable angina. J Am Coll Cardiol 19:1380, 1992
31. Singh BN (ed): Silent Myocardial Ischemia and Angina, pp 3–299. New York, Pergamon Press, 1988
32. Johnson SM, Mauritson DR, Willerson JT et al: A controlled trial of verapamil in Prinzmetal's variant angina. N Engl J Med 306:862, 1981
33. Robertson RH, Wood AJJ, Vaughan WK et al: Exacerbation of vasotonic angina pectoris by propranolol. Circulation 65:281, 1982
34. Falk E: Unstable angina with fatal outcome: Dynamic coronary thrombosis leading to infarction and/or sudden death. Circulation 71:699, 1985
35. Mizuno K, Satmura K, Miyamoto A et al: Angioscopic evaluation of coronary artery thrombi in acute coronary syndromes. N Engl J Med 326:287, 1992
36. Theroux P, Taeymans Y, Morissette D et al: A randomized study comparing propranolol and dilti-

azem in the treatment of unstable angina. J Am Coll Cardiol 5:717, 1985

37. HINT Research Group: Early treatment of unstable angina in the coronary care unit: A randomized, double-blind, placebo-controlled comparison of recurrent ischemia in patients with nifedipine or metoprolol or both. Br Heart J 56: 400, 1986

38. Hecht HS, Chew CYC, Burnam M et al: Radionuclide ejection fraction and regional wall motion during atrial pacing in stable angina pectoris: Comparison with metabolic and hemodynamic parameters. Am Heart J 101:726, 1981

39. Narahara KA: Hemodynamic effects of bepridil in patients with coronary artery disease. Am J Cardiol 69:17D, 1992

40. Yusuf S, Peto R, Lewis J et al: Beta-blockade during and after myocardial infarction: An overview of the randomized trials. Prog Cardiovasc Dis 17:335, 1985

41. Hamm CV, Opie LH: Protection of infarcting myocardium by slow channel inhibitors. Circ Res 54(Suppl I):129, 1983

42. Bussman WD, Seher W, Gruengras M: Reduction of creative kinase-MB indexes of infarct size by intravenous verapamil. Am J Cardiol 54:1224, 1984

43. Clark RE, Christlieb IY, Vanderwonder JC et al: Use of nifedipine to decrease ischemic-reperfusion injury in the surgical setting. Am J Cardiol 55:125B, 1985

44. Bersohn MM, Shine KL: Verapamil protection of ischemic isolated rabbit heart: Dependence on pre-treatment. J Mol Cell Cardiol 15:659, 1983

45. Held P, Yusuf S, Furberg C: Calcium channel blockers in acute myocardial infarction and unstable angina: An overview. Br Med J 299:1187, 1989

46. Gibson RS, Boden WE, Theroux P et al: Diltiazem and reinfarction in patients with non-Q wave myocardial infarction. N Engl J Med 315:423, 1986

47. Multicenter Diltiazem Post-Infarction Trial Research Group: The effect of diltiazem on mortality and reinfarction after myocardial infarction. N Engl J Med 319:385, 1988

48. The Danish Study Group on Verapamil in Myocardial Infarction: Secondary prevention with verapamil after myocardial infarction. Am J Cardiol 66:331, 1990

49. Lamas GA, Pfeffer MA, Hamm P et al: Do the results of randomized clinical trials of cardiovascular drugs influence medical practice? N Engl J Med 327:241, 1992

50. Parmley WW, Blumlein S, Sievers R: Modification of experiment atherosclerosis by calcium-channel blockers. Am J Cardiol 55:165B, 1985

51. Henry PD, Bentley KI: Suppression of atherogenesis in cholesterol-fed rabbit treated with nifedipine. J Clin Invest 6:1366, 1981

52. Lichten PR, Hugenholtz PG, Raffenbeul W et al: Retardation of angiographic progression of coronary artery disease by nifedipine. Results of the International Nifedipine Trial on Antiatherosclerotic Therapy (INTACT). Lancet 335:1109, 1990

53. Waters D, Lesperance J, Francetich M et al: A control trial to assess the effect of calcium-channel blocker upon the progression of coronary artery atherosclerosis. Circulation 82:1940, 1990

54. Singh BN: Control of cardiac arrhythmias by modulation of the slow myocardial channel. In Hurwitz L, Partridge LD, Leach JK (eds): Calcium Channels: Their Properties, Functions, Regulation and Clinical Relevance, pp 327–361. Boca Raton, CRC Press, 1992

55. Dougherty AH, Jackman WM, Nacarelli GV et al: Acute conversion of paroxysmal supraventricular tachycardia with intravenous diltiazem. Am J Cardiol 70:587, 1992

56. Camm AJ, Garratt CJ: Adenosine and supraventricular tachycardia. N Engl J Med 325:1621, 1992

57. Belhassen B, Horowitz LN: Use of intravenous verapamil for ventricular tachycardia. Am J Cardiol 54:1141, 1984

58. Buhler FR, Hulthen L: Calcium channel blockers: A pathophysiologically based antihypertensive treatment concept for the future. Eur J Clin Invest 2:1, 1982

59. Loutzenhiser RD, Epstein M, Hayashi K: Renal hemodynamics effects of calcium antagonists. Am J Cardiol 64:41F, 1969

60. Weber MA, Graettinger WF: Experiences with calcium channel blockers in the treatment of hypertension. In Hurwitz L, Partridge LD, Leach JK (eds): Calcium Channels: Their Properties, Functions, Regulations and Clinical Relevance, pp 309–326. Boca Raton, CRC Press, 1991

61. Weiss RJ, Bent B: Diltiazem-induced left ventricular mass regression in hypertensive patients. J Clin Hypertens 3:135, 1987

62. Rosing DR, Idanpaan-Heikkila U, Maron BJ et al: Use of calcium-channel blocking drugs in hypertrophic cardiomyopathy. Am J Cardiol 55:185B, 1985

62. Bonow RO, Dilsizian V, Rosing DR et al: Verapamil-induced improvement in left ventricular diastolic filling and increased exercise tolerance in patients with hypertrophic cardiomyopathy. Circulation 71:853, 1985

64. Packer M: Therapeutic application of calcium-channel antagonists for pulmonary hypertension. Am J Cardiol 55:196B, 1985

65. Landmark K, Refsum AM, Simonsen S et al: Verapamil and pulmonary hypertension. Acta Med Scand 204:299, 1978

66. Camerini F, Alberti E, Klugmann S et al: Primary pulmonary hypertension: Effect of nifedipine. Br Heart J 44:352, 1980

67. Polese A, Fiorentini C, Olvari MT et al: Clinical use of a calcium antagonist agent (nifedipine) in acute pulmonary edema. Am J Med 66:145, 1979

68. Gelmer HJ: Nimodipine: A new calcium antagonist in the prophylactic treatment of migraine. Headache 23:106, 1983

69. Triggle DJ: Calcium in the control of smooth muscle function and bronchial hyperreactivity. Allergy 38:1, 1983

70. Fanta CH: Calcium-channel blockers in the prophylaxis and treatment of asthma. Am J Cardiol 55:202B, 1985

71. Fox J, Daniel E: Role of Ca^{++} ions on genesis of lower esophageal sphincter tone and other active contractions. Am J Physiol 237:E163, 1979

72. Castell DO: Calcium-channel blocking agents for gastrointestinal disasters. Am J Cardiol 55:210B, 1985

73. Rodeheffer RJ, Rommer JA, Wigley F: Controlled double-blind trial of nifedipine in the treatment of Raynaud's phenomenon. N Engl J Med 308: 880, 1983

74. Terry RW: Nifedipine therapy in angina pectoris: Evaluation of safety and side effects. Am Heart J 104:681, 1982

ADDITIONAL READING

Hurwitz L, Partridge LD, Leach JK (eds): Calcium Channels: Their Properties, Functions, Regulations and Clinical Relevance. Boca Raton, CRC Press, 1991

Vanhoutte PM, Pasletti R, Govoni S: Calcium antagonists. Ann NY Acad Sci 552:1, 1988

Vasodilator Drugs in the Treatment of Heart Failure

William W. Parmley

This chapter discusses the principal vasodilator drugs that have been used in the treatment of acute and chronic heart failure. Although vasodilation has been used as a treatment of heart failure for more than three decades, it is clear that appreciation of its beneficial effects has occurred only within the past 15 years, and relatively routine use of this form of therapy has taken place only in the past 10 years.

Current studies suggest that vasodilators might be considered as first-line therapy, instead of digitalis. In most patients with congestive heart failure and fluid retention, diuretics will always be a part of the medical regimen irrespective of other drugs that are used. There are some circumstances, however, in which vasodilators may be good candidates for first-line therapy. For example, in patients with severe regurgitant lesions such as mitral or aortic regurgitation (in whom surgical therapy is not a current consideration), vasodilator drugs are extremely beneficial in reducing regurgitant fraction and increasing forward cardiac output. Under these circumstances they produce greater beneficial hemodynamic effects than digitalis and could be considered as first-line therapy. Consider, for example, patients with severe aortic or mitral regurgitation in whom ventricular contractility is preserved and there is no immediate consideration of valve replacement. The rationale for the use of these drugs would be to reduce regurgitant fraction and thus reduce the diastolic volume load on the heart. This might attenuate the rate of gradual cardiac dilation and irreversible decline in cardiac contractility. One might thus be able to treat the patient medically for a longer period until surgical therapy is required to replace the defective valve. It should be emphasized, however, that vasodilator therapy should not be used as a substitute for surgery under these circumstances. When an intrinsic decline in myocardial contractility is recognized, it is important to consider surgical therapy before further reductions in myocardial contractility occur. Vasodilators can also be considered if the heart failure is so severe that surgical therapy is not felt to be a reasonable option.

Another circumstance where vasodilators might be considered as first-line therapy is in patients with asymptomatic left ventricular dysfunction. The asymptomatic arm of the SOLVD trial showed benefit with enalapril. Similarly the SAVE trial in patients after an anterior myocardial infarction showed that captopril could slow the rate of ventricular dilation and prolong life in relatively asymptomatic patients.

Pathophysiologic Basis for the Use of Vasodilator Drugs

The neurohumoral response that accompanies congestive heart failure leads to peripheral vasoconstriction and an increase in calculated systemic vascular resistance. Many factors contribute to this increase in resistance.[1] These include an increase in sympathetic tone and circulating catecholamines, an increase in arginine vasopressin (ADH), and activation of the renin–angiotensin–aldosterone system. The arteriolar constriction thus produced is helpful in maintaining arterial pressure in the face of a fall in cardiac output. As Figure 7.1 suggests, however, this sets up a vicious cycle that can be deleterious to the patient with congestive heart failure. The increased systemic vascular resistance and increased impedance to ejection of blood may further reduce cardiac output by increasing afterload. Thus, patients spiral down this vicious cycle until they reach a new, low, steady-state level at which cardiac output is lower and systemic vascular resistance is higher than is optimal for the patient. Under these circumstances, the use of arteriolar vasodilator drugs can reduce resistance and improve forward cardiac output.

The rationale for the use of venodilators is closely related to the above argument. Venoconstriction is also produced by a marked increase in sympathetic tone and circulating catecholamines. Initially, this may help increase venous return and partially preserve cardiac function by the Frank-Starling mechanism. The peripheral veins serve as the capacitance reservoir of the circulation. Venoconstriction, therefore, will tend to shift more blood to the chest and thus increase right and left atrial filling pressures. Venodilators can attenuate this venoconstriction and redistribute blood away from the chest into the peripheral circulation. This produces a reduction in right and left atrial filling pressures and can help relieve the signs and symptoms of pulmonary and systemic congestion. It should be apparent from the above that in selecting vasodilators for the management of heart failure, it is frequently advisable to combine arteriolar and venodilators or to select therapy that will produce this combined effect.

The following discussion focuses on those drugs with arteriolar dilating properties, those with venodilating properties, and drugs with mixed effects, including the angiotensin-converting enzyme inhibitors. The

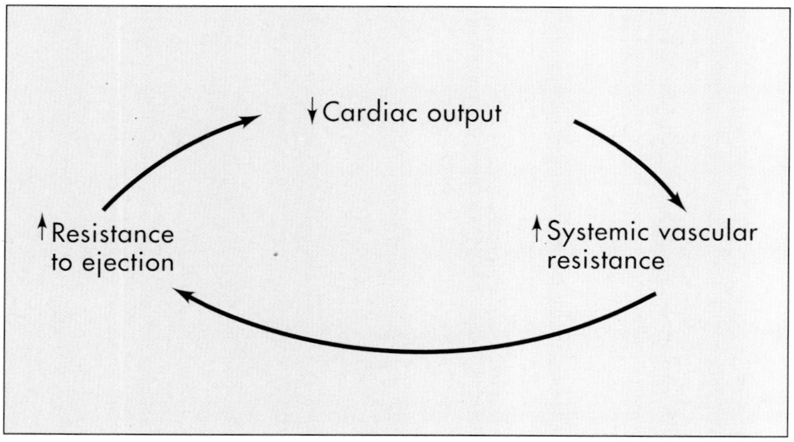

Figure 7.1 Vicious cycle in congestive heart failure. The decrease in cardiac output leads to a neurohumoral reflex increase in systemic vascular resistance. In turn, this further reduces ejection and leads to an additional reduction in cardiac output. Patients spiral down this cycle to a new steady-state level where cardiac output is lower and systemic vascular resistance is higher than is optimal for the patient.

α-adrenergic blocking drugs and the nitrates are discussed in more detail elsewhere in this volume.

Although the classification of drugs as arteriolar or venodilators has a theoretical basis, its pragmatic value has been questioned.[2] Nevertheless, this classification will generally be followed in this chapter.

Arteriolar Vasodilators
Hydralazine

Hydralazine is a potent, direct-acting vasodilator that causes smooth muscle relaxation of arteriolar resistance vessels.[3] It produces effective vasodilation of the renal and peripheral vasculature with little change in liver blood flow. It also has no major direct effect on coronary blood flow. Changes in coronary blood flow parallel changes in myocardial oxygen demand. Hydralazine has essentially no effect on the venous capacitance bed. In patients with hypertension and normal ventricular function, reflex tachycardia is frequent. In patients with hypertension and coronary artery disease, but normal ventricular function, hydralazine may worsen angina, presumably because of the reflex increase in heart rate and cardiac contractility produced by lowering the blood pressure. Although hydralazine has been alleged to have direct positive inotropic effects on the heart, it appears that its effects are mostly mediated by a reflex increase in sympathetic tone. In isolated heart muscle, hydralazine releases myocardial norepinephrine, but at doses that far exceed usual therapeutic doses.[4] With the depletion of myocardial norepinephrine stores and the blunted baroreceptor response in patients with congestive heart failure, it is less likely that hydralazine has a major impact on cardiac contractile state.

Although hydralazine is rapidly and almost completely absorbed from the gastrointestinal tract, its bioavailability depends on the degree of acetylation in the liver, which is an inherited trait. The United States population, in general, has about 50% rapid acetylators and 50% slow acetylators. Slow acetylators are more prone to develop the lupus syndrome and require lower doses for a pharmacologic effect. On the other hand, rapid acetylators have minimal risks for the lupus syndrome and require higher doses. Peak serum concentration is attained 30 minutes to 2 hours after an oral dose, which corresponds with its hemodynamic effects. Hydralazine is about 90% protein bound, and 2% to 15% of an administered dose is excreted unchanged in the urine.

In patients with chronic congestive heart failure,[3,5] hydralazine produces a marked decrease in systemic vascular resistance, with an approximate 50% or more increase in forward cardiac output (Fig. 7.2). In general, arterial pressure and heart rate are little altered. Pulmonary artery pressure and left ventricular filling pressure are little altered or in some cases may decrease slightly. Pulmonary vascular resistance decreases somewhat but generally less than with the nitrates. In patients with chronic mitral and aortic regurgitation, regurgitant fraction is reduced and forward stroke volume and cardiac output are increased.[6,7]

The usual administration of oral hydralazine is 200 to 400 mg daily in divided doses. In some patients, particularly those who are rapid acetylators, doses up to 1200 mg/d have been used. The lupus syndrome is seen in 15% to 20% of patients receiving more than 400 mg/d. Fluid retention is very common with hydralazine and must be treated with increased doses of diuretics or antialdosterone agents. The most frequent and troublesome side effects are nausea and other gastrointestinal symptoms. Rarely, polyneuropathy due to pyridoxine deficiency has been reported. Other very rare side effects include fever or a syndrome of flushing, sweating, and urticaria, perhaps secondary to inhibition of histamine.

Despite acute beneficial hemodynamic effects, there is usually no immediate increase in exercise tolerance. Chronic studies are more variable in attesting to the efficacy of hydralazine. Some studies suggest benefit with long-term administration,[8]

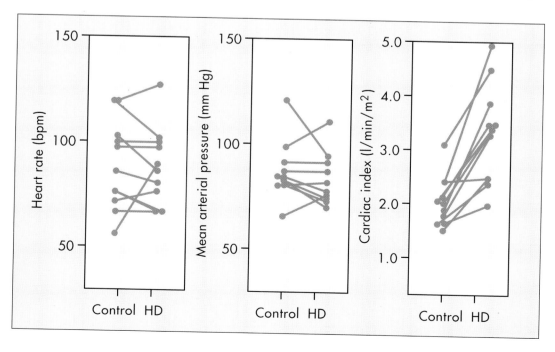

Figure 7.2 The hemodynamic effects of hydralazine (HD) in a group of patients with New York Heart Association Class III and IV heart failure who are doing poorly on digoxin and diuretics. Although there is some variability in response, there is no major change in heart rate or mean arterial pressure, whereas cardiac index increases by about 50%. (Modified from Chatterjee K, Parmley WW, Massie B et al: Oral hydralazine therapy for chronic refractory heart failure. Circulation 54:879, 1976. By permission of the American Heart Association, Inc)

while others have shown no sustained increase in exercise tolerance.[9] As is true of all vasodilators, tolerance may develop to the beneficial effects of hydralazine therapy in some patients. Hydralazine is usually combined with a venodilator such as isosorbide dinitrate, which will reduce pulmonary capillary wedge pressure.

Endralazine is a structural analogue of hydralazine; it has the advantage that its metabolism is independent of the patient's acetylator status and the lupus syndrome has not been observed.[10] Furthermore, the duration of action is longer and the hemodynamic effects appear to be similar. In 12 patients followed for an average of 3 months, there appeared to be sustained hemodynamic and functional improvement.[11]

Minoxidil

Minoxidil is a potent arteriolar vasodilator whose hemodynamic effects are quite similar to those of hydralazine. Minoxidil is almost completely absorbed after an oral dose, reaching a peak plasma concentration in 1 hour with a plasma half-life of 4 hours.

About 10% of a dose is excreted unchanged in the urine. The usual dose is 10 to 20 mg twice daily.

Minoxidil produces an increase in stroke volume and cardiac output (Fig. 7.3) with a striking reduction in systemic vascular resistance. In general, however, there is no change in arterial or pulmonary pressures or in heart rate.[12] Gastrointestinal symptoms are a limiting side effect of minoxidil. In addition, there is significant fluid retention, which almost invariably requires an increase in the dose of diuretics. Hair growth may be troublesome in female patients. Minoxidil is best considered as an alternative drug to hydralazine, perhaps in those who develop the lupus syndrome or intolerable side effects. It will also be more tolerable in patients who do not have considerable edema and can thus be appropriately controlled with increased doses of diuretics. One study did not show any improvement in exercise tolerance in a placebo-controlled trial of minoxidil, despite improved acute and chronic hemodynamics.[13] Data in general suggest that arteriolar vasodilators have far less beneficial effects on exercise tolerance than drugs with venodilating effects, such as the nitrates and angiotensin-converting enzyme inhibitors.

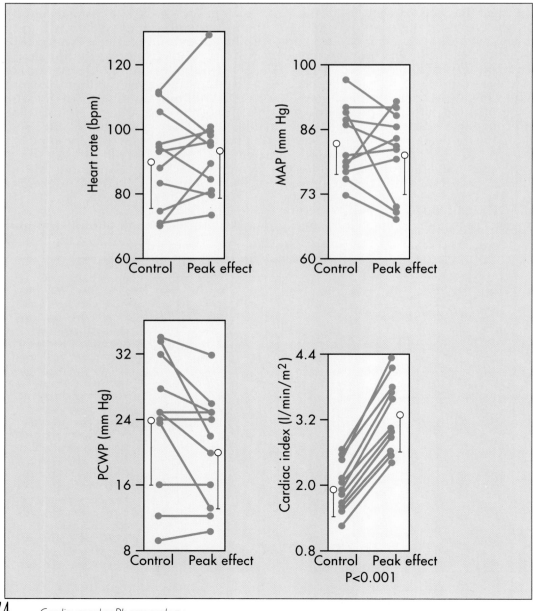

Figure 7.3 Peak hemodynamic effects of 10 to 30 mg of minoxidil in 11 patients with congestive heart failure. There are minimal effects on heart rate, mean arterial pressure (MAP), and pulmonary capillary wedge pressure (PCWP), but a substantial increase in cardiac index. (Modified from McKay C, Chatterjee K, Ports TA et al: Minoxidil in chronic congestive heart failure: A hemodynamic and clinical study. Am Heart J 104:575, 1982)

Calcium Entry Blockers

Calcium entry blocking agents have potent peripheral arteriolar vasodilating effects by interfering with calcium entry into peripheral smooth muscle. This reduction in systemic vascular resistance is effective in increasing cardiac output in patients with moderate congestive heart failure. The first three calcium entry blockers available in the United States were nifedipine, verapamil, and diltiazem. Nifedipine is the most potent arteriolar vasodilator of these three and is associated with the greatest tendency for reflex tachycardia. Verapamil has the greatest negative inotropic effect on the myocardium, and nifedipine, the least. Both verapamil and diltiazem depress atrioventricular conduction, while nifedipine has essentially no effect. Thus, of these three, nifedipine appears to have the most favorable profile for use in heart failure. Studies have been done with all three agents.[14–16] Representative effects with nifedipine are shown in Figure 7.4. There is a modest increase in stroke volume and cardiac output; arterial pressure decreases slightly, and there is no significant change in heart rate and pulmonary capillary wedge pressure. Right atrial pressure is unchanged or slightly reduced. An appropriate dose of nifedipine is 10 to 20 mg three times daily; 30 to 60 mg once daily of long acting nifedipine GITS may be preferable. The dose of diltiazem is 60 mg three times daily, and the dose of verapamil is 80 to 120 mg three times daily. Long-acting preparations of these two drugs are also available. A whole new series of dihydropyridine calcium blockers are now available.[17] These include nicardi-pine, isradipine, felodipine, amlodipine, and others. These agents are more vasoselective than nifedipine in that they have less direct action on the heart. Preliminary studies suggest that they may be effective in increasing cardiac output in patients with moderate heart failure.[18] Felodipine is being studied in the V-HEFT 3 trial to see if it will produce additive beneficial effects on top of ACE inhibitors. Amlodipine is undergoing similar evaluation in the PRAISE trial. Because of the potential for negative inotropic effects, it is unclear whether the calcium entry blockers will have a primary role in the treatment of congestive heart failure as arteriolar vasodilators. For example, in the MDPIT trial where diltiazem was given to patients post-myocardial infarction, there was an increased mortality in patients with pulmonary congestion and an ejection fraction less than 40%.[19] In patients with a higher ejection fraction and non-Q-wave infarction, diltiazem reduced mortality, presumably secondary to its anti-ischemic effects. Similar results were seen with verapamil in the DAVIT 2 trial.[20] In patients with LV dysfunction and hypertension or associated angina, calcium blockers may play a greater role. Adverse effects include hypotension, headache, flushing, palpitations, peripheral edema, and gastrointestinal side effects.[21] Increased atrioventricular block occurs with diltiazem and verapamil; flushing, hypotension, and ankle edema are more common with nifedipine and the other dihydropyridines. Patients with the sick sinus syndrome may also be at risk for bradycardia, especially with verapamil or diltiazem. Along with other arteriolar vasodilators, the calcium entry blockers have been used occasionally

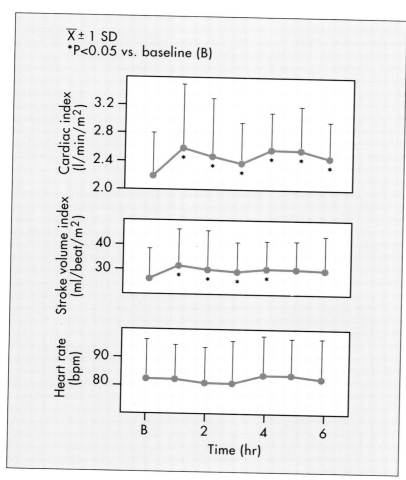

Figure 7.4 Hemodynamic effects of nifedipine (0.2 mg/kg orally) in 11 patients with congestive heart failure. There is a moderate increase in stroke volume and cardiac index in the supine position. (Modified from Leier CS, Patrick TS, Hemiller J et al: Nifedipine in congestive heart failure: Effects on resting and exercise hemodynamics and regional blood flow. Am Heart J 108:1461, 1984)

in the therapy of primary pulmonary hypertension.[22] Some patients may benefit from the calcium blockers or other arteriolar vasodilators, but the response to all vasodilator agents has been generally disappointing.[23]

VENODILATORS

Nitroglycerin and all the other nitrates are the prototype venodilator drugs.[24] The relative magnitude of their vasodilating effects is venous ≥ large arteries ≥ arterioles. Since the different nitrates are discussed in detail elsewhere in this volume, only pertinent facts related to the management of heart failure are discussed here. It appears that the mechanism of smooth muscle relaxation with the nitrates is due to an increase in cyclic guanosine monophosphate (GMP).[25] The nitrate ester is hydrolyzed (–SH dependent), and mononitrate stimulates the enzyme guanylate cyclase, perhaps through an intermediary (S-nitrosothiol), which increases cyclic GMP synthesis. Cyclic GMP in turn appears to decrease available calcium for smooth muscle contraction. This may occur through reduction of calcium release from intracellular stores and a decrease in the influx/efflux ratio across the cell membrane. The predominant effect of the nitrates is on venous capacitance,[26] with a striking reduction in systemic and pulmonary venous pressures (Fig. 7.5). In general, there is no major increase in cardiac output, although following high doses, especially with intravenous nitroglyc-erin,[27] the arteriolar vasodilating effect may become more prominent.

The duration of effect depends on the preparation used. Following sublingual nitroglycerin, the onset occurs within 2 to 3 minutes and lasts for about 20 to 30 minutes. Sublingual isosorbide dinitrate may last between 2 and 3 hours; topical nitroglycerin ointment may last for 4 to 6 hours; and orally administered isosorbide dinitrate may last up to 6 hours. Because oral nitrates are rapidly inactivated by first-pass metabolism in the liver, much larger doses must be given orally as compared with sublingual or transdermal preparations. Isosorbide dinitrate is metabolized more slowly than glycerol trinitrate. Its primary metabolites include mononitrates, which exhibit a

half-life of about 2.5 to 5.0 hours and markedly reduced potencies compared with the dinitrate. They may contribute, however, to the prolonged duration of action.[28] Usual therapeutic doses of oral isosorbide dinitrate are 20 to 80 mg, three or four times a day. Doses of the mononitrates are 20 mg twice a day.

Preliminary studies suggest that nitroglycerin patches are ineffective at usual doses in chronic congestive heart failure. Large doses up to 60 mg (six standard 10-mg patches) are required to produce a reduction in pulmonary capillary wedge pressure.[29] Recent information also suggests that tolerance to nitrates can develop with continuous exposure. There appears to be some correlation between the potency of nitrates and their ability to induce tolerance. The development of tolerance is assumed to be caused by conversion of SH to SS bonds, thus decreasing the available SH groups.[30] Therefore, a dose-free interval is required for the vasculature to regain responsiveness. Thus, intermittent dosing may be more effective than continuous nitrate delivery.

A continuous infusion of nitroglycerin can be effective, however, in certain clinical circumstances. When infused intravenously at the usual therapeutic doses of 10 to 100 μg/min, it has more pronounced arteriolar dilating effects and thus may increase cardiac output.[27] It generally is less effective than nitroprusside, however, in increasing cardiac output.[31] It is an effective drug in relieving ischemic pain, presumably by reducing blood pressure and pulmonary capillary wedge pressure, relieving vasoconstriction, and enhancing collateral flow. There is suggestive evidence that nitroglycerin might slightly reduce infarct size[32] and mortality[33] in patients with acute myocardial infarction. Its major hemodynamic benefit is the lowering of pulmonary capillary wedge pressure, and its major symptomatic benefits are the relief of dyspnea and rest angina.

Although oral nitrates can produce a striking reduction in pulmonary capillary wedge pressure, there may be no change in acute exercise tolerance. After several weeks of continued therapy with isosorbide dinitrate, however, exercise tolerance improves in patients with chronic congestive heart failure.[34]

Since nitrates have little effect on cardiac output,

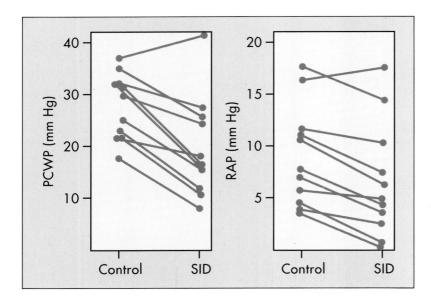

Figure 7.5 Hemodynamic effects of sublingual isosorbide dinitrate (SID) in 11 patients with congestive heart failure. In all but one instance, pulmonary capillary wedge pressure (PCWP) and right atrial pressure (RAP) were reduced.

they are frequently combined with an arteriolar vasodilator such as hydralazine.[35] This combined therapy can increase forward cardiac output and reduce pulmonary capillary wedge pressure, thus relieving the two major hemodynamic abnormalities in patients with chronic heart failure (Fig. 7.6). This combined therapy (hydralazine plus isosorbide dinitrate) was shown to prolong life in the V-HEFT 1 trial in patients with moderate heart failure already on digoxin and diuretics.[36] Nitrates may also produce beneficial hemodynamic effects in patients with mitral regurgitation, resulting in an increase in forward cardiac output and a decrease in regurgitant volume.[37]

The most common side effect of nitrate therapy is headache, to which tolerance frequently develops over a period of days. In some patients postural dizziness, hypotension, and weakness may occur, presumably because of too great a reduction in pulmonary capillary wedge pressure. Patients who are relatively hypovolemic because of high-dose diuretic therapy may be at risk for this hemodynamic side effect. Methemoglobinemia is a rare complication with long-term treatment using large doses of nitrates.

Molsidomine (N-ethoxycarbonyl-3-morpholinosydnonimine) belongs to the class of sydnonimines and has actions similar to the nitrates.[38] Thus, it is predominantly a venodilator and has been effective in angina pectoris and in heart failure with elevated atrial pressures. Its active metabolite (SIN-1A)

presumably depends on the presence of a free nitroso group, which stimulates guanylate cyclase, increases cellular levels of cyclic GMP, and initiates relaxation by removal of free calcium ions from smooth muscle cells. Although its side effect profile is similar to that of nitrates, it has been said to exhibit little or no tolerance during chronic administration, which may be an advantage over nitrates. It is not yet approved for use in the United States.

DRUGS WITH MIXED EFFECTS ON VEINS AND ARTERIES

Prazosin

Prazosin is a quinazoline derivative that is a relatively selective α_1 (postsynaptic)-blocker, which produces vasodilation.[39] It also can inhibit phosphodiesterase and cause smooth muscle relaxation. Prazosin produces a decrease in limb vascular resistance and hepatic resistance (at low doses) but does not influence renal vascular resistance significantly. Prazosin is rapidly and almost completely absorbed from the gastrointestinal tract, with a bioavailability ranging from 44% to 70%. About 6% of the drug is excreted unchanged in the urine, and the majority of the drug is excreted in the feces. The drug is more than 90% protein bound, with a mean elimination half-life of

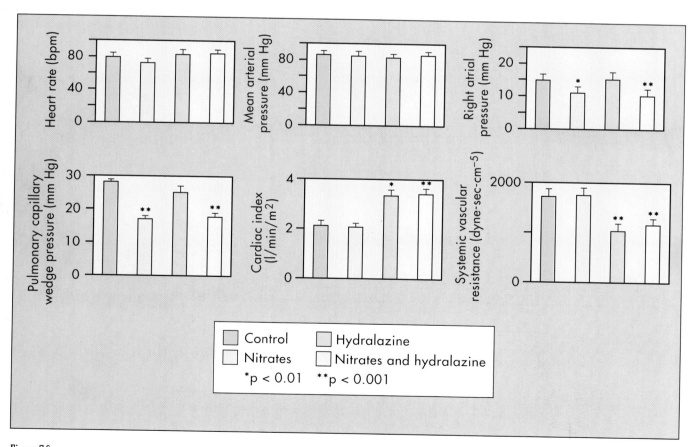

Figure 7.6 Hemodynamic effects of nitrates, hydralazine, and combination of nitrates plus hydralazine as compared with control in 12 patients with chronic congestive heart failure. Nitrates reduced right atrial and pulmonary capillary wedge pressures, and hydralazine decreased systemic vascular resistance and increased cardiac output. The combination of the two produced combined effects on filling pressures and cardiac output. (Modified from Massie B, Chatterjee K, Werner J et al: Hemodynamic advantage of combined oral hydralazine and nonparenteral nitrates in the vasodilator therapy of chronic heart failure. Am J Cardiol 40:794, 1977)

about 2 1/2 hours. Hemodynamic effects last approximately 6 hours. The usual dose is 3 to 5 mg administered three to four times daily.

The hemodynamic effects are relatively balanced between arteriolar dilation and venodilation. Thus, there is an increase in cardiac output associated with a decrease in systemic vascular resistance and arterial pressure. Venodilation produces a reduction in atrial pressures and in pulmonary artery pressure with some decline in pulmonary vascular resistance. Controlled studies have noted an increase in exercise tolerance after long-term therapy with prazosin hydrochloride.[40,41]

Despite these demonstrated long-term beneficial effects, however, there appears to be a rapid attenuation of its hemodynamic effects with long-term therapy.[42,43] The first dose produces the most dramatic effects, and subsequent doses show a marked attenuation (Fig. 7.7). Although the mechanism for this attenuation is unclear, plasma norepinephrine has been shown to increase during chronic therapy.[44] The increased vasoconstriction might therefore counteract some of the vasodilating effects of prazosin. Severe hypotension after a first dose is a potential problem, and 1 mg should be used as the first dose. Other side effects, such as gastrointestinal symptoms, palpitations, drowsiness, depression, and nervousness, are infrequent. This hemodynamic attenuation of its effects in congestive heart failure presumably led to the findings in the V-HEFT 1 trial, wherein mortality was similar in the placebo and prazosin treated groups.[36]

Trimazosin

Trimazosin is closely related to prazosin and appears to produce similar hemodynamic effects. Exercise tolerance has been reported to increase with long-term trimazosin therapy.[45] Another study produced beneficial hemodynamic effects during exercise but no change in resting hemodynamics or in exercise tolerance.[46] In some cases increased doses of diuretics

have been required. The beneficial hemodynamic dose varies between 25 and 100 mg three times daily. Data are too limited to determine its potential role in the management of chronic congestive heart failure.

Terazosin

Terazosin is another α_1-adrenoreceptor with hemodynamic effects similar to trimazosin. An increase in cardiac output and a decrease in atrial pressures occur both at rest and following exercise.[47] More data are required to assess its potential role in chronic heart failure.

Sodium Nitroprusside

Sodium nitroprusside is available intravenously and is a potent relaxant of both arterioles and veins. This direct-acting effect results in potent hemodynamic effects in patients with acute severe heart failure. These include a significant reduction of systemic vascular resistance together with an increase in cardiac output. In general, some decrease in arterial pressure accompanies the increase in cardiac output.[48] Potent venodilation leads to reduction of atrial and pulmonary artery pressures. The effects on renal function are variable. In some cases increased sodium and potassium excretion may occur, although decreased arterial pressure may worsen renal function and lead to increased plasma renin activity. Nitroprusside is most valuable in patients with high left ventricular filling pressures and reasonable arterial pressures (systolic pressure $\geq$ 100 mm Hg). In such patients there is a striking increase in cardiac output and a reduction in pulmonary capillary wedge and right atrial pressures. Nitroprusside is best given only in patients with an intra-arterial line and a balloon tip catheter in the pulmonary artery. Thus, one can avoid excessive reductions in arterial pressure while at the same time measuring the reduction in pulmonary capillary wedge pressure. The drug is initially

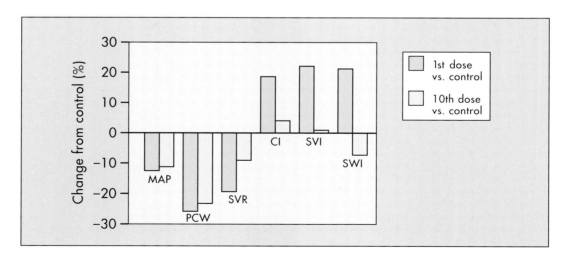

Figure 7.7 Comparison between the hemodynamic effects of the first and tenth doses of prazosin in 12 patients with chronic congestive heart failure. Although there is a persistent effect on reduction of mean arterial pressure (MAP) and pulmonary capillary wedge pressure (PCWP) there is marked attenuation of the effect on systemic vascular resistance (SVR) cardiac index (CI), stroke volume index (SVI), and stroke work index (SWI). (Modifed from Arnold SB, Williams RL, Ports TA et al: Attenuation of prazosin effect on cardiac output in chronic heart failure. Ann Intern Med 91:345, 1979)

administered at a dose level of about 15 μg/min, with a gradual titration upward until pulmonary capillary wedge pressure is reduced and cardiac output increased. At the same time, the fall in arterial pressure must be minimized. In patients with significant mitral or aortic regurgitation, sodium nitroprusside is effective in increasing forward cardiac output and reducing regurgitant volume.[49,50] In general, it is used in patients with acute severe heart failure who have a reasonable blood pressure and a high filling pressure. It might also be helpful in patients with acute severe mitral or aortic regurgitation or for the short-term therapy of patients with severe chronic heart failure in whom oral therapy is going to be subsequently initiated.

The effects of nitroprusside in patients with acute severe heart failure following myocardial infarction[51] are shown in Figure 7.8. Group II and III patients with the most severe heart failure following myocardial infarction showed an increase in stroke volume together with a decrease in left ventricular filling pressure. Group I patients, who had an initial left ventricular filling pressure less than 15 mm Hg, had a reduction in stroke volume as they moved down the ascending limb of their ventricular function curve.

This was accompanied by hypotension and tachycardia. Thus, nitroprusside should be limited to patients with a high left ventricular filling pressure, and care should be taken not to reduce filling pressure much below the optimal range of 15 to 18 mm Hg. If this occurs, volume loading to bring the filling pressure up to a higher level can still retain the beneficial effects of nitroprusside. In two controlled studies in patients with acute myocardial infarction, nitroprusside reduced mortality in one study[52] and had no effect in the other.[53] In the latter study, it was most beneficial several hours after the infarct and in patients with high filling pressures. Some studies have suggested that nitroprusside may cause a coronary steal syndrome[54] and thus be less beneficial than intravenous nitroglycerin. No significant deleterious effects of nitroprusside have been found in other studies.[55]

The most serious side effect of nitroprusside is hypotension. This can be managed by temporarily discontinuing the drug. Rare complications include decreased arterial oxygen, cyanide toxicity, hypothyroidism, methemoglobinemia, lactic acidosis, vitamin B_{12} deficiency, inhibition of platelet function, and gastrointestinal symptoms.

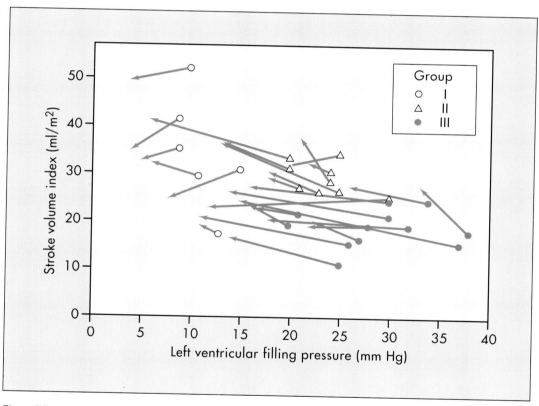

Figure 7.8 Hemodynamic effects of nitroprusside on left ventricular function in patients with acute myocardial infarction. Group I patients had an initial filling pressure less than 15 mm Hg. Group II and III patients had left ventricular failure with filling pressures greater than 15 mm Hg. In Group III, the stroke work index was less than 20 g-m/m², and in Group II it was greater than 20 g-m/m.² In Groups II and III, nitroprusside produced an increase in stroke volume, together with a reduction in left ventricular filling pressure. In Group I patients, the effects on stroke volume were more variable, but tended to decrease because of the reduction in filling pressure down the ascending limb of the ventricular function curve. (Modified from Chatterjee K, Parmley WW: The role of vasodilator therapy in heart failure. Prog Cardiovasc Dis 19:301, 1977)

Phentolamine

Phentolamine is an α-adrenergic blocker with relatively balanced effects on arteries and veins.[56] It produces an increase in cardiac output together with a reduction in pulmonary capillary wedge pressure. It reduces arterial pressure and has a greater tendency to cause reflex tachycardia than does sodium nitroprusside. It is restricted to parenteral administration and is infused continuously at a dose of 0.1 to 2.0 mg/min. It does not appear to have any advantages over nitroprusside and has been used far less frequently.

ANGIOTENSIN-CONVERTING ENZYME INHIBITORS
Captopril

The renin-angiotensin-aldosterone system is activated in chronic congestive heart failure.[1] Decreased perfusion pressure, adrenergic stimulation, and reduced sodium all stimulate the juxtaglomerular apparatus around the afferent arteriole in the renal glomerulus to release renin. Renin converts angiotensinogen (which is produced in the liver) to angiotensin I, an inactive decapeptide. Angiotensin I is then changed by converting enzyme to angiotensin II, a potent vasoconstrictor. Angiotensin II has three effects that may be deleterious to the patient with heart failure. First of all, it is a potent vasoconstrictor that can directly increase systemic vascular resistance. Second, it facilitates sympathetic outflow and may worsen the sympathetic-mediated increase in systemic vascular resistance. Third, it stimulates the production and release of aldosterone, which leads to further sodium retention. Theoretically, therefore, if one could prevent the formation of angiotensin II, one might benefit patients with heart failure.

Converting enzyme, which alters angiotensin I to angiotensin II, is located everywhere in the body, but appears to predominate in pulmonary capillary endothelial cells. Inhibition of this enzyme leads to reduced levels of angiotensin II, even though there is a feedback increase in renin levels. Converting enzyme is also responsible for the degradation of bradykinin, a potent vasodilator.[57] Thus, inhibition of converting enzyme may produce vasodilation both by decreasing angiotensin II levels and increasing bradykinin levels. Captopril is the first orally available angiotensin-converting enzyme inhibitor to be used in chronic congestive heart failure. Its hemodynamic effects[58] include a substantial fall in systemic vascular resistance with a fall in arterial pressure. Despite the fall in arterial pressure, there may be a slight decrease in heart rate (Fig. 7.9). Presumably this occurs because of a reduction in sympathetic tone to the sinoatrial node. After a single oral dose, these effects last for up to 8 hours. Together with the decrease in systemic resistance, there is an increase in forward cardiac output (Fig. 7.10). There is also considerable venodilation, with a reduction in pulmonary capillary wedge pressure and right atrial pressure. The precise reason for a decrease in pulmonary capillary wedge pressure is unclear. Angiotensin II is not a potent venoconstrictor. It is more likely that withdrawal of sympathetic tone plays a more prominent role in the venodilation than does a reduction in angiotensin II levels. Furthermore, a reduction in arterial pressure enhances ejection of blood and in and of itself can reduce end-diastolic volume. There is frequently a concordant change in arterial pressure and pulmonary capillary wedge pressure.[59]

Vasodilators also increase the apparent compliance

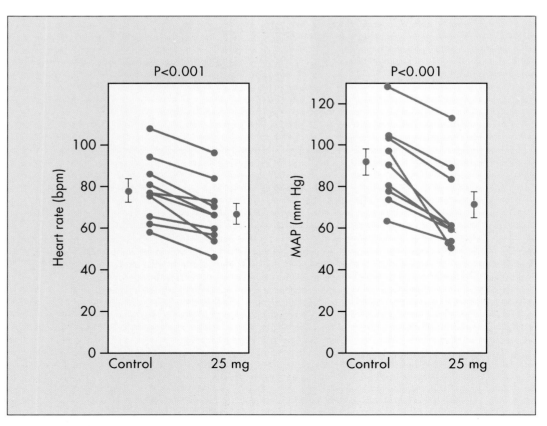

Figure 7.9 Effects of 25 mg of captopril on the hemodynamics of nine patients with congestive heart failure. Despite a reduction in mean arterial pressure (MAP), there is no reflex increase in heart rate. In fact, heart rate tends to slow slightly. (Modified from Ader R, Chatterjee K, Ports T et al: Immediate and sustained hemodynamic and clinical improvement in chronic heart failure by an oral angiotensin-converting enzyme inhibitor. Circulation 61:931, 1980)

of the left ventricle. This is not due to a change in the intrinsic stiffness properties of the myocardium, but rather to a reduction in intrapericardial pressure, due to a reduction in the intrapericardial volume.[60] All of these effects may contribute to the fall in diastolic pressure of the heart.

There are important dose response considerations[61] to the use of captopril in chronic congestive heart failure. In general, there may be a potent first-dose hypotensive effect, so it is wise to begin at an extremely low dose. One can begin with 6.25 mg three times a day and gradually work up to a dose of 25 to 50 mg three times a day, or 50 mg twice a day. Since the major effect of captopril is to block converting enyme, when that has occurred higher doses produce no greater effect (Fig. 7.11). In general, 25 mg three times a day is an effective dose in approximately 90% of patients with chronic congestive heart failure. The responsiveness to captopril depends on several factors. In patients with a low serum sodium, there is a more dramatic response to captopril, presumably because of the increased renin levels.[62] There is a generally increased response in patients with higher renin levels and a clear-cut increased

response in patients with higher systemic vascular resistance.

Controlled randomized clinical trials have shown that captopril causes an improvement in exercise tolerance.[63,64] In addition, there appears to be a sense of well-being associated with the administration of captopril, which is maintained despite low arterial pressures. In patients with mild heart failure, captopril was compared to digoxin as first-line therapy. Captopril increased exercise tolerance more than digoxin, whereas digoxin increased ejection fraction more.[65]

A number of side effects have been noted. Severe hypotension is the most important hemodynamic effect, particularly following the first dose. Skin rash is relatively common, but may go away with continued use of captopril. A change in taste, nausea, anorexia, or diarrhea may occur in some patients. Proteinuria, neutropenia, and hemolytic anemia are very infrequent side effects. Since smaller doses have been used in the treatment of heart failure as compared with the treatment of hypertension, it appears that the side effect profile in patients with congestive heart failure may not be as high as those treated for hypertension.

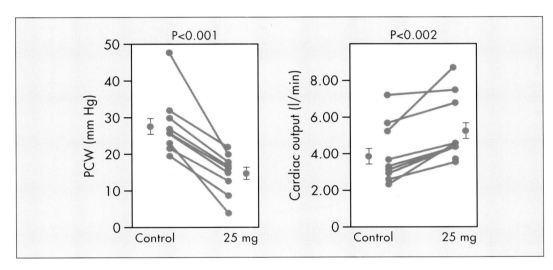

Figure 7.10 In the same group of patients as listed in Figure 7.9, 25 mg of captopril produced a substantial reduction in pulmonary capillary wedge pressure (PCWP) and a modest increase in forward cardiac output. (Modified from Ader R, Chatterjee K, Ports T et al: Immediate and sustained hemodynamic and clinical improvement in chronic heart failure by an oral angiotensin-converting enzyme inhibitor. Circulation 61:931, 1980)

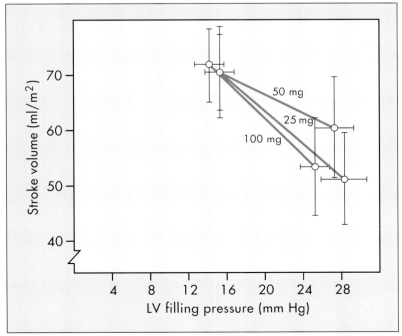

Figure 7.11 In the same group of patients listed in Figure 7.9, the sequential effects of 25 mg, 50 mg, and 100 mg of captopril are illustrated. Patients were allowed to return to control levels between doses. The shift up and to the left produced by captopril, with an increase in stroke volume and reduction in left ventricular filling pressure, was similar with each of the three doses. At this dose range, therefore, patients were on the plateau of responsiveness, presumably due to maximal inhibition of converting enzyme. (Modified from Ader R, Chatterjee K, Ports T et al: Immediate and sustained hemodynamic and clinical improvement in chronic heart failure by an oral angiotensin converting enzyme inhibitor. Circulation 61:931, 1980)

The effects on renal function are variable.[66] In some cases there is direct improvement in renal function. At the same time, renal function may deteriorate in some patients, perhaps related to the reduction in blood pressure. The counterbalancing of these two adverse effects will tend to have variable effects on renal function in individual patients. In a double-blind study of the effects of captopril on renal function, modest reductions in renal function occurred despite improvement in the symptoms of congestive heart failure.[67] It was postulated that loss of the direct compensatory effects of angiotensin II led to the decline in renal function. Angiotensin-converting enzyme inhibitors tend to increase serum potassium levels. This presumably occurs because of the reduction in angiotensin II and aldosterone levels and the resultant reduction in renal potassium excretion. Thus, one should not combine these drugs with potassium-sparing diuretics, since serious hyperkalemia may result. In the SAVE trial, captopril was effective in reducing mortality in patients after an anterior myocardial infarction.[68] This presumably occurred because of the ability of captopril to reduce wall stress and thus reduce thinning of the infarct segment and the subsequent ventricular remodeling and dilatation that ensues.[69]

Enalapril

Enalapril is a longer-acting angiotensin-converting enzyme inhibitor than captopril. It can be administered twice daily, with a usual dose of 5 to 10 mg. It appears to be devoid of problems with skin rash, proteinuria, and metallic taste. Data suggest that the hemodynamic and clinical profiles are similar to those of captopril.[70] A multicenter study of 73 patients showed improved exercise capacity and hemodynamics with chronic treatment. The dose used was 10 to 20 mg/d in either single or divided doses.[71] A direct comparison of captopril and enalapril suggested that the longer-acting enalapril could produce more hypotension and syncope or near-syncope than captopril.[72] Because large fixed doses of enalapril (40 mg/d) were used, however, it is probable that enalapril and captopril can produce similar beneficial effects at appropriate doses.

Enalapril is the most widely studied ACE inhibitor in mortality trials of patients with congestive heart failure. In the CONSENSUS trial conducted in northern Scandinavia, enalapril prolonged life in patients with severe congestive heart failure, as compared with placebo.[73] In the V-HEFT 2 trial[74] enalapril was compared with hydralazine-isosorbide dinitrate. Enalapril was slightly superior by producing a modest reduction in mortality (sudden death), although hydralazine-isosorbide dinitrate tended to increase ejection fraction and exercise tolerance slightly more. In the symptomatic arm of the SOLVD trial in patients with moderate heart failure, enalapril reduced mortality compared to placebo.[75] In the asymptomatic arm of the SOLVD trial, enalapril was also better than placebo,[76] a result similar to the benefit of captopril in the SAVE trial.[68] An overview of all these trials suggests that ACE inhibitors are effective over the entire spectrum of heart failure from asymptomatic left ventricular dysfunction to severe failure.

A number of other ACE inhibitors have become available for the treatment of hypertension. These include lisinopril, benazepril, quinapril, fosinopril, and ramipril. Although not specifically approved for the treatment of heart failure, it is likely that they would be similarly efficacious. The longer half-life of some of these agents allows them to be given once daily.

COMBINATION THERAPY

In considering the application of vasodilator drugs for the management of heart failure, it is clear that combination therapy may be more valuable than any single drug alone. For example, the combination of hydralazine and nitrates has been very effective in producing the desired hemodynamic effects of both arteriolar dilation and venodilation.[35] In a similar fashion, combinations of hydralazine and captopril are useful in individual patients.[77] Although captopril is effective in reducing pulmonary capillary wedge pressure, its arteriolar dilating effects are relatively modest, resulting in only minor increases in forward cardiac output. The addition of hydralazine can dramatically increase forward cardiac output in patients already on captopril. These two combinations of vasodilator drugs appear to be the most effective ones studied, although other combinations will undoubtedly emerge in the future that may be useful in the management of patients with chronic heart failure.

It should also be noted that vasodilators and inotropic agents are generally synergistic in their hemodynamic effects.[78,79] This occurs because these work by different mechanisms. Inotropic agents increase the contractility of the myocardium, while vasodilators reduce the load against which the heart works. Several combinations of these two classes of drugs can be helpful in individual patients.

EFFECTS ON LEFT VENTRICULAR COMPLIANCE

All vasodilators that lower atrial pressures appear to increase the compliance of the left ventricle in patients with congestive heart failure. That is, the passive pressure–volume relationship is shifted downward.[80,81] An example of this phenomenon is seen in Figure 7.12. When the left ventricular diastolic pressure is displayed on a log scale, the exponential passive pressure–volume relationship becomes a straight line. The top line represents early and late diastolic pressure and volume in a patient with heart failure. Following sublingual nitroglycerin, the passive pressure–volume relationship is shifted downward. In particular, note that there is a reduction in left ventricular end-diastolic pressure, with no change in end-diastolic volume.

Several mechanisms have been postulated to explain this phenomenon. Since ischemia can stiffen muscle and decrease left ventricular compliance, one could speculate that relief of ischemia with vasodilator therapy might be responsible.[82] Although this hypothesis might explain changes in some instances of ischemia, it can't explain similar changes in patients without ischemic heart disease. It seems clear that the usual cause of this change in compliance is not relief of ischemia. In addition, vasodilators apparently do not have a direct significant effect on the diastolic properties of heart muscle.

Two other effects appear to account for this phenomenon: the influence of a stiff pericardial sac and the interaction of the left and right heart chambers.[83] The pericardium has a stiff passive pressure–volume relationship, which becomes manifest in heart failure as a restraining influence on the dilated heart. The transmural pressure, which fills the left ventricle, is the left ventricular diastolic pressure minus the intrapericardial pressure (assuming the intrathoracic pressure is near zero). When one gives a vasodilator drug that lowers right and left atrial pressures by decreasing heart volume, there is a decrease in intrapericardial pressure. Because the pericardium is such a stiff structure, it takes very little reduction in intrapericardial volume to produce a substantial fall in intrapericardial pressure. If there is a similar fall in left ventricular diastolic and intrapericardial pressures, there is little change in the transmural filling pressure of the left ventricle. Hence, diastolic pressure falls with little change in left ventricular volume. It is obviously not possible to measure intrapericardial pressure in the routine clinical situation. However, experimental studies have shown that under most circumstances, mean right atrial pressure is a reasonable approximation of intrapericardial pressure.[84] Thus, one can quantitate the potential importance of this mechanism by noting changes in right atrial pressure produced by vasodilator drugs.

The second mechanism responsible for this shift in the left ventricular pressure–volume relationship is closely related. Within the pericardial sac are the four heart chambers, which can interact with each other.[85] As one decreases intrapericardial pressure and volume, it appears that left ventricular volume increases in relation to the other chambers. Perhaps the decrease in right-sided pressures diminishes the potential interactive effect of the right ventricle on the left ventricle.

Overall, it is clear that the pericardium has an important effect on the diastolic properties of the failing left ventricle and that vasodilator drugs produce beneficial effects on left ventricular compliance. By lowering diastolic pressures, there is a reduction in pulmonary congestion. Preservation of end-diastolic volume preserves stroke volume at a given ejection fraction. Reduction of systemic vascular resistance then enhances stroke volume at a given end-diastolic volume.

This phenomenon probably occurs with any intervention that reduces atrial pressures. It has also recently been noted with the new potent inotropic–vasodilator drugs, which can dramatically alter resting hemodynamics.[86]

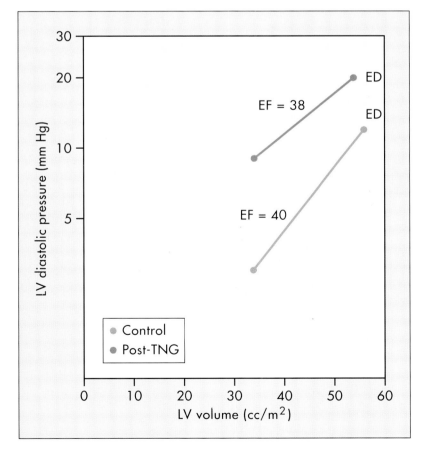

Figure 7.12 Representative changes in the passive pressure–volume relationship of the the ventricle following nitroglycerin in a patient with chronic coronary artery disease and digestive heart failure. Early and late diastolic pressure and volume points are plotted on a log scale, such that the exponential passive–pressure volume relationship tends to become a straight line. Following the administration of 0.4 mg of nitroglycerin sublingually there was a reduction in end-diastolic pressures at approximately the same end-diastolic volume. There was no change in ejection fraction. (Modified from Parmley WW, Chunk L, Chatterjee K et al: Acute changes in the diastolic pressure-volume relationship of the left ventricle. Eur J Cardiol 4:105, 1976)

Vasodilator Drugs and Mechanical Lesions

In patients with acute myocardial infarction and acute severe mitral regurgitation due to papillary muscle dysfunction, vasodilators such as nitroprusside can be dramatic in reversing the deleterious hemodynamic consequences (Fig. 7.13). When this was first described, it was not clear whether or not the beneficial effect was due only to relief of ischemia.[87] Subsequent studies in patients with chronic mitral regurgitation unrelated to ischemia[49] demonstrated similar beneficial effects: decreased pulmonary capillary wedge pressure and regurgitant fraction and increased cardiac output (Fig. 7.14). The beneficial effect of arteriolar dilation is the enhancement of forward output. The beneficial effect of venodilation is probably a reduction in left ventricular size with an improvement in mitral valve competence.

It should be noted that vasoconstrictor drugs can potentially worsen mitral regurgitation. In the setting of acute heart failure and severe mitral regurgitation, preference should be given to vasodilator drugs. This problem is compounded because in very low flow states in acute heart failure, there may not be a characteristic murmur,[88] and the mitral regurgitation can then be detected only by abnormal *v* waves in the pulmonary capillary wedge pressure trace.

Aortic regurgitation is a clinical situation in which arteriolar vasodilators such as hydralazine can enhance forward cardiac output and decrease regurgitant volume.[7] There are several clinical situations in which they might be useful. In the patient with severe acute aortic regurgitation, due for example to a ruptured cusp, hydralazine can help stabilize the hemodynamics while more definitive surgical therapy is being considered. In patients with chronic aortic regurgitation and heart failure in whom surgical therapy is considered inadvisable because of high risk or other problems, vasodilator therapy would be extremely important. A more difficult clinical question concerns the asymptomatic patient with moderately severe aortic or mitral regurgitation. An attractive hypothesis is that vasodilator therapy might be able to unload the left ventricle and reduce the rate of cardiac dilatation.[89] This might retard the rate at which cardiac contractility declines and thus delay surgical replacement of the valve. A controlled trial with hydralazine supports this hypothesis.[90]

Another mechanical lesion that can be helped with vasodilator therapy is a ruptured interventricular septum following acute myocardial infarction. The degree of left-to-right shunting in this circumstance depends on the size of the defect and the relative magnitude of pulmonary and systemic vascular resistance. A drug such as sodium nitroprusside usually decreases systemic vascular resistance more than pulmonary vascular resistance and thus decreases the magnitude of the left-to-right shunt.[91] In some cases, however, the reverse can occur and the shunt will

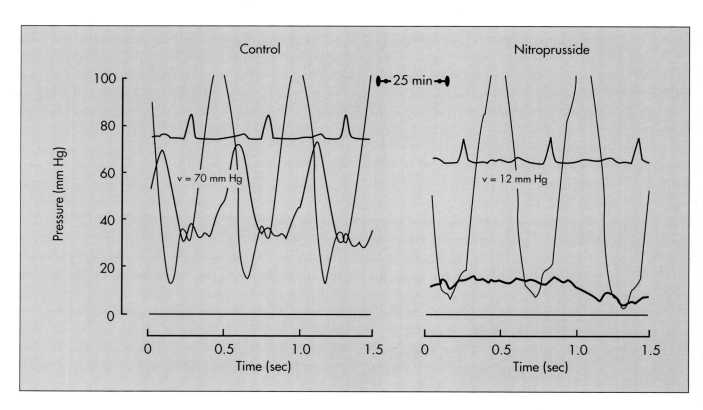

Figure 7.13 Hemodynamic effects of sodium nitroprusside in a patient with acute severe mitral regurgitation following acute myocardial infarction. Pulmonary capillary wedge pressure and left ventricular pressure are illustrated before and after nitroprusside infusion. Note the large *v* waves, up to 70 mm Hg, and elevated diastolic pressures prior to nitroprusside administration. During nitroprusside there was a dramatic reduction in diastolic pressures and disappearance of the *v* waves. This was accompanied by disappearance of the murmur of mitral regurgitation. (Chatterjee K, Parmley WW: The role of vasodilator therapy in heart failure. Prog Cardiovasc Dis 19:301, 1977)

worsen. With a balloon-tip catheter in the pulmonary artery, one can measure the step up in oxygen content of blood from the right atrium to the pulmonary artery. Changes in the oxygen content reflect changes in the degree of shunting. For example, a decrease in oxygen content following nitroprusside administration reflects a decrease in the left-to-right shunt. In children with a congenital ventricular septal defect, data suggest that vasodilator therapy can worsen the shunting owing to a greater reduction in pulmonary vascular resistance, especially with a low baseline systemic vascular resistance.[92]

Another potential adverse effect of vasodilator therapy is a reduction in arterial oxygen in patients with initially high filling pressures.[93] This occurs because of a ventilation–perfusion mismatch. With high filling pressures, perfusion is preferentially shifted toward the upper lobes where ventilation is also better. Vasodilators that lower left ventricular filling pressure lead to better perfusion of the lower lobes in areas of poor ventilation. Thus, shunting of poorly oxygenated blood across the lungs leads to a reduction in arterial oxygen content. This is rarely deleterious and in fact is generally accompanied by clinical improvement in dyspnea due to a reduction in pulmonary capillary wedge pressure.

SELECTION OF A VASODILATOR IN CHRONIC CONGESTIVE HEART FAILURE

Because of the benefits of the ACE inhibitors over the entire spectrum of heart failure, it seems reasonable to start one of these agents in all patients. Diuretics should be used when there is retention of salt and water, as manifested by weight gain. Digitalis is effective in the presence of atrial fibrillation and moderate to severe heart failure. A combination of the above three agents is more effective than either drug alone in improving left ventricular function. ACE inhibitors improve clinical class and exercise tolerance. They will be especially beneficial in patients who have a low serum sodium and a high renin level.[89] If blood pressure is too low to consider initiating angiotensin-converting enyme inhibitors, hydralazine or hydralazine plus nitrates can be considered in such patients. The calcium blockers can be considered in patients with hypertension and heart failure. These agents might also be effective in patients with associated coronary artery disease and angina pectoris. The ability of the calcium blockers to reduce myocardial oxygen consumption and relieve vasoconstriction should be effective in this setting.

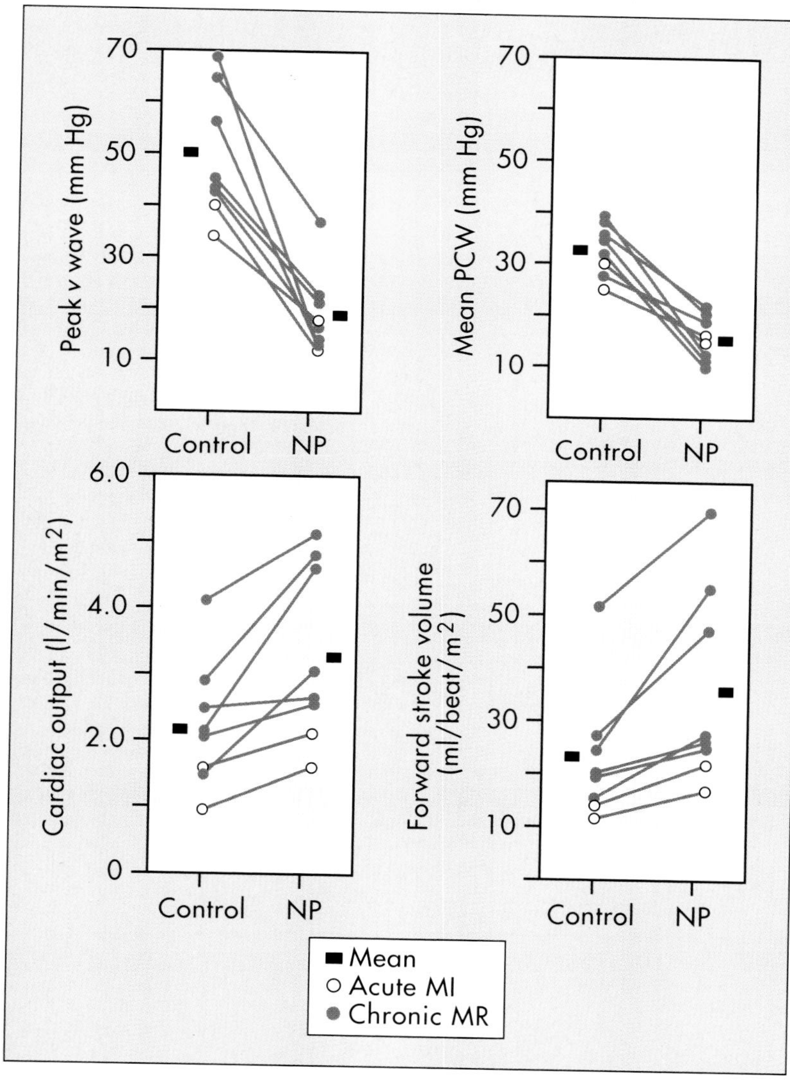

Figure 7.14 Hemodynamic effects of sodium nitroprusside (NP) in 8 patients with mitral regurgitation. Two patients had mitral regurgitation on the basis of acute myocardial infarction (acute MI), and 6 patients had chronic mitral regurgitation. Note that sodium nitroprusside (NP) produced a dramatic reduction in peak v wave and mean pulmonary capillary wedge (PCW) pressure in all patients. Similarly, nitroprusside produced an increase in cardiac output and forward stroke volume. (Modified from Chatterjee K, Parmley WW, Swan HJC et al: Beneficial effects of vasodilator agents in severe mitral regurgitation due to dysfunction of subvalvar apparatus. Circulation 48:684, 1973)

One difficulty in patients with chronic heart failure is assessing the chronic response to vasodilators. Studies have noted that the acute hemodynamic response will not necessarily correlate with the chronic clinical response.[94] Similarly, there has been great difficulty in using objective measures, such as echocardiography or radionuclide angiography, to follow the response to vasodilator therapy.[95] Clinical response and an increase in exercise tolerance are the most important markers of improvement in patients treated for congestive heart failure. Several ways of monitoring this improvement have been used. Increase in exercise time on a treadmill is useful, but it also depends considerably on the motivation of the patient and the interaction with the physician conducting the test. Total body oxygen consumption (Vo_2) provides useful quantitative information, although it is also subject to the same pitfalls as time on the treadmill.

"Anaerobic threshold," as monitored by a rise in lactate and an alteration in the respiratory exchange ratio, provides important biochemical information about the adequacy of oxygen delivery to exercising skeletal muscles.[96] It appears that limited flow to skeletal muscle is extremely important as a mechanism for producing fatigue in heart failure patients.

Some improvement in exercise tolerance in such patients can be achieved by exercise conditioning. Although the degree of such exercise training is obviously limited in symptomatic patients, it may be an important factor in the beneficial long-term response to vasodilator drugs. Such drugs may increase the cardiovascular capacity and thus allow patients to exercise more and benefit from the training effects thus obtained.

Although many of these drugs can be started in outpatients, it appears prudent to hospitalize patients with severe heart failure and use invasive hemodynamic monitoring to select an appropriate dose. Although the acute response may not necessarily predict the chronic clinical response of the patient, it is helpful in selecting an appropriate dose of the drug and documenting a beneficial hemodynamic effect and avoid lowering left ventricular filling presssure too much. Tolerance may potentially develop with all of the drugs that have been mentioned,[97] although it probably is least common with the angiotensin-converting enzyme inhibitors.

Besides improving symptoms, vasodilators also have a favorable effect on long-term survival. Furberg and Yusuf[98] analyzed evidence from a number of short-term studies using different vasodilator drugs. They noted some favorable trends, especially with the angiotensin-converting enzyme inhibitors. More importantly, the multicenter V-HEFT trial provided direct evidence of benefit.[36] Heart failure patients on digitalis and diuretics were randomized into three treatment groups: placebo, prazosin, and hydralazine-nitrates. At 3 years, the mortality rates of the placebo and prazosin groups were similar (47%), while that of the hydralazine-isosorbide dinitrate group was 36%, representing a risk reduction of 36%. Since prazosin has shown hemodynamic tachyphylaxis,[42,43] its lack of long-term efficacy is understandable.

In the CONSENSUS trial carried out in northern Scandinavia,[73] enalapril was effective in prolonging life in patients with class IV congestive heart failure (Fig. 7.15). This important study helped establish angiotensin-converting enzyme inhibitor therapy as the premier vasodilator therapy for patients with congestive heart failure. Not only does this therapy increase exercise tolerance and prolong life, it also appears to improve well-being and the quality of life better than other vasodilator drugs. Since enalapril was better than hydralazine-isosorbide dinitrate in the V-HEFT 2 trial, this further established the preeminence of ACE inhibitors. The ability of ACE inhibitors to reduce mortality in the SOLVD and SAVE trials further confirmed this fact.

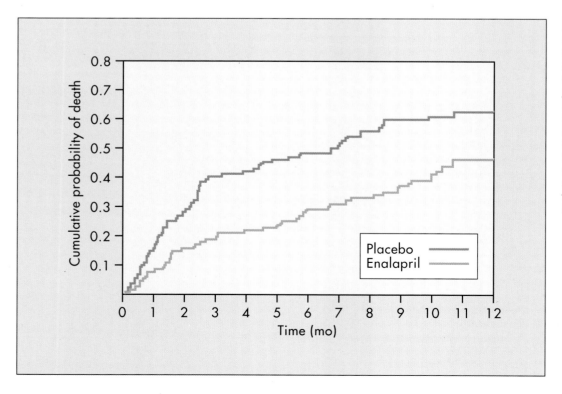

Figure 7.15 Cumulative mortality in the CONSENSUS Trial. The reduction in mortality in the enalapril-treated group was evident at 3 months, with relatively parallel curves thereafter. (Modifed from CONSENSUS Trial Study Group: Effects of enalapril on mortality in severe congestive heart failure. N Engl J Med 316:1429, 1987)

REFERENCES

1. Chatterjee K, Parmley WW: Vasodilator therapy for acute myocardial infarction and chronic heart failure. J Am Coll Cardiol 1:133, 1983

2. Packer M: Conceptual dilemmas in the classification of vasodilator drugs for severe chronic heart failure. Advocacy of a pragmatic approach to the selection of a therapeutic agent. Am J Med 76:3, 1984

3. Chatterjee K, Parmley WW, Massie B et al: Oral hydralazine therapy for chronic refractory heart failure. Circulation 54:879, 1976

4. Koch-Weser J: Myocardial inactivity of therapeutic concentrations of hydralazine and diazoxide. Experientia 30:170, 1974

5. Franciosa JA, Pierpont C, Cohn J: Hemodynamic improvement after oral hydralazine in left ventricular failure. Ann Intern Med 86:388, 1977

6. Greenberg BH, Massie BM, Brundage BH et al: Beneficial effects of hydralazine in severe mitral regurgitation. Circulation 58:273, 1978

7. Greenberg B, DeMot H, Murphy E et al: Beneficial effects of hydralazine on rest and exercise hemodynamics in patients with severe aortic insufficiency. Circulation 62:49, 1980

8. Chatterjee K, Ports TA, Brundage BH et al: Oral hydralazine in chronic heart failure: Sustained beneficial hemodynamic effects. Ann Intern Med 92:600, 1980

9. Franciosa JA, Weber KT, Levine TB et al: Hydralazine in the long term treatment of chronic heart failure: Lack of difference from placebo. Am Heart J 104:587, 1982

10. Quyyumi M, Wagstaff D, Evans TR: Acute hemodynamic effects of endralazine: A new vasodilator for chronic refractory congestive heart failure. Am J Cardiol 51:1353, 1983

11. Quyyumi M, Wagstaff D, Evans TR: Long-term beneficial effects of endralazine, a new arteriolar vasodilator at rest and during exercise capacity in chronic congestive heart failure. Am J Cardiol 54:1020, 1984

12. McKay C, Chatterjee K, Ports TA et al: Minoxidil in chronic congestive heart failure: A hemodynamic and clinical study. Am Heart J 104:575, 1982

13. Franciosa JA, Jordan RA, Wilen MM et al: Minoxidil in patients with chronic left heart failure: Contrasting hemodynamic and clinical effects in a controlled trial. Circulation 70:63, 1984

14. Leier CS, Patrick TS, Hermiller J et al: Nifedipine in congestive heart failure: Effects on resting and exercise hemodynamics and regional blood flow. Am Heart J 108:1461, 1984

15. Ferlinz J, Citron PD: Hemodynamic and myocardial performance characteristics after verapamil use in congestive heart failure. Am J Cardiol 51:1339, 1983

16. Walsh RW, Porter CB, Starling MR et al: Beneficial hemodynamic effects of intravenous and oral diltiazem in severe congestive heart failure. J Am Coll Cardiol 3:1044, 1984

17. Parmley, WW: Efficacy and safety of calcium channel blockers in hypertensive patients with concomitant left ventricular dysfunction. Clin Cardiol 15:235–242, 1992

18. Ryman KS, Kubo SH, Lystash J et al: The effect of nicardipine on rest and exercise hemodynamics in chronic congestive heart failure. Am J Cardiol 58:583, 1986

19. Multicenter Diltiazem Postinfarction Trial Research Group: The effect of diltiazem on mortality and reinfarction after myocardial infarction. N Engl J Med 319:385–392, 1988

20. Danish Study Group on Verapamil in Myocardial Infarction: Effect of verapamil on mortality and major events after acute myocardial infarcton (The Danish Verapamil Infarction Trial II DAVIT II). Am J Cardiol 66:779–785, 1990

21. McAllister RC Jr: Clinical pharmacology of slow channel blocking agents. Prog Cardiovasc Dis 25:83, 1982

22. Camerini F, Alberti E, Klugmann S et al: Primary pulmonary hypertension: Effects of nifedipine. Br Heart J 44:352, 1980

23. Packer M, Medina N, Yushak M: Adverse hemodynamic and clinical effects of calcium channel blockade in pulmonary hypertension secondary to obliterative pulmonary vascular disease. J Am Coll Cardiol 4:890, 1984

24. Packer M: New perspectives on therapeutic application of nitrates as vasodilator agents for severe chronic heart failure. Am J Med (Suppl) 74:61, 1983

25. Ignarro W, Lippton H, Edwards JC et al: Mechanism of vascular smooth muscle relaxation by organic nitrates, nitrites, nitroprusside and nitrate oxide: Evidence for the involvement of S-nitrothols as active intermediates. J Pharmacol Exp Ther 218:739, 1981

26. Franciosa JA, Nordstrom LA, Cohn JN: Nitrate therapy for congestive heart failure. JAMA 240:443, 1978

27. Herling IM: Intravenous nitroglycerin: Clinical pharmacology and therapeutic considerations. Am Heart J 108:141, 1984

28. Bogaert MG: Clinical pharmacokinetics of organic nitrates. Clin Pharmacokinet 8:410, 1983

29. Rajfer S, Demma FJ, Goldberg LI: Sustained beneficial hemodynamic responses to large doses of transdermal nitroglycerin in congestive heart failure and comparison with intravenous nitroglycerin. Am J Cardiol 54:120, 1984

30. Needleman P, Johnson EM Jr: Mechanism of tolerance development to organic nitrates. J Pharmacol Exp Ther 184:709, 1973

31. Armstrong PW, Walker DC, Burton JR et al: Vasodilator therapy in acute myocardial infarction: A comparison of sodium nitroprusside and nitroglycerin. Circulation 52:118, 1975

32. Flaherty JT, Becker LC, Bulkley BH et al: A randomized prospective trial of intravenous nitroglycerin in patients with acute myocardial infarction. Circulation 68:576, 1983

33. Derrida JR, Sal R, Chiche P: Effects of prolonged nitroglycerin infusion in patients with acute myocardial infarction. Am J Cardiol 41:407, 1978

34. Franciosa JA, Goldsmith SR, Cohn JN: Contrasting immediate and long-term effects of isosorbide dinitrate on exercise capacity in congestive heart failure. Am J Med 69:559, 1980

35. Massie B, Chatterjee K, Werner J et al: Hemodynamic advantage of combined oral hydralazine and nonparenteral nitrates in the vasodilator therapy of chronic heart failure. Am J Cardiol 40:794, 1977

36. Cohn JN, Archibald DG, Ziesche S et al: Effect of vasodilator therapy on mortality in chronic congestive heart failure. N Engl J Med 314:1547, 1986

37. Sniderman AD, Marpole DGT, Palmer WH et al: Response of the left ventricle to nitroglycerin in patients with and without mitral regurgitation. Br Heart J 36:357, 1974

38. Denolin H (ed): International symposium on Molsidomine. Am Heart J 109:625, 1985

39. Miller RR, Awan NA, Maxwell KS et al: Sustained reduction of cardiac impedance and preload in congestive heart failure with the antihypertensive vasodilator, prazosin. N Engl J Med 297:303, 1977

40. Markham RV, Corbett JR, Gilmore A et al: Efficiency of prazosin in the management of chronic congestive heart failure: A six month randomized double blind placebo controlled study. Am J Cardiol 51:1346, 1983

41. Colucci WS, Wynne J, Holman BL et al: Long-term therapy of heart failure with prazosin: A randomized double blind trial. Am J Cardiol 45:337, 1980

42. Packer M, Meller J, Gorlin R et al: Hemodynamic and clinical tachyphylaxis to prazosin-mediated afterload reduction in severe chronic congestive heart failure. Circulation 59:531, 1979

43. Arnold SB, Williams RL, Ports TA et al: Attenuation of prazosin effect on cardiac output in chronic heart failure. Ann Intern Med 91:345, 1979

44. Colucci WS, Williams CH, Braunwald E: Increased plasma norepinephrine during prazosin therapy for severe congestive heart failure. Ann Intern Med 93:452, 1980

45. Weber KT, Kinasewitz GA, West JS et al: Long term vasodilator therapy with trimazosin in chronic cardiac failure. N Engl J Med 303:242, 1980

46. Kirlin PC, Das S, Pitt B: Chronic alpha-adrenoreceptor blockade with trimazosin in congestive heart failure. Int J Cardiol 8:89, 1985

47. Leier CV, Patterson SE, Huss P et al. The hemodynamic and clinical responses to terazosin, a new alpha blocking agent in congestive heart failure. Am J Med Sci 292:128, 1986

48. Franciosa JB, Guiha NM, Limas CJ et al: Improved left ventricular function during nitroprusside infusion in acute myocardial infarction. Lancet 1:650, 1972

49. Chatterjee K, Parmley WW: The role of vasodilator therapy in heart failure. Prog Cardiovasc Dis 19:301, 1977

50. Bolen JL, Alderman EL: Hemodynamic consequences of afterload reduction in patients with chronic aortic regurgitation. Circulation 53:879, 1976

51. Chatterjee K, Parmley WW, Ganz W et al: Hemodynamic and metabolic responses to vasodilator therapy in acute myocardial infarction. Circulation 48:1183, 1973

52. Durrer JD, Lie KL, VanCapelle FRJ et al: Effect of sodium nitroprusside on mortality in acute myocardial infarction. N Engl J Med 306:1121, 1982

53. Cohn JN, Franciosa JA, Francis CS et al: Effect of short term infusion of sodium nitroprusside on mortality rate in acute myocardial infarction complicated by left ventricular failure. N Engl J Med 306:1129, 1982

54. Chiarello M, Gold HK, Leinbach RC et al: Comparison between the effects of nitroprusside and nitroglycerin on ischemic injury during acute myocardial infarction. Circulation 54:766, 1976

55. daLuz PL, Forrester JS, Wyatt LH et al: Hemodynamic and metabolic effects of sodium nitroprusside on the performance and metabolism of regional ischemic myocardium. Circulation 52:400, 1975

56. Walinsky P, Chatterjee K, Forrester JS et al: Enhanced left ventricular performance with phentolamine in acute myocardial infarction. Am J Cardiol 33:37, 1974

57. Witzball H, Hirsch F, Scherer B et al: Acute hemodynamic and hormonal effects of captopril are diminished by indomethacin. Clin Sci 62:611, 1982

58. Ader R, Chatterjee K, Ports T et al: Immediate and sustained hemodynamic and clinical improvement in chronic heart failure by an oral angiotensin converting enyme inhibitor. Circulation 61:931, 1980

59. Franciosa JA, Guiha NH, Limas CJ et al: Arterial pressure as a determinant of left ventricular filling pressure after acute myocardial infarction. Am J Cardiol 34:506, 1974

60. Glantz SA, Parmley WW: Factors which affect the diastolic pressure-volume curve. Circ Res 32:171, 1978

61. Chatterjee K, Rouleau JL. Parmley WW: Hemodynamic and myocardial metabolic effects of captopril in chronic heart failure. Br Heart J 47:233, 1982

62. Packer M, Medina N, Yushak M: Relation between serum sodium concentration and the hemodynamic and clinical responses to converting enzyme inhibition with captopril in severe heart failure. J Am Coll Cardiol 3:1035, 1984

63. Kramer BL, Massie BM, Topic N: Controlled trial of captopril in chronic heart failure: A rest and exercise hemodynamic study. Circulation 67:807, 1983

64. Captopril Multicenter Research Group: A placebo controlled trial of captopril in refractory chronic congestive heart failure. J Am Coll Cardiol 2:755, 1983

65. Captopril Digoxin Multicenter Research Group: Comparative effects of therapy with captopril and digoxin in patients with mild to moderate heart failure. JAMA 259:539–544, 1988

66. Dzau VJ, Colucci WS, Williams GH et al: Sustained effectiveness of converting-enzyme inhibition in patients with severe congestive heart failure. N Engl J Med 302:1373, 1980

67. Cleland JG, Dargie HJ, Gillen G et al: Captopril in heart failure: A double blind study of the effects on renal function. J Cardiovasc Pharmacol 8:700, 1986

68. Pfeffer MA, Braunwald E, Moye LA et al: The effect of captopril on mortality and morbidity in patients with left ventricular dysfunction following myocardial infarction. N Engl J Med, 327: 669-677, 1992

69. Pfeffer MA, Lamas GA, Vaughan DE et al: Effect of captopril on progressive ventricular dilatation after anterior myocardial infarction. N Engl J Med 319:80–86, 1988

70. DiCarlo L, Chatterjee K, Parmley WW et al: Enalapril: A new angiotensin-converting enzyme inhibitor in chronic heart failure: Acute and chronic hemodynamic evaluations. J Am Coll Cardiol 2:865, 1983

71. Gomez HJ, Cirillo VJ, Davies RO et al: Enalapril in congestive heart failure: Acute and chronic invasive hemodynamic evaluation. Int J Cardiol 1:37, 1986

72. Packer M, Lee WH, Yushak M, Medina N: Comparison of captopril and enalapril in patients with severe chronic heart failure. N Engl J Med 315:847, 1986

73. CONSENSUS Trial Study Group. Effects of enalapril on mortality in severe congestive heart failure. N Engl J Med 316:1429, 1987

74. Cohn JN, Johnson G, Ziesche S et al: A comparison of enalapril with hydralazine-isosorbide dinitrate in the treatment of chronic congestive heart failure. N Engl J Med 325:303–310, 1991

75. The SOLVD Investigators. Effect of enalapril on survival in patients with reduced left ventricular ejection fractions and congestive heart failure. N Engl J Med 325–302, 1991

76. The SOLVD investigators. Effects of enalapril on mortality and the development of heart failure in asymptomatic patients with reduced left ventricular ejection fractions. New Engl J Med 327:685-691, 1992

77. Massie BM, Packer M, Hanlon JT et al: Hemodynamic responses to combined therapy with captopril and hydralazine in patients with severe heart failure. J Am Coll Cardiol 2:338, 1983

78. Parmley WW, Chatterjee K: Combined vasodilator and inotropic therapy: A new approach in the treatment of heart failure. In Mason D (ed): Advances in Heart Disease, p 45. New York, Grune & Stratton, 1977

79. Verma SP, Silke B, Nelson GF et al: Hemodynamic advantages of a combined inotropic/venodilator regimen over inotropic monotherapy in acute heart failure. J Cardiovasc Pharmacol 7:943, 1985

80. Alderman EL, Glantz SA: Acute hemodynamic interventions shift the diastolic pressure-volume curve in man. Circulation 54:662, 1976

81. Parmley WW, Chuck L, Chatterjee K et al: Acute changes in the diastolic pressure-volume relationship of the left ventricle. Eur J Cardiol 4:105, 1976

82. Mann T, Goldberg S, Mudge GH et al: Factors contributing to altered left ventricular diastolic properties during angina pectoris. Circulation 59:14, 1979

83. Tyberg JV, Misbach GA, Glantz SA et al: The mechanism for shifts in the diastolic left ventricular pressure-volume curve: The role of the pericardium. Eur J Cardiol (Suppl)7:1963, 1978

84. Smith ER, Smiseth OA, Kingma I et al: Mechanism of action of nitrates: Role of changes in venous capacitance and in the left ventricular diastolic pressure-volume relation. Am J Med 76(6A):14,:1984

85. Visner MS, Araentzen CE, O'Connor MJ et al: Alterations in left ventricular three-dimensional dynamic geometry and systolic function during acute right ventricular hypertension in the conscious dog. Circulation 67:353, 1983

86. Kereiakes DJ, Viquerat C, Lanzer P et al: Mechanisms of improved left ventricular function following intravenous MDL in 17,043 patients with severe chronic heart failure. Am Heart J 108:1278, 1984

87. Chatterjee K, Parmley WW, Swan HJC et al: Beneficial effects of vasodilator agents in severe mitral regurgitation due to dysfunction of subvalvar apparatus. Circulation 48:684, 1973

88. Forrester JS, Diamond C, Freedman S et al: Silent mitral insufficiency in acute myocardial infarction. Circulation 44:877, 1971

89. Greenberg BH, Rahimtoola SH: Usefulness of vasodilator therapy in acute and chronic valvular regurgitation. Curr Probl Cardiol 9:1, 1984

90. Greenberg B, Massie B, Bristow JD et al: Long term vasodilator therapy of chronic aortic insufficiency: A randomized, double-blinded, placebo controlled clinical trial. Circulation 78:92–103, 1988

91. Tecklenberg PL, Fitzgerald J, Allaire BI et al: Afterload reduction in the management of postinfarction ventricular septal defect. Am J Cardiol 38:956, 1976

92. Zakazawa M, Atsuyoshi T, Chon T et al: Significance of systemic vascular resistance in determining the hemodynamic effects of hydralazine on large ventricular septal defects. Circulation 68:420, 1983

93. Benowitz HZ, LeWinter M, Wagner PD: Effect of sodium nitroprusside on ventilation-perfusion mismatching in heart failure. J Am Coll Cardiol 4:918, 1984

94. Franciosa JA, Dunkman B, Leddy CL: Hemodynamic effects of vasodilators and long-term response in heart failure. J Am Coll Cardiol 3:1521, 1984

95. Franciosa JA, Park M, Levine B: Lack of correlation between exercise capacity and indices of resting left ventricular performance in heart failure. Am J Cardiol 47:33, 1981

96. LeJemtel TH, Mancini D, Gumbardo D et al: Pitfalls and limitations of maximal oxygen uptake as an index of cardiovascular functional capacity in patients with chronic heart failure. Heart Failure 1:112, 1985

97. Packer M: Tolerance to vasodilator therapy. Cardiovasc Rev Rep 4:903, 1983

98. Furberg CD, Yusuf S: Effect of vasodilators on survival in chronic congestive heart failure. Am J Cardiol 55:1110, 1985

Hypolipidemic Agents

8

Mary J. Malloy

John P. Kane

Atherosclerosis is a complicated process that is initiated by certain circulating lipoproteins that enter the subintimal space and are endocytosed by macrophages and transformed smooth muscle cells.[1,2] Lipoproteins that have been identified in the artery wall and are thought to be atherogenic include low density lipoproteins (LDL), intermediate density lipoproteins (IDL), very low density lipoproteins (VLDL), and the Lp(a) lipoproteins. A large body of epidemiologic evidence supports a relationship between the levels of these atherogenic lipoproteins in plasma and the risk of atherosclerotic disease.[3,4] These observations are the basis for what is termed the lipid hypothesis: the rate at which atherogenic lipoproteins reach the subintima is directly related to their concentrations in plasma. A major corollary of this hypothesis is that reducing levels of such lipoproteins in plasma will decrease the rate of progression of coronary artery disease or induce its regression. The lipid hypothesis was solidly supported by research in animals such as the rhesus monkey[5] as early as the 1970s. However, it was only in 1990 that evidence was adduced in human coronary arteries that validates this hypothesis for the human species. The advent of quantitative coronary angiography has permitted the demonstration of highly significant regression in coronary lesions following treatment with diet and potent combined drug regimens that result in marked reduction of LDL levels in plasma.[6-8] Another study employing consensus panel assessment of coronary lesions also strongly supports the ability of these regimens to induce re-gression.[9] Thus, the treatment of atherogenic hyperlipidemia to retard the development of atherosclerotic coronary artery disease or induce its regression has a strongly established rationale. That these benefits extend to other arterial systems is supported by quantitative evidence for regression of femoral artery disease.[10,11]

Because atherosclerosis is a truly multifactorial disease process, the therapeutic approach must also encompass interventions directed at other prominent risk factors such as cigarette smoking, hypertension, and diabetes.

Still other aspects of the process of atherogenesis hold promise of new venues of treatment. It is now recognized that covalent modifications of LDL and other atherogenic lipoproteins can lead to uptake by scavenger receptors on macrophages and smooth muscle cells, transforming them into foam cells.[12] Oxidation of lipoprotein lipids with subsequent covalent chemical alteration of apolipoprotein B is probably the most important mechanism leading to endocytosis by this pathway. The availability of natural antioxidants may thus be an important factor in the development of coronary disease. Likewise, the use of antioxidant medications is of potential value in regression regimens. This antioxidant hypothesis is currently being examined in several clinical trials.

Epidemiologic evidence also indicates that the level of total high density lipoprotein (HDL) cholesterol in plasma is inversely related to risk of coronary artery disease, suggesting a protective effect of HDL against atherogenesis.[13] HDL exerts an antioxidant effect on other lipoproteins and may protect endothelium but the most likely mechanism of protection involves the participation of HDL in the retrieval of cholesterol from peripheral tissues in the centripetal transport system.[14] Data from several intervention trials have demon-strated an independent contribution of increasing HDL cholesterol levels to regression of coronary disease during treatment.[6,9] Because recent studies show that HDL comprises as many as eight discrete species, strategies of intervention directed at increasing HDL cholesterol levels cannot be evaluated fully until effects on levels of individual species and on specific mechanisms of centripetal transport are known. Empirically, it is important to note that in the Coronary Drug Project, niacin treatment was correlated with increased survival. This drug is known to increase levels of total HDL.

In some kindreds, hypertriglyceridemia appears to contribute to the risk of coronary artery disease. Elevated levels of VLDL and IDL should be treated in patients with overt coronary disease and those with affected relatives. Severe hypertriglyceridemia is also an important cause of acute pancreatitis. Because the risk of pancreatitis appears to be related to levels of circulating triglyceride-rich lipoproteins, aggressive treatment of the hyperlipidemia by diet, abstinence from alcohol, and the application, if necessary, of drug treatment can be expected to effect material reduction in risk.

Before treatment with any drug is initiated in the management of hyperlipidemia, modification of diet should be attempted. Successful dietary control often makes the use of drugs unnecessary. The recommended diet restricts the patient's intake of saturated fat and cholesterol and controls calories and alcohol consumption in selected persons. Although patients vary with respect to the degree of effect of cholesterol and saturated fat intake on levels of LDL, both tend to raise LDL. Excess caloric intake increases synthesis and secretion of VLDL, especially in obese persons. Alcohol tends to increase levels of HDL cholesterol, but it appears, from ultracentrifugal analysis at least, that the species of HDL affected are not those associated with the greatest inverse risk relationship with respect to coronary heart disease. Because it is a major determinant of secretion rates of VLDL triglycerides, alcohol should be avoided by patients with hypertriglyceridemia.

A panel of experts sponsored by the National Institutes of Health[15] has published revised guidelines for treatment of patients with elevated levels of LDL, based on either total cholesterol or LDL-cholesterol level in serum. These new guidelines also take into account levels of HDL cholesterol. A level of HDL cholesterol below 35 mg/dl is classified as a major risk factor for coronary heart disease (CHD) and determines follow-up for primary prevention in individuals without evidence of CHD. The desirable level of LDL cholesterol is less than 160 mg/dl in a person without CHD who has fewer than two risk factors, less than 130 mg/dl in a person without CHD who has two or more risk factors, or 100 mg/dl or less in a person with CHD. Clearly an appreciation of an individual's potential risk for developing CHD should shape the physician's clinical judgement regarding that patient's management.

If drug therapy is prescribed, the diet should be continued. It has been observed that, at least in the majority of patients, hyperlipidemia is better controlled, and sometimes at lower drug dosage, when the patient also follows the suggested diet.

Drugs used to treat hyperlipidemia should not be used in women who are pregnant or likely to become pregnant or during lactation. Familial hypercholesterolemia is the only primary hyperlipidemia for which drug treatment should be considered in children. Persons homozygous for this disease should be treated early and aggressively. Drug treatment of heterozygous children, however, remains experimental and should probably not be started before age 7 or 8, at which time myelination of the central nervous system is nearly complete. Such factors as the level of LDL in plasma, other lipoprotein risk factors, the child's special circumstances, and the natural history of disease in the family should be considered before initiating drug treatment. The drug of choice is a bile acid binding resin.

AVAILABLE AGENTS
Bile Acid Binding Resins
MECHANISMS OF ACTION

The two available resins, colestipol and cholestyramine, are high molecular weight polymers that bind the anionic bile acids in the intestinal lumem.[16] The resins are not absorbed from the intestine and hence carry the bile acids out into the stool. They are capable of binding some nonionic hydrophobic substances, but apparently do not interfere significantly with the absorption of fat-soluble vitamins in persons with normal gastrointestinal tracts. Binding of some cationic molecules, such as iron, probably involves bridging with a polyanion, such as the phosphate ion. Again, this is not of clinical significance in patients with normal iron economies.

The bile acids, which are formed from cholesterol, are normally reabsorbed from the intestine with over 95% efficiency. The blockade of reabsorption results in up to a tenfold increase in the rate of bile acid synthesis by liver from cholesterol via the 7α-hydroxylase reaction and subsequent steps. This draft on cholesterol pools results in increased expression of high-affinity LDL receptors on hepatocyte membranes, drawing on circulating LDL for cholesterol to meet the in-creased requirements of bile acid production. However, de novo synthesis of cholesterol in the liver also occurs. Suppression of this compensatory increase in sterol biosynthesis is an important site of action for agents that are synergistic with the bile acid binding resins.

The bile acid sequestrants are of use only in those forms of hyperlipidemia involving elevations of LDL. Hypertriglyceridemia, if present in addition to elevated LDL levels, may be aggravated significantly by resin therapy. The addition of another agent, such as niacin, is indicated in such situations. Bile acid binding resins are contraindicated in treatment of primary hypertriglyceridemias without elevated LDL levels.

SIDE EFFECTS

Most patients complain of constipation and bloating, both of which are usually easy to control if adequate amounts of dietary fiber or psyllium seed preparations, which may be mixed with the resin, are used. Occasionally, diarrhea or even steatorrhea occurs. The latter and rare cases of bowel obstruction have only been reported in patients who have cholestasis or pre-existing bowel disease. Prothrombin time should be measured more frequently in patients who are also

taking coumarin or indandione anticoagulants. There is a theoretical risk of increased formation of gallstones, particularly in obese patients, although this risk appears to be very small in practice. The resins may impair the absorption of other drugs. Some known to be affected are digitalis glycosides, thiazide diuretics, warfarin, thyroxine, iron salts, folic acid, phenylbutazone, and tetracyclines. Hence, it is recommended that any medication except niacin be given 1 hour before or at least 3 hours after the resin is given.

DOSAGE

Colestipol is available in 5-g packets or in bulk. Most patients tolerate the drug better if the dose is increased over several weeks from 5 g two or three times daily to the maximum dose of 10 g three times daily. Some of the milder forms of hypercholesterolemia respond well to a total dose of 15 to 20 g daily. The granules are mixed with water or juice and should hydrate for at least 10 seconds. Colestipol should be taken with meals in two or three daily doses. To avoid irritation of the pharynx by residual granules, it is advisable to follow the medication with a small amount of soft food. Cholestyramine is available in 4-g packets and in bulk, has a usual maximum dose of 24 to 32 g/d, and should be taken in similar fashion.

USES

The resins are used to treat patients with heterozygous familial hypercholesterolemia, in whom a reduction in LDL of about 20% may be expected in compliant patients. In combination with niacin and/or a reductase inhibitor, however, levels of LDL are normalized in most of these patients. Greater reductions, often at lower dosages, are seen in persons with milder forms of hypercholesterolemia. They are also useful drugs in patients with familial combined hyperlipidemia. If hypertriglyceridemia is also present, the resins often cause further increases in VLDL that require the addition of a second agent, such as niacin.

Niacin (Nicotinic Acid)
MECHANISM OF ACTION

Niacin, which decreases levels of both LDL and VLDL, is a water-soluble B vitamin. Although the amide of nicotinic acid (niacinamide) functions normally in the role of vitamin cofactor, it completely lacks effect on lipid metabolism. Physicians should thus be alert to substitution of niacinamide for niacin, a frequent error in dispensing the medication. Niacin probably acts primarily by inhibiting secretion of VLDL, thus decreasing production of LDL as well.[17] There is also increased clearance of VLDL via the lipoprotein lipase pathway, and cholesterogenesis is inhibited.[18] Excretion of neutral sterols in bile is increased, but that of bile acids is not.[19] Catabolism of HDL is decreased, and concentrations of HDL, chiefly HDL$_2$ and apolipoprotein A-I, the chief protein species of HDL, rise in plasma.[20] Levels of circulating fibrinogen are reduced, and levels of tissue plasminogen activator rise, perhaps influencing thrombolysis. Niacin may reduce VLDL production through its potent inhibitory effect on the intracellular lipase system of adipose tissue. Inhibition results in a decreased flux of free fatty acid precursors to liver, but it has not been established that this effect is sustained during long-term treatment.

SIDE EFFECTS

When niacin treatment is begun and when dosage is increased, almost all patients complain of a warm sensation, usually accompanied by a flush. This prostaglandin-mediated phenomenon, a harmless vasodilation, can be blunted if the patient takes 0.3 g of aspirin 20 to 30 minutes before the niacin. This should only be needed in the first few days or weeks. Itching and a transient rash are also common. Liver function should be assessed prior to starting the drug and at regular intervals thereafter, since niacin may cause mild-to-moderate elevations of transaminase levels. This effect is reversible and is minimized if the dose is increased slowly. It is probably due in most cases to microsomal enzyme induction rather than to hepatic parenchymal toxicity. Serious hepatic toxicity occurs rarely. However, if transaminase levels exceed three to four times normal, the drug should be discontinued or the dose reduced. Such patients require careful observation. Severe hepatic dysfunction, including acute necrosis, has been associated with sustained release preparations of niacin, contraindicating their use. More severe pruritus, prolonged rash, dry skin, and acanthosis nigricans have been observed. Nausea and abdominal discomfort are experienced by some patients. These symptoms are minimized by taking the medications with meals and by the use of nonaluminum-based antacids, if necessary. They are rarely encountered if niacin is taken at the same time as colestipol or cholestyramine because of the buffering properties of the resins. The drug should not be given to persons with severe peptic disease, however. Moderate impairment of carbohydrate tolerance has occurred, but is reversible except in some patients who appear to have latent diabetes. Hyperuricemia is a relatively common side effect, but is unlikely to become symptomatic unless the patient has preexisting gout. Atrial arrhythmias have been encountered rarely. Another, very rare, toxic effect is macular edema, which is usually first manifested by blurring of vision. Again, if the niacin is stopped in timely fashion, this lesion is completely reversible.

DOSAGE

The starting dose should be 100 mg two to no more than three times daily with meals. The patient should be told to expect the common side effects and warned not to take the drug on an empty stomach. The dose should be increased slowly by 100-mg increments as tolerated. The daily dose should not exceed 2.5 g by the end of the first month. The maximum dose should never exceed 7.5 g. Patients with heterozygous familial hypercholesterolemia or familial combined hyperlipidemia vary greatly in the dose of niacin required in combination with a resin to normalize their levels of LDL. The usual range, however, is 4 to 6 g/d. Patients with other forms of hypercholesterolemia or with hypertriglyceridemia may require much lower doses (1.5 g to 3.5 g/d).

USES

Niacin, in combination with a bile acid binding resin[21] or a reductase inhibitor normalizes levels of LDL in most patients with heterozygous familial hypercholesterolemia and familial combined hyperlipidemia. Also, these combinations are useful in the treatment of some patients with the hyperlipidemia of nephrosis. In patients with severe mixed lipemias who have incomplete response to diet therapy, and in those with familial dysbetalipoproteinemia, small doses of niacin are often effective.

Gemfibrozil

MECHANISM OF ACTION

Gemfibrozil, like the first-generation fibric acid derivative clofibrate,[22] appears to increase clearance of triglyceride-rich lipoproteins by enhancing the activity of lipoprotein lipase and perhaps also by decreasing synthesis of VLDL. There is a decreased flux of free fatty acids to the liver since this drug decreases lipolysis in adipose tissue. Levels of LDL may be modestly reduced or increased and levels of HDL cholesterol are moderately increased.[23] There is also a moderate increase in HDL protein.

SIDE EFFECTS

Gemfibrozil may cause muscular, gastrointestinal, and cutaneous side effects. An increased incidence of gallstones, increased transaminase activity, arrhythmias, and decreased white blood cell count and hematocrit have been reported. Because metabolites of this drug are excreted by the kidneys, it should be avoided in patients with renal insufficiency and nephrosis, who are at increased risk for the toxic effects. Doses of coumarin and indanedione anticoagulants should be reduced and monitored closely when gemfibrozil is prescribed. The likelihood of myopathy with increased plasma levels of creatine kinase is increased if gemfibrozil is given with HMG-CoA reductase inhibitors. If this combination is used, the dosage of those drugs must be limited and the patient's creatine kinase level monitored closely.

DOSAGE

Although the usual dose is 600 mg twice daily, some patients have a good lipid-lowering effect with half this amount.

USES

Marked reduction of triglyceride-rich lipoproteins in patients with familial dysbetalipoproteinemia can often be achieved. Some cases of severe endogenous hypertriglyceridemia unresponsive to diet can be ameliorated by gemfibrozil. Although men who took gemfibrozil in the Helsinki Heart Study had a 34%

decrease in the incidence of coronary events compared to those taking placebo,[24] increases in noncoronary deaths observed in the trial suggest that this agent should be used cautiously. It is not recommended for patients with overt coronary disease based on the secondary prevention component of the Helsinki trial. It is also not indicated in patients whose only lipid abnormality is a low level of HDL cholesterol.

Other Fibric Acid Derivatives

Other, somewhat more potent, congeners are available in Europe. One is fenofibrate, given in doses of 100 mg three times a day. It is secreted virtually entirely as the anion by the kidneys. Another is bezafibrate, given in doses of 200 mg three times daily.

Neomycin

Neomycin has been used for 20 years for treatment of hypercholesterolemia. Although very useful as a secondary therapeutic choice in certain instances, it has not yet been approved by the Food and Drug Administration for this indication.

MECHANISM OF ACTION

Levels of LDL in serum are reduced by this aminoglycoside antibiotic. Poorly absorbed itself, it inhibits absorption of cholesterol, increases excretion of bile acids, and decreases the total body pool of cholesterol.[25]

SIDE EFFECTS

Even low doses of neomycin may occasionally cause nausea, cramping, diarrhea, and malabsorption. Enterocolitis has occurred secondary to overgrowth of resistant bacteria. Patients with preexisting bowel disease may have enhanced absorption of the drug and a greater incidence of the well-known otic, nephric, hematopoietic, and hepatic toxicity. These effects are otherwise extremely rare when the daily dose is no greater than 2 g. Neomycin should be avoided in patients with kidney disease and is known to decrease absorption of digitalis glycosides. Because high-frequency hearing loss is the earliest manifestation of neomycin ototoxicity, patients with previous high-frequency loss probably should not be treated with this drug. Audiometry should be done yearly in patients receiving long-term treatment.

DOSAGE

The usual dose is 0.5 to 2 g/d. It should be given with meals in two divided doses.

USES

Neomycin alone can achieve approximately a 20% reduction in cholesterol levels in patients with familial hypercholesterolemia when they are unable to tolerate other agents.[26,27] It is also likely to be beneficial in other disorders with elevated levels of LDL. Its complementarity with bile acid binding resins is variable and limited, probably because the principal modes of action of the drugs, interference with bile acid reabsorption, are redundant. However, complementarity with niacin appears to exist. Neomycin has no value in the treatment of isolated hypertriglyceridemia.

Probucol

MECHANISM OF ACTION

Probucol treatment is associated with increased fractional clearance of LDL[28] and increased excretion of bile acids.[29] Some inhibition of cholesterol biosynthesis also occurs. Unlike the time course of most other agents, probucol may cause LDL levels in plasma to decrease continuously for 4 months or more, achieving a reduction of 15% to 20% in most cases. Decreases of up to 27% have been described in patients with homozygous familial hypercholesterolemia, a more striking effect than that obtained with most agents. Impressive decreases in the diameters of tendon xanthomas have been observed in patients with homozygous and heterozygous familial hypercholesterolemia and in the corresponding animal model, the Watanabe heritable hyperlipidemic (WHHL) rabbit. This suggests that the most important action of probucol may be at the level of the uptake of LDL by the macrophage. Reports of amelioration of atheromatous disease in patients homozygous for familial hypercholesterolemia and in homozygous WHHL rabbits suggest that this effect extends to arterial plaques as well.[30,31] Potent inhibition of the endothelial cell-mediated oxidation of LDL resulting in decreased uptake of LDL by the scavenger pathway of macrophages is consistent with such an effect on both tendons and atherosclerotic plaques.[32] Thus, probucol may inhibit atherogenesis by a mechanism independent of its ability to lower LDL levels.

Levels of HDL in plasma are frequently decreased proportionately even more than those of LDL.[33] This effect includes levels of apolipoprotein A-I as well as the lipid constituents of HDL. Because low HDL-cholesterol levels are correlated epidemiologically with an increased risk of coronary heart disease, it remains to be determined whether decreases in plasma levels of HDL resulting from treatment with probucol are inimical. However, preliminary results suggest that centripetal transport of cholesterol may be enhanced by probucol. This hydrophobic drug partitions into adipose tissue from which it reenters plasma slowly after treatment is stopped. Thus, substantial plasma levels of the drug may be present for up to several months.

SIDE EFFECTS

Serious ventricular arrhythmias and prolonged QT intervals have been reported in animals receiving high doses of probucol. Increases in the QT interval of 20 to 25 msec are commonly observed in humans treated with probucol. This is apparently unassociated with increased frequency of premature ventricular contractions. It remains unknown whether more serious problems with cardiac rhythmicity might occur in the presence of acid–base or electrolyte disturbances or during myocardial ischemia in humans. Patients may experience diarrhea, nausea, and abdominal pain.

DOSAGE
The usual dose is 500 mg twice daily.

USES
The inhibition of foam cell formation with its attendant impact on atherogenesis provides an attractive potential rationale for the use of this agent. The available data suggest that it may be the most useful drug for treatment of patients with homozygous familial hypercholesterolemia. However, further evidence of its safety and a better understanding of its effects on HDL will be required before broad application in the prevention of atherosclerosis is warranted, especially in the less severe forms of hyperlipidemia.

Dextrothyroxine

MECHANISM OF ACTION
Dextrothyroxine is a synthetic isomer of thyroxine that is alleged to have little of the calorigenic property of its naturally occurring isomer, levothyroxine, while retaining the effects of thyroid hormone on lipid metabolism. However, it appears that substantial calorigenic activity remains. Thyroxine appears to exert its primary influence on lipid metabolism by stimulating the conversion of cholesterol to bile acids and by increasing the number of high-affinity LDL receptors on cell membranes. Neutral sterol excretion in the stool is increased, and a modest decrease in circulating levels of LDL is observed.

SIDE EFFECTS
Because some of the calorigenic and related adrenergic effects of levothyroxine are retained, arrhythmias and increased angina are frequently encountered.

USES
Because other agents are more effective in lowering levels of LDL cholesterol, and because of the apparent risk of ventricular arrhythmia, there is no indication for use of this drug in the treatment of hyperlipidemia.

HMG-CoA Reductase Inhibitors

MECHANISM OF ACTION
HMG-CoA reductase inhibitors are structural analogs of hydroxymethylglutaryl CoA, an obligatory intermediary in the biosynthesis of sterols and other isoprenoid substances.[16] These agents act by competitive inhibition of HMG-CoA reductase, leading to reduced production of mevalonic acid. The original compounds, compactin (released abroad) and its methylated derivative, lovastatin, are soluble products formed by *Penicillium* and *Aspergillus* organisms, respectively. A number of synthetic congeners have been developed. Pravastatin and simvastatin are also available for use in the United States. The reductase inhibitors probably do not significantly suppress synthesis of nonsterol isoprenoids, such as ubiquinone and dolichol, because the enzymes in the initial reactions leading to these products have a high affinity for mevalonate.[34]

In humans, the primary effect of these drugs is induction of increased numbers of LDL receptors, leading to increased fractional clearance of LDL[35] and a decrease of 20% to 50% in levels of LDL cholesterol in plasma. A decrease in the production rate of LDL may also result from an increased endocytotic flux of VLDL remnants into liver via the LDL receptor, resulting in diminished conversion of these precursor lipoproteins to LDL. Small increases in total HDL cholesterol also occur.

SIDE EFFECTS
A number of minor side effects of the reductase inhibitors, such as headache, minimal gastroenteric symptoms, rash, muscle cramps, and insomnia, have been described that do not frequently preclude use of the drugs. Two potentially serious side effects have appeared in clinical experience: a myopathic syndrome and a chemical hepatitis. The myopathy is characterized by painful, tender and/or weak muscles, high levels of serum creatine kinase, and, in extreme cases, myolysis with myoglobinemia, myoglobinuria, and the risk of renal shutdown. Marked elevations of creatine kinase can occur in the absence of painful muscles. When these drugs are used alone, myopathy probably occurs in less than 1% of patients and is completely reversible on cessation of the drug but tends to recur with resumption of treatment. It can appear with doses as small as 20 mg/day. Risk of the myopathy is increased by the concomitant administration of drugs that compete with the reductase inhibitors for catabolism. The most important of these is cyclosporine. Research in progress suggests that very small doses of lovastatin (10 mg or less per day) may be compatible with this drug. However, the combination of these agents must be monitored with extreme care. Other drugs that may increase the incidence of myopathy when given with the reductase inhibitors include the fibric acid derivatives gemfibrozil and clofibrate, erythromycin, and possibly niacin. In all cases, it is important to follow creatine kinase levels closely if these agents are used in combination. In practice, modest elevations of creatine kinase activity, up to two times the upper limit of normal, may occur in some patients, particularly after strenuous exercise, without signaling a signi-ficant myopathy. Pravastatin is more hydrophilic than lovastatin or simvastatin and some studies show a preferential distribution to the liver. These properties may be associated with a lower incidence of myositis. Further clinical experience will be needed to validate this. Severe hepatic dysfunction associated with reductase inhibitors may occur and may accompany the myopathic syndrome. It is characterized by marked elevations in transaminase enymes in serum, often with symptoms of malaise and nausea. It is reversible on cessation of the drug, but tends to recur if it is reinstituted. In practice, many patients

taking reductase inhibitors have elevations of serum transaminase levels up to three times the upper limit of normal with no apparent deleterious effect in contrast to the marked elevations encountered in the chemical hepatitis described above. Current experience suggests that therapy may be continued with frequent monitoring of liver function in the patients with the lesser elevations of transaminase activity. In all patients taking a reductase in-hibitor transaminase levels should be monitored at 8-week intervals during the first year of therapy and at about 3- to 5-month intervals thereafter. HMG-CoA reductase inhibitors should not be given to persons with overt hepatic dysfunction and should be used with great caution in those with a history of hepatic dysfunction or heavy alcohol use.

DOSAGE

Dosage ranges, according to the biological response, are between 10 to 80 mg/d of lovastatin, 10 to 40 mg/d of pravastatin, and 5 to 40 mg/d of simvastatin. On a mass basis, simvastatin is about twice as potent as the other two drugs. The drugs may be given in one evening dose or twice daily. Diminished dosage and close monitoring are required if they are given with agents that may precipitate the myopathic syndrome.

USES

HMG-CoA reductase inhibitors are primarily used in disorders involving elevated levels of LDL in serum. There is no indication for their use in severe forms of hypertriglyceridemia, despite the fact the serum cholesterol levels may be elevated, because LDL levels tend to be low in these disorders. In patients with mild elevations of LDL, lovastatin or pravastatin in doses of 20 to 40 mg/d may reduce serum cholesterol levels from 20% to 40%. In patients with heterozygous familial hypercholesterolemia, similar decreases in levels of LDL cholesterol may be achieved with doses of 40 to 60 mg/d of lovastatin.[36,37] Usually there is a diminished incremental effect with increases to 80 mg/d. The effectiveness of reductase inhibitors in severe primary hypercholesterolemia is greatly increased when it is combined with other agents (see below). Reductase inhibitors are effective in treating familial dysbetalipoproteinemia in some persons. They are also effective in familial combined hyperlipoproteinemia, especially when given with niacin.

DRUG COMBINATIONS

Treatment with two or more drugs in combination may be necessary in the following circumstances: (1) when a bile acid binding resin fails to normalize levels of LDL, (2) when both VLDL and LDL are elevated, and (3) when levels of VLDL increase significantly during treatment of hypercholesterolemia with a resin.

Those combinations which have been found to offer significant complementarity are niacin with resin and combinations of niacin or bile acid seques-

trant with HMG-CoA reductase inhibitors.

The combination of bile acid binding resin with niacin is the first combination of choice for treatment of heterozygous familial hypercholesterolemia,[21,38] reflecting the combined effects of the individual drugs. A significant increase in levels of HDL due to the niacin is also observed. This may prove to be of additional benefit if centripetal transport of cholesterol is shown to be enhanced. There are no additional toxic effects and, in fact, the acid-neutralizing property of the resin relieves the gastric irritation experienced by some patients who take niacin. The absorption of niacin is not impeded by the resin so the drugs may be taken together. To achieve normalization of LDL in heterozygous familial hypercholesterolemia, a full dose of resin with 4 g to 6.5 g of niacin is usually required. A few patients with this disorder do not normalize their LDL even at these doses.

The combination of a resin with an HMG-CoA reductase inhibitor is as effective as the resin with niacin regimen in lowering LDL levels, although the former does not appear to raise HDL-cholesterol levels substantially.[35,38] An HMG-CoA reductase inhibitor with niacin is an especially useful combination in the treatment of familial combined hyperlipidemia.

Maximum effectiveness in treatment of hypercholesterolemia is afforded by the ternary regimen consisting of a reductase inhibitor, a bile acid binding resin, and niacin.[39] In patients with severe heterozygous familial hypercholesterolemia, total serum cholesterol levels were reduced from a mean of 433 mg/dl on diet alone to 183 mg/dl on this regimen.

Drug combinations also may be of use in treating severe endogenous or mixed hypertriglyceridemia in which the combination of niacin and gemfibrozil appears to be more effective than either agent alone.

TREATMENT OF HOMOZYGOUS FAMILIAL HYPERCHOLESTEROLEMIA

Patients with homozygous familial hypercholesterolemia are rare, but the fulminant nature of the atherosclerosis demands the most aggressive treatment regimens. In the totally receptor-negative patient, bile acid binding resins and reductase inhibitors have essentially no effect. The drugs indicated in this disorder are probucol and niacin. Many patients have some residual receptor activity, however, affording the opportunity for a small effect of resins and HMG-CoA reductase inhibitors. The most effective means of lowering levels of LDL appears to be extracorporeal immunophoresis. When niacin, probucol, or neomycin are used in concert with this approach, reaccumulation of LDL is significantly delayed. Patients with severe hypercholesterolemia due to various genetic compound states are much more common than those with homozygous hypercholesterolemia. Often they have combinations of tuberous or planar cutaneous xanthomas with tendinous xanthomas. Because many of these patients tend to develop atherosclerotic lesions at a very rapid rate, they, too, should receive aggressive multiple drug therapy.

REFERENCES

1. Fuster V, Badimon L, Badiman JJ et al: The pathogenesis of coronary artery disease and the acute coronary syndromes. N Engl J Med 326: 242, 1992

2. Schwartz CJ, Valente AJ, Sprague EA et al: The pathogenesis of atherosclerosis: An overview.Clin Cardiol 14 (2 Suppl 1):1, 1991

3. Carlson LA, Bottinger LE, Ahfeldt PE: Risk factors for myocardial infarction in the Stockholm prospective study: A 14-year followup focusing on the role of plasma triglycerides and cholesterol. Acta Med Scand 206:351, 1979

4. Kannel WB, Castelli WP, Gordon T: Cholesterol in the prediction of atherosclerotic disease: New perspectives based on the Framingham Study. Ann Intern Med 90:85, 1979

5. Armstrong ML, Warner ED, Connor WE: Regression of coronary atheromatosis in rhesus monkeys. Circ Res 27:59, 1970

6. Brown G, Albers JJ, Fisher LD et al: Regression of coronary artery disease as a result of interim lipid-lowering therapy in men with high levels of apolipoprotein B. N Engl J Med 323:1289, 1990

7. Kane JP, Malloy MJ, Ports TA et al: Regression of coronary atherosclerosis during treatment of familial hypercholesterolemia with combined drug regimens. JAMA 264:3007, 1990

8. Watts GF, Lewis B, Brunt JNH et al. Effects on coronary artery disease of lipid-lowering diet, or diet plus cholestyramine, in the St. Thomas atherosclerosis regression study (STARS). Lancet 339:563, 1992

9. Cashin-Hemphill L, Mack WJ, Pogoda JM, et al: Beneficial effects of colestipol-niacin on coronary atherosclerosis—a 4 year follow up. JAMA 264: 3013, 1990

10. Barndt R, Blankenhorn DH, Crawford DW, Brooks SH: Regression and progression of early atherosclerosis in treated hyperlipoproteinemic patients. Ann Intern Med 86:139, 1977

11. Blankenhorn DH: Reversibility of latent atherosclerosis: Studies by femoral angiograpy in humans. Mod Concepts Cardiovasc Dis 47:79, 1978

12. Parthasarathy S, Steinberg D, Witztum JL: The role of oxidized low-density lipoproteins in the pathogenesis of atherosclerosis. Annu Rev Med 43:219, 1992

13. Castelli GT, Hjortland W, Kannel W, et al: High density lipoprotein as a protective factor against coronary heart disease: The Framingham study. Am J Med 66:707, 1977

14. Fielding PE, Fielding CJ, Havel PJ et al: Cholesterol net transport, esterification and transfer in human hyperlipidemic plasma. J Clin Invest 71:449, 1983

15. Summary of second report of the National Cholesterol Education Program (NCEP) Expert Panel on Detection, Evaluation, and Treatment of High Blood Cholesterol in Adults (Adult Treatment Panel II). JAMA 269:3015, 1993

16. Kane JP, Malloy MJ. Treatment of hyperlipidemia. Annu Rev Med 41:471, 1990

17. Grundy SM, Mok HYI, Zech L, Berman M: Influence of nicotinic acid on metabolism of triglycerides and cholesterol in man. J Lipid Res 22:24, 1981

18. Miettinen TA: Effect of nicotinic acid on catabolism and synthesis of cholesterol in man. Clin Chim Acta 20:43, 1968

19. Einarsson K, Hellstrom K, Leijd B: Bile acid kinetics and steroid balance during nicotinic acid therapy in patients with hyperlipoproteinemia types II and IV. J Lab Clin Med 90:618, 1977

20. Shepherd J, Packard CJ, Patsch JP et al: Effects of nicotinic acid therapy on plasma high density lipoprotein subfraction distribution and composition and on apolipoprotein A metabolism. J Clin Invest 63:858, 1979

21. Kane JP, Malloy MJ, Tun P et al: Normalization of low density lipoprotein levels in heterozygous familial hypercholesterolemia with a combined drug regimen. N Engl J Med 304:251, 1981

22. Grundy SM, Ahrens EH Jr, Salen G et al: Mechanisms of action of clofibrate on cholesterol metabolism in patients with hypertriglyceridemia. J Lipid Res 13:531, 1972

23. Lewis JE: Long term use of gemfibrozil (Lopid) in the treatment of dyslipidemia. Angiology 33:603, 1982

24. Frick MH, Elo O, Haapa K et al: Helsinki Heart Study: Primary prevention trial with gemfibrozil in middle-aged men with dyslipidemia. N Engl J Med 317:1237, 1987

25. Thompson GR, Barrowman J, Gutierrez L: Action of neomycin on the intraluminal phase of lipid absorption. J Clin Invest 50:319, 1971

26. Miettinen TA: Effects of neomycin alone and in combination with cholestyramine on serum cholesterol and fecal steroids in hypercholesterolemic subjects. J Clin Invest 64:1485, 1979

27. Samuel P: Treatment of hypercholesterolemia with neomycin—a time for reappraisal. N Engl J Med 301:595, 1979

28. Kesaniemi YA, Grundy SM: Influence of probucol on cholesterol metabolism in man. J Lipid Res 25:780, 1984

29. Nestel PJ, Billington T: Effects of probucol on low density lipoprotein removal and high density lipoprotein synthesis. Atherosclerosis 38: 203, 1981

30. Kita T, Nagano Y, Yokode M et al: Probucol prevents the progression of atherosclerosis in Watanabe heritable hyperlipidemic rabbit: An animal model for familial hypercholesterolemia. Proc Natl Acad Sci USA 84:5928, 1978

31. Yamamoto A, Matsuzawa Y, Yokoyama S et al: Effects of probucol on xanthomata regression in familial hypercholesterolemia. Am J Cardiol 57: 29H, 1986

32. Parthasarathy S, Young SG, Witztum JL et al: Probucol inhibits oxidative modification of low density lipoprotein. J Clin Invest 77:641, 1986

33. Mellies MJ, Gartside PS, Glatfelter L et al: Effects of probucol on plasma cholesterol high and low density lipoprotein cholesterol and apolipoproteins A-I and A-II in adults with primary hypercholesterolemia. Metabolism 29:956, 1980

34. Brown MS, Goldstein JL: Multivalent feedback regulation of HMG CoA reductase, a control mechanism coordinating isoprenoid synthesis and cell growth. J Lipid Res 21:505, 1980

35. Bilheimer DW, Grundy SM, Brown MS et al: Mevinolin and colestipol stimulate receptor mediated clearance of low density lipoprotein from plasma in familial hypercholesterolemia heterozygotes. Proc Natl Acad Sci USA 80:4124, 1983

36. Illingworth DR, Sexton GJ: Hypocholesterolemic effects of Mevinolin in patients with heterozygous familial hypercholesterolemia. J Clin Invest 74:1972, 1984

37. Havel RJ, Hunninghake DB, Illingworth DR et al: Lovastatin (Mevinolin) in the treatment of heterozygous familial hypercholesterolemia: A multicenter study. Ann Intern Med 107:609, 1987

38. Illingworth DR, Phillipson BE, Rapp JH et al: Colestipol plus nicotinic acid in treatment of heterozygous familial hypercholesterolemia. Lancet 1:296, 1981

39. Malloy MJ, Kane JP, Kunitake ST, Tun P: Complementarity of colestipol, niacin, and lovastatin in treatment of severe familial hypercholesterolemia. Ann Intern Med 107:616, 1987

Antithrombotic Therapy in Cardiac Disease

9

Valentin Fuster

John H. Ip

Ik-Kyung Jang

William P. Fay

James H. Chesebro

Thrombosis within the circulatory system has been recognized as the principal mechanism responsible for cardiovascular morbidity and mortality.[1-3] The pathogenic process leading to thrombosis in various disease states such as in the coronary arteries, cardiac chambers, and prosthetic heart valves appear to be different.[3-5] Thrombosis in the coronary arteries depends on the activation of both platelets and the clotting system. On the other hand, thrombus formation in dilated cardiac chambers depends mainly on the clotting system and platelets may play a minor role, whereas prosthetic valve thrombosis depends on the activation primarily of the coagulation system, and secondarily of the platelets. Thus, understanding of these pathogenic mechanisms is essential in the formulation of therapeutic and preventive strategies in these disease entities.

In this chapter we address the role of platelet activation and fibrin formation in thrombogenesis; the pharmacology of antithrombotic agents; the pathogenesis and risk of thrombosis and embolism in coronary arteries, cardiac chambers, and prosthetic valves; and the role of antithrombotic therapy in cardiac disease.

ROLE OF PLATELET ACTIVATION AND FIBRIN FORMATION IN THROMBOGENESIS

Platelets are fragments of membrane-enclosed megakaryocytic cytoplasm that travel in the periphery of the circulating blood and do not adhere to intact endothelium. When endothelial injury is superficial, only a monolayer of platelets adheres to the exposed subendothelium. When endothelial damage is more severe, exposure of collagen and other elements of the vessel wall stimulates activation of platelets and the coagulation system, leading to thrombus formation. In this section we will examine the processes of platelet adhesion, platelet aggregation, and activation of the clotting system, as well as endogenous inhibitors of thrombosis.

Platelet Adhesion: Role of Collagen Fibers and von Willebrand Factor

Platelets do not attach to the intact endothelium but firmly adhere to a disrupted or damaged endothelial surface.[6] After removal of the endothelial lining of a normal blood vessel by a mild or superficial injury, the subendothelium becomes coated by a layer of adherent platelets.[6] Platelet receptors are essential in the process of adhesion and aggregation (Fig. 9.1). Glycoprotein Ib in the platelet membrane appears to be important for normal initial contact of platelets with von Willebrand factor in the subendothelial surface. Glycoprotein Ia, which binds directly to exposed endothelial collagen, may also be important. Glycoprotein IIb/IIIa in the platelet membrane is the receptor for variety of circulating proteins, including von Willebrand factor and fibronectin and, aside from being important in platelet aggregation (see later), also favors platelet adhesion.[6] In the clinical context, subtle injury of the endothelial cell layer, for example that produced by flowing blood at arterial branch points or through stenoses, may trigger platelet adhesion. The release of platelet and endothelial cell growth factors may contribute to the early process of atherogenesis. On the other hand, in the acute coronary syndromes, severe vascular injury (plaque rupture) exposes components of the arterial media, particularly fibrillar collagen (with type I being more prevalent in diseased vessels and type III in normal vessels), which in addition to other mediators discussed later, induce platelet adhesion, aggregation, and thrombus formation.[6-8]

Platelet adhesion is determined not only by the degree of vascular injury as described previously but also by transport of the platelets to the injured area. This transport is determined by the wall shear rate, which is a measure of the difference in blood velocity between the center of the vessel and along the wall. At higher wall shear rates, characteristic of medium-sized stenotic arteries, initial platelet deposition rate and maximum extent of deposition are significantly higher.[9,10]

On artificial surfaces, the process of platelet adhesion is less understood. A film of adsorbed plasma proteins forms immediately after exposure of the surface to blood, and apparently different surfaces become coated with different proteins, which, by means of their surface charge, react differently with platelets.[11] Among the adsorbed plasma proteins that have been studied are fibrinogen, which tends to increase platelet adherence, and albumin, which tends to have the opposite effect.

Platelet Aggregation and Release: Role of Collagen, Thrombin, Thromboxane A₂, Adenosine Diphosphate, and Serotonin

In this second stage, platelets adhere to each other and the platelet mass builds. This platelet aggregation seems to depend primarily on an increase in cytoplasmic calcium, which appears to be mediated by three pathways. First, concomitant with the process of platelet adhesion there is an activation of platelets by extrinsic stimuli, specifically collagen and thrombin; second, during such platelet activation there is the release of platelet intracytoplasmic granule constituents, particularly adenosine diphosphate (ADP), which further activate neighboring platelets, causing aggregation; and third, also during such platelet activation there is synthesis and release

of the platelet prostanoid thromboxane A$_2$ (TXA$_2$), which also activates neighboring platelets, causing aggregation.

In certain pathologic situations, such as when an atherosclerotic plaque ruptures, there are extrinsic factors that may be very potent in triggering calcium release and platelet aggregation, specifically exposed collagen from the vessel wall and thrombin generated from the activation of the intrinsic and extrinsic

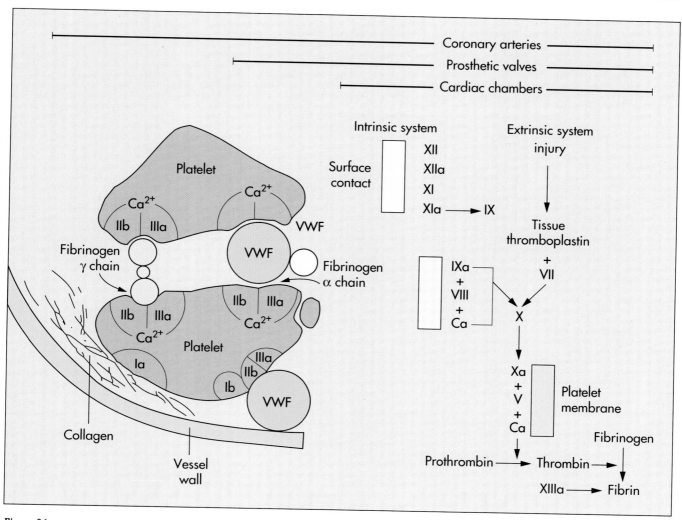

Figure 9.1 **Left** Schematic representation of the interactions among platelet membrane receptors (glycoproteins Ia, Ib, and IIb–IIIa), adhesive macromolecules, and the disrupted vessel wall. Numbers indicate the different pathways of platelet activation, dependent on (1) collagen, (2) thrombin, (3) adenosine diphosphate (ADP) and serotonin, and (4) thromboxane A$_2$ (TXA$_2$). **Right** The intrinsic and extrinsic systems of the coagulation cascade. Note the interaction between clotting factors and the platelet membrane. (Ca = calcium; VWF = von Willebrand factor) (Modified from Fuster V, Stein B, Badimon L, Chesebro JH: Antithrombotic therapy after myocardial reperfusion in acute myocardial infarction. J Am Coll Cardiol 12(Suppl A):78A, 1988)

clotting systems (Fig. 9.2; see Fig. 9.1). Through the actions of these extrinsic activators, calcium is then released from the dense tubular system into the cytoplasm, which in turn is associated with the activation of the actin–myosin system. These reactions in the adherent platelets and in the circulating neighboring platelets cause platelet contraction and the release of ADP and serotonin (see second pathway); also, TXA$_2$ synthesis then takes place followed by its release (see third pathway).[6,12] In addition, collagen and thrombin may also have a direct effect on platelets, possibly through a platelet-activating factor (PAF; see Fig. 9.2)

that may expose the platelet membrane receptor IIb–IIIa to fibrinogen and von Willebrand factor, thus promoting aggregation.[6,12–15] For the purpose of this discussion, these reactions, which are dependent on collagen and thrombin, constitute the first pathway of platelet activation and aggregation.

After the adherent platelets and circulating neighboring platelets have been exposed to collagen and thrombin, the second pathway may be activated. This pathway is mediated by ADP and serotonin, which are released from the platelet-dense granules after contraction (see Figs. 9.1 and 9.2). ADP is a potent

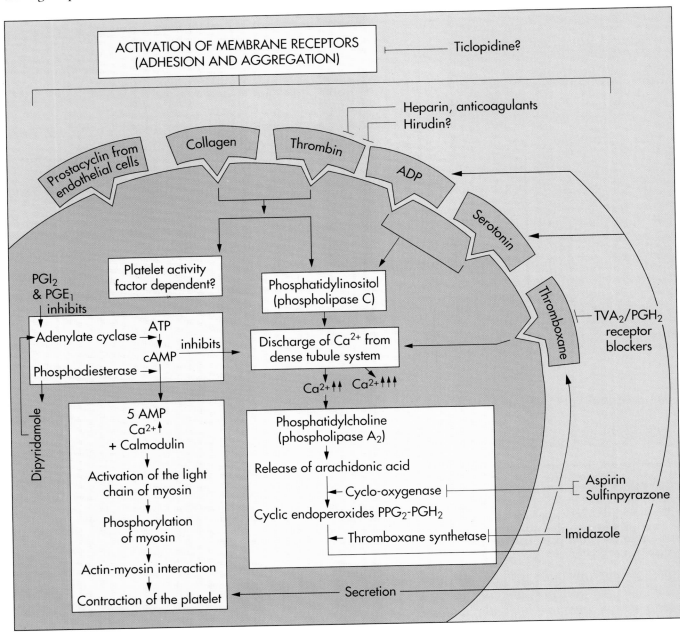

Figure 9.2 Mechanisms of platelet activation and presumed sites of action of various platelet inhibitor agents. Platelet agonists lead to the mobilization of calcium (Ca^{2+}), which functions as a mediator of platelet activation through metabolic pathways dependent on adenosine diphosphate (ADP), thromboxane A$_2$ (TXA$_2$), thrombin, and collagen. Cyclic adenosine monophosphate (cAMP) inhibits calcium mobilization from the dense tubular system. Note that thrombin and collagen may independently activate platelets by means of platelet activating factor. Asterisk indicates a platelet inhibitor. Dashed line indicates a presumed site of drug action. (ATP = adenosine triphosphate; EPA = eicosapentaenoic acid; PGE$_1$ = prostaglandin E$_1$; PGH$_2$ = prostaglandin H$_2$; PGI$_2$ = prostaglandin I$_2$) (Modified from Fuster V, Stein B, Badimon L, Chesebro JH: Antithrombotic therapy after myocardial reperfusion in acute myocardial infarction. J Am Coll Cardiol 12(Suppl A): 78A, 1988)

inducer of platelet aggregation in the presence of calcium and fibrinogen. It stimulates neighboring platelets and, most importantly, exposes their binding sites IIb–IIIa to fibrinogen and von Willebrand factor,[6,12–15] thus promoting aggregation. Furthermore, the turbulence present in stenotic areas and at branching points within the arterial tree promotes red blood cell lysis, with the subsequent release of ADP, which in turn activates platelets and promotes their aggregation.

Again, after the adherent platelet and neighboring platelets have been exposed to collagen and thrombin, a third pathway of TXA_2 synthesis may be activated (see Figs. 9.1 and 9.2). This pathway is mediated by arachidonic acid, which is released from the platelet membrane by the action of phospholipase A_2 on phosphatidylcholine.[16] Cyclo-oxygenase converts arachidonic acid into the proaggregating prostaglandin endoperoxide intermediates (prostaglandins G_2 and H_2); TXA_2 is formed by the action of thromboxane synthetase, particularly on prostaglandin H_2. TXA_2 is both a potent platelet aggregating substance and a vasoconstrictor. It stimulates platelet aggregation by promoting the mobilization of intracellular calcium and, most importantly, causes a conformational change in the glycoprotein IIb/IIIa complex, which results in the exposure of previously occult fibrinogen and von Willebrand factor binding sites, thus promoting aggregation.[6,12–15]

In summary, collagen that becomes exposed after vessel injury, thrombin generated by activation of the coagulation system, and products of platelet secretion such as ADP and TXA_2 can enhance the thrombotic process by stimulating adjacent platelets and also facilitating the exposure of their membrane receptors to fibrinogen and von Willebrand factor. These reactions, in turn, promote further platelet aggregation and thrombus growth.

Activation of the Clotting Mechanism: Role of Thrombin and Fibrin Formation

In addition to adhering to the injured vessel wall, activated platelets markedly accelerate the generation of thrombin.[16] Perhaps by rearranging their surface lipoproteins during contraction, activated platelets promote the interaction of clotting factors.[16] It is on the platelet surface that the interactions between factors IX and VIII and factors X and V occur.[16]

Classic and didactic schematization requires a division to be made between the intrinsic and extrinsic pathways of activation (see Fig. 9.1).[17] In the intrinsic pathways, all necessary factors are present in the circulating blood itself and the initial reaction is set off by contact of the blood with a negatively charged surface (e.g., subendothelial collagen) or with a foreign surface (e.g., the glass wall of a test tube). In the extrinsic pathway it is not a plasma component but tissue fluid that initiates the blood coagulation process: following vessel damage, this tissue factor, called tissue thromboplastin, mixes with the blood and starts the coagulation process. After activation of factor X the two pathways merge into one. Both appear to be equally necessary to ensure normal hemostasis. More specifically, and as outlined in Figure 9.2, in the intrinsic system coagulation is initiated by the adsorption of factor XII onto a foreign surface or collagen. Both kallikrein and high-molecular-weight kininogen are required for the rapid surface activation of factor XII. In addition, high-molecular-weight kininogen increases the reactivity of factor XIIa in the conversion of factor XI to XIa. Factor XIa converts factor IX to the activated protease factor IXa, whereupon factors VIII and IXa form a complex activating factor X. Both platelet phospholipid, made available by aggregated platelets, and calcium are essential for maximal activation of factor X. In the presence of factor V, calcium, and platelet phospholipid, factor Xa subsequently converts prothrombin (factor II) to thrombin. As mentioned, the extrinsic system is triggered by the release of the tissue thromboplastin, a protein-phospholipid mixture that activates factor VII or VIIa. Together they serve as cofactors for the activation of both factor IX and factor X. Once factor Xa is formed, thrombin production proceeds as described previously. Thrombin cleaves fibrinogen to fibrin, activates factor XIII, which stabilizes fibrin, and also, as previously mentioned, induces platelet aggregation.

It should be emphasized that platelet aggregation and the subsequent generation of thrombin may be activated by circulating catecholamines. This may be of major importance because there may be a link between conditions of stress and the development of arterial thrombosis. Of no less importance is the increasing evidence of an enhanced thrombogenicity in cigarette smokers and in patients with a strong family history of coronary disease,[1,18] as well as in patients with hyperlipidemia and in patients with diabetes mellitus.[1]

Endogenous Inhibitors of Thrombosis: Role of Prostacyclin, Protein C, Fibrinolysis, and Antithrombin III

During platelet activation and fibrin formation there are endogenous mechanisms that tend to limit thrombus formation. The most important of these are prostacyclin, antithrombin III, protein C, and the fibrinolytic system.

Prostacyclin (PGI_2), a compound discovered by Moncada and colleagues,[19] seems to be the main prostaglandin metabolite in vascular tissue, being most highly concentrated on the intimal surface, particularly the endothelium, and progressively decreasing in activity toward the adventitial surface. PGI_2 is a potent systemic vasodilator and also a potent inhibitor of platelet aggregation. The platelet-inhibitory action of PGI_2 seems to be related to an activation of the platelet membrane adenylate cyclase enzyme, which leads to an increase in platelet cyclic adenosine monophosphate (AMP) and a decrease in the activation of platelet calcium and therefore of platelet function. Presumably, like the synthesis of the prostanoid TXA_2 by the platelet, as previously discussed, the vessel wall synthesizes PGI$_2$ from its own precursors (Fig. 9.3). That is, arachidonic acid is converted into cyclic endoperoxides by means of the cyclo-oxygenase enzyme, and such endoperoxides are subsequently converted into PGI$_2$ synthetase enzyme. It has been claimed that PGI$_2$ can be produced by the cells of the vessel wall in response to stimulation by endothelial injury or thrombin; most importantly, the platelets adhering to sites of vascular damage not only release TXA$_2$, which promotes the aggregation of platelets, but also concomitantly release endoperoxides, which potentiate PGI$_2$ synthesis by the arterial wall. Thus, the process of platelet aggregation and thrombosis may be limited or prevented. In this context, Greenland Inuit, who have a bleeding tendency but in whom thrombosis or atherosclerosis does not develop, seem to have little platelet TXA$_2$ (or rather a biologically low active TXA$_3$) and a substantial amount of a prostacyclin-type substance (prostaglandin I$_3$), all of these factors presumably related to diet.[20,21] Indeed, it has been suggested that an imbalance between platelet proaggregating and disaggregating activity of both prostaglandin systems (TXA$_2$ and PGI$_2$) may be an important factor leading to thrombosis and vascular disease.[16] Thus, it has been suggested that some of the so-called risk factors of atherosclerosis and thrombosis may promote vascular disease by altering this TXA$_2$–PGI$_2$ equilibrium system.[1]

Antithrombin III is another important endogenous anticoagulant that inhibits thrombin and activated factors IX, X, XI, and XII. Its inhibitory action is markedly increased by heparin.[22] A deficiency in antithrombin III is associated with thrombosis, which is evidence of the clinical relevance of this control mechanism.[23]

Protein C is activated by the association of thrombin with thrombomodulin (see Fig. 9.3). In addition to being a potent anticoagulant, protein C initiates fibrinolysis by activating plasminogen and neutralizing a circulating inhibitor of tissue plasminogen activator.[24] Once activated, plasminogen is converted to plasmin, which hydrolyzes fibrin into soluble fragments and degrades fibrinogen, prothrombin, and factors VIII and V.[25] The proteolytic activity of plasmin remains localized to the fibrin surface; as fibrin degradation proceeds to completion, plasmin is rapidly inactivated by α_2 plasmin inhibitor. A specific plasminogen activator inhibitor has been identified in human platelets[26] and in the extracellular matrix of cultured endothelial cells.[27] Recent findings underscore the importance of the fibrinolytic system in maintaining normal hemostasis and suggest that the balance between plasminogen activators and inhibitors may be important in both arterial and venous thrombotic disorders. Indeed, patients who are congenitally deficient in protein C and persons who have low fibrinolytic response are prone to recurrent thrombosis.[28,29]

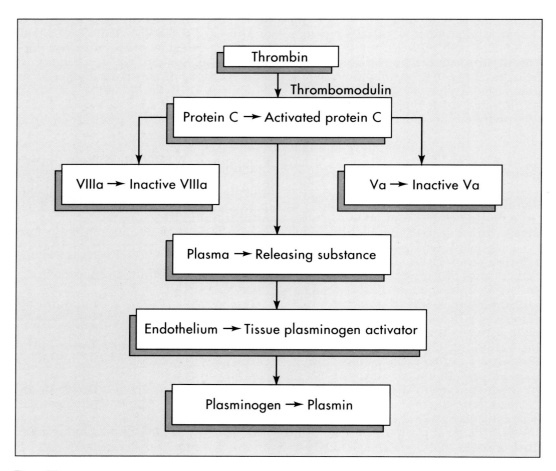

Figure 9.3 Activation of protein C and fibrinolysis. (Modified from Wessler S, Gitel SN: Warfarin from bedside to bench. N Engl J Med 311:645, 1984)

PHARMACOLOGY OF THE ANTITHROMBOTIC AGENTS

In this section we present a review of the pharmacology of platelet inhibitors, heparin, oral anticoagulants, and thrombolytic agents.

Platelet Inhibitors

Assessment of the pharmacologic actions that inhibit platelet function can be considered in three broad categories: drugs that inhibit the platelet arachidonate pathway; drugs that increase platelet cyclic AMP levels; and drugs that specifically block thrombin-mediated platelet activation.

INHIBITORS OF ARACHIDONIC ACID PATHWAY

Inhibitors of Platelet Cyclo-oxygenase—Aspirin
MECHANISM OF ACTION The cyclo-oxygenase enzyme, which is important in the conversion of arachidonic acid into the cyclic endoperoxides prostaglandin G_2 and prostaglandin H_2, can be blocked by numerous nonsteroidal anti-inflammatory drugs such as aspirin, indomethacin, ibuprofen, and naproxen. Acetylsalicylic acid, or aspirin (Fig. 9.4), inhibits cyclo-oxygenase in platelets by acetylating it, which inhibits the formation of TXA_2. Aspirin only partially inhibits platelet aggregation induced by ADP, collagen, or thrombin (at low concentrations). The adherence of the initial layer of platelets to the subendothelium and the release of granule contents are not inhibited by aspirin.[30] Consequently, the effects of platelet-derived growth factor and other mitogens on smooth muscle cell proliferation may still occur in the presence of cyclo-oxygenase inhibitors.[31] In contrast, these drugs inhibit platelet aggregate formation of the layer of adherent platelets, presumably by blocking TXA_2 synthesis.

The acetylation of cyclo-oxygenase on platelets exposed to aspirin is permanent,[32] and thus the effects of the drug persist for the life of the platelets. The long-term administration of 1 mg/kg/d of aspirin effectively inhibits platelet cyclo-oxygenase and TXA_2 formation. In contrast, aspirin inhibition of vascular endothelial cyclo-oxygenase is not irreversible because these cells are capable of synthesizing new enzyme, although they may require several hours to do so. Although earlier studies suggested that platelet cyclo-oxygenase is more sensitive to the inhibitory effects of low-dose aspirin than is vascular wall cyclo-oxygenase, more recent experimental data[33] challenge this concept.

IDEAL DOSE Beneficial effects of aspirin on cyclo-oxygenase-dependent platelet aggregation may be approximately equivalent over a dose range of at least 100 to 1500 mg daily. Numerous clinical studies have demonstrated the protective effects of aspirin in this dose range in patients with unstable angina and acute myocardial infarction, as well as in primary and secondary prevention of cardiovascular disease.[34–39] For example, two randomized clinical trials[34,35] using

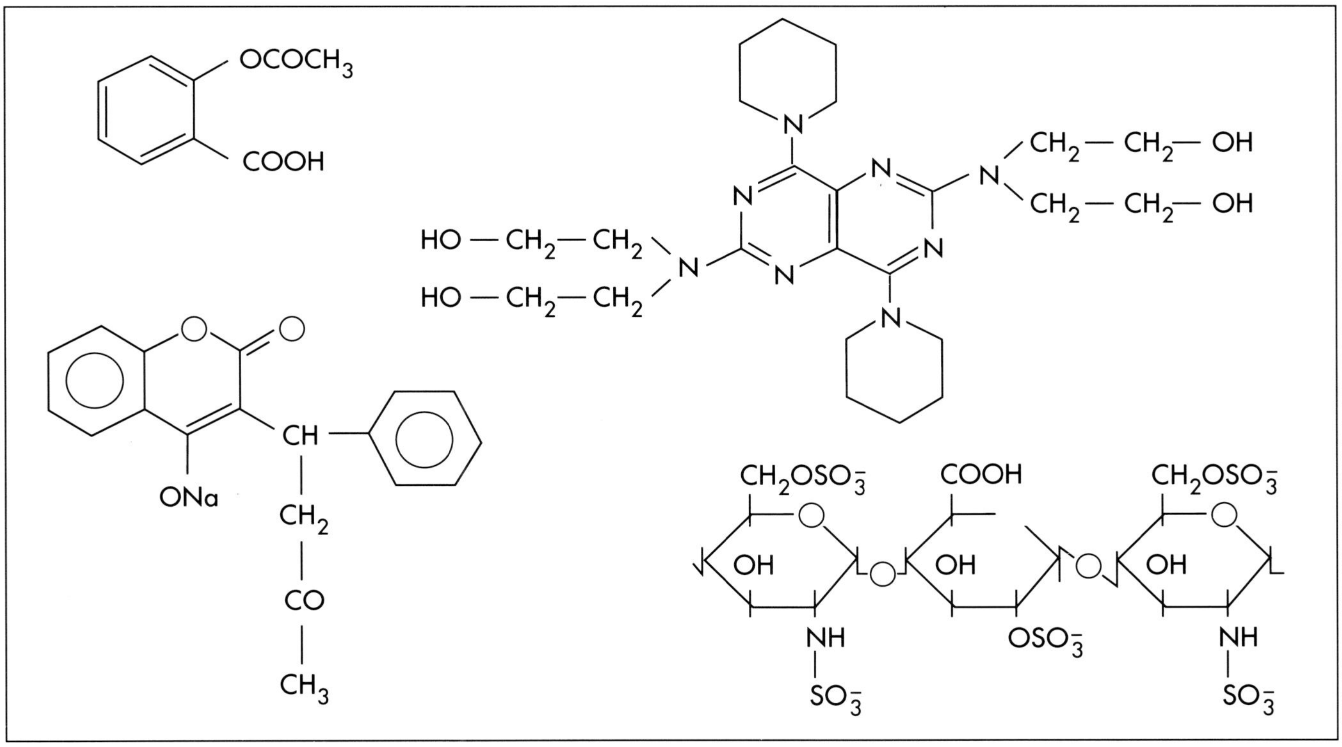

Figure 9.4 Chemical structure of the antithrombotic agents most commonly used in the United States: (clockwise) acetylsalicylic acid (aspirin), dipyridamole (Persantine), heparin, and warfarin sodium.

aspirin in doses of 324 and 1300 mg daily in patients with unstable angina showed similar reduction in mortality and nonfatal myocardial infarction. Similarly, in a recent overview of 25 clinical trials[38] using antiplatelet agents in the secondary prevention of cardiac disease, it was shown that aspirin used in doses ranging from 100 to 1500 mg/d reduced vascular mortality by 13%, nonfatal myocardial infarction by 31%, nonfatal stroke by 42%, and all important vascular events by 25%. There was no evidence that doses of 900 to 1500 mg of aspirin daily were any more effective in avoiding cardiovascular events than a lower dose of 300 mg, or one standard aspirin tablet, per day. This observation is pharmacologically plausible because doses lower than 300 mg/d would be sufficient to produce virtually complete inhibition of cyclo-oxygenase-dependent platelet aggregation. However, direct evidence of the effects of aspirin in doses lower or less frequent than 300 mg/d is not available from these trials of secondary prevention. At present, the best studied, most inexpensive, and least toxic dose range is 160 to 325 mg/d.

SIDE EFFECTS Aspirin side effects are mainly gastrointestinal and dose related.[39] Aspirin rarely causes significant generalized bleeding unless it is combined with anticoagulant therapy. There is evidence that aspirin affects the gastric mucosa by inhibiting synthesis of prostaglandins.[39,40] The effect of aspirin on gastric mucosa is reduced by treatment with cimetidine or antacid and by the use of enteric-coated aspirin.[39–41] Most of the side effects of aspirin are dose related. The recently completed UK-TIA trial tested two daily dosages of aspirin versus placebo among 2345 patients with a history of transient ischemic attacks or mild ischemic stroke.[42] It was therefore possible to compare directly the frequencies of side effects reported at 300 mg/d and at 1200 mg/d. For each category of symptom, including indigestion, nausea or heartburn, constipation, any gastrointestinal hemorrhage, and serious gastrointestinal hemorrhage, the percentage of participants reporting it was lowest in the placebo group, somewhat higher in the group receiving 300 mg/d, and highest among those receiving 1200 mg/d. Moreover, for symptoms of gastrointestinal distress as well as for any gastrointestinal hemorrhage, the differences between the low- and high-dose groups were statistically significant. Since there is no evidence that the higher doses are any more effective than the lower doses, an aspirin dose of 160 to 325 mg/d for the prevention of thromboembolic disease is currently recommended.

OTHER INHIBITORS OF PLATELET CYCLO-OXYGENASE Although nonsteroidal anti-inflammatory drugs reversibly inhibit cyclo-oxygenase, the antithrombotic activity of these compounds has not been properly tested in large randomized trials and therefore their use cannot be recommended.[43] Furthermore, one of the nonsteroidal anti-inflammatory agents, indomethacin, has been found to increase coronary vascular resistance and exacerbate ischemic attacks in patients with coronary disease.[44]

Drugs That Alter Platelet Membrane Phospholipids (Omega-3-Fatty Acids)

Both eicosapentaenoic acid and docosahexaenoic acid are present in high concentration in most saltwater fish and may account for the lower incidence of coronary heart disease in Greenland Inuit and populations who consume large amounts of fish.[45,46] Eicosapentaenoic acid competes with arachidonic acid for platelet cyclo-oxygenase. This leads to the formation of two endoperoxidases (prostaglandins G_3 and H_3) and TXA_3, which have minimal biologic activity.[47] Furthermore, eicosapentaenoic acid not only produces endothelial cell prostacyclin but also stimulates the formation of prostaglandin I_3, which has antiplatelet activity. The net result is a shift in the hemostatic balance toward an antiaggregative and vasodilative state. Docosahexaenoic acid also has platelet inhibitory effects and undergoes retrocoversion to eicosapentaenoic acid.[48] Although fish consumption may decrease the incidence of coronary artery disease, fish oils are associated with some potentially adverse events, such as increased bleeding diathesis and reduced inflammatory and immune responses.[48] Before fish oils are recommended for the prevention of atherosclerosis, more properly designed and controlled human trials are necessary.[47] The role of fish oils in the prevention of restenosis after coronary angioplasty is reviewed later in this chapter.

Inhibitors of Thromboxane Synthetase

Imidazole-analogue thromboxane synthetase inhibitors have been developed with the expectation of not only suppressing TXA_2 biosynthesis but also sparing or even enhancing the formation of prostacyclin by the vascular endothelium.[49] The rationale behind this hypothesis was that, in the presence of a thromboxane synthetase inhibitor, platelet-derived prostaglandin G_2 would be transferred to the endothelial cells and used in the production of prostacyclin. Although thromboxane synthetase inhibitors have shown some benefits in experimental models,[50] their effects in clinical trials[51,52] in patients with coronary artery disease have been debatable. This may be a result of two factors: (1) TXA_2 may not be completely suppressed by the available compounds, and (2) the prostaglandin endoperoxide intermediates that result from thromboxane synthetase inhibition have significant proaggregating effects themselves.

Blockers of Thromboxane and Prostaglandin Endoperoxide Receptors

A promising approach to the inhibition of the proaggregating and vasoconstrictive effects of TXA_2 is the pharmacologic blockade of the receptors for both TXA_2 and the prostaglandin endoperoxidases.[53] However, it remains to be demonstrated that such agents will offer an advantage over aspirin in suppressing TXA_2-dependent platelet function. The combination of a thromboxane synthetase inhibitor (which potentiates prostacyclin synthesis) and a TXA_2-prostaglandin H_2-receptor blocker (which prevents the proaggregative effects of these compounds) may offer a unique approach to platelet inhibition[54] but requires further testing.

DRUGS THAT INCREASE PLATELET CYCLIC AMP LEVELS

Dipyridamole

MECHANISM OF ACTION Dipyridamole (see Fig. 9.4) increases platelet cyclic AMP by three mechanisms: (1) it blocks breakdown by inhibiting phosphodiesterase; (2) it activates adenylate cyclase by a prostacyclin-mediated effect on the platelet membrane[55]; and (3) it increases the levels of plasma adenosine by inhibiting its uptake by vascular endothelium and red blood cells.[56,57] Adenosine, in turn, enhances platelet adenylate cyclase activity. In addition, the vasodilative effects of dipyridamole also appear to be related to the elevation in plasma adenosine levels. Although there are in vitro data to support dipyridamole's mechanisms of action on the platelet, there is no firm clinical evidence that such mechanisms contribute to a significant antithrombotic effect in humans.[40,57]

In contrast to aspirin, the antithrombotic effects of dipyridamole are more evident on prosthetic materials (artificial heart valves[58,59] and arteriovenous cannulas) than on biologic surfaces. Although one study[60] showed that aspirin potentiates the efficacy of dipyridamole in experimental thromboembolism on prosthetic surfaces, other studies[57] have shown conflicting results with regard to the pharmacologic interaction between these two agents. Furthermore, aspirin alone was as effective as the combination of aspirin and dipyridamole in recent antithrombotic trials[61-65] in patients with myocardial infarction, saphenous vein graft disease, and stroke. On the basis of these findings, there is little evidence to support the use of dipyridamole as an antithrombotic agent except in combination with warfarin in high-risk patients with a mechanical prosthesis[66-70] and perhaps in the preoperative period for coronary artery bypass surgery,[71,72] to prevent platelet activation by the extracorporeal pump; however, this last indication has not been properly tested.

SIDE EFFECTS Epigastric discomfort or nausea occurs in more than 10% of patients; however, these symptoms tend to subside after a few days, particularly if a low dose is used initially and it is given with meals. In addition, and in contrast with aspirin, when dipyridamole is given alone or in combination with anticoagulants, it does not seem to increase the incidence of gastritis, gastroduodenal ulcer, or the tendency to bleed. Because dipyridamole is a vasodilator, headaches occur in almost 10% of patients, but they become major problems in only 3% of those patients. Allergy, particularly skin rash, occurs infrequently.

Prostaglandin E₁ and Prostacyclin (PGI₂)

Prostaglandin E_1 and prostacyclin are powerful systemic vasodilators and inhibitors of platelet aggregation by virtue of their ability to increase platelet cyclic AMP. Intravenous infusions of prostaglandin E_1 are commonly used in neonates with congenital heart disease, who depend on the persistence of a patent ductus arteriosus until surgical correction is done. These agents have also been used to improve myocardial function in patients with acute myocardial infarction and to treat peripheral vascular disease.[73]

Prostacyclin is a potent, naturally occurring platelet inhibitor. Its clinical use has been limited by its instability at neutral pH and its propensity to cause significant systemic hypotension at the doses required for platelet inhibition. Its duration of action is very short, and the pharmacologic effects disappear in 30 minutes. Infusion of prostacyclin strongly limits platelet interaction with artificial surfaces and preserves platelet number and function during cardiopulmonary bypass.[74,75] The effects of prostacyclin in patients with ischemic heart disease and peripheral vascular insufficiency are controversial.[73] Emerging data, however, suggest that these prostanoids may improve the results of intracoronary thrombolysis in acute myocardial infarction.[76,77] Further research in this area is needed.

PROSTACYCLIN ANALOGUES Iloprost, a new synthetic prostacyclin analogue, is chemically stable at neutral pH. In an in vitro comparison with equimolar concentrations of prostaglandin E_1 and prostacyclin, iloprost was found to be more potent in increasing the levels of cyclic AMP and inhibiting platelet aggregation by various agonists, particularly thrombin.[78] Another prostacyclin analogue, ciprostene, was found to reduce the rate of ischemic events in patients after coronary angioplasty and was associated with a beneficial trend toward a lower rate of restenosis.[79] Therefore, clinically stable analogues of prostacyclin may be effective for temporary control of platelet activity in the management of thromboembolic disorders. These compounds are undergoing clinical testing.

OTHER PLATELET INHIBITORS

Ticlopidine

Ticlopidine hydrochloride is a novel platelet antiaggregant that functions primarily as an inhibitor of the adenosine diphosphate pathway of platelet aggregation.[80] In contrast to aspirin, ticlopidine inhibits most of the known stimuli to platelet aggregation when they are tested at physiologic concentrations. Ticlopidine does not inhibit the cyclo-oxygenase pathway, nor does it block the production of thromboxane by platelets or the production of prostacyclin by endothelial cells. Like aspirin, ticlopidine alters platelet function for the normal life span of the platelet.[81] Optimal efficacy is reached 3 days after its administration, and its effects last for several days after administration of the drug has been stopped.

Clinical evaluation of this drug is now underway.[39,40] Preliminary evidence from an Italian multicenter trial[82] suggests that it is effective in patients with unstable angina for the prevention of myocardial infarction and cardiovascular death. Another recent study[83] showed a reduction in the incidence of acute occlusion and thrombosis after coronary angioplasty in patients treated with ticlopidine. In addition, this agent was found to be effective in reducing vein graft closure in patients after aortocoronary bypass surgery.[84] Recent published data[85,86] suggest that ticlopidine reduces cardiovascular morbidity and mortality in patients with stroke and appears more effective than aspirin in patients with transient ischemic attacks. However, ticlopidine is associated with occasional side effects, including rash and neutropenia.

Sulfinpyrazone

Sulfinpyrazone is structurally related to phenylbutazone but has minimal anti-inflammatory activity. In contrast to aspirin, sulfinpyrazone is a competitive inhibitor of platelet cyclo-oxygenase, but the exact mechanism of its antithrombotic activity is not well understood.[60] It inhibits the formation of thrombus on the subendothelium and protects the endothelium from chemical injury in vitro and possibly in vivo. In addition, sulfinpyrazone produces a dose-dependent inhibition of experimental thromboembolism in artificial cannulas,[60] reduces the rate of thrombotic events in patients with arteriovenous cannulas,[87] and normalizes platelet survival in patients with artificial heart valves.[88] Overall, beneficial effects have been more consistent on prosthetic than biologic surfaces. Thus, despite a beneficial trend in decreasing vascular events after myocardial infarction[89] and reducing the occlusion rates in saphenous vein coronary grafts,[65,90] sulfinpyrazone was found to have no additional benefit in unstable angina[35] and stroke.[91] Side effects of sulfinpyrazone include increased sensitivity to warfarin, hypoglycemia when combined with sulfonylureas, exacerbation of peptic ulcer, and precipitation of uric acid stones.

Dextran

Dextran of a molecular weight of 65,000 to 80,000 daltons prolongs the bleeding time after intravenous infusion of more than 1 liter. The mechanism of action is unclear. It may involve some alteration of platelet membrane function[92] or interference with factor VIII–von Willebrand factor complex.[93] Although some experimental studies[94] have shown an antithrombotic effect of dextran, no effect was found in a randomized trial[95] in patients undergoing coronary angioplasty. Furthermore, dextran has been associated with a low but disturbing incidence (0.6%) of anaphylactoid reactions.[96] Data supporting the role of dextran as an antithrombotic agent on foreign materials (i.e., arterial stents and vascular grafts) are emerging.

By inhibiting thrombin formation with heparin, oral anticoagulant agents, or other thrombin inhibitors, the effects of thrombin on platelet activation can be partially prevented.

Peptide Blockers of Thrombin

An emerging strategy in antithrombotic therapy involves the synthesis of peptides that specifically block thrombin-mediated platelet activation.[97] A number of these agents have been studied in vitro and in experimental animals; however, no clinical experience is yet available. Another potent selective thrombin inhibitor, hirudin, initially isolated from the salivary secretions of the medicinal leech, was recently synthesized by DNA recombinant technology. Hirudin prevents the activation of clotting factors V, VIII, and XIII. In addition, by being a powerful thrombin inhibitor, it blocks the metabolic pathway of platelet activation dependent on thrombin. Hirudin has been shown to prevent thrombosis in an animal model of carotid angioplasty and was found to have a more potent antithrombotic effect than heparin.[98] Because these agents may effectively inhibit platelet activation by blocking thrombin, their potential for clinical use is enormous. Intensive research in this area is underway.

Heparin
MECHANISMS OF ACTION

Heparin is a complex mucopolysaccharide of variable molecular weight (Fig. 9.4). The term *heparin* refers not to a single structure but rather to a family of mucopolysaccharide chains of varying length and composition. The heparin used clinically is derived from porcine intestinal mucosa or bovine lung and is composed of molecules of molecular weights ranging from 4,000 to 40,000 daltons. The effect of heparin as an anticoagulant is essentially direct and immediate and depends on its ability to accelerate the action of the naturally occurring plasma inhibitor antithrombin III; indeed, absence or near absence of antithrombin III renders heparin useless for antithrombotic therapy. Antithrombin III inhibits thrombin as well as several of the proteases of the coagulation cascade, including factors Xa, IXa, XIa, and XIIa, by the formation of 1:1 protease–inhibitor complexes. The interaction of heparin with antithrombin III leads to a conformational change in the inhibitor, which greatly accelerates its interaction with coagulation proteases, particularly thrombin and factor Xa.[99] For example, the inactivation of thrombin by antithrombin III is accelerated approximately 1000-fold by heparin. However, the efficiency of antithrombin III in inhibiting blood clotting may be more dependent on inhibition of factor Xa activity than on inhibition of thrombin.[100] This is because inhibiting earlier steps in the blood coagulation system (see Fig. 9.1) should have a more potent antithrombotic effect than inhibiting subsequent steps, owing to the amplification process inherent in the coagulation cascade; that is, a single factor Xa molecule can lead to the generation of multiple thrombin molecules.[100–102] Heparin-enhanced inactivation of factor Xa by antithrombin III is believed to be the mechanism by which relatively low doses of subcutaneous heparin prevent venous thrombosis in high-risk patients.

In platelet-rich arterial thrombus, heparin appears able to reduce markedly the risk of total occlusion (the central core of the thrombus) but incapable of totally preventing mural thrombus after deep arterial injury. This can be explained by the natural inhibitors of heparin that are released during thrombosis (platelet factor 4 and fibrin II monomer), the difficulty with heparin–antithrombin III of inhibiting factor Xa when it is bound within an activator complex, the masking of antithrombin III and heparin cofactor II receptors on thrombin when fibrin is bound to thrombin, and the exquisite sensitivity of platelets for activation by thrombin.

Pharmaceutical-grade heparin preparations can be fractionated into distinct subpopulations on the basis of either molecular weight or affinity for antithrombin III. Low-molecular-weight heparin (molecular weight 5000 to 7000 daltons) effectively catalyzes the inactivation of factor Xa by antithrombin III, yet does not prolong the activated partial thromboplastin time (APTT) (i.e., less antithrombin effect) nor interact with platelets to the extent that high-molecular-weight heparin does.[100,103,104] Therefore, it has been suggested that low-molecular-weight heparin may be an effective antithrombotic agent with a relatively low risk of hemorrhagic side effects in patients with venous thrombosis.[105]

Dose, Administration, and Control of Therapy

The major aim of heparin administration is to prevent the formation and extension of thrombi while minimizing the risk of bleeding. Since even at low plasma concentration heparin is antithrombotic, the appropriate amount of anticoagulation depends on the intensity of the thrombogenic stimulus. Heparin is not absorbed by the gastrointestinal mucosa and must be given parenterally. It may be given continuous intravenously, intermittent intravenously, or subcutaneously into the fat of the subcutaneous tissue over the lower abdominal wall near the iliac crest or into the chest wall below the clavicle. Absorption from these depot sites is erratic, and hematomas are common at sites of intramuscular injection; hence, the intramuscular route should be avoided. Both calcium and sodium salts of heparin seem to be equally safe and effective. The volume of distribution of heparin seems largely confined to the intravascular space, reflecting its strong binding to protein. After intravenous injection, the average half-life in humans is about 90 minutes when average doses are used (5000 units every 4 hours).[106] After subcutaneous injection, the half-life is longer. Heparin's half-life is, however, variable, and clinicians must be aware that dose requirements are not identical for all patients. In addition, correlation between heparin's anticoagulant effect and the dose is poorer in patients with disease states than in normal volunteers. For example, in patients with pulmonary embolism, heparin clearance is accelerated, which necessitates higher dosage early in the treatment course.

At present, no test is completely satisfactory for monitoring heparin effect. What is needed is a test that directly monitors the generation of thrombin as well as the blood levels of antithrombin III. In the absence of such information at this time, only general guidelines can be recommended. The test most commonly used to monitor heparin therapy is the APTT,[100,103,107,108] which measures the effect of heparin on the intrinsic and common coagulation pathways (see Fig. 9.1). The protamine sulfate neutralization assay, which measures the amount of protamine sulfate (a heparin inactivator) necessary to normalize the thrombin clotting time, can also be used to monitor heparin therapy.[100,103,109,110] The anticoagulation effect of heparin should be maintained at a level that is equivalent to 0.1 to 0.5 units of heparin per milliliter (using protamine sulfate titration standard curve). This heparin level corresponds to an APTT of 1.5 to 2.5 times control. The activated clotting time (ACT), which measures the effect of heparin on whole blood clotting, allows rapid determination of the anticoagulant effect of heparin and has been used to regulate heparin therapy during cardiopulmonary bypass and percutaneous transluminal coronary angioplasty, where larger heparin doses are needed (it is less sensitive at lower heparin levels).[111,112]

When used to treat patients with active thrombosis, heparin should be administered in a dose sufficient to prolong an appropriate coagulation test to within a defined level. In most cases, it is desirable to achieve an anticoagulant effect rapidly and to sustain it throughout the period of treatment. This is achieved by an initial intravenous bolus injection of heparin, which can be followed either by continuous infusion or by intermittent intravenous injections. A moderately large bolus dose of heparin of between 5,000 and 10,000 units is injected intravenously, producing heparin levels immediately after injection considerably higher than the therapeutic range. This is followed by a dose between 25,000 and 50,000 units of heparin over 24 hours (depending on the patient's response), which maintains the majority of patients within a therapeutic range (Fig. 9.5).[100,103,113] If a patient with active thrombosis is at risk of bleeding (e.g., early postoperative period), heparin should be given by continuous intravenous infusion; and if the risk is very high, a lower dose of heparin may be used. If patients are not at high risk of bleeding, heparin can be administered by 4-hourly intermittent intravenous injections in full therapeutic doses. Therapeutic levels of heparin can also be achieved with subcutaneous injections. In addition, subtherapeutic levels of heparin achieved by injecting a low dose subcutaneously may be used in prophylaxis of venous thrombosis.

Continuous Infusion

Continuous heparin infusion (Fig. 9.6, see Fig. 9.5) is commonly used in patients with acute coronary syndromes, cardiac-chamber thrombosis, and ongoing venous thrombosis. Heparin is given as an initial bolus injection followed by a maintenance infusion with an automatic infusion pump.[100,103,113] The laboratory test used for monitoring heparin is performed approximately 6 hours after the bolus injection and then at least once more in the first 24 hours. Monitoring is continued twice daily until the desired effect is achieved and the dose–response relationship is stable. Monitoring is then continued on a once-daily basis.

An initial bolus injection of 5000 units should be followed by a maintenance infusion of 30,000 units/24 h, which can then be adjusted according to the results of the test used to monitor heparin therapy. In patients with major pulmonary embolism, an initial bolus dose of 10,000 units of heparin should be given, both because of the urgency of obtaining a marked anticoagulant effect and because heparin clearance is accelerated in patients with pulmonary embolism. The anticoagulant effect of heparin should then be maintained at a level that is equivalent to 0.3 to 0.4 units/ml of heparin (using protamine sulfate titration), since this is the heparin concentration that prevents the extension of experimental thrombi. This heparin level corresponds to an APTT of 1.5 to 2 times control. In patients with pulmonary embolism, it is most desirable that the regimen used achieve levels of about 0.4 to 0.5 units/ml of heparin, corresponding to an APTT of 2 to 2.5 times control; this may require infusion of nearly 50,000 units of heparin/24 h. If the APTT (or corresponding test) is above the therapeutic range, the dose of heparin should be reduced, usually between 2000 and 4000 units/24 h, and the APTT be repeated 4 to 6 hours later. If the results of the monitoring test are below the therapeutic range, a second bolus of 2000 units can be given and the dose of heparin increased by 3000 units/24 h. It should be noted that the dosage requirements may change after the first 2 to 3 days of treatment, but thereafter the dose–response relationship in any patient is usually stable.

Lower doses of heparin may be given in a patient with calf vein or even proximal vein thrombi in the early postoperative period or in a patient who has a hemostatic defect. In these patients, the initial bolus dose should be 2000 units followed by a maintenance dose of 15,000 to 20,000 units for 24 hours, and the laboratory effect of heparin should be monitored more frequently than usual to maintain the heparin level at between 0.1 and 0.2 units/ml.[100,103,113] This corresponds to an APTT of 1.25 to near 1.5 times control.

FIGURE 9.5 HEPARIN REGIMENS

Dosage (units/24 h)	Route	Clinical Indications	Therapeutic Range (APTT Ratio)
Low (10,000–15,000)	Subcutaneous (continuous intravenous)	Elective general surgery (not including major orthopedic procedures)	
Intermediate (20,000–30,000)	Subcutaneous (continuous intravenous)	Orthopedic procedures Acute myocardial infarction, heart failure, and immobilization After acute venous thromboembolism	1.5
Average or "therapeutic" (25,000–50,000)	Intravenous (continuous, intermittent, or subcutaneous)	Acute thromboembolism	1.5–2
High (40,000–60,000)	Intravenous (continuous or intermittent)	Massive acute venous thromboembolism	2–2.5

Intermittent Intravenous Injection

When infusion pumps are not readily available or cannot be adequately supervised or early ambulation is desired, there are some practical advantages of using a heparin lock with an intermittent intravenous protocol (see Figs. 9.5 and 9.6). In addition, with such intermittent intravenous injection the need for careful monitoring is less important. For these reasons many physicians prefer separate injections of 5000 units intravenously every 4 hours or 10,000 units intravenously every 6 hours. However, this approach has been reported to produce more bleeding in patients who have a high risk of hemorrhage.[100,103,114,115] Nevertheless, it should be noted that in these studies about 25% higher daily doses of heparin were used in the groups given intermittent intravenous injections, so that the increased rate of bleeding could have been related to the dose rather than the method of administration. Although it is sometimes recommended that the dose be adjusted to produce an APTT of approximately 1.5 times control immediately before the next injection is due, in practice laboratory monitoring with intermittent heparin is difficult and is not performed routinely in many institutions.

Subcutaneous Injection

Subcutaneous heparin injections can be given in low, intermediate, or full therapeutic doses (see Figs. 9.5 and 9.6).[100,103,113] When heparin is used prophylactically in patients subjected to elective abdominal or thoracic surgery, it is usually given by subcutaneous injection in doses of 5000 units every 8 or 12 hours.[100,103,116–118] The first dose is given 2 hours preoperatively and thereafter every 8 or 12 hours for the first 7 days, preferably until 2 days after complete mobilization.[102] For this purpose, 0.2 ml of concentrated heparin containing 5000 units is used. Monitoring is not required as long as the patient does not have a history of abnormal bleeding.

An intermediate heparin regimen of about 10,000 units given every 12 hours is of prophylactic value in patients at very high risk of venous thromboembolism and can also be used for the secondary prevention of venous thrombosis after a 7- to 10-day course of full-dose heparin.[100,103,118] A dose of 10,000 to 15,000 units given every 12 hours has been successful in acute myocardial infarction for prevention of recurrence[100,103,119] and for prevention of left ventricular thrombi.[100,103,120] The dosage requirement should first be determined by adjusting the APTT for 2 or 3 days, and then outpatient laboratory monitoring is no longer required. The dose is adjusted so that the APTT 6 hours after injection is about 1.5 times control (heparin level, 0.2 to 0.3 units/ml).

HEPARIN NEUTRALIZATION AND HEPARIN SIDE EFFECTS

Many reported episodes of major bleeding are related to risk factors for hemorrhage more overriding than dose or route of administration. These risk factors include lack of hemostatic competence prior to heparinization, invasive procedures, aspirin use, bodily trauma, and recent surgery while on therapy. In general, heparin should not be used in patients with hemorrhagic diathesis, hypertension with a diastolic pressure persistently over 105 mm Hg, cerebrovascular hemorrhage, major trauma, acute ulceration, or overt bleeding from gastrointestinal, genitourinary, or respiratory tracts.[121]

With continuous infusion, the anticoagulant effect of heparin is gone within hours of discontinuation of the drug, so minor bleeding is not a threat. When

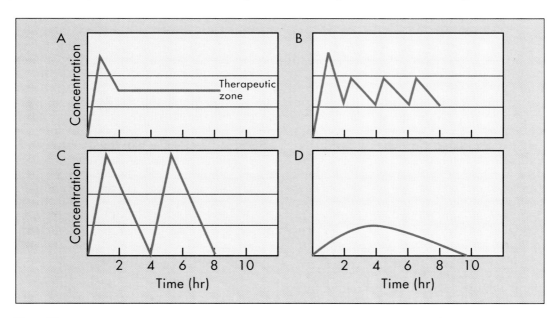

Figure 9.6 Blood concentration of heparin after **A** bolus injection followed by continuous intravenous infusion, **B** and **C** intermittent intravenous injections, and **D** subcutaneous injection. The risk of bleeding is higher when high-dose intermittent intravenous injection **C** is used and lower with subcutaneous injection **D**. (Modified from Verstraete M, Vermylen J: Antithrombotic and fibrinolytic agents and substances which lower blood viscosity. In Thrombosis, pp 76–112. New York, Pergamon Press, 1985)

heparin is given as a bolus dose, the duration of the effect depends on dose size (i.e., 3 to 4 hours with 5,000 units and 6 hours with 15,000 units). Heparin given subcutaneously produces low peak blood levels of the drug but sustains these for up to 12 hours. When bleeding is more severe, protamine sulfate (1% solution) is the drug of choice to neutralize heparin. The protamines are low-molecular-weight proteins rich in arginine and therefore strongly basic; they combine quickly with heparin to form salts devoid of anticoagulant activity. One milligram of protamine sulfate neutralizes about 100 units of heparin. Only 50% of the calculated protamine sulfate dose should be administered, and only 25% of the calculated dose should be given if it has been 2 hours since heparin was administered. No more than 50 mg of protamine sulfate should be given in any 10-minute period, since severe toxic reactions, including hypotension and anaphylaxis, may occur (epinephrine and corticosteroids should be available when protamine is used), especially if protamine has been previously used.

Heparin can cause thrombocytopenia (platelet count under 100,000/mm³) in 3% to 10% of patients.[100,122,123] This appears to be an immune-mediated phenomenon that typically occurs from 6 to 12 days after initiation of heparin therapy and is unique among the drug-induced thrombocytopenias in that it can be complicated by arterial thromboembolism. The diagnosis of heparin-induced thrombocytopenia is confirmed by rapid normalization of the platelet count on discontinuation of heparin. It is not necessarily prevented by substituting low-molecular-weight heparin.

Other complications of heparin therapy include osteoporosis, urticaria, alopecia, elevation of hepatic transaminases, and development of painful nodules at sites of subcutaneous injection.

OVERLAPPING OF COUMARIN WITH HEPARIN

When patients are being converted from heparin to warfarin, heparin should be continued for at least 24 hours after a therapeutic prothrombin time has been achieved since the anticoagulant effect of warfarin can be delayed relative to its effect on prothrombin time.[124] This is because factor VII has a half-life (5 hours) that is shorter than the other vitamin K-dependent clotting factors (factors II, IX, and X). Consequently, early in the course of coumarin therapy the prothrombin time, which assesses the extrinsic coagulation pathway (see Fig. 9.1), can be prolonged while the intrinsic and common coagulation pathways are still "intact." In addition, the half-life of protein C, an endogenous vitamin K-dependent anticoagulant, is similar to that of factor VII, and antithrombin III levels are transiently depressed after a course of heparin therapy. Therefore, a relative prothrombotic state due to protein C and antithrombin III deficiency could potentially be created by discontinuing heparin as soon as the prothrombin time becomes therapeutic.

Oral Anticoagulants

MECHANISM OF ACTION

Coagulation factors II, VII, IX, and X, protein C, and protein S are vitamin K-dependent proteins that are synthesized in hepatocytes. Post-translational modification of these proteins is necessary in order to yield biologically active molecules and involves the γ-carboxylation of glutamic acid residues located near the carboxy terminus of each protein. Coumarin anticoagulants inhibit vitamin K-2,3-epoxide reductase within hepatic microsomes and thus prevent recycling of vitamin K, which is necessary for the synthesis of γ-carboxyglutamic acid (Gla) residues.[124]

The clotting factors in blood are normally in a state of dynamic equilibrium, with the level of each individual factor not changing much over time. With a dose of coumarin sufficiently large to completely block hepatic synthesis, each factor disappears from the blood in accord with its half-life. With discontinuance of the drug, the clotting factors return to normal depending on their intrinsic synthesis rates. Thus, after a latent period peculiar to each type of oral anticoagulant, the prothrombin time becomes prolonged, mainly from the effect of lowering of the concentration of factor VII, the vitamin K-dependent factor with the shortest half-life (5 hours). Plasma concentration of the other vitamin K-dependent coagulation factors will decrease more slowly because their half-life is longer (20 to 60 hours for factor IX and X, and 80 to 100 hours for prothrombin). After 3 to 5 days of coumarin treatment, the lowered blood levels of the affected coagulation factors become virtually uniform. For effective treatment of thrombosis, the levels of factors II, VII, IX, and X should remain at approximately 25% of normal.

In North America, warfarin sodium is preferred among the coumarin drugs, and the indanedione drugs are seldom used for oral anticoagulant therapy since they are more prone to side effects and more difficult to control. Although the various coumarin congeners do differ in speed of induction of effect and in their individual metabolism, they all induce quantitatively similar effects on the clotting mechanism. Warfarin is extremely soluble in an aqueous medium and is completely absorbed from the gastrointestinal tract. It is almost totally bound to plasma proteins, which may be partially responsible for its long plasma half-life. The biologic half-life of warfarin ranges from 35 to 45 hours and is independent of the size of the dose.[106,124] Warfarin is metabolized by hepatic microsomal enzymes. It can cross the placental barrier, but there is no firm evidence that the drug appears in breast milk in significant amounts. In one study involving mothers and infants, no warfarin was found either in the mother's milk or in the plasma of the breast-fed infant.[125]

DOSE, ADMINISTRATION, AND CONTROL OF THERAPY

Treatment with warfarin is usually begun by the oral route. O'Reilly and Aggeler were the first to suggest that in order to decrease the danger of hemorrhage in sensitive patients, warfarin therapy should be started without large loading doses.[124,126] As suggested by the guidelines of the American Heart Association, warfarin therapy can be instituted with daily doses of 10 to 15 mg/d for the first 2 to 3 days.[101] Subsequent doses can be tailored according to the prothrombin time. Maintenance doses are usually less than 10 mg/d. To establish the optimum regimen for each patient, the prothrombin time should be monitored two to three times each week during the first several weeks of therapy. After the therapeutic range is achieved, the interval between prothrombin time determinations may be increased to 2 weeks. In some patients this interval may be increased to 3 or 4 weeks, but it is inadvisable to obtain a prothrombin time assay at intervals of more than 1 month.

Oral anticoagulants are contraindicated in patients with a hemorrhagic diathesis, poorly controlled hypertension, cerebrovascular hemorrhage, major trauma, active peptic ulcer disease, or overt bleeding from the gastrointestinal, genitourinary, or respiratory tracts. Inadequate laboratory facilities or unsatisfactory patient cooperation should also be considered as contraindications. Relative contraindications to oral anticoagulation include concomitant use of aspirin in a dose causing gastric erosion (over 325 mg/d), vasculitis, bacterial endocarditis, pericarditis complicating acute myocardial infarction, renal or liver disease, and thyrotoxicosis treated with radioactive iodine because of the possibility of gland hemorrhage. Adequate preparation before administration of oral anticoagulants may reduce the hazard of bleeding in disorders such as ulcerative colitis, sprue, steatorrhea, and pancreatitis. Among diabetic patients requiring long-term warfarin therapy, the question often arises whether anticoagulation would create the risk of vitreous or retinal hemorrhage.[101,127] Advanced age has been considered a relative contraindication to long-term oral anticoagulation due to potentially lethal side-effects and the frequent use of other drugs that may interact with warfarin.[127,128] Nevertheless, clear evidence concerning the risk–benefit ratio of oral anticoagulation in elderly patients is not available, and age alone should not proscribe the use of warfarin in patients at high risk of thromboembolism.[121,129–131]

Numerous medications interact with warfarin.[130] Therefore, it is vital to instruct all patients on warfarin therapy to report promptly when any drug is deleted from or added to their therapeutic regimen, including nonprescription compounds. Frequent prothrombin time determinations will permit dose adjustments that can prevent either underanticoagulation or overanticoagulation. Similarly, any major change in diet (e.g., leafy vegetables, green beans, and liver contain large amounts of vitamin K) should be reported so that drug dosage can be adjusted based on more frequent determinations of the prothrombin time. Drugs that interact with warfarin can do so by altering warfarin absorption, plasma protein binding, and metabolism, consequently causing significant potentiation or inhibition of the drug's anticoagulant effect. A list of the more important interactions is presented in Figure 9.7.

The prothrombin time is the test most frequently used to monitor warfarin therapy. It is performed by adding calcium and thromboplastin to citrated plasma and then measuring the time to fibrin formation. Thromboplastin is an extract of brain, lung, or placenta that contains tissue factor and phospholipid, which are necessary for the activation of factor X by factor VII.[124,132] Thromboplastins extracted from different organs or species or by different methods (saline versus acetone) can vary significantly in their sensitivity to reductions in levels of vitamin K-dependent factors; that is, a single plasma sample from a patient on coumarin could yield significantly different prothrombin times if assayed in two different laboratories that used different commercial thromboplastins. Approximately 90% of the thromboplastins used in North America are extracted from rabbit brain. However, major variations in prothrombin times between laboratories may occur. However, thromboplastins used in the United Kingdom are significantly more sensitive to reductions in vitamin K-dependent factors than most North American thromboplastins. Therefore, in order to properly interpret the laboratory test and clinical literature concerning

FIGURE 9.7 DRUGS AFFECTING ANTICOAGULANT ACTIVITY

Enhanced Effect		Decreased Effect
Chloramphenicol	Disulfiram	Vitamin K
Cimetidine	Sulfonamides	Oral contraceptives
Anabolic steroids	Chloral hydrate	Rifampin
D-Thyroxine	Alcohol (abuse only)	Griseofulvin
Clofibrate	Allopurinol	Glutethimide
Metronidazole	Amiodarone	Cholestyramine
Phenylbutazone	Antibiotics	Barbiturates
Sulfinpyrazone	Methyldopa	Phenytoin
Quinidine	Aspirin (in high doses)	

oral anticoagulation, the reader must bear in mind the thromboplastin used (Fig. 9.8).

In an effort to standardize prothrombin time determinations and thus allow direct comparison of assays performed with different thromboplastins, the World Health Organization (WHO) has recommended the use of an international normalized ratio (INR), which is defined as the prothrombin time (PT) ratio (i.e., PT observed/PT mean control) results that would be obtained if WHO primary international reference thromboplastin (IRP) were used to test the plasma sample.[124,132] This is based on the determination of the international sensitivity index (ISI) of the thromboplastin used in the local laboratory. The ISI is a measure of the responsiveness of a given thromboplastin to reduction of the vitamin K-dependent coagulation factors. For a PT ratio with a thromboplastin with an ISI value of C, INR = (observed ratio)^C. For example, for a thromboplastin with an ISI of 1.4, a PT ratio of 2.5 is equivalent to $2.5^{1.4} = 3.6$ with the IRP. Today it is recommended that all laboratories report INR measurements and the PT.

The intensity of oral anticoagulation necessary to properly treat or prevent intravascular thrombosis varies depending on the clinical situation. The American College of Chest Physicians Conference on Antithrombotic Therapy has offered the following recommendations concerning oral anticoagulant therapy.[132]

1. A less intense degree of oral anticoagulation (INR 2.0 to 3.0, corresponding to a PT ratio of 1.3 to 1.5 using a typical North American thromboplastin with an ISI = 2.4) should be used in the following clinical situations:

a. Prevention of venous thromboembolism in high-risk patients

b. Treatment of venous thrombosis and pulmonary embolism (after an initial course of heparin)

c. Prevention of systemic embolism in patients with tissue cardiac valve prostheses and in selected patients with atrial fibrillation, acute transmural anterior wall myocardial infarction, or valvular heart disease

2. A more intense degree of oral anticoagulation (INR = 2.5 to 3.5, corresponding to a PT ratio of 1.4 to 1.7 using a typical North American thromboplastin with an ISI = 2.4) should be used in patients with mechanical cardiac valve prostheses, in patients with recurrent systemic thromboembolism, and in patients with recent arterial thrombosis.

SIDE EFFECTS

The most important side effect of oral anticoagulation is bleeding. The risk of bleeding varies from patient to patient depending on the intensity of anticoagulation, the indication for its use, and the presence of co-morbid conditions. Hull and colleagues have shown that in patients with venous thrombosis, those randomized to more intense anticoagulant therapy (INR 2.5 to 4.5) have a risk of bleeding over five times greater (22% versus 4%) than those randomized to less intense anticoagulation (INR 2.0).[133] Levine and colleagues pooled data from 171 studies dealing with rates of bleeding in patients on long-term oral anticoagulant therapy.[121,129,134] The risk of major bleeding (intracranial or retroperitoneal bleeding or bleeding leading directly to death, hospitalization, or transfusion) was 8.1% in patients anticoagulated because of venous thromboembolism, 7% in ischemic cerebrovascular disease, 4.7% in ischemic heart disease, and 2.4% in patients with prosthetic cardiac valves. The incidence of major bleeding is best expressed in terms of rate per 100 patient-years of therapy. It ranges from 2 to 22/100 patient-years in ischemic cerebrovascular disease and from 0 to 7.7/100 patient-years in myocardial infarction and is 0.8/100 patient-years in patients with prosthetic cardiac valves. Levine and colleagues[121,129,134] concluded that the reason for the relatively high incidence of bleeding complications in patients with ischemic cerebrovascular disease and venous thromboembolism is the frequent presence of co-morbid conditions such as hypertension, malignancy, and recent surgery.

Bleeding in patients on oral anticoagulants may occur at unusual sites. Hemorrhage into the bowel lumen, the intestinal wall, the mesentery, the rectus muscle, or the corpus luteum may simulate an acute abdominal crisis. Similar conditions apply to genitourinary bleeding, which may mimic a renal tumor. Hematomas may cause carpal tunnel compression, and, rarely, there may be pericardial, adrenal, or retroperitoneal hemorrhage. When to search for the cause of an episode of spontaneous bleeding, such as from the genitourinary or gastrointestinal tracts, can be decided if the prothrombin time is obtained within 24 hours of hemorrhage. Experience has shown that when the prothrombin time ratio is in the range of 1.5 to 2.0, the likelihood of finding a localized lesion is greater than if the prothrombin time is in excess of 2.5. In the former situation, further efforts to identify the bleeding source should be undertaken promptly.

FIGURE 9.8 THERAPEUTIC RANGES FOR VARIOUS THROMBOPLASTINS EQUIVALENT TO THE CONVENTIONAL RANGE WITH THE BRITISH COMPARATIVE THROMBOPLASTIN (RATIO 2.0 – 4.0)

Reagent	Range of Ratios
British Comparative Thromboplastin	2.0–4.0
Thrombotest	2.0–3.5
Rabbit thromboplastin (brain–lung)	1.5–2.0
Rabbit thromboplastin (brain)	1.3–1.7

Minor bleeding in patients with prolonged prothrombin times can be treated by withholding warfarin temporarily. Major bleeding will necessitate discontinuing the drug and administration of vitamin K_1 or blood products, when appropriate. The dose of vitamin K_1 depends not only on the endpoint desired but also on the intensity of warfarin effect. A common mistake is the administration of a high dose of vitamin K_1 in an effort to return the prothrombin time to normal more rapidly. Larger doses of vitamin K_1 do not increase the rate of synthesis of the individual vitamin K-dependent clotting factors; rather, vitamin K_1 restores extrinsic synthesis rates for a period that is dose dependent. The route of vitamin K_1 administration may be intravenous, subcutaneous, or oral, depending on the nature and urgency of the clinical situation. Some correction of the prothrombin time is noted within 6 hours, and full correction occurs within 24 hours. If the patient is to remain on warfarin, the dose should be limited to 0.5 to 1.0 mg. Higher amounts, up to 10 mg, may be indicated if the patient is not to be maintained on therapy after the hemorrhage is controlled. Large doses of vitamin K_1 may make the patient resistant to warfarin for many days, preventing effective anticoagulant therapy for that time period. An immediate reversal of the clotting defect can be achieved by transfusion of blood, plasma, or plasma concentrates rich in the vitamin K-dependent clotting factors. Because these factors are relatively stable, they remain fully potent in ordinary banked blood or lyophilized plasma. Three units or 15 ml/kg of blood or plasma should suffice for an initial effect, providing time for concomitant vitamin K_1 administration to exert its action.[101] In patients with limited cardiac reserve, the recommended volumes of blood or plasma may precipitate pulmonary edema unless significant blood loss has occurred. Plasma concentrates rich in factors II, VII, IX, and X obviate the hazard of hypervolemia but carry with them the risk of thrombosis, hepatitis, and AIDS.

Nonhemorrhagic side effects of warfarin include coumarin embryopathy and coumarin-induced skin necrosis. Coumarin readily crosses the placenta and has been found to be teratogenic, particularly during the first trimester of pregnancy.[135] Fetal bone and cartilage development seems to be sensitive to warfarin, as evidenced by the best described abnormalities of coumarin embryopathy: nasal deformity and stippling of the bony epiphyses. This effect may be mediated by deficiency of osteocalcin, a vitamin K-dependent protein.[136] An increased incidence of fetal wastage and central nervous system defects has also been observed with exposure to warfarin during pregnancy.[137] For this reason, the majority of experts advise substitution of subcutaneous heparin (e.g., approximately 10,000 to 15,000 units subcutaneously every 12 hours with target APTT 1.5 to 2 times control) for coumarin at least during the first trimester of pregnancy as well as for several weeks prior to delivery.[138] Indeed, high-dose subcutaneous heparin has been advocated all throughout the pregnancy by many.[135,136] Therefore, fertile women receiving warfarin must be warned of the risks of teratogenicity and should be advised to notify their physicians at the earliest suspicion of pregnancy.

Coumarin-induced necrosis of the skin and subcutaneous tissues is a rare but striking complication of warfarin therapy that has been associated with hereditary protein C deficiency.[139] The lesion appears within 3 to 10 days of drug administration, usually in the lower half of the body. It occurs particularly in women and in areas of abundant subcutaneous fat, such as the buttocks, breasts, thighs, and abdomen. The initial manifestation of coumarin-induced skin necrosis is an erythematous patch. Frank hemorrhagic necrosis may develop within 24 hours. Coumarin necrosis should not be confused with purple toes syndrome,[140] in which painful, blue toes develop, often with livedo reticularis to the knees or to the iliac crest; this is believed to represent atheromatous embolization to the extremities, perhaps accentuated by warfarin.[141] When coumarin-induced necrosis occurs, warfarin should be discontinued. If further anticoagulation is indicated, heparin therapy should be initiated.[101]

Thrombolytic Agents

The acute coronary syndromes, including acute myocardial infarction, unstable angina, and sudden death, are caused by thrombotic occlusion of critically situated blood vessels. Timely pharmacologic dissolution of blood clots therefore might abort the evolution of these syndromes with preservation of the myocardium and reduction of mortality. This can be achieved with intravenous infusion of thrombolytic agents, which convert plasminogen, the inactive proenzyme of the fibrinolytic system, to the proteolytic enzyme plasmin, which lyses the fibrin of blood clots (see Fig. 9.3).[142] Plasminogen can be converted to plasmin by several different types of plasminogen activator.[142-144] Plasmin is a serine protease that digests fibrin to soluble degradation products. Natural inhibition of the fibrinolytic system occurs both at the level of the plasminogen and also at the level of the plasmin. Plasminogen is a single-chain glycoprotein consisting of 790 amino acids that is converted to plasmin by cleavage of the Arg560–Val561 peptide bond. The plasminogen molecule contains structures, called lysine-binding sites, that mediate its binding to fibrin and accelerate the interactions between plasmin and its physiologic inhibitor α_2-antiplasmin. The lysine binding plays a critical role in the regulation of fibrinolysis. Plasminogen activators are serine proteases with a high specificity for plasminogen, which hydrolyze the Arg560–Val561 peptide bond.

Currently, five thrombolytic agents are either approved for clinical use or under clinical investigation in patients with acute myocardial infarction: streptokinase, recombinant tissue-type plasminogen activator (rt-PA), acylated plasminogen streptokinase activator complex (APSAC), urokinase, and single-chain urokinase-type plasminogen activator (scu-PA, prourokinase).[142-144] Readers should bear in mind that the field of thrombolysis is progressing rapidly and the goal of this section is to present a brief overview of the current status of thrombolysis.

STREPTOKINASE

Mechanism of Action

Streptokinase is a nonenzymatic antigenic protein produced by Lancefield group-C strains of β-hemolytic streptococci. It forms a 1:1 stoichiometric complex with plasminogen, a process that exposes the active site of the light chain of plasminogen. This complex is converted spontaneously to a streptokinase-plasmin complex, which is a powerful activator of plasminogen. Streptokinase, however, does not discriminate between circulating and fibrin-bound plasminogen. Circulating plasmin is initially neutralized by α-antiplasmin, but when the antiplasmin level is significantly reduced, plasmin exerts its proteolytic effects on several plasma proteins, including fibrinogen and factors V and VIII; this last reaction contributes to the bleeding risk of streptokinase. The half-life of streptokinase in the blood is approximately 30 minutes.[142]

Reperfusion

Many factors influence the success of thrombolytic therapy: some relate to the nature of the occlusion, such as the age and location and the concentration of plasminogen and plasmin inhibitors on the thrombus; others relate to the therapeutic regimen, such as the dosage of the agent used, the duration of the therapy, and the speed with which treatment is begun.[142–146] Rentrop and co-workers pioneered the use of intracoronary streptokinase in patients with acute myocardial infarction.[147] The enthusiasm stemmed in part from the anticipated greater incidence of thrombolysis with the drug delivered directly in the vicinity of the clot, the potential for efficacy with a lower dose, and the advantage of confirmation of the presence of an occlusive thrombus prior to treatment and angiographic assessment of its response to lytic therapy. Although these advantages are real, the delay associated with intracoronary administration and the relatively limited immediate availability of cardiac catheterization facilities for most patients presenting with acute infarction have led to virtual abandonment of the intracoronary route as the primary or sole approach for most patients. The collective experience from numerous earlier studies of intracoronary streptokinase with a dose of 250,000 units in patients with acute myocardial infarction indicates that thrombolysis with reperfusion occurs in about 85% of patients.[148–150]

The reported patency rate of intravenous streptokinase in patients with acute myocardial infarction is lower than that achieved with intracoronary streptokinase. The cumulative database from angiographic studies indicates that the infarct vessel patency rate at 60 to 120 minutes was approximately 48% with the use of 1.5 million units infused over 1 hour.[151–162] However, a definite "catch-up" phenomenon for streptokinase has been documented by serial angiography performed up to 24 hours after symptom onset. By the time of late follow-up cardiac catheterization, the patency rate of arteries treated with streptokinase approaches 80%. An increased recanalization rate (above 80%) without increased bleeding complications has recently been reported with a different lytic approach: "front-loaded t-PA regimen."[163]

Complications

The complications of administration of intracoronary streptokinase are related to the catheterization and angiographic procedures, the thrombolytic agent, the adverse effects of reperfusion, and the consequences of reocclusion. The major risk of either intracoronary or intravenous streptokinase is hemorrhage.[164] A systemic lytic state with fibrinogenolysis is induced even when the subtherapeutic or low-dose intracoronary streptokinase is administered. Bleeding occurs most frequently at the site of vascular puncture. However, systemic hemorrhage, including cerebral, gastrointestinal, mediastinal, and urinary tract bleeding, may be encountered, particularly when occult predisposing causes are present. The reported prevalence of hemorrhage requiring transfusion after intracoronary or intravenous streptokinase has ranged from 1.3% to 18%, but most studies report an incidence of 10% or less. Fortunately, the incidence of intracerebral bleeding is rare, occurring in less than 1% of patients.[144–146] Transient hypotensive episodes have also been reported in approximately 9% of patients given intracoronary streptokinase and in 17% of patients given intravenous streptokinase.[164] However, hypotension has generally responded to transient interruption of the infusion of streptokinase and administration of fluids or atropine. Another side effect of streptokinase is related to its antigenicity. Overt allergic reactions are not common. Frank anaphylaxis is extremely rare, and rash, swollen lips, and urticaria occur in less than 2% of patients.[164]

RECOMBINANT TISSUE-TYPE PLASMINOGEN ACTIVATORS

Mechanism of Action

Native tissue-type plasminogen activator (t-PA) is a trypsin-like serine protease composed of 527 amino acids and produced by recombinant DNA technology.[142,144–146] As a consequence of limited plasmin action on the fibrin surface, native t-PA is rapidly converted to a two-chain activator. The heavy chain (A) of this molecule contains two regions that share a high degree of homology with the five kringles of plasminogen, while the catalytic site is located on the light chain (B).[142,144–146] The one-chain and two-chain forms of t-PA have different amidolytic activities in vitro, but have virtually the same fibrinolytic activity. t-PA is a poor plasminogen activator in the absence of fibrin, but it binds specifically to fibrin and activates plasminogen at the fibrin surface several hundred times more efficiently than in the circulation. The underlying principle of this phenomenon is that both plasminogen and t-PA bind to fibrin and form a cyclic ternary complex. Thus, fibrin serves as a cofactor for plasminogen activation by lowering the K_m of t-PA for plasminogen. As a consequence of these kinetic characteristics, plasmin is predominately generated on the fibrin surface.[144–146] This in turn results in a relative sparing of circulating fibrinogen and other plasma proteins to plasmin-mediated degradation. Recombinant tissue-type plasminogen activator (rt-PA) is produced through complex biologic techniques, is predominately single-chain t-PA, and is the only one currently on the market for clinical use.

The optimal regimen of rt-PA has not yet been established. The use of a high dosage (150 mg) appears to yield a higher patency rate but is associated with a significantly higher incidence of intracerebral hemorrhage. Thus, a dose of 100 mg is currently recommended.[144–146] Other approaches like a "front-loaded rt-PA regimen" are promising.[163]

Reperfusion

The cumulative data from numerous angiographic studies[151–163] in patients with acute myocardial infarction indicate that the infarct vessel patency rate is approximately 80% at 120 minutes after 100 mg of rt-PA. Controversy exists as to whether the fibrin specificity of rt-PA confers an advantage over streptokinase in terms of reperfusion and myocardial salvage. As discussed previously, although the patency rate at early phase appears to be higher in patients receiving rt-PA, a "catch-up" phenomenon has been demonstrated for streptokinase. At 24 hours after thrombolytic therapy, the patency rate of arteries treated with agents lacking fibrin selectivity is similar to that of patients treated with rt-PA. Thus, although rt-PA holds promise for improved early coronary thrombolytic action, it has not yet been demonstrated whether this effect translates into superior preservation of left ventricular function or a reduction of mortality.[165]

Complications

Speculation has ranged from a prediction that rt-PA would be associated with less bleeding because of the absence of a systemic lytic state[166,167] to fear that it would result in an increased risk of bleeding secondary to augmented fibrinolytic potency.[145,168] Direct comparative trial data with streptokinase showed little difference in extracranial bleeding complications.[151,169–171] In the Thrombolysis in Myocardial Infarction-II (TIMI-II) trial,[172] the incidence of intracranial hemorrhage was 0.5% in 2742 patients treated with 100 mg. As opposed to other large mortality trials,[173–176] this overall low frequency was established with detailed data collection and routine computed axial tomographic scanning for any new neurologic deficit. In contrast to streptokinase, rt-PA is nonantigenic and lacks hypotensive effect.

ACYLATED PLASMINOGEN STREPTOKINASE ACTIVATOR COMPLEX

Mechanism of Action

Acylated plasminogen-streptokinase-activator complex (APSAC) is an equimolar complex of streptokinase and Lys-plasminogen that is rendered inactive by acylation of the catalytic center of the plasminogen portion.[142,144–146,177] When introduced in the systemic circulation, APSAC can attach itself to fibrin-bound plasminogen without being inactivated by α_2-antiplasmin. Deacylation occurs spontaneously and results in sustained activity. Activation of APSAC bound to the fibrin of clot theoretically confers a fibrin specificity to the drug. In fact, when the drug is administered intravenously to patients at therapeutic dose (30 units), systemic fibrinogenolysis is constant. Progressive deacylation after injection confers a prolonged half-life to the drug, averaging 90 minutes compared with 23 minutes for streptokinase. This prolonged half-life results in long-lasting thrombolytic effects. Because the intravenous injection of the complex does not cause profound hemodynamic effects, the drug can be administered in a bolus injection.[144–146,177]

Reperfusion

Results of several clinical studies[177–179] indicate that the patency rate of infarct-related artery at 90 minutes after intravenous APSAC (30 units) is approximately 69%. A direct comparison of intravenous APSAC and streptokinase was made in a French randomized, open-designed, multicenter study and demonstrated a slightly higher patency rate in patients receiving APSAC as compared with streptokinase (72% versus 55%).[179] A larger, more definitive trial of intravenous APSAC versus streptokinase has just been completed in the United States, but the results have not yet been presented.

Complications

The bleeding complication rate produced by APSAC is remarkably similar to that of other thrombolytic agents with or without fibrin specificity. In a French multicenter trial involving 231 patients, a bleeding complication was observed in 6.5% of the APSAC-treated patients, and only half of these patients required blood transfusion.[179]

UROKINASE AND SINGLE-CHAIN UROKINASE-TYPE PLASMINOGEN ACTIVATOR

Mechanism of Action

Urokinase is a double-chain glycoprotein that acts as a trypsin-like protease.[142–144] It occurs in two molecular forms—S1 (32 kd) and S2 (54 kd)—the former being a proteolytic degradation product of the latter. Urokinase isolated from human urine or cultured embryonic kidney cells is nonantigenic. It is a direct activator of plasminogen and generates plasmin by cleaving the Arg560–Val561 bond of the plasminogen molecule. Urokinase does not have fibrin specificity and activates fibrin-bound as well as circulating plasminogen; therefore, it also induces a systemic activation of the fibrinolytic system as soon as the α_2-antiplasmin level is reduced. The half-life of urokinase is about 10 minutes, and thus the persistence of thrombolysis may be less than with streptokinase. Single-chain urokinase-type plasminogen activator (scu-PA) or prourokinase is a single-chain glycoprotein containing 411 amino acids, which is converted to urokinase by hydrolysis of the Lys158–Ile159 peptide bond. scu-PA has very little activity toward low-molecular-weight substrate but has intrinsic plasminogen-activating potential, although with a catalytic efficiency that is two orders of magnitude lower than that of urokinase. The half-life of scu-PA is about 8 minutes.[142–144]

Reperfusion

Two reports[180,181] have indicated that the patency rate at 60 minutes in patients with acute myocardial infarction given either intracoronary or intravenous urokinase is about 60%. This moderately fibrin-selective thrombolytic agent can be given intravenously with a reduced systematic lytic state and predictably lower bleeding risk than intravenous streptokinase. The recanalization rate of scu-PA in patients with acute myocardial infarction is about 78% as reported by Van de Werf and co-workers[182] using 70 mg of scu-PA infused over 1 hour. The potential value of these two agents may relate to synergistic effects on clot lysis and reperfusion when combined with other thrombolytic agents. Topol and colleagues[183] have demonstrated that although the patency rates in patients with acute myocardial infarction given the combination of t-PA and urokinase were not significantly higher than those achieved by t-PA alone, the reocclusion rate was substantially lower. Similarly, some beneficial effects in terms of bleeding complications and reocclusion were observed when the combination of t-PA and scu-PA was used.[184] Other combinations such as t-PA and streptokinase are currently being evaluated. These synergistic combinations of thrombolytic agents may offer better cost–benefit and risk–benefit ratios than single-agent therapy. However, in order to reach valid conclusions, continued investigation of synergism should be carried out using investigational procedures with respect to both experimental design and data analysis

PATHOGENESIS OF THROMBOSIS AND EMBOLISM IN CORONARY ARTERIES, CARDIAC CHAMBERS, AND PROSTHETIC VALVES

The pathogenic mechanisms leading to thrombosis and embolism appear to differ among coronary arteries, cardiac chambers, and prosthetic heart valves. The pathogenesis of arterial thrombosis involves damage to the vessel wall and exposure of a thrombogenic substrate leading to platelet activation and fibrin formation. Intracavitary thrombosis mainly occurs in situations of blood stasis, which favor the activation of the coagulation system and the generation of fibrin. Platelet activation may play a role in the presence of endocardial injury. Prosthetic heart valves mainly promote activation, primarily of the coagulation system and secondarily of the platelets.

Coronary Arteries: Platelets and Fibrin

THE CONCEPT OF VASCULAR INJURY: PLATELETS AND FIBRIN

Vascular injury and thrombus formation represent the key events in the progression of atherosclerosis, in the pathogenesis of acute coronary syndromes, and in various vascular diseases. We have previously proposed a pathologic classification of vascular injury and its pathophysiologic cellular responses in an attempt to help to understand the pathogenesis of various vascular diseases and formulate therapeutic strategies in the prevention of these diseases.[185,186] We proposed the classification of vascular injury into three types (Fig. 9.9):

Type I: functional alterations of endothelial cells without significant morphologic changes

Type II: endothelial denudation and intimal injury but with intact internal elastic lamina and media

Type III: endothelial denudation with damage of intima and media

In type I endothelial injury no significant platelet deposition or thrombus formation can be demonstrated, although there is some recent evidence that a few platelets interact with such subtly injured endothelium and contribute, by the release of growth factors, to some intimal hyperplasia; this may be the basis of the initiation of the atherosclerotic process. In contrast, with type II injury, an obvious monolayer or a few layers of platelets with or without thrombus formation can be seen; the release of platelet growth factors may contribute to an accelerated intimal hyperplasia as it occurs in the coronary vein graft within the first postoperative year. In type III injury with exposure of components of the medial layer, particularly the fibrillar collagen, marked platelet aggregation with mural thrombus formation follows. Vascular injury of this magnitude also stimulates thrombin formation through both the intrinsic (surface-activated) and extrinsic (tissue factor–dependent) coagulation pathways, in which the platelet membrane facilitates interactions between clotting factors (see Fig. 9.1). And as discussed above, thrombin promotes the formation and polymerization of fibrin, which stabilizes the expanding thrombotic mass, allowing it to resist dislodgement by the forces of arterial blood flow. Like collagen, thrombin is also a powerful activator of platelet aggregation. Platelets and the coagulation system are therefore clearly interrelated in the genesis of arterial thrombosis following deep type III injury as it is seen in the acute coronary syndromes or following coronary angioplasty.

LABILE VERSUS FIXED THROMBUS

Delivery and activation of platelets at the site of vascular injury are dependent both on shear rate, which is a measure of the difference in blood velocity between the center and the periphery of the vessel, and on the degree of vessel injury (type II versus type III). In areas of luminal stenosis, a high shear rate promotes contact between blood elements and the vessel wall[10] and favors platelet activation. Most importantly, the influence of the severity of vascular injury on thrombus formation has been demonstrated in perfusion chamber experiments[9] in which different tissue substrates were exposed to blood at various shear rates. With type II vascular injury, platelet deposition and thrombus formation may occur, but the phenomenon is usually transient; with type III injury, platelet aggregation is considerably increased, leading to fixation of thrombus and persistent vascular occlusion.

CLINICAL CORRELATIONS OF VASCULAR INJURY AND THROMBOSIS

The concepts of vascular injury and thrombosis are important in the understanding of the pathogenesis of various vascular diseases, including the initiation and progression of atherosclerosis, the acute coronary syndromes, vein graft disease, and restenosis following coronary angioplasty.

Initiation and Progression of Atherosclerosis

The process of type I vascular injury followed by intermittent deposition of a few platelets and monocytes, lipid accumulation, smooth muscle cell proliferation, and resultant plaque formation represents the prevalent view of the initiation of spontaneous atherogenesis.[2,186,187] However, the precise nature of the injury remains unknown; that is, whether it is the turbulence of blood flow that injures the endothelium or whether it is injured from inside the vessel wall by means of toxic lipids (oxidized cholesterol) is controversial.

Accumulating evidence suggests that repetitive type II injury of soft fatty plaques (see later in section on acute coronary syndromes) with thrombus formation and incorporation represents a major mechanism for the progression of atherosclerosis.[186,188,189] In an autopsy study[190] of coronary arteries of 129 patients with atheromatous disease who died of noncardiac causes, Davies and co-workers demonstrated that 16% of the arteries studied revealed the presence of fissure in atherosclerotic plaque (type II

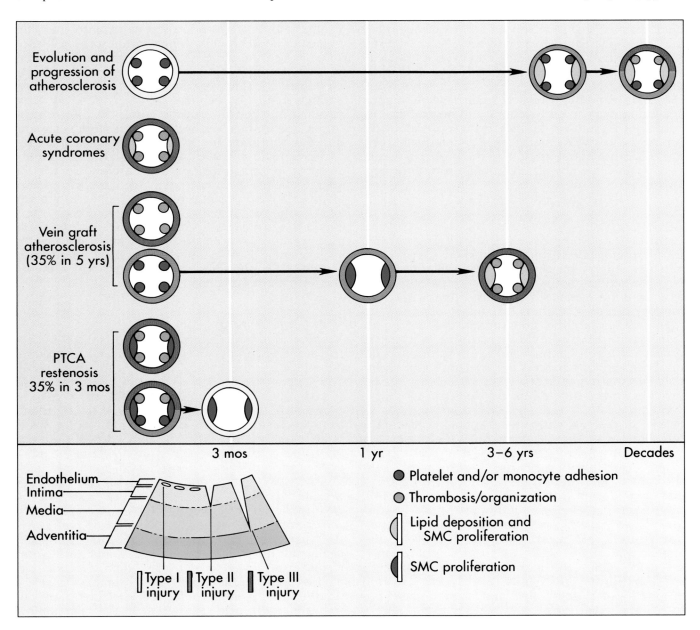

Figure 9.9 The role of vascular injury and various cellular interactions in the pathogenesis of atherosclerosis, acute coronary syndromes, acute and chronic vein graft occlusion, and PTCA restenosis. (PTCA = percutaneous transluminal coronary angioplasty; SMC = smooth muscle cells)

injury) and, in some cases, overlying thrombi. This degree of frequency of plaque fissure (type II injury) in a static pathologic evaluation probably suggests that a single plaque may undergo many fissures, with subsequent thrombus formation and organization, during the evolution and progression into an advanced lesion. Indeed, analysis of coronary trees in patients dying of ischemic heart disease showed morphologic appearance consistent with previously healed fissures with various stages of thrombus incorporation and organization to be almost ubiquitous and suggested that most fissures probably reseal with incorporation of overlying thrombus without manifestation of clinical symptoms.[8,189] Further evidence supporting thrombosis and thrombus incorporation as part of plaque progression is provided by a study using monoclonal antibodies in identifying fibrin, fibrinogen, and their degradation products.[191] It was demonstrated that in advanced fibrous plaque, fibrin and fibrin-related products were detected in the intima, neointima, and subintima and even in the deeper medial layer, especially around thrombus, collagen, and smooth muscle cells; on the other hand, these fibrin and fibrin-related products were found in small quantities in early lesions and normal arteries. Although it is as yet unknown how prevalent this process is, its clinical significance is potentially enormous because mural thrombi in the region of fissures may be prevented by platelet inhibitors or anticoagulant agents.

Acute Coronary Syndromes

Pathologic,[8,192] angioscopic,[193] and angiographic[194,195] data have firmly established that type III vascular injury—major plaque and plaque rupture, with formation of mural and/or occlusive thrombus as a common mechanism—leads to the acute coronary syndromes, namely, unstable angina, acute myocardial infarction, and sudden death. In addition, accumulating evidence indicates that the process of type III injury and the resulting intraluminal thrombotic process are dynamic and repetitive, and this dynamic process has been suggested to provide a physiologic link between these clinical syndromes.[2,7,196] Indeed, pathologic studies by Falk[192] in patients with unstable angina leading to infarction or sudden death revealed the presence of layers of thrombi of different age in the majority of cases, suggesting that recurrent episodes of mural thrombosis and organization, rather than a single episode of abrupt thrombotic event, occurred in the transition between these syndromes. Similarly, studies[195,197] in patients with unstable angina have demonstrated both a rapid progression of stenosis angiographically as well as clinical deterioration to myocardial infarction in a significant percentage of these patients. This again reflects the dynamic process of intraluminal thrombosis and organization in these clinical syndromes. In addition, there is increasing evidence suggesting that the coronary lesion responsible for unstable angina and acute myocardial infarction is frequently only mildly to moderately stenotic. For example, Ambrose and co-workers[195,197,198] demonstrated that over 70% of the lesions responsible for unstable angina have a prior

stenosis of less than 50%, while about one half of the lesions leading to acute myocardial infarction have nonsignificant narrowing. This strongly supports the idea that type III injury of a small plaque with superimposed thrombosis is the primary determinant of acute occlusion, rather than the severity of the underlying lesion, in a significant proportion of patients presenting with acute coronary syndromes. Similar pathogenic mechanisms of sudden death can also be inferred from the pathologic data. For example, Davies and colleagues[190] reported that over 70% of sudden cardiac death cases have evidence of recent mural and/or occlusive intraluminal thrombus overlying the sites of plaque fissure and rupture at autopsy.

Thus, type III vascular injury—plaque rupture—with thrombus formation appears to be the major mechanism leading to the acute coronary syndromes.[2] In a proportion of patients with unstable angina, type III vascular injury in the form of fissure may lead to transient vessel occlusion and ischemia by labile thrombus; in some of these patients, a more permanent occlusion may lead to infarction or sudden death. Indeed, myocardial infarction may result from type III vascular injury in the form of an ulcer, and thus be associated with more persistent and fixed thrombotic coronary occlusion in the face of inadequate collateral flow. In addition, spontaneous or pharmacologic lysis of thrombus occurs in some patients, placing them at high risk of reocclusion.[2,7,196] Why a plaque ruptures, leading to growth of the atherosclerotic plaque or acute coronary syndromes, is unclear. Thus far, it appears that the small plaques that rupture are soft because they have a high content of fat (vulnerable plaques); in addition they contain numerous macrophages, which favors the formation of an abscess.[2,186,199]

Vein Graft Disease

Vascular injury also appears to be the critical initiating event in coronary vein graft disease. Vein grafts are subject to mechanical injury, which may occur when the veins are harvested or in handling during the operation, resulting in a transient predominantly type III injury; this injury may lead to acute thrombotic occlusion, but in most cases the vessel wall heals quickly.[200,201] With the exposure of the vein grafts to a relatively high pressure flow and the presence of various biologic risk factors such as hypercholesterolemia and smoking, this may induce and perpetuate type II injury and hinder the process of reendothelialization, which might otherwise occur under normal conditions. During the first postoperative year, the most notable and consistent histologic change in the vein graft is marked intimal thickening characterized by smooth muscle cell proliferation and an increase in hyaline matrix.[201] Lie and associates[202] reported that even within 3 weeks after the operation, smooth muscle cells appear in the subendothelial portion of the intima, followed by proliferation and fibrointimal thickening. Beyond the first year after operation, there is further connective tissue synthesis from smooth muscle cells and fibroblasts, followed by incorporation of lipid into the lesions. In the presence of various biologic risk factors, such as hyperlipidemia and smoking, this process can be accelerated and enhanced, leading to vascular occlusion. Thus, graft specimens from patients between 1 and 5 years after operation show typical histologic features of atherosclerosis: a mixture of fibrous plaque with intimal hyperplasia, ulceration, cholesterol clefts, foam cells, and in some areas, calcification with disruption of the medial layer.[203] In addition, because of the predisposition of the fatty plaques to rupture (type III injury), occlusive or nonocclusive thrombus formation may also occur during this late stage of graft disease as documented in surgical specimens and autopsy studies.[202,203] In a recent report, two thirds of the vein grafts removed during a second coronary artery bypass operation showed evidence of mural or occlusive thrombus.[204]

Postangioplasty Restenosis

Type III vascular injury, associated with intense platelet aggregation and mural thrombus formation, also results in the release of various cellular growth factors and subsequent hyperplastic response[205]; this appears to be the pathogenic mechanism for coronary restenosis after percutaneous transluminal coronary angioplasty (PTCA). In a study of restenosis in pigs, it was demonstrated that immediately after balloon injury to the carotid arteries, type III injury was induced with marked platelet aggregation and mural thrombus formation.[206] Necrosis of the medial smooth muscle cells was evident at 24 hours, and the process of progressive intimal proliferation of smooth muscle cells and reorganization and incorporation of thrombi finally led to partial or total occlusion of the lumen. Type III changes in the vessel wall seen in patients who died several days after angioplasty included denudation of the endothelium, intimal necrosis, medial tear, adventitial hemorrhage, and thrombosis.[206–208] Coronary angioscopy studies[209,210] have also described mural thrombi, intimal flaps, dissection, and ruptured atheroma as common findings. In contrast to these acute morphologic features, specimens obtained weeks to months after successful angioplasty have shown marked circumferential fibrointimal thickening and organized thrombi at sites where chronic restenosis occurred.[205,207,208] Similarly, tissues removed from restenotic segments via atherectomy also have been composed mainly of smooth muscle cells and collagen.[211] The mitogenic stimuli appear to be due to the release of growth factors from aggregating platelets and possibly endothelial cells and smooth muscle cells.

Cardiac Chambers: Predominance Of Fibrin Component

Intracavitary mural thrombi develop frequently in patients with acute myocardial infarction, chronic left ventricular aneurysm, dilated cardiomyopathy, and atrial fibrillation.[3–5] The pathogenesis of thrombosis may be outlined along the lines established more than a century ago by the pathologist Rudolf Virchow, who defined a triad of precipitating factors: (1) endothelial injury, (2) a zone of circulatory stasis, and (3) a hypercoagulable state.[212] In addition to these factors, the clinical significance derives from the potential for systemic embolism, which also depends on dynamic forces of the circulation.

ENDOTHELIAL INJURY

In the first few days after acute myocardial infarction, leukocytic infiltration separates endothelial cells from their basal lamina.[213] The resulting exposure of subendothelial tissue to intracavitary blood serves as the nidus for thrombus development. Specific endocardial abnormalities have also been identified histologically in surgical and postmortem specimens from patients with left ventricular aneurysms[214] and at autopsy in patients with idiopathic dilated cardiomyopathy.[215]

BLOOD STASIS

Both experimental[216] and clinical studies[217,218] have emphasized the importance of wall motion abnormalities in the development of left ventricular thrombi, and it seems clear that stasis of blood in regions of akinesis or dyskinesis is the essential factor. Similarly, stasis is important in the development of atrial thrombi,[219] when effective mechanical atrial activity is impaired, as occurs in atrial fibrillation, atrial enlargement, mitral stenosis, and cardiac failure. Stasis is paramount to conditions of low shear rate, in which activation of the coagulation system rather than of platelets leads to fibrin formation and constitutes the predominant pathogenetic mechanism in the development of intracavitary thrombi (see Fig. 9.1).

HYPERCOAGULABLE STATE

One study of patients with acute myocardial infarction found a significantly greater incidence of thromboembolism in cases of elevated serum fibrinogen levels,[220] suggesting a hypercoagulable tendency in this condition. Although this limb of Virchow's triad is controversial, it is conceivable that a systemic procoagulant tendency arises during the acute stage of myocardial infarction and predisposes to thromboembolic events. More relevant is experimental evidence that suggests that the surface of a fresh thrombus is itself highly thrombogenic, producing at least a local if not a systemic hypercoagulable state.[7]

DYNAMIC FORCES OF THE CIRCULATION

The problems of thromboembolism originating from the cardiac chambers prompt consideration of the balance between the effects of regional injury, stasis, and procoagulant factors, which favor thrombus formation, and dynamic forces of the circulation, which are responsible for the migration of thrombotic material into the systemic circulation. Even though stasis favors thrombus formation within the sac of a left ventricular aneurysm, isolation from dynamic circulatory forces protects against embolic migration.[221,222] In diffusely dilated cardiomyopathy, on the other hand, mural thrombus is not isolated from the circulation and the embolic risk is higher. Thus, factors leading to thrombus formation are not the same as those that produce systemic embolism, and this paradox must not be neglected in the selection of therapeutic options.

Prosthetic Valves: Fibrin and Platelets
MECHANICAL PROSTHESIS

Once circulation is restored after implantation of a prosthetic cardiac valve, platelet deposition begins almost immediately both on the prosthetic surface itself—particularly on the endocardium-suture-prosthesis interfaces—and on damaged perivalvular tissues.[223,224] The prosthetic surface area exposed to the circulation is the major factor leading not only to platelet deposition but, more importantly, to activation of factor XII, initiating the coagulation cascade.[225] In addition, the flow stasis and abnormal hemodynamic characteristics of the prosthetic devices promote mainly fibrin generation and, less importantly, platelet activation (see Fig. 9.1). Finally, the process of fibrin thrombus formation can be facilitated in areas with stasis and decreased blood flow, such as in the left atrium during atrial fibrillation and in the left ventricle during low cardiac output state secondary to left ventricular dysfunction.

BIOLOGIC PROSTHESIS

Bioprosthetic valves are considerably less thrombogenic,[226] mainly because of the natural or biologic properties of the material used in their construction and also because of their characteristic axial flow profile, leaflet pliability, and cyclic sinusoidal washout.[225,227]

ROLE OF ANTITHROMBOTIC THERAPY IN CARDIAC DISEASE

We established in the foregoing sections the importance of pathogenesis at the site of thrombosis: platelet and fibrin components in arterial disease, predominance of fibrin in cardiac chambers, and predominance of fibrin over platelet component in prosthetic valves. We can also classify the various clinical heart disease syndromes according to absolute and relative risk of developing thromboembolic events (Fig. 9.10).[228] We shall discuss three general risk categories: the highest involving more than six episodes per 100 patients per year, a medium risk range of 2% to 6% annually, and a lower risk rate of less than two events per 100 patients per year. Persons without overt evidence of heart disease have a comparable annual event rate below 1%. The concept of pathogenesis and the concept of risk stratification define the therapeutic role and intensity of the various antithrombotic strategies in preventing thromboembolism in coronary arteries, cardiac chambers, and prosthetic heart valves.

Coronary Arteries
ACUTE CORONARY SYNDROMES

Type III vascular injury with recurrent thrombosis is the major mechanism linking the acute coronary syndromes. During the early phase of the acute

---

FIGURE 9.10 EMERGING ANTITHROMBOTIC APPROACH TO CARDIAC DISEASE BASED ON PATHOGENESIS AND THROMBOEMBOLIC RISK

	Thromboembolic Risk		
Pathogenesis	**High (> 6% per year)**	**Medium (2%–6% per year)**	**Low (<2% per year)**
Arterial system	Unstable angina Acute MI MI: after thrombolysis PTCA: early phase SVBG: early phase	Chronic stable angina Chronic phase after MI PTCA: chronic phase SVBG: chronic phase	Primary prevention of cardio-vascular disease
Platelets = Fibrin	Platelet inhibitor plus anticoagulant*	Platelet inhibitor or anticoagulant (INR 2.0–3.0)†	Platelet inhibitor‡
Cardiac chambers	A-fib: prior embolism A-fib: mitral stenosis	A-fib: other forms of organic heart disease Early phase after anterior MI Dilated cardiomyopathy	A-fib: idiopathic Chronic LV aneurysm
Fibrin > Platelets	Anticoagulant (INR 2.5–3.5 in prior embolism or 2.0–3.0 in mitral stenosis)	Anticoagulant (INR 2.0–3.0) Platelet inhibitor	Usually no need for therapy
Prosthetic valves	Old mechanical prostheses Mechanical prostheses: prior embolism	Recent mechanical prostheses Bioprostheses: A-fib	Bioprostheses: normal sinus rhythm
Fibrin > Platelets	Anticoagulant (INR 2.5–3.5 plus platelet inhibitor)	Anticoagulant (INR 2.5–3.5 in mechanical prostheses or 2.0–3.0 in bioprostheses)	Usually no need for therapy

*Heparin may be used in acute phase.
†Although both are beneficial, platelet inhibitor therapy is recommended based on lower toxicity, cost, and ease of administration.
‡Only to be considered for persons at high risk for coronary disease.
MI = Myocardial infarction; PTCA = Percutaneous transluminal coronary angioplasty; SVBG = Saphenous vein bypass graft; INR = International normalized ratio of prothrombin suppression; A-fib = Atrial fibrillation; LV = Left ventricular

coronary syndromes of unstable angina and acute myocardial infarction, the risk of developing thrombotic occlusion (or reocclusion after vessel reperfusion) is substantial, varying between 5% and 20%.[168] This high risk of thrombotic occlusion or reocclusion makes antithrombotic therapy mandatory in patients with unstable angina and myocardial infarction.

Unstable Angina

There have been three large, randomized, placebo-controlled, double-blind studies of aspirin in unstable angina. In the Veterans Administration Cooperative Study,[34] 1266 men with unstable angina were randomized to buffered aspirin (324 mg/d) or placebo for 12 weeks. During the treatment period, the incidence of death and acute myocardial infarction was reduced from 10.1% to 5.0% in the treated group (p = 0.0005). More importantly, the benefits of aspirin were maintained in the 1-year follow-up period. No increase in the gastrointestinal side effects was seen. In the Canadian Multicenter trial,[35] 555 patients (73% men) with unstable angina were randomized to receive aspirin (1300 mg/d), sulfinpyrazone (800 mg/d), a combination of both, or placebo. After 2 years, the incidence of death and myocardial infarction was reduced in the aspirin-treated groups from 17% to 8.6%, a risk reduction of 51% (p = 0.008). Sulfinpyrazone conferred no benefit and did not interact with aspirin. Gastrointestinal side effects were more frequently seen in the aspirin-treated groups, probably because of the high dosages used.

In the recently published Montreal Heart Institute Study,[229] 479 patients with unstable angina were randomized to aspirin (325 mg twice daily), intravenous heparin, a combination of both, or placebo. The study was ended after a mean of 6 days, when a final therapeutic decision for the individual patient was made. Aspirin significantly reduced the rate of myocardial infarction by 72% compared with placebo. Further support for the use of antiplatelet agents in unstable angina comes from the recently completed Italian Study of Ticlopidine in Unstable Angina (STAI).[82] Preliminary evidence from this study showed that the ticlopidine, at a dose of 250 mg twice daily for 6 months, reduced the incidence of mortality and myocardial infarction by more than 50%.

ANTICOAGULANTS Evidence of the beneficial effects of heparin in unstable angina was suggested by Telford and Wilson,[230] who demonstrated an 80% reduction in the incidence of myocardial infarction in patients with unstable angina treated with heparin for 7 days. Deficiencies in patient recruitment, however, left the conclusions of this study less convincing. The strongest support for immediate anticoagulation in unstable angina comes from the Montreal Heart Institute Study.[229] Heparin decreased the rate of infarction by 89% and the incidence of refractory angina by 50%. Although no statistically significant difference among aspirin, heparin, or their combination was found, there was a trend favoring heparin over aspirin.

There is already strong evidence supporting the use of either intravenous heparin or aspirin in the management of patients with unstable angina beginning as soon as after onset. Because a substantial proportion of these patients develop myocardial infarction despite treatment with one agent or the other, there is a pressing need to test combinations of low-dose aspirin and heparin in larger clinical trials. Indeed, preliminary reports from a randomized, placebo-controlled trial in patients with unstable angina demonstrated that combination use of intravenous heparin and aspirin significantly reduced the risk of myocardial infarction during the follow-up period of 90 days.[231] Further clinical trials and longer follow-up are needed to confirm the beneficial effects. Otherwise, beyond the acute phase, we recommend aspirin in a dose of 325 mg/d.

THROMBOLYTIC THERAPY The role of thrombolytic therapy in unstable angina is uncertain.[232] There are nine reported studies using thrombolytic therapy in patients with unstable angina. These studies[233–244] were all relatively small, and the data were inconclusive. As yet, there is no consensus on which patients with unstable angina will have clinical or angiographic benefit from thrombolytic therapy. Part of the problem in reaching a consensus is that these studies have differed in patient populations, timing of angiography after episodes of rest pain, baseline medications, dose, route, and duration of thrombolytic therapy, angiographic end points, and use of control groups for analysis of clinical outcome after thrombolytic therapy. More importantly, significant differences in coronary substrates leading to unstable angina as compared with those leading to acute myocardial infarction probably explain why the success in thrombolytic therapy in myocardial infarction cannot be duplicated in unstable angina.[232] First, of patients who present with an acute myocardial infarction with ST segment elevation, 70% to 90% have total occlusion of the infarct-related artery on angiography. In unstable angina, the frequency of total occlusion of the ischemic-related artery is significantly less, as low as 8%.[197] Second, the thrombus formation in unstable angina develops slowly after type III injury and much of the thrombus present in these lesions may be partially organized by the time of clinical presentation. This partial organization may explain the pathologic finding by Falk,[192] who showed layering of thrombus in most of the patients who died after an episode of unstable angina. Therefore, in such patients only small amounts of thrombus would be present and amenable to thrombolysis. In addition, thrombus formation in patients with unstable angina may occur not within the lumen but beneath the fibrous cap of the plaque. Moreover, after type III injury, there may be a geometric change in the shape of the plaque without significant intraluminal thrombus formation. In both situations, little thrombus would be available for thrombolysis.[232] Finally, the extent of type III injury in unstable angina is probably less than in acute myocardial infarction and may thus result in a smaller amount of intraluminal thrombus formation.[2,186]

Thus, at present, the data are insufficient to yield a definite conclusion. The future of thrombolysis in unstable angina is dependent on the results of large randomized trials similar to those in acute myocardial infarction. Both angiographic and clinical trials are required to assess the efficacy. The risks and benefits of thrombolysis will also need to be determined. Preliminary, unpublished information from a large trial

(TIMI Group) using rt-PA in unstable angina has been negative overall on both angiographic and clinical end points.[245]

Acute Myocardial Infarction

As in unstable angina, type III vascular injury and superimposed thrombotic occlusion play major roles in the development of acute myocardial infarction.[8] In some patients, particularly those with non-Q-wave infarction, spontaneous early vessel reperfusion occurs as a result of thrombus lysis or resolution of vasospasm, limiting myocardial necrosis[246,247] but setting the stage for subsequent ischemic events. The more extensive necrosis that occurs in Q-wave infarction probably results from persistent thrombotic coronary occlusion in the face of inadequate collateral flow. In addition, because spontaneous vessel recanalization seems to occur in both non-Q and Q-wave infarction, an aggressive antithrombotic approach using thrombolytic agents and antithrombotic drugs to these patients is beginning to emerge for achieving both successful lysis and the prevention of thrombotic reocclusion.

THROMBOLYTIC THERAPY AND RETHROMBOSIS[173,174] The use of thrombolytic therapy in acute myocardial infarction has been discussed elsewhere. We therefore will concentrate on one of the major problems we face currently in patients following successful thrombolytic therapy: rethrombosis.

Reocclusion after successful recanalization is a frequent problem that precludes improvement in left ventricular function and increases mortality. Serial coronary angiography is necessary before, during, and after therapy to assess the reperfusion of the artery. Thus, few studies have systemically determined the incidence of reocclusion. Some studies have defined nonangiographic clinical reperfusion and reocclusion, which is unreliable because of spasm or silent reocclusion with or without collaterals. In this context, early reocclusion is defined as the angiographic closure of a reperfused or patent artery within the first 24 hours of thrombolytic therapy and late occlusion as angiographic closure usually assessed just before hospital discharge. The rate of early reocclusion is quite variable; it ranges from 0% to 45% and usually is 6% to 18%. Late reocclusion ranges from 11% to 24%. Both processes are due to rethrombosis, which in turn appears to depend on two main factors[173]: (1) the pathologic substrate, namely, type III vascular injury with exposure of collagen and lipid gruel and the thrombogenic surface of the residual thrombus on the atherosclerotic plaque, and (2) the rheologic factors or the increase in shear rate and turbulent flow created by the residual stenosis.[9,10]

As discussed in the previous section, type III vascular injury with the exposure of various thrombotic elements creates a strong stimulus for thrombosis. Potent thrombotic stimuli include the release of tissue thromboplastin, depletion of factors that inhibit tissue factor, and the activation of platelets by collagen, fatty gruel, and smooth muscle cells.[2,186] In addition, deep medial structures such as the fibrillar collagen can activate the coagulation system. The intrinsic pathway is activated by the negatively charged collagen, while the extrinsic pathway is activated by the thromboplastin released from the damaged tissue. This leads to mural thrombosis. Furthermore, during lysis (endogenous or exogenous) there is release of active thrombin from within the dissolving thrombus and activation of platelets by the active surface of the thrombus. Thus, theoretically, the use of both an antiplatelet agent and an anticoagulant following thrombolysis appears to be advisable.

Thus, prevention of reocclusion requires inhibition of mechanisms involved in rethrombosis and includes two basic principles: (1) thorough lysis and (2) antithrombotic therapy. The first principle involves the use of the newer generation of, and synergistic combination of, thrombolytic agents. This area is under active investigation. Preliminary results with scu-PA[182-184] seem to be promising, especially in reducing the reocclusion rate. In addition, studies using a combined infusion of rt-PA and urokinase[183] appear to reduce the reocclusion rate as compared with that of rt-PA alone. Similarly, the use of streptokinase and half the usual dose of rt-PA revealed a late reocclusion rate of only 6%.[143,144] However, the data are still insufficient to conclude which combinations will provide the best therapeutic results; large randomized clinical trials are currently underway. The role of antiplatelet therapy and anticoagulant therapy is discussed below.

ANTIPLATELET THERAPY[39,248] The strongest evidence supporting the use of platelet inhibitors in the acute stage of myocardial infarction comes from the recently published Second International Study of Infarct Survival (ISIS-2).[36] Patients with suspected myocardial infarction treated within 24 hours had a 23% reduction in 5-week vascular mortality compared with those given placebo. This dramatic benefit was possibly related to prevention of reinfarction in patients with spontaneous vessel recanalization. Indeed, aspirin reduced the rate of nonfatal reinfarction by almost half.[36]

As discussed previously, patients with acute myocardial infarction treated with thrombolytic agents are at high risk of early reocclusion, which approaches 5% to 20%.[173,174,249] The importance of concomitant platelet inhibitor therapy in patients undergoing thrombolysis was emphasized by the results of the ISIS-2 trial,[36] in which streptokinase alone decreased early cardiovascular mortality by 25%, while the combination of aspirin and streptokinase decreased the death rate by 42% compared with placebo. The benefits of these agents appeared independent of one another, and the addition of aspirin to streptokinase reduced the clinical reinfarction rate by 50%. Thus, we advocate aspirin (160 to 325 mg daily) as early as possible in the treatment of acute myocardial infarction, whether or not thrombolytic agents are given. Daily aspirin therapy should be continued on discharge.

ANTICOAGULANT THERAPY[248,250] The role of anticoagulants in patients with acute infarction for the prevention of coronary rethrombosis, infarct extension, and death has not been settled. Of the large number of studies conducted, only three randomized trials[251-253] have been large enough to be able to detect a significant effect of therapy. Although all three studies showed a beneficial trend toward reduced incidence of death and reinfarction, only the Bronx Municipal Hospital trial[252] found a significant reduction (30%) in the case fatality rate. In addition, anticoagulation therapy has been clearly shown to reduce pulmonary and systemic embolism after myocardial infarction.[251-253] When the results of the only six published randomized trials were pooled,[254] a significant 21% reduction in mortality in treated patients emerged. Despite the limitation inherent in retrospective meta-analysis of heterogeneous trials, short-term anticoagulation in acute myocardial infarction appears to provide a modest reduction in early mortality. Because of the high risk of reinfarction, however, the combination of aspirin and an anticoagulant may prove beneficial and deserves clinical testing. The role of heparin in patients with acute myocardial infarction treated with thrombolytic therapy is unresolved. The reports from the large International TPA Versus Streptokinase Mortality Trial[173] and the ISIS-3 trial[174] demonstrated no significant improvement in mortality and reinfarction rate in patients treated with both thrombolytic therapy and high-dose subcutaneous heparin compared to patients treated with thrombolytic therapy only. In addition, the bleeding complication rate was significantly higher in the heparin group. The administration of heparin subcutaneously began 4 to 12 hours after thrombolysis, however, so it is possible that adequate anticoagulation was not achieved during the acute period of clot lysis. Thus, given the marked thrombogenicity of residual thrombus following vessel recanalization, and while awaiting results of further clinical trials, use of high-dose subcutaneous heparin as early as possible (17,000 units q 12 hours) at the time of lytic therapy has been advocated.[173]

CHRONIC PHASE AFTER MYOCARDIAL INFARCTION

Survivors of acute myocardial infarction are at medium risk of recurrent infarction or cardiac death.[255] Because cardiac morbidity and mortality during the period may be related to a number of factors, including left ventricular dysfunction, ventricular arrhythmias, and recurrent myocardial infarction, proving that antithrombotic therapy is beneficial in these patients has been difficult and has generated controversy for several decades.

PLATELET INHIBITORS With respect to the use of antiplatelet agents for secondary prevention of vascular events, no less than 10 randomized, placebo-controlled, double-blind trials in postmyocardial infarction patients have been conducted.[38] Despite the large total number of patients studied (>17,000), no clear evidence of benefit from therapy was shown in any single study. Reduction in cardiac mortality rate varied from 12% to 57%. An extensive meta-analysis of these studies was recently published.[38] Despite the inherent problems of pooled data, this overview concluded that among survivors of myocardial infarction, platelet inhibitors reduced vascular mortality by 13%, nonfatal reinfarction by 31%, nonfatal stroke by 42%, and all important vascular events by 25%. Aspirin alone was at least as effective as the combination of aspirin and dipyridamole and more effective than sulfinpyrazone. Available data do not justify the additional cost and frequency of administration of drugs other than aspirin in this group of patients.[38]

ANTICOAGULANTS[248,250,256] Numerous studies have assessed the usefulness of long-term anticoagulation in the secondary prevention of cardiovascular disease after myocardial infarction, but few randomized con-

trolled trials were large enough to be able to detect a significant effect from therapy. A pooled analysis[257] of nine trials of anticoagulation in postinfarction patients showed that this therapy decreased overall mortality by about 20%. However, because not all trials were properly controlled, the conclusion of this collective analysis must be interpreted with caution. Emerging evidence from a Norwegian trial[258] supports the use of warfarin after myocardial infarction for the prevention of reinfarction and reduction of mortality.

Considering the above data, the evidence supporting the use of aspirin in the secondary prevention of cardiovascular morbidity and mortality beyond the acute phase of myocardial infarction is at least as strong as that supporting anticoagulation. At a daily dose of 325 mg, aspirin offers several advantages over long-term anticoagulants in cost, ease of administration, and side effects. Thus, to survivors of myocardial infarction, daily aspirin is recommended.

CHRONIC STABLE CORONARY ARTERY DISEASE

Patients with a remote history of myocardial infarction (beyond 2 years) and those with chronic stable angina are at medium risk of coronary ischemic events, which varied between 2.5% and 5% per year.[255] In patients with remote myocardial infarction, recurrent thrombotic events are probably the main cause of mortality. Most studies of platelet inhibitors in survivors of myocardial infarction have shown a beneficial trend toward lower mortality and reinfarction, which became significant only when the data derived from all available trials were pooled.[38]

For anticoagulant therapy, in the Sixty-Plus Reinfarction Study,[259] patients older than 60 and treated for a median of 6 years with warfarin after myocardial infarction were randomly assigned to continue anticoagulant or substitute placebo. The design was double-blinded, and anticoagulant dosage was tightly controlled for a period of 2 more years, at which point anticoagulated patients had a 26% lower mortality rate (p = 0.07) and 55% lower incidence of reinfarction (p = 0.0005) when compared with patients treated with placebo. It appears, therefore, that both aspirin and anticoagulants are effective in prevention of reinfarction and reduction in mortality in asymptomatic patients after remote myocardial infarction, but the former is associated with lower cost and risk.

Although no prospective randomized trial of antithrombotic therapy in chronic stable angina has been published, the sustained beneficial effects of aspirin after initial therapy for patients with unstable angina suggest a role for aspirin in stable coronary disease.[34,35] A dose of 160 to 325 mg daily is associated with minimal gastrointestinal toxicity and should be considered in these patients.

PRIMARY PREVENTION OF CORONARY EVENTS[39,248,250]

Results from a double-blind, placebo-controlled trial[37] of more than 22,000 male physicians in the United States assigned to receive aspirin (325 mg every other day) for 5 years revealed a 44% reduction in the incidence of myocardial infarction from approximately 0.4% to 0.2% per year (p = 0.00001). Before advising the widespread use of aspirin in apparently healthy people, three issues need to be addressed. First, there was a slight increase in the incidence of hemorrhagic stroke in the aspirin-treated group. Second, in a randomized British primary prevention trial[260] involving more than 5000 male physicians, the use of aspirin (500 mg/d) did not reduce the rate of myocardial infarction, but did increase the incidence of disabling stroke. Finally, the long-term effects of aspirin blockade of the prostaglandin system in various tissues, particularly the central nervous system, are unknown.

Even though these studies were done in healthy volunteers and, admittedly, their conclusions should be applied only to "healthy individuals," the increased incidence of hemorrhagic stroke is disconcerting. Aspirin therefore should be recommended for primary prevention only to individuals at high risk for coronary artery disease, those for whom the benefits of therapy outweigh its risks. Further analysis of the United States Physicians' Health Study[261] suggests that aspirin exerts a greater impact on patients at higher risk for coronary events, namely those with cardiovascular risk factors or evidence of cerebral or peripheral vascular disease.

PROGRESSION OF ATHEROSCLEROSIS

As discussed earlier, repetitive type II injury of soft fatty plaques with thrombus formation and incorporation represents a major mechanism for the progression of atherosclerosis.[188,189] This concept is based on the pathologic finding of old, organized coronary thrombi difficult to distinguish from atherosclerotic changes in the arterial wall. A more recent study[191] demonstrated the presence of fibrinogen, fibrin, and their degradation products in areas of advanced atherosclerotic plaques. On the basis of these observations, recurrent episodes of plaque disruption and thrombosis may lead not necessarily to acute ischemic syndromes but to progressive narrowing of the coronary arteries. Although it is still unclear how prevalent this process is, its clinical significance is enormous because thrombotic episodes may be prevented by platelet inhibitors or anticoagulants. In this context, a 5-year trial of platelet-inhibitor therapy in the angiographic progression of coronary disease in patients with stable angina was recently completed at the Mayo Clinic. Preliminary evidence suggests that platelet inhibitors reduce the incidence of myocardial infarction and new lesion formation.[262]

CORONARY INTERVENTIONS

Vein Graft Disease Following Bypass Surgery

Coronary vein graft disease is the most important contributor to cardiac mortality and morbidity after coronary artery surgery. Occlusion rates are 8% to 18% per distal anastomosis at 1 month postoperatively, and 16% to 26% at 1 year. At the end of 5 years, up to 35% of vein grafts will be occluded.[200,201] Vein graft disease can be divided into 3 stages: an early postoperative stage of thrombotic occlusion related to type III injury; a second stage of intimal hyperplasia that occurs within the first year and is probably due to repetitive type II injury, platelet aggregation, and mitogen release. Beyond the first year, lipid accumulation, further smooth-muscle cell proliferation, and thrombus incorporation resembling that of spontaneous atherosclerosis constitute the final stage of atheroma formation.[200,201]

EARLY GRAFT OCCLUSION[263,264] As discussed in previous sections, early occlusion seems to be related to a type III vascular injury caused by surgical manipulation and exposure of the graft to high rates of arterial blood flow.[200] This process is mainly thrombotic in origin, and platelets play a major pathogenetic role. Antithrombotic therapy is most effective in reducing the rate of early postoperative thrombotic occlusion.

Several trials[265–267] have documented that aspirin, with or without dipyridamole, or ticlopidine reduces the incidence of early vein graft occlusion. Antiplatelet therapy should be instituted preoperatively or in the immediate postoperative period, because benefit is lost if therapy is initiated more than 3 days after surgery. Administration of aspirin before surgery carries the risk of increased postoperative bleeding,[267] so we prescribe dipyridamole preoperatively, followed by aspirin alone (325 mg daily) beginning immediately after surgery. Whether the addition of preoperative dipyridamole offers any real value over postoperative aspirin alone is unknown. Because extracorporeal circulation activates the coagulation system and platelets, the routine use of heparin intraoperatively may be important in the prevention of thrombus formation and early graft occlusion. Thus, the combination of intraoperative heparin and perioperative platelet inhibitor drugs effectively reduces the incidence of graft occlusion in this high-risk population.

Two studies[268,269] have addressed the effect of anticoagulation on vein graft patency. In one,[268] there was a trend toward higher patency rate with warfarin, started 3 to 4 days postoperatively. In another,[269] this drug offered no advantage over placebo. These studies were compromised by incomplete angiographic follow-up, small sample size, or late implementation of antithrombotic therapy. Although no comparative studies have been published, it is difficult to advocate the use of anticoagulants because of the impressive success of aspirin after saphenous vein graft surgery.

LATE GRAFT OCCLUSION[263,264] The beneficial effect of antiplatelet therapy is less apparent, however, in late graft occlusion, as a different pathologic process supervenes. This process includes smooth muscle cell proliferation, lipid accumulation, and recurrent thrombus formation and organization, a process similar to that of spontaneous atherosclerosis.[200] Although the beneficial effects of antiplatelet agents in reducing late occlusion are less striking, these patients are at a medium risk of developing thrombotic and ischemic events and long-term aspirin therapy appears sensible.

Coronary Angioplasty

Coronary angioplasty has been an important alternative to surgical revascularization in suitable patients with coronary artery disease since its introduction by Andreas Gruntzig in 1977,[270] and its use has been greatly expanded in the last few years. Despite improvement in equipment and technique, however, acute reocclusion after successful angioplasty occurs in about 5% of patients, whereas late restenosis, generally within 3 to 6 months, occurs in 25% to 35% of patients.[185,271] As discussed in previous sections, acute occlusion appears to be secondary to a type III vascular injury with resultant thrombus formation, while the process of late restenosis is due to intimal hyperplasia and thrombus organization.

ACUTE OCCLUSION[264,272] Several studies[273–276] have clearly shown that pretreatment of patients with aspirin, aspirin plus dipyridamole, or ticlopidine (all in association with heparin) significantly reduces the rate of acute thrombotic complications after angioplasty. The role of heparin alone in prevention of acute vessel occlusion during angioplasty has not been properly tested clinically, but there is experimental evidence that suggests an inverse relation between the dose of heparin and both platelet deposition and mural thrombosis.[277] In addition, uncontrolled preliminary studies in patients with unstable angina have demonstrated that pretreatment with heparin for 1 to 8 days reduces the incidence of acute thrombotic occlusion during and after angioplasty.[278–280] Therefore, high-dose heparin is widely used during and after intervention. Given the substantial risk of acute thrombotic complication associated with angioplasty, pretreatment with aspirin combined with adequate heparization throughout the procedure is strongly recommended. The angiographic appearance of intraluminal thrombus or vessel dissection usually dictates the duration of heparin therapy on completion of the procedure.

LATE RESTENOSIS[264,272] The effects of antithrombotic therapy on late restenosis have been disappointing. Clinical trials[274–276] using different platelet-inhibiting regimens have shown no impact on the restenotic rate. Similarly, anticoagulation with heparin[281] or warfarin[282] was of no benefit when compared with aspirin. However, long-term aspirin therapy is recommended to these patients, on the basis of favorable experience in chronic coronary artery disease for secondary prevention of ischemic complications.[262]

Cardiac Chambers
ATRIAL FIBRILLATION[283,284]

Systemic embolism is a common and potentially devastating complication of atrial fibrillation associated with both mitral valve disease and certain other forms of organic heart disease. Blood stasis appears to play a predominant pathogenetic role in thrombus formation in patients with atrial fibrillation. Patients at highest risk are those with a history of systemic embolism in the previous 2 years; in this group, the embolic risk approaches 10% to 20% in the first 1 or 2 years.[285] Although no prospective randomized trials of anticoagulants are available, the current recommendation is for long-term anticoagulant therapy aimed at prolonging prothrombin time to 1.5 to 2 times control (standard INR of prothrombin suppression, 3.0 to 4.5) in these patients.

Patients at somewhat lower but nevertheless substantial risk of embolism (which approaches 6% per year) are those with atrial fibrillation associated with mitral stenosis. Data from numerous nonrandomized and uncontrolled trials have suggested that anticoagulation reduces the rates of embolism and death in patients with rheumatic valvular disease by 25%.[283] Based on known embolic risk and on results of clinical trials, chronic anticoagulation to prolong prothrombin time to 1.3 to 1.5 times control (INR 2.0 to 3.0) is recommended for these patients. In addition, patients with uncontrolled hyperthyroidism and heart failure appear to be at increased risk of embolism.[283] Although anticoagulation in these patients has not been evaluated by prospective randomized trials, this therapy is recommended until the patients become euthyroid and reversion to sinus rhythm has been achieved.

At the lower end of the spectrum of embolic risk in patients with atrial fibrillation are those without evidence of associated organic heart disease. The natural history of lone atrial fibrillation was addressed by the Framingham investigators,[286] who followed 30 of these patients for more than 10 years and found a fourfold increase in the incidence of stroke as compared with matched controls. Aside from the small sample size, other limitations of the analysis were the relatively advanced age of the subjects (mean, 70 years) and the inclusion of patients with hypertension. In another study,[287] 97 normotensive patients younger than 60 years with lone atrial fibrillation were followed for a mean of 17 years at the Mayo Clinic. Anticoagulants were used in just a few subjects. Only eight embolic events were identified, an overall incidence well below 1% per year. These data suggest that for patients younger than 60 years with atrial fibrillation but no evidence of organic heart disease, the hazards of chronic anticoagulation outweigh its potential benefits.

Between these two poles exists a large group of patients with an intermediate but incompletely defined risk of embolism: those with nonvalvular atrial fibrillation associated with various forms of cardiovascular disease. The embolic risk in these patients lies between 4% and 6% per year[283,284] and accounts for almost one half of cardioembolic strokes. Given the severe functional deficits that often follow embolic stroke and the fact that these events are usually unheralded by warning signs, preventive therapy is the only rational approach. In a retrospective study at the Montreal Heart Institute, nonanticoaguted patients had an incidence of systemic embolism of 5.5% per year, whereas anticoagulated patients had a significantly lower embolic rate of 0.7% per year.

Based on five prospective studies on patients with nonvascular atrial fibrillation,[288–292] the third ACCP conference on antithrombotic therapy has made the following recommendations: "It is strongly recommended that long-term oral warfarin therapy (INR 2.0 to 3.0) be used in patients with atrial fibrillation who are eligible for anticoagulation, except in patients less than 60 years of age who have no associated cardiovascular disease (lone atrial fibrillation). Patients with atrial fibrillation who are poor candidates for anticoagulation therapy should be treated with aspirin at a dose of 325 mg/day."[283] This is based on one study (SPAF[289]), but not on two others—AFASAK[288] and BAATAF.[290]

ACUTE MYOCARDIAL INFARCTION[248,284]

Approximately one third of patients with acute anterior myocardial infarction and less than 5% of those with inferior infarction develop left ventricular mural thrombi.[293] These thrombi tend to occur in the first week and particularly in the first 2 days. Thrombi are more likely to form in cases of large infarcts (peak serum creatine kinase > 2000 units/liter). Systemic embolism, which occurs in about 10% of cases in which left ventricular thrombi are echocardiographically apparent, is the most important complication, affecting 2% to 5% of victims of myocardial infarction.[293] Echocardiographically, thrombi that protrude into the left ventricular cavity and have increased mobility are more likely to embolize than those without these characteristics.[293]

Because the incidence of embolism is highest in the first 1 to 3 months after myocardial infarction and short-term anticoagulation has been demonstrated to reduce the embolic rate by 25% to 75%,[248,284] the following approach is recommended: patients with increased embolic risk, namely, those with large anterior infarcts, congestive heart failure, or atrial fibrillation, should receive heparin on admission (aimed at prolonging the APTT to 1.5 to 2 times control). A study by Turpie and colleagues[294] demonstrated that high-dose subcutaneous heparin (12,500 units every 12 hours) significantly reduced the incidence of mural thrombosis in patients with anterior infarcts as compared with low-dose heparin (5000 units twice daily). Heparin therapy may be followed by warfarin to prolong the prothrombin time to 1.3 to 1.5 times control (INR 2.0 to 3.0) in patients with echocardiographic evidence of mural thrombi or large akinetic regions. Warfarin may be stopped after 1 to 3 months unless there is the risk of heart failure or impaired left ventricular function or persistent echocardiographic evidence of mural thrombi. The optimal duration of anticoagulation in this group has not been determined.

CHRONIC LEFT VENTRICULAR ANEURYSM[248,284]

In contrast to the prevalence of thromboembolism in acute myocardial infarction, the incidence of embolism in chronic left ventricular aneurysm is significantly lower (0.35% per year).[295] The reason for this difference is probably twofold. First, thrombi formed after acute myocardial infarction are usually mobile, are friable, and protrude into the ventricular cavity, whereas thrombi in chronic aneurysms are laminated and more adherent to the endocardium.[214,293] Second, thrombi located within an aneurysmal sac, which is devoid of contractile fibers, are less prone to propulsion into the left ventricular outflow tract.[222] Although some investigators have found a persistent risk of embolism in postinfarction patients, it was not the presence of an aneurysm but rather the mobility and protrusion of thrombus that predicted embolic events. Given available data, patients with remote infarction and chronic left ventricular aneurysm are at low risk of embolism and need not receive anticoagulants. Whether these drugs should be given to patients with echocardiographic evidence of mobile and protruding thrombi, however, remains to be established.

DILATED CARDIOMYOPATHY[284]

Pathologic studies[215] have found a high prevalence of right and left ventricular mural thrombi in patients with idiopathic dilated cardiomyopathy. Blood stasis and low shear rate present in a dilated, hypocontractile ventricle lead to activation of coagulation processes. Because the mural thrombus is not mechanically isolated, as occurs in a ventricular aneurysm, embolism of thrombotic materials may occur. In a retrospective study,[296] patients treated with anticoagulants had no evidence of systemic embolism, whereas those not anticoagulated had an embolic rate of 3.5% per year. Lacking any prospective trial of antithrombotic therapy in these patients at medium risk for embolism, this evidence supports chronic warfarin administration,[296] particularly in those with overt heart failure or atrial fibrillation.

Prosthetic Valves

MECHANICAL PROSTHESES[225,297]

Prosthetic surfaces are thrombogenic by virtue of their ability to activate both the intrinsic coagulation system and platelets. Increased shear rate, blood stasis (particularly in high-profile prosthetic devices), and associated disturbances of the cardiac chambers predispose to thromboembolism.[225] Patients with history of embolism and valves manufactured before the mid 1970s are at highest risk, which exceeds six events per 100 patients per year.[226,227] Atrial fibrillation and left ventricular thrombus contribute additional risk. Patients with newer mechanical valves have a risk of thromboembolism that ranges between 1% and 5% per year despite anticoagulation.

Anticoagulants

Warfarin, at a dose sufficient to prolong the prothrombin time to slightly less than 1.5 to 2 times control (INR 2.5 to 3.5), is the most important agent for prevention of thromboembolism.[225,297] Studies in patients with mechanical prostheses have consistently shown that anticoagulation significantly reduces the incidence of valvular thrombosis and embolism.[226,227] In fact, inadequate anticoagulation increases the thromboembolic risk twofold to sixfold,[226,227] whereas excessive anticoagulation (prothrombin time more than 2.5 times control) increases the risk of bleeding complications fourfold to eightfold.

Anticoagulants Plus Platelet Inhibitors

Platelet inhibitors alone have not been found to confer protection against embolism in patients with mechanical prostheses. Indeed, studies of aspirin plus dipyridamole in these patients have shown an incidence of thromboembolism as high as 10% per year.[298,299] Patients with mechanical valves treated with warfarin had significantly fewer thromboembolic events compared with those treated with aspirin combined with either dipyridamole or pentoxifylline.[299] It seems clear, therefore, that patients with mechanical prostheses should receive anticoagulant therapy indefinitely, aimed at a prothrombin time of slightly less than 1.5 to 2 times control (INR 2.5 to 3.5).[225,297] However, the addition of a platelet inhibitor such as dipyridamole (300 to 400 mg daily) to warfarin may reduce the thromboembolic risk below that of warfarin alone. Indeed, the antithrombotic effects of dipyridamole are more evident on prosthetic materials such as artificial heart valves than on biologic surfaces. Therefore, we suggest supplementing warfarin with dipyridamole (300 to 400 mg/d) in patients with mechanical valves and prior embolism and in those with older prosthetic devices. The combination of an oral anticoagulent (INR 2.0 to 3.5) and low-dose aspirin (100 to 325 mg/d) has recently been shown to be of benefit in patients who are at high risk but without bleeding.

BIOLOGICAL PROSTHESES[225,297]

Although bioprosthetic valves are less thrombogenic than mechanical valves, thromboembolism may occur with an incidence of two to three per 100 patients per year, particularly in the first 3 months after surgery, and more often in those patients with mitral than aortic prostheses and in those with atrial fibrillation or prior embolism.[225,226,297] Patients with mitral bioprostheses should receive warfarin postoperatively, aimed at a prothrombin time of 1.3 to 1.5 times control (INR 2.0 to 3.0) for 1 to 3 months, unless atrial fibrillation persists, in which case warfarin should be used indefinitely.[225,226,297] Although aortic bioprostheses are associated with a lower incidence of embolism, the concomitant presence of atrial fibrillation may warrant the use of chronic warfarin therapy in these patients as well.

Patients who maintain normal sinus rhythm postoperatively without left ventricular dysfunction or prior embolism are at low risk. In these patients there may be no need for sustained anticoagulant therapy. This is particularly true for patients with aortic bioprostheses, in whom even platelet inhibitor may be unnecessary.[225,226,297] No randomized controlled studies of platelet inhibitors in patients with bioprostheses have been reported. In an uncontrolled trial, longterm aspirin therapy was associated with a low incidence of embolism in these patients.

SPECIAL SITUATIONS[225,297]

Four special situations should be considered in prescribing anticoagulant therapy for patients with prosthetic heart valves[226]: noncardiac surgery, prosthetic valve endocarditis, anticoagulation after a thromboembolic event, and anticoagulation during pregnancy.

Noncardiac Surgery

Temporary discontinuation of anticoagulation for 7 to 10 days appears to be of minimal risk for patients undergoing a noncardiac operation. To keep this risk to a minimum and unless contraindicated, however, it is recommended to discontinue the warfarin 4 to 5 days before operation and to start heparin administration (to maintain the activated partial thromboplastin time at two times control) and dipyridamole

(300 to 400 mg/d). The heparin infusion should be continued 4 to 5 hours before the operation. Subcutaneous heparin (15,000 units per day given in two or three divided doses) can be considered during and early after operation. Warfarin therapy should be restarted as soon as safe after the operation.

Prosthetic Valve Endocarditis

Of patients with prosthetic valve endocarditis who are not receiving anticoagulant therapy, thromboembolism to the central nervous system occurs in about 50%. Three nonrandomized clinical trials[300–302] in patients with prosthetic valve endocarditis who were receiving anticoagulant therapy suggest that the thromboembolic rate can be decreased sixfold to ninefold with adequate anticoagulation. It should be noted, however, that the risk of intracranial hemorrhage is substantial and may approach 14%.[301,302] Although the benefits and the risks of anticoagulation in patients with native or bioprosthetic valve endocarditis are not well defined, it is currently recommended that anticoagulant therapy not be given to patients with uncomplicated infective endocarditis involving a native valve or a bioprosthetic valve in patients with normal sinus rhythm. This is based on the increased incidence of hemorrhage in these patients and the lack of demonstrated efficacy of anticoagulation in this setting.

Anticoagulation After Thromboembolic Event[303,304]

The appropriate time to start anticoagulation after thromboembolism to the brain has been controversial. A second embolism can occur early after the initial event, so that immediate anticoagulation appears rational. Caution should be exercised, however, because anecdotal reports and experimental studies suggest that immediate anticoagulation, especially in patients with a large embolic infarct, can result in secondary hemorrhage with increased morbidity. Data from 15 prospective and retrospective studies[303,304] suggest that approximately 12% of patients with aseptic embolism to the brain from a cardiac source experience a second embolic event within 2 weeks. Immediate anticoagulation with heparin appears to decrease the risk of recurrent embolism. Several nonrandomized studies suggested that there was a reduction in risk of early recurrent embolism within 14 days to about one third of that in patients who did not receive anticoagulation.[303,304]

There are wide variations in the reported risk of symptomatic brain hemorrhage after immediate anticoagulation for embolic stroke. One group of studies showed no hemorrhage worsening in 162 patients who received anticoagulation immediately, but others have reported hemorrhage worsening in 1% to 24% of these patients.[303,304] A lack of reporting about the details of anticoagulant administration does not allow analysis of these discrepant results.

Patients with a large infarct appear to be at greater risk of hemorrhagic worsening after immediate anticoagulation of embolic stroke. Spontaneous hemorrhagic transformation may be delayed for several days, but appears most likely to occur within 48 hours. Thus, it is recommended that immediate anti-coagulation be started in patients who are nonhypertensive and have small or moderately sized embolic strokes and in whom a CT scan of the head can be done within 48 hours after the stroke to exclude hemorrhagic transformation. The same principles appear to apply for the continuation of anticoagulant therapy in patients with a prosthetic valve who experience an embolic stroke during long-term anticoagulant therapy. Because patients with a large embolic infarct or severe hypertension appear to be at special risk for delayed hemorrhagic transformation, anticoagulation should be postponed for 5 to 7 days. This allows time to document that a repeat tomographic scan of the head does not show hemorrhagic transformation. In patients with hemorrhagic complications, anticoagulation should be postponed 8 to 10 days.

Antithrombotic Therapy During Pregnancy [135,136]

For pregnant patients with prosthetic heart valves, the use of heparin and oral anticoagulation is problematic because neither the safety of oral anticoagulant therapy during pregnancy nor the efficacy of heparin therapy for prophylaxis of systemic embolism is established. Patient education is critical for women of childbearing age who have a prosthetic cardiac valve. Ideally pregnancy should be carefully planned and the regimen of anticoagulant therapy should be modified to avoid the teratogenic effects of warfarin, since fetal wastage is approximately 60% in women who receive warfarin therapy at the time of conception and during the first trimester. In addition, warfarin exposure in the first trimester and possibly thereafter may predispose to congenital anomalies, especially nasal hypoplasia, stippling of bones, mental retardation, optic atrophy, and microcephaly. Furthermore, because the coumarin derivatives cross the placental barrier, hemorrhagic complications can occur in the fetus, especially at the time of delivery. In contrast, heparin does not cross the placental barrier.

Two approaches have been recommended: the first is to use heparin therapy throughout pregnancy, administered every 12 hours by subcutaneous injection in doses adjusted to keep APTT at 1.5 to 2 times control (may need 15,000 units twice daily or more). This regimen should be continued until 1 week before delivery, when the patients should be hospitalized and switched to heparin infusion, which is continued until the induction of labor. Since the beneficial effect of subcutaneous heparin with mechanical prosthetic valves during pregnancy is not fully proven, however, a bioprosthetic heart valve is preferred for women of childbearing age, because many of them do not need chronic anticoagulation. Nevertheless, the risk of bioprosthetic calcification and need for reoperation in very young women has to be kept in mind.

The second approach is to use heparin until the 13th week, change to warfarin until the middle of the third trimester, then restart heparin therapy until delivery. Although the latter approach might avoid warfarin embryopathy, other fetopathic effects (e.g., central nervous system abnormalities) are still possible. Before this approach is recommended, therefore,

the potential risks should be explained to the patient. In addition, the use of warfarin at any time during pregnancy carries significant medicolegal implications, because the manufacturer explicitly states that warfarin usage in pregnancy is contraindicated. Thus, this approach is not recommended in the United States.

Antiplatelet agents should be avoided during pregnancy because aspirin may cause premature closure of the ductus arteriosus, and dipyridamole and sulfinpyrazone have indeterminate effects on the fetus and are not approved for use during pregnancy. In addition, platelet-inhibitor drugs do not appear to offer significant protection against thromboembolism during pregnancy.

In summary, activation of the coagulation system and, secondarily, of platelets occurs in patients with prosthetic valves. For those at high risk, combination of anticoagulation and a platelet inhibitor is suggested. Medium-risk patients can be managed with an anticoagulant alone and those at low risk may not require antithrombotic treatment.

CONCLUSIONS

An approach to antithrombotic therapy in various cardiovascular diseases has emerged based on the evolving concept of vascular injury and thrombosis, and with the knowledge of pathophysiology and an appreciation of differential clinical features determining morbid risk. The essential parameters of this approach form the framework of Figure 9.10.

In the arterial circulation, type II and III injury leads to both platelet activation and production of thrombin and fibrin, suggesting a combined therapeutic approach with a platelet inhibitor, an anticoagulant, or a combination of both (acutely and short term). The propensity to thrombosis determines the intensity of antithrombotic therapy. High-risk patients with unstable angina and evolving acute myocardial infarction should be treated aggressively with a platelet inhibitor and perhaps acutely with an anticoagulant as well, although the final recommendation awaits the results of several ongoing clinical trials. Patients undergoing coronary angioplasty or saphenous bypass surgery should receive platelet inhibitors and adequate anticoagulation during the procedure. Coronary disease patients are at more moderate risk in the chronic phase of stable angina, after myocardial infarction, of angioplasty, and of bypass surgery; such patients are best managed with a platelet inhibitor rather than an anticoagulant for reasons of convenience, safety, and economy. In low-risk patients in whom prevention of complications of atherosclerosis is desired, aspirin may be prescribed to those with certain risk factors, such as diabetes, family history, tobacco exposure, and hypercholesterolemia. However, a hint that long-term aspirin administration may be associated with an elevated risk of intracerebral hemorrhage militates against its indiscriminate use; furthermore, the long-term effects (benefits or risks) of aspirin therapy are unknown.

Within the cardiac chambers, stasis of blood flow causes coagulation to predominate over platelet activation as the principal mechanism of thrombus formation, and anticoagulant therapy alone seems most appropriate in management of these patients. At highest risk are patients with atrial fibrillation and prior embolism; at somewhat lower yet substantial risk are those patients with atrial fibrillation associated with mitral stenosis or uncontrolled hyperthyroidism. In all such patients at high risk, high-intensity anticoagulation is recommended. Patients at medium risk are those immediately after large anterior myocardial infarction and uncompensated dilated cardiomyopathy; for these patients, evidence suggests a need for moderately intense chronic anticoagulation. Some patients with nonvalvulopathic atrial fibrillation associated with other forms of cardiac disease benefit from warfarin therapy, but subgroups in this population have not yet been identified. At lowest risk are patients with lone atrial fibrillation without overt heart disease and those with chronic left ventricular aneurysm in whom anticoagulants are not required.

The thrombogenicity of prosthetic heart valves involves both fibrin formation and, to a lesser extent, platelet activation and is considerably greater for mechanical than biologic devices. Patients at highest risk—those with older mechanical prostheses or prior embolism—should be treated with a combination of an anticoagulant and a platelet inhibitor; either dipyridamole or aspirin may be beneficial. At medium risk are patients with modern mechanical valves and those with bioprostheses in the presence of atrial fibrillation, who can be successfully managed with an anticoagulant alone. When bioprostheses are in place along with normal sinus rhythm, the embolic risk is low enough that antithrombotic therapy may not be needed.

REFERENCES

1. Fuster V, Chesebro JH: Current concepts of thrombogenesis: Role of platelets. Mayo Clin Proc 56:102, 1981
2. Fuster V, Badimon L, Badimon JJ, Chesebro JH: The pathogenesis of coronary disease and the acute coronary syndromes (part two). N Engl J Med 326:310, 1992
3. Badimon L, Badimon JJ, Fuster V: Pathogenesis of thrombosis. In Fuster V, Verstraete M (eds): Thrombosis in Cardiovascular Disorders, pp 17–40. Philadelphia, WB Saunders, 1992
4. Stein B, Fuster V: Decision making based on risk. In Fuster V, Verstraete M (eds): Thrombosis in Cardiovascular Disorders, pp 491–500. Philadelphia, WB Saunders, 1992
5. Halperin JL, Petersen P: Thrombosis in the cardiac chambers: Ventricular dysfunction and atrial fibrillation. In Fuster V, Verstraete M (eds): Thrombosis in Cardiovascular Disorders, pp 215–236. Philadelphia, WB Saunders, 1992
6. Hawiger J: Formation and regulation of platelet and fibrin hemostatic plug. Hum Pathol 18:111, 1987
7. Fuster V, Badimon L, Cohen M et al: Insights into the pathogenesis of acute ischemic syndromes. Circulation 77:1213, 1988
8. Davies MJ, Thomas AC: Plaque fissuring—the cause of acute myocardial infarction, sudden ischemic death and crescendo angina. Br Heart J 53:363, 1985
9. Badimon L, Badimon JJ, Galvez A et al: Influence of arterial damage and wall shear rate on platelet deposition: Ex vivo study in a swine model. Arteriosclerosis 6:312, 1986
10. Badimon L, Badimon JJ: Mechanism of arterial thrombosis in nonparallel streamlines; platelet thrombi grew on the apex of stenotic severely injured vessel wall: Experimental study in the pig model. J Clin Invest 84:1134, 1989
11. Lindon JN, Collins REC, Coe NP et al: In vivo assessment in sheep of thromboresistant materials by determination of platelet survival. Circ Res 46:83, 1971
12. Stein B, Fuster V, Israel DH et al: Platelet inhibitor agents in cardiovascular disease: An update. J Am Coll Cardiol 14:813, 1989

13. Peerschke EB: The platelet fibrinogen receptor. Semin Hematol 22:241, 1985
14. Shattil SJ, Brass LP: Induction of the fibrinogen receptor on human platelets by intracellular mediators. J Biol Chem 262:992, 1987
15. Coller BS: Activator effects access to the platelet receptor for adhesive glycoproteins. J Cell Biol 103:451, 1986
16. Moncada S, Vane JR: Arachidonic acid metabolite and the interactions between platelet and vessel wall. N Engl J Med 300:1142, 1979
17. Verstraete M, Vermylen J: Cellular, chemical and rheological factors in thrombosis and fibrinolysis. In Thrombosis, pp 1–54. New York, Pergamon Press, 1985
18. Fuster V, Chesebro JH, Frye RL et al: Platelet survival and the development of coronary artery disease in the young: The effects of cigarette smoking, strong family history, and medical therapy. Circulation 63:546, 1981
19. Moncada S, Gryglewski R, Bunting S et al: An enzyme isolated from arteries transforms prostaglandin endoperoxides to an unstable substance that inhibits platelet aggregation. Nature 263:1976
20. Dyerberg J, Bang HO, Stoffersen E et al: Eicosapentaenoic acid and prevention of thrombosis and atherosclerosis. Lancet 2:117, 1978
21. Kromhout D, Bosschieter EB, Coulander CDL: The inverse relation between fish consumption and 20-year mortality from coronary heart disease. N Engl J Med 312:1205, 1985
22. McNeely TB, Griffith MJ: The anticoagulant mechanism of action of heparin in contact-activated plasma: Inhibition of factor X activation. Blood 65:1226, 1985
23. Egeberg O: Inherited antithrombin deficiency causing thrombophilia. Thromb Haemost 13:516, 1965
24. van Hinsberg VWM, Bertina RM, van Wijngaarden A et al: Activated protein C decreases plasminogen activator-inhibitor activity in endothelial cell conditioned media. Blood 65:444, 1985
25. Collen D: On the regulation and control of fibrinolysis. Thromb Haemost 43:77, 1980

26. Erikson LA, Ginsberg MH, Loskutoff DJ: Detection and partial characterization of an inhibitor of plasminogen activator in human platelets. J Clin Invest 74:1465, 1984

27. Minuro J, Schleef RR, Loskutoff DJ: Extracellular matrix of cultured bovine aortic endothelial cells contain functionally active type I plasminogen activator inhibitor. Blood 70:721, 1987

28. Griffin JH, Evatt B, Zimmerman TS et al: Deficiency of protein C in congenital thrombotic disease. J Clin Invest 68:1370, 1980

29. Dreyer NA, Pizzo SV: Blood coagulation and idiopathic thromboembolism among fertile women. Contraception 22:123, 1980

30. Tschopp TB: Aspirin inhibits platelet aggregation, but not adhesion to collagen fibrils: An assessment of platelet adhesion and platelet deposited mass by morphometry and ^{51}Cr-labelling. Thromb Res 11:619, 1977

31. Clowes AW, Karnovsky MJ: Failure of certain antiplatelet drugs to affect myointimal thickening following arterial endothelial injury in the rat. Lab Invest 36:452, 1977

32. Roth CL, Majerus PW: The mechanism of the effects of aspirin on human platelets: I. Acetylation of a particulate fraction protein. J Clin Invest 56:624, 1975

33. Kyrle PA, Eichler HC, Jagh V, Lechner K: Inhibition of prostacyclin and thromboxane A_2 generation by low-dose aspirin at the site of plug formation in man in vivo. Circulation 75:1025, 1987

34. Lewis HD, Davies JW, Archibald DG et al: Protective effects of aspirin against acute myocardial infarction and death in man with unstable angina: Results of a Veterans Administration Cooperative Study. N Engl J Med 309:396, 1983

35. Cairns JA, Gent M, Singer J et al: Aspirin, sulfinpyrazone, or both in unstable angina. N Engl J Med 313:1369, 1985

36. ISIS-2 (Second International Study of Infarct Survival) Collaborative Group: Randomized trial of intravenous streptokinase, oral aspirin, both or neither among 17,187 cases of suspected acute myocardial infarction: ISIS-2. Lancet 2:349, 1988

37. Final report of the aspirin component of the ongoing Physician Health Study. N Engl J Med 321:129, 1989

38. Antiplatelet Trialists' Collaborative: Secondary prevention of vascular disease by prolonged antiplatelet treatment. Br Med J 296:320, 1988

39. Fuster V, Dyken ML, Vokonas PS, Hennekens CH: Aspirin as a therapeutic agent in cardiovascular disease. Circulation 1993 (in press)

40. Hirsh J, Dalen JE, Fuster V et al: Aspirin and other platelet-active drugs: The relationship between dose, effectiveness and side effects. Chest 104(Suppl):327S, 1992

41. MacKerchner PA, Ivery KL, Baskin WN et al: Protective effects of cimetidine on aspirin-induced gastric mucosal damage. Ann Intern Med 87:676, 1977

42. UK-TIA Study Group: United Kingdom Transient Ischemic Attack (UK-TIA) aspirin trial: Interim result. Br Med J 296:316, 1988

43. Neri Serneri GG, Castellani S: Platelet and vascular prostaglandins: Pharmacological and clinical implication. In Born GVR, Neri Serneri GG (eds): Antiplatelet Therapy, Twenty Years' Experience, pp 37–51. Amsterdam, Elsevier, 1987

44. Friedman PL, Brown EJ, Cunther S et al: Coronary vasoconstrictor effect of indomethacin in patients with coronary artery disease. N Engl J Med 305:1171, 1981

45. Kromhout D, Bosschieter EB, Coulander CDL et al: The inverse relation between fish consumption and 20-year mortality from coronary heart disease. N Engl J Med 312:1205, 1985

46. Shekelle RB, Missel L, Paul O et al: Letter: Fish consumption and mortality from coronary heart disease. N Engl J Med 313:549, 1985

47. Goodnight SH, Cairns JA, Fisher M et al: Assessment of the therapeutic use of n-3 fatty acids in vascular disease and thrombosis. Chest 104(Suppl):347S, 1992

48. Leaf A, Weber PC: Cardiovascular effects of n-3 fatty acids. N Engl J Med 318:549, 1988

49. Fitzgerald GA, Reilly LA, Perderson AK: The biochemical pharmacology of thromboxane synthetase inhibition in man. Circulation 72:1194, 1985

50. Mullane KM, Fornabaio D: Thromboxane synthetase inhibitors reduce infarct size by a platelet-dependent, aspirin-sensitive mechanism. Circ Res 62:668, 1988

51. Rueben SR, Kuan P, Cairns T, Cysle OH: Effects of dazoxiben and exercise performance in chronic stable angina. Br J Clin Pharmacol 15(Suppl):83, 1983

52. Thaulow E, Dale J, Myhre E: Effects of a selective thromboxane synthetase inhibitor, dazoxiben, and of acetylsalicylic acid on myocardial ischemia in patients with coronary artery disease. Am J Cardiol 53:1255, 1984

53. Saussy DL Jr, Mais DE, Knapp DR et al: Thromboxane A_2 and prostaglandin endoperoxide receptors in platelets and vascular smooth muscle. Circulation 72:1202, 1985

54. Cresele P, Van Houtte E, Arnout J et al: Thromboxane synthetase inhibition combined with thromboxane receptor blockade: A step forward in antithrombotic therapy. Thromb Haemost 52:364, 1984

55. Moncada S, Korbut R: Dipyridamole and other phosphodiesterase inhibitors act as antithrombotic agents by potentiating endogenous prostacyclin. Lancet 1:1286, 1978

56. Crutchley DJ, Ryan US, Ryan JW: Effects of aspirin and dipyridamole on the degradation of adenosine diphosphate by cultured cells derived from bovine pulmonary artery. J Clin Invest 66:29, 1980

57. Fitzgerald CA: Dipyridamole. N Engl J Med 316:1247, 1987

58. Harker LA, Slichter SJ: Studies of platelet and fibrinogen kinetics in patients with prosthetic heart valves. N Engl J Med 283:1302, 1970

59. Weily HS, Steele PP, Davies H et al: Platelet survival in patients with substitute heart valves. N Engl J Med 290:534, 1974

60. Hanson SR, Harker LA, Bjornsson TD: Effects of platelet-modifying drugs of arterial throboembolism in baboons: Aspirin potentiates the antithrombotic effects of dipyridamole and sulfinpyrazone by mechanisms independent of platelet cyclo-oxygenase inhibition. J Clin Invest 75:1591, 1985

61. The Persantine-Aspirin Reinfarction Study Group: Persantine and aspirin in coronary artery disease. Circulation 62:449, 1980

62. Bousser MC, Eschwege E, Haugenau M et al: "AICLA" controlled trial of aspirin and dipyridamole in the secondary prevention of atherothrombotic cerebral ischemia. Stroke 14:5, 1983

63. American-Canadian Cooperative Study Group: Persantine-aspirin trial in cerebral ischemia: II. Endpoint results. Stroke 16:406, 1985

64. Brown BC, Cukingnan RA, DeRouen T et al: Improved graft patency in patients treated with platelet-inhibiting therapy after coronary bypass surgery. Circulation 72:138, 1985

65. Goldman S, Copeland J, Mortiz T et al: Improvement in early saphenous vein graft patency after coronary artery bypass surgery with antiplatelet therapy: Results of a Veterans Administration Cooperative Study. Circulation 77:1324, 1988

66. Sullivan JM, Harken DE, Gorlin R: Pharmacologic control of thromboembolic complications of cardiac valve replacement. N Engl J Med 284:1391, 1971

67. Kasahara T: Clinical effect of dipyridamole ingestion after prosthetic heart valve replacement—especially on the blood coagulation system. J Jpn Assoc Thorac Surg 25:1007, 1977

68. Groupe de Récherche PACTE: Prevention des accidents thromboemboliques systemiques chez les porteurs de prosthesis valvulaires artificielles: Essai cooperatif controlé du dipyridamole. Coeur 9:915, 1978

69. Rajah SM, Sreeharan N, Joseph A et al: A prospective trial of dipyridamole and warfarin in heart valve patients (abstr). Acta Ther 6(Suppl 93):54, 1980

70. Chesebro JH, Fuster V, Elveback LR et al: Trial of combined warfarin plus dipyridamole or aspirin therapy in prosthetic heart valve replacement: Danger of aspirin compared with dipyridamole. Am J Cardiol 51:1537, 1983

71. Chesebro JH, Clements IP, Fuster V et al: A platelet-inhibiter drug trial in coronary artery bypass operation: Benefit of perioperative dipyridamole and aspirin therapy on early postopertive vein graft patency. N Engl J Med 307:73, 1982

72. Chesebro JH, Fuster V, Elveback LR et al: Effect of dipyridamole and aspirin in late vein graft patency after coronary artery bypass surgery. N Engl J Med 310:209, 1984

73. Weksler BB: Prostaglandin and vascular function. Circulation 70(Suppl III):III-63, 1984

74. Coppe D, Sobel M, Seavans L et al: Preservation of platelet function and number by prostacyclin during cardiopulmonary bypass. J Thorac Cardiovasc Surg 81:274, 1981

75. Smith MC, Danviriyasup K, Crow JW et al: Prostacyclin substitution for heparin in long-term hemodialysis. Am J Med 81:274, 1982

76. Uchida Y, Hanai T, Hasewaga K et al: Recanalization of obstructed coronary artery by intracoronary administration of prostacyclin in patients with acute myocardial infarction. Adv Prostaglandin Thromboxane Leukotriene Res 11:377, 1983

77. Sharma B, Wyeth RP, Heinemann FM, Bissett JK: Addition of intracoronary prostaglandin E_1 to streptokinase improves thrombolysis and left ventricular function in acute myocardial infarction (abstr). J Am Coll Cardiol 11(Suppl A):104A, 1988

78. Fisher CA, Kappa JR, Sinha AK et al: Comparisons of equimolar concentrations of iloprost, prostacyclin, and prostaglandin E_1 on human platelet function. J Lab Clin Med 109:184, 1987

79. Raizner A, Hollman J, Demke D, Wakefield L: Beneficial effects of ciprostene in PTCA: A multicenter, randomized, controlled trial (abstr). Circulation 78(Suppl II):II-290, 1988

80. Lee H, Paton RC, Ruan C: The in vivo effect of ticlopidine on fibrinogen and factor VIII binding to human platelets (abstr). Thromb Haemost 46:67, 1981

81. O'Brien JR: Ticlopidine, a promise for the prevention and treatment of thrombosis and its complications. Haemostasis 13:1, 1983

82. Violi F, Scrutini D, Cimminielli C et al: STAI (Study of Ticlopidine in Unstable Angina) (abstr). J Am Coll Cardiol 13(Suppl A):238A, 1989

83. White CA, Chaitman B, Lasser TA et al: Antiplatelet agents are effective in reducing the immediate complications of PTCA: Results from the multicenter trial of ticlopidine (abstr). Circulation 76(Suppl IV):IV-400, 1987

84. Limet R, David JL, Magotteaux P et al: Prevention of aorto-coronary bypass graft occlusion. J Thorac Cardiovasc Surg 94:773, 1987

85. Gent M, Blakeley JA, Easton JD et al: The Canadian American Ticlopidine Study (CATS) in thromboembolic stroke. Lancet 1:1215, 1989

86. Hass WK, Easton JD, Adams HP et al: A randomized trial comparing ticlopidine hydrochloride with aspirin for the prevention of stroke in high risk patients. N Engl J Med 321:501, 1989

87. Kaegi A, Pineo GF, Shimizu A et al: Arteriovenous venous shunt thrombosis: Prevention by sulfinpyrazone. N Engl J Med 290:304, 1974

88. Steele PP, Rainwater J, Vogel R: Platelet suppressant therapy in patients with prosthetic heart valves: Relationship of clinical effectiveness to alteration of platelet survival time. Circulation 60:910, 1979

89. Report from the Anturane Reinfarction Italian Study: Sulfinpyrazone in post-myocardial infarction. N Engl J Med 290:304, 1974

90. Baur HR, Van Tassel RA, Pierach CA, Gobel RL: Effects of sulfinpyrazone on early graft occlusion after myocardial revascularization. Am J Cardiol 49:420, 1982

91. Canadian Cooperative Study Group: A randomized trial of aspirin and sulfinpyrazone in threatened stroke. N Engl J Med 299:53, 1978

92. Harker LA, Fuster V: Pharmacology of platelet inhibitors. J Am Coll Cardiol 8(Suppl B):21B, 1986

93. Oberg M, Hedner U, Bergentz SE: Effect of dextran-70 on factor VIII and platelet function in von Willebrand's disease. Thromb Res 12:629, 1978

94. Weiss HJ: The effect of clinical dextran on platelet aggregation, adhesion and ADP release in man: In vivo and in vitro studies. J Lab Clin Med 69:37, 1967

95. Swanson KT, Vlietstra RE, Holmes DR et al: Efficacy of adjunctive dextran during PTCA. Am J Cardiol 54:447, 1984

96. Brown RIG, Aldridge HE, Schwartz L et al: The use of dextran-40 during PTCA: A report of three cases of anaphylactoid reactions—one near fatal. Cathet Cardiovasc Diagn 11:591, 1985

97. Hanson SR, Harker LA: Interruption of acute platelet-dependent thrombosis by the synthetic antithrombin D-phenylalanyl-L-prolyl-L-arginylchloromethyl ketone. Proc Natl Acad Sci USA 85:3184, 1988

98. Stein B, Fuster V. Clinical pharmacology of platelet inhibition. In Fuster V, Verstraete M (eds): Thrombosis in Cardiovascular Disorders, pp 99–120. Philadelphia, WB Saunders, 1992

99. Rosenberg RD: Biochemistry of heparin antithrombin interactions and the physiologic role of this natural anticoagulant mechanism. Am J Med 87:3, 1989

100. Hirsh J, Dalen JE, Deykin D, Poller L: Heparin: Mechanisms of action, pharmacokinetics, dosing considerations, monitoring, efficacy and safety. Chest 104(Suppl):337S, 1992

101. Wessler S: A Guide to Anticoagulant Therapy, pp 1–28. Washington, DC, American Heart Association, 1984

102. Verstraete M, Vermylen J: Antithrombotic and fibrinolytic agents and substances which lower blood viscosity. In Thrombosis, pp 76–112. New York, Pergamon Press, 1985

103. Hirsh J: Heparin. N Engl J Med 324:1565, 1991

104. Hirsh J: Optimal therapeutic ranges for unfractionated heparin and low molecular weight heparins. In Fuster V, Verstraete M (eds): Thrombosis in Cardiovascular Disorders, pp 147–160. Philadelphia, WB Saunders, 1992

105. Samama B, Boissel JP, Combe-Tazali S, Leizorovicz A: Clinical studies with low molecular weight heparins in the prevention and treatment of venous thromboembolism. Ann NY Acad Sci 556:386, 1989

106. Wessler S, Gitel SN: Pharmacology of heparin and warfarin. J Am Coll Cardiol 8:10B, 1986

107. Basu D, Gallus A, Hirst J et al: A prospective study of the value of monitoring heparin treatment with the activated partial thromboplastin time. N Engl J Med 287:324, 1972

108. Schriever HG, Epstein SE, Mintz MD: Statistical correlation and heparin sensitivity of activated partial thromboplastin time, whole blood coagulation time and automated coagulation time. Am J Clin Pathol 60:323, 1973

109. Perkins HA, Osborn JJ, Hurt R et al: Neutralization of heparin in vivo with protamine: A simple method of estimating the required dose. J Lab Clin Med 48:223, 1956

110. Chiu HM, Hirsh J, Yung WL et al: Relationship between anticoagulant and antithrombotic effects of heparin in experimental venous thrombosis. Blood 49:171, 1977

111. Esposito RA, Culliford AT, Colvin SB et al: The role of the activated clotting time in heparin administration and neutralization for cardiopulmonary bypass. J Thorac Cardiovasc Surg 85:174, 1983

112. Ogilby JD, Kopelman HA, Klein LW, Agarwal JB: Adequate heparinization during PTCA: Assessment using activated clotting time. J Am Coll Cardiol 11:237A, 1988

113. Hirsch J: Pharmacology, monitoring and administration of heparin: Proceedings of the ACCP-NHLBI International Conference on Antithrombotic Therapy. Chest 89:26S, 1986

114. Salzman EW, Deykin D, Shapiro RM et al: Management of heparin therapy: Controlled prospective trial. N Engl J Med 292:1046, 1975

115. Glazier RL, Crowell EB: Randomized prospective trial of continuous vs intermittent heparin therapy. JAMA 236:1365, 1976

116. Salzman EW: Heparin for prophylaxis of venous thromboembolism. Ann NY Acad Sci 556:371, 1989

117. Kakkar VV: Current recommendations in prevention of thrombosis in surgery. Lancet 1:237, 1987

118. Gold EW: Prophylaxis of deep venous thromboembolism: Literature review. Orthopedics 11:1197, 1988

119. The SCATI Group: Randomized controlled trial of subcutaneous calcium-heparin in acute myocardial infarction. Lancet 2:182, 1989

120. Turpie AGG, Robinson JG, Doyle DJ et al: Comparison of high-dose with low-dose subcutaneous heparin to prevent left ventricular mural thrombosis in patients with acute transmural anterior myocardial infarction. N Engl J Med 320:352, 1989

121. Levine MN, Hirsh J, Landefeld S, Raskob G: Hemorrhagic complication of anticoagulant therapy. Chest 102(Suppl):352S, 1992

122. Miller ML: Heparin-induced thrombocytopenia. Cleve Clin J Med 56:483, 1989

123. Warkentin TE, Kelton JG: Heparin-induced thrombocytopenia. Annu Rev Med 40:31, 1989

124. Hirsh J, Dakn JE, Deykin D, Poller L: Oral anticoagulants: Mechanism of action, clinical effectiveness and optimal therapeutic range. Chest 102(Suppl):312S, 1992

125. Batty JD, Breckenridge A, Lewis PJ et al: May mothers taking warfarin breast feed their infants? Br J Clin Pharmacol 3:969, 1976

126. O'Reilly RA, Aggeler PM: Studies on coumarin anticoagulant drugs: Initiation of warfarin therapy without a loading dose. Circulation 47:2657, 1968

127. Scott PJW: Anticoagulant drugs in the elderly: The risks usually outweigh the benefits. Br Med J 297:1261, 1988

128. Hirsh J: Oral anticoagulation. N Engl J Med 1991

129. Levine MN, Hirsh J: Hemorrhagic complications of long term antithrombotic therapy. In Fuster V, Verstraete M (eds): Thrombosis in Cardiovascular Disorders, pp 515–522. Philadelphia, WB Saunders, 1992

130. Verstraete M, Wessler S: Drug interference with heparin and oral anticoagulants. In Fuster V, Verstraete M (eds): Thrombosis in Cardiovascular Disorders, pp 141–146. Philadelphia, WB Saunders, 1992

131. Lowe GD: Anticoagulant drugs in the elderly: Valuable in selected patients. Br Med J 297:1261, 1988

132. Poller L, Hirsh JL: Optimal therapeutic ranges for oral anticoagulation. In Fuster V, Verstraete M (eds): Thrombosis in Cardiovascular Disorders, pp 161–174. Philadelphia, WB Saunders, 1992

133. Hull R, Hirsh J, Jay R et al: Different intensities of oral anticoagulant therapy in the treatment of proximal-vein thrombosis. N Engl J Med 307:1676, 1982

134. Levine MN, Raskob G, Hirsh J: Hemorrhagic complications of long-term anticoagulant therapy. Chest 95:26S, 1989

135. Ginsberg JS, Hirsh J: Anticoagulants during pregnancy. In Fuster V, Verstraete M (eds): Thrombosis in Cardiovascular Disorders, pp 485–490. Philadelphia, WB Saunders, 1992

136. Ginsberg JS, Hirsh J: Use of antithrombotic agents during pregnancy. Chest 102(Suppl): 385S, 1992

137. Sareli P, England MJ, Berk MR et al: Maternal and fetal sequelae of anticoagulation during pregnancy in patients with mechanical heart valve prostheses. Am J Cardiol 63:1462, 1989

138. Howie PW: Anticoagulants in pregnancy. Clin Obstet Gynecol 13:349, 1986

139. McGehee WC, Klotz TA, Epstein DJ, Rappaport SI: Coumarin necrosis associated with hereditary protein C deficiency. Ann Intern Med 101: 59, 1984

140. Feder W, Auerback R: "Purple toes": An uncommon sequela of oral coumarin drug therapy. Ann Intern Med 55:911, 1976

141. Kazmier FJ, Sheps SC, Bernatz PE et al: Livedo reticularis and digital infarcts: A syndrome due to cholesterol emboli arising from atheromatous abdominal aortic aneurysm. Vasc Dis 3:12, 1966

142. Verstraete M, Collen D: Thrombolytic agents. In Fuster V, Verstraete M (eds): Thrombosis in Cardiovascular Disorders, pp 175–190. Philadelphia, WB Saunders, 1992

143. Collen D, Cold HK: Fibrin specific thrombolytic agents and new approaches to coronary arterial thrombolysis. In Julian D, Kubler W, Norris RM et al (eds): Thrombolysis in Cardiovascular Disease, pp 45–67. New York, Marcel Dekker, 1989

144. Collen D, Stump DC, Gold HK: Thrombolytic therapy. Annu Rev Med 39:405, 1988

145. Marder VT, Sherry S: Thrombolytic therapy: Current status: Part I. N Engl J Med 318:1512, 1988

146. Marder VT, Sherry S: Thrombolytic therapy: Current status: Part II. N Engl J Med 318:1585, 1988

147. Rentrop KP, Feit F, Blanke H et al: Effects of intracoronary streptokinase and intracoronary nitroglycerin on coronary angiographic patterns and mortality in patients with acute myocardial infarction. N Engl J Med 319:1457, 1984

148. Kennedy JW, Ritchie JL, Davies KB, Fritz JK: Western Washington randomized trial of intracoronary streptokinase in acute myocardial infarction. N Engl J Med 309:1477, 1983

149. Simoons ML, Serruys PW, Band MVD et al: Improved survival after thrombolysis in acute myocardial infarction: A randomized trial conducted by the ICI in the Netherlands. Lancet 1:578, 1985

150. Rentrop KP: Thrombolytic therapy in patients with acute myocardial infarction. Circulation 71:627, 1985

151. Verstraete M, Bory M, Collen D et al: Randomized trial of intravenous recombinant tissue type plasminogen activator resists intravenous streptokinase in acute myocardial infarction. Lancet 1:842, 1985

152. Verstraete M, Brower RW, Collen D et al: Double-blind randomized trial of intravenous tissue type plasminogen activator versus placebo in acute myocardial infarction. Lancet 2:965, 1985

153. Verstraete M, Arnold AER, Brower RW et al: Acute coronary thrombolysis with recombinant tissue type plasminogen activator: Initial patency and influence of maintained infusion on reocclusion rate. Am J Cardiol 60:231, 1987

154. Simoons ML, Arnold AER, Betriu W et al: Thrombolysis with rt-PA in acute myocardial infarction: No beneficial effects of immediate PTCA. Lancet 1:197, 1988

155. Topol EJ, Morris DC, Smalling RW et al: A multicentered, randomized, placebo-controlled trial of a new form of intravenous rt-PA (Activase) in acute myocardial infarction. J Am Coll Cardiol 9:1205, 1987

156. Topol EJ, Califf RM, George BS et al: A randomized trial of immediate versus delayed elective angioplasty after intravenous TPA in acute myocardial infarction. N Engl J Med 317:581, 1987

157. Topol EJ, George BS, Kereiakes DJ et al: A randomized controlled trial of intravenous TPA and early intravenous heparin in acute myocardial infarction. Circulation 79:281, 1989

158. Gold HK, Leinbach RC, Garabedian HD et al: Acute coronary reocclusion after thrombolysis with recombinant human tissue type plasminogen activator: Prevention using a maintenance infusion. Circulation 73:347, 1986

159. TIMI Research Group: Immediate versus delayed catheterization and angioplasty following thrombolytic therapy for acute myocardial infarction. JAMA 260:2849, 1988

160. Johns JA, Gold HK, Leinbach RC et al: Prevention of coronary artery occlusion and reduction in late coronary artery stenosis after thrombolytic therapy in patients with acute myocardial infarction. Circulation 78:546, 1988

161. Stack RS, O'Conner CM, Mark DB et al: Coronary perfusion during acute myocardial infarction with a combined therapy of coronary angioplasty and high dose intravenous streptokinase. Circulation 77:151, 1988

162. Brochier ML, Quillet L, Kulbertus H et al: Intravenous anisoylated plasminogen streptokinase in evolving myocardial infarction. Drugs 3(Suppl 3):140, 1987

163. Neuhaus KL, von Essen R, Tebbe U et al: Improved thrombolysis in acute myocardial infarction with front-loaded administration of alteplase: Results of the rt-PA-APSAC patency rate (TAPS). J Am Coll Cardiol 19:885, 1992

164. Bono DD: Problems with thrombolysis. In Julian D, Kubler W, Norris RM (eds): Thrombolysis in Cardiovascular Disease, pp 279–292. New York, Marcel Dekker, 1989

165. Topol E, Califf RM: Tissue type plasminogen activator: Why the backlash? J Am Coll Cardiol 13:1477, 1989

166. Collen D, Topol E, Tiefenbrumd AJ et al: Coronary thrombolysis with r-TPA: A prospective randomized controlled trial. Circulation 70:1012, 1984

167. Collen D: Human tissue type plasminogen activator: From the laboratory to the bed side. Circulation 72:18, 1985

168. Pitt B: Clot specific thrombolytic agents: Is there an advantage? J Am Coll Cardiol 12:588, 1988

169. Magnani B, for the PAIMS investigators: Plasminogen Activator Italian Multicenter Study (PAIMS): Comparison of intravenous rt-PA with intravenous streptokinase in acute myocardial infarction. J Am Coll Cardiol 13:19, 1989

170. White HD, Rivers JT, Maslowski AH et al: Effects of intravenous streptokinase as compared with that of tissue type plasminogen activator on left ventricular function after first myocardial infarction. N Engl J Med 320:817, 1989

171. Chesebro JH, Knatterud G, Roberts R et al: Thrombolysis in Myocardial Infarction (TIMI) Trial, phase I: A comparison between intravenous tissue type plasminogen activator and intravenous streptokinase. Circulation 76:142, 1987

172. TIMI Study Group: Comparison of invasive and conservative strategies after treatment with intravenous tissue type plasminogen activator in acute myocardial infarction: Results of the TIMI-II trial. N Engl J Med 320:618, 1989

173. Cairns JA, Fuster V, Kennedy JS: Coronary thrombolysis. Chest 102(Suppl):482, 1992

174. Sobel BE: Thrombolysis in the treatment of acute myocardial infarction. In Fuster V, Verstraete M (eds): Thrombosis in Cardiovascular Disorders, pp 289–326. Philadelphia, WB Saunders, 1992

175. Gruppo Italiano per lo Studie della Sopravivenza nell'Infarto Miocardico: GISSI-2: A factorial randomised trial of alteplase versus streptokinase and heparin versus no heparin among 12,490 patients with acute myocardial infarction. Lancet 336:65, 1990

176. Third International Study of Infarct Survival Collaborative Group: ISIS-3: A randomised comparison of streptokinase vs tissue-plasminogen activator vs anistreplase and of aspirin plus heparin vs aspirin alone among 41,299 cases of suspected acute myocardial infarction. Lancet 339:753, 1992

177. Monk JP, Heel RC: Anisoylated plasminogen streptokinase activator complex (APSAC): A review of its mechanism of action, clinical pharmacology and therapeutic use in acute myocardial infarction. Drugs 34:25, 1987

178. AIMS Trial Study Group: Effects of intravenous APSAC on mortality after myocardial infarction: Preliminary report of a placebo-controlled clinical trial. Lancet 1:545, 1988

179. Bassand JP, Machecourt J, Cassagnes J et al: Multicenter trial of intravenous anisoylated activator complex (APSAC) in acute myocardial infarction: Effects on infarct size and left ventricular function. J Am Coll Cardiol 13:988, 1989

180. Mathey DC, Schofer J, Sheehan EH et al: Intravenous urokinase in acute myocardial infarction. Am J Cardiol 55:878, 1985

181. Tennant SN, Dixon J, Venable TC et al: Intracoronary thrombolysis in patients with acute myocardial infarction: Comparison of the efficacy of urokinase with streptokinase. Circulation 69:756, 1984

182. Van der Werf F, Vanhaecke J, de Grost H et al: Coronary thrombolysis with recombinant single chain urokinase-type plasminogen activator in patients with acute myocardial infarction. Circulation 74:1066, 1986

183. Topol EJ, Califf RM, George BS et al: Coronary arterial thrombolysis with combined infusion of r-TPA and urokinase in patients with acute myocardial infarction. Circulation 77:1100, 1988

184. Collen D, Van der Werf F: Coronary thrombolysis with low dose synergistic combinations of r-TPA and recu-PA in man. Am J Cardiol 60:431, 1987

185. Ip JH, Fuster V, Badimon L et al: Syndromes of accelerated atherosclerosis: Role of vascular injury and smooth muscle cell proliferation. J Am Coll Cardiol 15:1667, 1990

186. Fuster V, Badimon L, Badimon JJ, Chesebro JH: The pathogenesis of coronary disease and the acute coronary syndromes (part one). N Engl J Med 326:242, 1992

187. Ross R: The pathogenesis of atherosclerosis: An update. N Engl J Med 314:488, 1986

188. Schwartz CJ, Valente AJ, Kelly JL et al: Thrombosis and the development of atherosclerosis: Rokitanski revisited. Semin Thromb Hemost 14:189, 1988

189. Woolf N, Davies MJ: Interrelationship between atherosclerosis and thrombosis. In Fuster V, Verstraete M (eds): Thrombosis in Cardiovascular Disorders, pp 99–120. Philadelphia, WB Saunders, 1992

190. Davies MJ, Bland MJ, Hartgartner WR et al: Factors influencing the presence or absence of acute coronary thrombi in sudden ischemic death. Eur Heart J 10:203, 1989

191. Bini A, Fenoglia JJ, Mesa-Tejada R et al: Identification and distribution of fibrinogen, fibrin and fibrin degradation products in atherosclerosis: Use of monoclonal antibody. Atherosclerosis 1:109, 1989

192. Falk E: Unstable angina with fatal outcome, dynamic coronary thrombosis leading to infarction and/or sudden death: Autopsy evidence of recurrent mural thrombosis with peripheral embolization culminating in total vascular occlusion. Circulation 71:699, 1985

193. Sherman CT, Litvak F, Grundfest W et al: Coronary angioscopy in patients with unstable angina. N Engl J Med 315:913, 1986

194. Levin DC, Fallon JT: Significance of the angiographic morphology of localized coronary stenosis: Histopathological correlates. Circulation 66:316, 1982

195. Ambrose JA, Winters SL, Stern A et al: Angiographic morphology and the pathogenesis of unstable angina. J Am Coll Cardiol 5:609, 1985

196. Gorlin R, Fuster V, Ambrose JA: Anatomic-physiologic link between the acute coronary syndromes. Circulation 74:2, 1986

197. Ambrose JA, Tennebaum MA, Alexopoulos D et al: Angiographical progression of coronary artery disease and the development of myocardial infarction. J Am Coll Cardiol 12:256, 1988

198. Ambrose JA, Hjendale-Monsen CE, Borrico S et al: Angiographic demonstration of a common link between unstable angina pectoris and non Q wave myocardial infarction. Am J Cardiol 61: 244, 1988

199. Richardson PD, Davies MJ, Born GVR: Influence of plaque configuration and stress distribution on fissuring of coronary atherosclerotic plaques. Lancet 2:941, 1989

200. Fuster V, Chesebro JH: Role of platelets and platelet inhibitor in coronary artery vein graft bypass disease. Circulation 73:227, 1986

201. Ip JH, Fuster V, Badimon L, Chesebro JH: Interactions between blood and coronary arterial wall. Curr Opin Cardiol 4:0772, 1989

202. Lie JT, Lawrie WM, Morris GC: Aortocoronary bypass saphenous vein graft atherosclerosis. Am J Cardiol 40:906, 1977

203. Atkinson JB, Forman BB, Vaugh WK et al: Morphologic changes in long term saphenous vein bypass grafts. Chest 88:341, 1985

204. Solymoss BC, Nadeau P, Millette D, Campeau L: Late thrombosis of saphenous vein coronary bypass grafts related to risk factors. Circulation 7:1140, 1988

205. Ip JH, Fuster V, Israel D, Badimon L, Badimon J, Chesebro JH: The role of platelets, thrombin, and hyperplasia in restenosis after coronary angioplasty. J Am Coll Cardiol 17(Suppl B):77B, 1991

206. Steele PM, Chesebro JH, Stanson AW et al: Balloon angioplasty in natural history of pathophysiological responses to injury in a pig model. Circ Res 57:105, 1985

207. Waller BF: "Crackers, breakers, stretchers, drillers, scrapers, shavers, welders and melters": The future treatment of atherosclerotic coronary artery disease? A clinical-morphological assesment. J Am Coll Cardiol 13:969, 1989

208. Block PC, Myler RK, Stertzer S, Fallon JT: Morphology after transluminal angioplasty in human beings. N Engl J Med 305:382, 1981

209. Uchida Y, Hasegawa K, Kawamura K, Shibuya I: Angioscopic observation of the coronary luminal changes induced by percutaneous coronary angioplasty. Am Heart J 117:769, 1989

210. Mizuno K, Mugamoto A, Shibuya T et al: Changes in angioscopic macromorphology following coronary angioplasty (abstr). Circulation 78(Suppl II):II-289, 1988

211. Leclerc G, Isner JM, Kearney M et al: Evidence implicating nonmuscle myosin in restenosis. Circulation 85:543, 1992

212. Virchow R: Gesammelte Abhandlunger zum wissenschaftlichen Medicine, pp 219–732. Frankfurt, Medinger Son & Co, 1856

213. Johnson RC, Crissman RS, Didio LA: Endocardial alteration in myocardial infarction. Lab Invest 40:183, 1979

214. Hochman JJ, Platia EB, Bulkley BH: Endocardial abnormalities in left ventricular aneurysm: A clinical pathologic study. Ann Intern Med 100: 29, 1984

215. Roberts WC, Seigel RJ, McNanus BM: Idiopathic dilated cardiomyopathy: Analysis of 152 necrosy patients. Am J Cardiol 60:1340, 1987

216. Mikell FL, Asinger RW, Elsperger KJ et al: Regional stasis of blood in the dysfunctional left ventricle: Echocardiographic detection and differentiation from early thrombosis. Circulation 66:755, 1982

217. Asinger RW, Mikell FL, Elsperger KJ, Hodges M: Incidence of left ventricular thrombosis after acute myocardial infarction: Serial evaluation by two-dimension echocardiogram. N Engl J Med 305:297, 1981

218. Weinrich DJ, Burke JF, Pauletto FJ: Left ventricular mural thrombi complicating acute myocardial infarction: Long term follow-up with serial echocardiography. Ann Intern Med 100:789, 1984

219. Shresta NK, Moreno FL, Narciso FV et al: Two-dimensional echocardiographic diagnosis of left atrial thrombus in rheumatic heart disease: A clinicopathologic study. Circulation 67:341, 1983

220. Fulton RM, Duckett K: Plasma-fibrinogen and thromboemboli after myocardial infarction. Lancet 2:1161, 1976

221. Fuster V, Halperin JL: Left ventricular thrombi and cerebral embolism. N Engl J Med 320:392, 1989

222. Cabin HS, Roberts WC: Left ventricular aneurysm, intra-aneurysmal thrombus and systemic embolus in coronary heart disease. Chest 320: 392, 1980

223. Dewanjee MK, Fuster V, Rao SA et al: Noninvasive radioisotopic technique for detection of platelet deposition in mitral valve prosthesis and quantification of visceral microembolism in dogs. Mayo Clin Proc 58:307, 1983

224. Acar J, Vahanian V, Fauchet M et al: Detection of prosthetic valve thrombosis using indium-111 platelet imaging (abstr). Eur Heart J 20:261, 1989

225. Chesebro JH, Fuster V: Valvular heart disease and prosthetic heart valves. In Fuster V, Verstraete M (eds): Thrombosis in Cardiovascular Disorders, pp 161–174. Philadelphia, WB Saunders, 1992

226. Fuster V, Badimon L, Badimon JJ, Chesebro JH: Prevention of thromboembolism induced by prosthetic heart valves. Semin Thromb Hemost 14:50, 1988

227. Edmunds HC Jr: Thrombosis and bleeding complications of prosthetic heart valves. Ann Thorac Surg 44:430, 1987

228. Stein B, Fuster V, Halperin JL, Chesebro JH: Antithrombotic therapy in cardiac disease: An emerging approach based on pathogenesis and risk. Circulation 80:1501, 1989

229. Theroux P, Ouimet H, McCanu T et al: Aspirin, heparin or both to treat acute unstable angina. N Engl J Med 319:1105, 1988

230. Telford AM, Wilson C: Trial of heparin versus atenolol in prevention of myocardial infarction in intermediate coronary syndrome. Lancet 1: 1225, 1981

231. The RISC Group: Risk of myocardial infarction and death during treatment with low-dose aspirin and intravenous heparin in men with unstable coronary artery disease. Lancet 336: 827, 1990

232. Ambrose JA, Alexoupoulous D: Thrombolysis in unstable angina: Will the beneficial effects of thrombotic therapy in myocardial infarction apply to patients with unstable angina? J Am Coll Cardiol 13:1666, 1989

233. Lawrence JR, Shephard JT, Bone I et al: Fibrinolytic therapy in unstable angina: A controlled clinical trial. Thromb Res 17:767, 1980

234. Rentrop P, Blanke H, Karsch KP et al: Selective intracoronary thrombolysis in acute myocardial infarction and unstable angina. Circulation 63:307, 1981

235. Vetrovec GW, Leinbach RC, Gold HK, Crowley MJ: Intracoronary thrombolysis in syndromes of unstable ischemia: Angiographic and clinical results. Am Heart J 104:946, 1982

236. Mandelkorn JB, Wolf NM, Singh S et al: Intracoronary thrombus in nontransmural myocardial infarction and in unstable angina pectoris. Am J Cardiol 52:1, 1983

237. Ambrose JA, Hjemdahl-Monsen C, Borrico S et al: Quantitative and qualitative effects of intracoronary streptokinase in unstable angina and non-Q wave myocardial infarction. J Am Coll Cardiol 9:1156, 1987

238. Gold HK, Johns JA, Leinbach RC et al: A randomized, blinded placebo-controlled trial of recombinant human TPA in patients with unstable angina. Circulation 9:1156, 1987

239. Gotoh K, Minamino T, Katoh O et al: The role of intracoronary thrombus in unstable angina: Angiographic assessment and thrombolytic therapy during ongoing angina attacks. Circulation 77:526, 1988

240. DeZwaan C, Bar FW, Janssen JHA et al: Effects of thrombolytic therapy in unstable angina: Clinical and angiographic results. J Am Coll Cardiol 12:301, 1988

241. Topol EJ, Nicklas JM, Kandler NH et al: Coronary revascularization after intravenous TPA for unstable angina pectoris: Results of a randomized double-blind, placebo-controlled trial. Am J Cardiol 62:368, 1988

242. Schreiber TL, Macina G, McNulty A et al: Urokinase plus heparin versus aspirin in unstable angina and non-Q-wave myocardial infarction. Am J Cardiol 64:840, 1989

243. Williams DO, Topol EJ, Califf RM et al: Intravenous recombinant tissue-type plasminogen activator in patients with unstable angina pectoris. Circulation 82:376, 1990

244. Ardissino D, Barberis P, De Servi S et al: Recombinant tissue-type plasminogen activator followed by heparin compared with heparin alone for refractory unstable angina pectoris. Am J Cardiol 66:910, 1990

245. Braunwald E: The TIMI trial on unstable angina. Presented at American Heart Association Meeting, Nov. 1992

246. Gibson RS, Beller GA, Gheorghiade M et al: The prevalence and clinical significance of residual myocardial ischemia 2 weeks after uncomplicated non-Q wave infarction: A prospective natural history study. Circulation 73:1186, 1986

247. Timmis AD, Griffin B, Crick JCP et al: The effects of early coronary patency on the evolution of myocardial infarction: A prospective arteriographic study. Br Heart J 58:345, 1987

248. Cairns JA, Hirsh J, Lewis D et al: Antithrombotic therapy in coronary artery disease. Chest 102(Suppl):456S, 1992

249. Ross AM: Myocardial infarction: Adjunctive antithrombotic therapy in thrombolysis. In Fuster V, Verstraete M (eds): Thrombosis in Cardiovascular Disorders, pp 327–342. Philadelphia, WB Saunders, 1992

250. Hebert P, Fuster V, Hennekens CH: In Fuster V, Verstraete M (eds): Thrombosis in Cardiovascular Disorders, pp 261–274. Philadelphia, WB Saunders, 1992

251. Report of the Working Party on Anticoagulation Therapy in Coronary Thrombosis to the Medical Research Council: Assessment of short term anticoagulation administration after cardiac infarction. Br Med J 1:335, 1969

252. Drapkin A, Merskey C: Anticoagulation therapy after myocardial infarction: Relation of therapeutic benefit to patient's age, sex and severity of infarction. JAMA 222:541, 1977

253. Veterans Administration Hospital Investigators: Anticoagulation in acute myocardial infarction: Results of a cooperative clinical trial. JAMA 225:724, 1973

254. Chalmers TC, Matta RJ, Smith H, Kunzler AM: Evidence favoring the use of anticoagulation in the hospital phase of acute myocardial infarction. N Engl J Med 297:1091, 1977

255. Kannel WB, Wolf PA, Garrison RJ: Survival following initial cardiovascular events: Framingham Study: Section 35, publication No. PB 88-204049. US Department of Health and Human Services, National Institutes of Health, US Department of Commerce. Washington, DC, US Government Printing Office, 1988

256. Smith P: Antithrombotic therapy in the chronic phase of myocardial infarction. In Fuster V, Verstraete M (eds): Thrombosis in Cardiovascular Disorders, pp 343–362. Philadelphia, WB Saunders, 1992

257. International Anticoagulation Review Group: Collaborative analysis of long-term anticoagulation administration after acute myocardial infarction. Lancet 1:203, 1970

258. Smith P, Arnesen H: Oral anticoagulant reduces mortality, reinfarction and cerebral vascular event alter myocardial infarction: WARIS study (abstr). Eur Heart J 30:264, 1989

259. Report of the Sixty-Plus Reinfarction Study Research Group: A double-blind trial to assess long-term oral anticoagulation therapy in elderly patients after myocardial infarction. Lancet 2:989, 1980

260. Peto R, Gray R, Collins R et al: A randomized trial of the effects of prophylactic daily aspirin among British male doctors. Br Med J 296:313, 1988

261. Fuster V, Cohen M, Halperin J: Aspirin in the prevention of coronary disease. N Engl J Med 321:129, 1989

262. Chesebro JH, Webster MW, Smith HC et al: Antiplatelet therapy in coronary disease progression—reduced infarctions and even lesion progression (abstr). Circulation 80(Suppl II):II-266, 1989

263. Chesebro JH, Goldman S: Coronary artery bypass surgery: Antithrombotic therapy. In Fuster

V, Verstraete M (eds): Thrombosis in Cardiovascular Disorders, pp 375–388. Philadelphia, WB Saunders, 1992

264. Stein PD, Dalen JE, Goldman S et al: Antithrombotic therapy in patients with saphenous vein and internal mammary artery bypass graft following and following percutaneous transluminal coronary angioplasty. Chest 102(Suppl): 508S, 1992

265. Chesebro JH, Clements IP, Fuster V et al: A platelet inhibitor trial in coronary artery bypass operations: Benefit of perioperative dipyridamole and aspirin therapy on early postoperative vein-graft patency. N Engl J Med 307:73, 1982

266. Limet R, David JL, Magotteauz P et al: Prevention of aorta-coronary bypass graft occlusion. J Thorac Cardiovasc Surg 94:773, 1987

267. Goldman S, Copeland J, Mortiz T et al: Improvement in early saphenous vein graft bypass surgery with antiplatelet therapy: Results of a Veterans Administration Cooperative Study. Circulation 77:1324, 1988

268. McEnany MT, Salzman FW, Mundth ED et al: The effect of antithrombotic therapy on the patency rates of saphenous vein bypass grafts. J Thorac Cardiovasc Surg 83:81, 1982

269. Pantley GA, Goodnight SH, Rahimtoola SH et al: Failure of antiplatelet and anticoagulant therapy to improve patency of grafts after coronary artery operation: A controlled randomized study. N Engl J Med 301:962, 1979

270. Gruntzig AR, Senning A, Suganthalan WE: Nonoperative dilation of coronary artery stenosis: Percutaneous transluminal coronary angioplasty. N Engl J Med 301:61, 1979

271. McBride W, Lange RA, Hillls DC: Restenosis after successful coronary angioplasty: Pathophysiology and prevention. N Engl J Med 318: 1734, 1988

272. Calipp RM, Willerson JT: Percutaneous transluminal coronary angioplasty: Prevention of occlusion and restenosis. In Fuster V, Verstraete M (eds): Thrombosis in Cardiovascular Disorders, pp 389–408. Philadelphia, WB Saunders, 1992

273. Barnathan ES, Schwartz JS, Taylor L et al: Aspirin and dipyridamole in the prevention of acute coronary thrombosis complicating coronary angioplasty. Circulation 76:125, 1987

274. Schwartz L, Bourassa MC, Lesperance J et al: Aspirin and dipyridamole in the prevention of restenosis after percutaneous transluminal coronary angioplasty. N Engl J Med 318:1714, 1988

275. White CW, Chaitman B, Lassar TA et al: Antiplatelet agents are effective in reducing the immediate complication of PTCA: Results from the Ticlopidine Multicenter Trial. Circulation 76 (Suppl IV):400, 1987

276. White CW, Knudson M, Schmidt D et al: Neither ticlopidine nor aspirin-dipyridamole prevents restenosis post PTCA: Results from a randomized placebo-controlled multicenter trial (abstr). Circulation 76:IV-213, 1987

277. Heras M, Chesebro JH, Penny WJ et al: Importance of adequate heparin dosage in arterial angioplasty in a porcine model. Circulation 78: 654, 1988

278. Lukas MA, Deutsch E, Laskey WK: Beneficial effect of heparin therapy on PTCA outcome in unstable angina (abstr). J Am Coll Cardiol 11 (Suppl A):132A, 1988

279. Douglas JS, Lutz JF, Clements SD et al: Therapy of large intracoronary thrombi in candidates for PTCA (abstr). J Am Coll Cardiol 11(Suppl A): 238A, 1988

280. Pow TK, Varricchione TR, Jacobs AK et al: Does pretreatment with heparin prevent abrupt closure following PTCA (abstr)? J Am Coll Cardiol 11(Suppl A):238A, 1988

281. Ellis SG, Roubin GS, Wilente J et al: Results of a randomized trial of heparin and aspirin versus aspirin alone for prevention of acute closure and restenosis after PTCA (abstr). Circulation 76(Suppl):IV-213, 1987

282. Thorton MA, Gruntzig AR, Hollman J et al: Coumadin and aspirin in the prevention of restenosis after PTCA: A randomized study. Circulation 69:721, 1984

283. Laupacis A, Albers G, Dunn MI, Feinberg WM: Antithrombotic therapy in atrial fibrillation. Chest 102(Suppl):426S, 1992

284. Halperin JL, Petersen P. Thrombosis in the cardiac chambers: Ventricular dysfunction and atrial fibrillation. In Fuster V, Verstraete M (eds): Thrombosis in Cardiovascular Disorders, pp 215–236. Philadelphia, WB Saunders, 1992

285. Halperin JL, Hart RC: Atrial fibrillation and stroke: New ideas and persisting dilemmas. Stroke 19:937, 1988

286. Brand FN, Abbott RD, Kannel WB, Wolf PA: Characteristic and prognosis of lone atrial fibrillation: 30-year follow-up in the Framingham Study. JAMA 254:3449, 1985

287. Kopecky SL, Gersh BJ, McGoon MD et al: The natural history of lone atrial fibrillation: A population-based study over three decades. N Engl J Med 317:669, 1987

288. Petersen P, Boysen G, Godtfredsen J et al: Placebo-controlled, randomised trial of warfarin and aspirin for prevention of thromboembolic complications in chronic atrial fibrillation: The Copenhagen AFASAK study. Lancet 1:175, 1989

289. The Stroke Prevention in Atrial Fibrillation Investigators: The Stroke Prevention in Atrial Fibrillation Trial: Final results. Circulation 84:527, 1991

290. The Boston Area Anticoagulation Trial for Atrial Fibrillation Investigators: The effect of low-dose warfarin on the risk of stroke in patients with nonrheumatic atrial fibrillation. N Engl J Med 323:1505, 1990

291. Connolly SJ, Laupacis A, Gent M et al: Canadian Atrial Fibrillation Anticoagulation (CAFA) Study. J Am Coll Cardiol 18:349, 1991

292. Ezckowitz MD, Bridger SL, James KE et al: Warfarin in the prevention of stroke associated with nonrheumatic atrial fibrillation. N Engl J Med 327:1406, 1992

293. Meltzer RS, Visser CA, Fuster V: Intracardiac thrombi and systemic embolization. Ann Intern Med 104:689, 1986

294. Turpie AGG, Robinson JG, Doyle DJ et al: Comparison of high dose and low dose subcutaneous heparin to prevent left ventricular mural thrombosis in patients with acute transmural myocardial infarction. N Engl J Med 320:352, 1989

295. Lapeyre AC, Steele PP, Kazmier FJ et al: Systemic embolism in chronic left ventricular aneurysm: Incidence and role of anticoagulation. J Am Coll Cardiol 6:534, 1985

296. Fuster V, Gersh BJ, Giuliani ER et al: The natural history of idiopathic dilated cardiomyopathy. Am J Cardiol 47:525, 1981

297. Stein PD, Alpert JS, Copeland J et al: Antithrombotic therapy in patients with mechanical and biological prosthetic heart valves. Chest 102(Suppl):445S, 1992

298. Meyers ML, Lawrie GM, Crawford ES et al: The St. Jude valve prosthesis: Analysis of the clinical results in 815 implants and the need for systemic anticoagulation. J Am Coll Cardiol 13:57, 1989

299. Mok CY, Boey J, Wang R et al: Warfarin versus dipyridamole-aspirin and pentoxylline-aspirin for the prevention of prosthetic valve thromboembolism: A prospective randomized clinical trial. Circulation 72:1059, 1985

300. Altman R, Boullon F, Rouvier J, Raca R, de la Fuente L, Favaloro R: Aspirin and prophylaxis of thromboembolic complications in patients with substitute heart valves. J Thorac Cardiovasc Surg 72:127, 1976

301. Turpie AGG, Gent M, Laupacis A et al: Reduction in mortality by adding aspirin (100 mg) to oral anticoagulants in patients with heart valve replacement (abstr). J Am Coll Cardiol 19(Suppl A):103A, 1992

302. Karchmer AW, Dismukes WE, Buckley MJ et al: Late prosthetic valve endocarditis—clinical features influencing therapy. Am J Med 64:199, 1978

303. Sherman DG, Dyken ML, Fisher M et al: Antithrombotic therapy for cerebrovascular disease. Chest 102(Suppl):529S, 1992

304. Sherman DG, Hart RG: Stroke and transient ischemic attack: Thromboembolism and antithrombotic therapy. In Fuster V, Verstraete M (eds): Thrombosis in Cardiovascular Disorders, pp 409–422. Philadelphia, WB Saunders, 1992

Cardiovascular Drug Interactions

Neal L. Benowitz

General Considerations

Multiple drug therapy is common in patients with cardiovascular disease. In one teaching hospital survey[1] the median number of drugs administered to hospitalized patients was 12 (range 8 to 25). A patient receiving ten drugs simultaneously is exposed to approximately 10 million possible interactions. Most of these interactions are inconsequential. Some interactions are beneficial and are used to therapeutic advantage. Other drug interactions may have adverse or even lethal consequences. These are the subject of this chapter. Physicians can and should be able to anticipate significant adverse drug interactions and adjust the types or doses of medications so as not to injure the patient.

Characteristics of drug interactions that are likely to lead to significant consequences include (1) an interaction of substantial magnitude and (2) a steep dose-response relationship so that slight or moderate decrease in drug action leads to therapeutic failure or (3) a narrow therapeutic index such that a small or moderate increase in drug action leads to toxicity. Many of the drugs fitting this description are those used in treating patients with cardiovascular disease. Adverse drug interactions in such patients are often not recognized because it is difficult to distinguish adverse drug effects from worsening of the underlying disease. Awareness of the potential for drug interactions combined with an understanding of the pharmacology of the agents and careful observation when new drugs are started are the key elements to preventing adverse drug interactions.

Drug interactions may occur because of altered pharmacokinetics or pharmacodynamics. Examples of various mechanisms of interaction are given in discussion of individual drugs. Case examples are presented to place interactions in a clinical context.

Cardiac Glycosides (Figure 10.1)

Interactions Affecting Bioavailability

Case Example A 71-year-old woman with chronic congestive heart failure developed a respiratory tract infection associated with cough and wheezing. To her customary drug regimen of hydralazine, furosemide, isosorbide dinitrate, and digoxin, 0.25 mg/d, erythromycin and theophylline were added. Her usual serum digoxin concentration was 1.4 ng/ml. Four days later, she developed nausea and vomiting with an atrioventricular junctional rhythm. Her serum digoxin concentration was 2.6 ng/ml.[2]

Digoxin tablets, because of slow absorption, are variably absorbed; absorption is more complete from elixir (capsule) preparations. Absorption from tablets may be reduced in patients with rapid gastrointestinal transit. Accelerating gastrointestinal transit with metoclopramide may decrease bioavailability, and slowing transit with propantheline (and other drugs with anticholinergic activity) may increase bioavailability, leading to significant changes in digoxin levels.[3] Such interactions are not usually noted when patients are taking elixir preparations because absorption is more rapid.

Treatment with cancer chemotherapeutic agents and irradiation injures the intestinal epithelial cells and results in reduced absorption of drugs, including digoxin.[4] The magnitude of the effect is substantial, with an average reduction of bioavailability of 50%. The rate of dissolution of the tablets seems to be an important factor in that antineoplastic therapy does not significantly impair the bioavailability of the solution-in-capsule or elixir preparations.

Digoxin that is not absorbed in the upper gastrointestinal tract or that is excreted into the bile may be reductively metabolized by anaerobic bacteria *(Eubacterium alantum)* in the colon. Reduced digoxin metabolites such as dihydrodigoxin, which are not believed to be pharmacologically active, may account for up to 40% of eliminated digoxin in a minority (about 10%) of patients. In such patients, administration of antibiotics such as erythromycin or tetracycline can lead to substantially increased bioavailability of digoxin and may result in clinical toxicity as illustrated in the case example.[5] Patients who excrete a major fraction of digoxin as reduced metabolites are typically those who require a higher than usual daily digoxin dose. This is an example of an uncommon but potentially predictable interaction.

Cholestyramine and colestipol, drugs used in treating hypercholesterolemia, as well as some antacids and kaolin-pectin, may bind digoxin in the gut and reduce absorption. The magnitude of the effect when digoxin is given with cholestyramine is a 20% to 30% reduction in bioavailability, but can be minimized by spacing digoxin dosing at least an hour before that of the resins.[6] Enterohepatic recirculation occurs to a small extent with digoxin and to a much larger extent with digitoxin. Cholestyramine or charcoal binds cardiac glycosides in the gut and reduces the extent of enterohepatic recycling. As a consequence, elimination half-life may be substantially shortened.[7,8] This interaction has been used successfully in the therapy of digitoxin poisoning.[9]

Interactions Resulting in Altered Distribution

Case Example A 50-year-old man was taking digoxin, 0.25 mg/d, and quinidine sulfate, 300 mg every 6 hours. The morning predosing serum digoxin concentration was 1 ng/ml. Two hours after the afternoon quinidine dose, PR interval prolongation was noted and his serum digoxin concentration was 2.5 ng/ml.

Cardiac glycosides are extensively distributed to body tissues. There appear to be both specific and nonspecific digitalis binding sites. Quinidine, some of the calcium entry blockers, and cyclosporine may displace digoxin from nonspecific binding sites (Fig.

FIGURE 10.1 DRUG INTERACTIONS AFFECTING DIGOXIN

Interacting Drug	SDC	Type of Interaction	Possible Mechanism	Recommendations
Amiodarone	↑	Decreased clearance	Inhibits metabolism or renal excretion	Decrease digoxin dose; monitor SDC
Antacids	↓	Decreased absorption		Do not give antacids within 1 hour of digoxin
Antineoplastic drugs	↓	Decreased absorption	Damage to intestinal epithelium	Monitor SDC, increase dose as necessary; substitute capsule for tablet
Bepridil	↑	Decreased clearance	Unknown	Monitor SDC, decrease dose as necessary
Captopril	↑	Decreased clearance	Inhibits renal excretion	Monitor SDC, decrease dose as necessary
Cholestyramine, colestipol	↓	Decreased absorption, increased clearance	Binds digoxin in intestine; interferes with entero-hepatic recirculation	Do not give cholestyramine within 1 hour of digoxin; monitor SDC
Cyclosporine	↑	Decreased clearance, reduced distribution volume	Inhibits renal excretion	Monitor SDC, decrease dose as necessary
Diltiazem	↑	Decreased clearance	Inhibits metabolism and renal excretion	Reduce digoxin dose; monitor SDC
Erythromycin	↑	Increased bioavailability, decreased clearance	Decreases gut metabolism (significant in only small % of patients)	Monitor SDC, adjust dose in affected patients
Furosemide (and other diuretics)	↑	Decreased renal clearance, increased toxicity	Overdiuresis reduces tubular secretion; hypokalemia, hypomagnesemia	Observe carefully; monitor SDC; monitor potassium and magnesium levels
Hydralazine	↓	Increased renal clearance	Increases filtration and secretion (heart failure patients)	Uncertain
Indomethacin	↑	Decreased clearance	Inhibits renal excretion	Interaction described in premature infants; reduce dose by 50%; monitor SDC
Methimazole, propylthiouracil	↑	Decreased renal clearance, increased myocardial sensitivity	Conversion from hyperthyroid to euthyroid state	Decrease digoxin dose; monitor SDC
Metoclopramide	↓	Decreased absorption	Increased gastrointestinal motility (significant for tablet but not capsule or elixir formulations)	Monitor SDC, increase dose as necessary; subsitute capsule for tablet
Nitroprusside	↓	Increased renal clearance	Increases filtration and secretion (heart failure patients)	Uncertain
Propafenone	↑	Decreased clearance	Inhibition of renal and non-renal clearance	Decrease digoxin dose; monitor SDC
Rifampin	↓	Increased clearance	Accelerates metabolism or biliary secretion	Monitor SDC, increase dose as necessary
Quinidine, quinine	↑	Decreased clearance, reduced distribution volume	Inhibits metabolism, biliary secretion, and renal excretion; displacement from tissue binding sites	Reduce dose by 50%; monitor SDC
Spironolactone	↑	Decreased clearance	Inhibits renal tubular secretion	Monitor SDC, decrease dose as necessary
Tetracycline	↑	Increased bioavailability, decreased clearance	Decreases gut metabolism (significantly in only small % of patients)	Monitor SDC, adjust dose in affected patients
Thyroid hormones	↓	Increased clearance, reduced myocardial sensitivity	Conversion from hypothyroid to euthyroid state	Monitor SDC, increase dose as necessary
Verapamil	↑	Decreased clearance	Inhibits metabolism and renal excretion	Reduce digoxin dose; monitor SDC

SDC = Serum digoxin concentration

10.2). This displacement results in transient elevation of serum digoxin concentrations, so that digoxin levels rise and fall in parallel with rising and falling quinidine concentrations.[10] The transient rise in serum digoxin concentration may be associated with manifestations of digitalis toxicity, although the overall clinical significance of this phenomenon is unknown. Alteration in distribution kinetics per se does not affect steady-state digoxin levels and does not require dosage adjustment.

INTERACTIONS RESULTING IN ALTERED ELIMINATION

Case Example A 74-year-old woman was hospitalized with new-onset atrial fibrillation. On digoxin, 0.25 mg/d for 8 days, her serum digoxin concentration was 0.8 ng/ml and she had a ventricular response rate of 80 beats per minute. The following day she was started on quinidine, 300 mg every 6 hours, and discharged in hope of pharmacologic cardioversion. Five days later, she developed abdominal pain and nausea. One week later she was admitted with high-degree atrioventricular block and frequent premature ventricular contractions. Her serum digoxin concentration was 5.8 ng/ml, and quinidine, 2.3 μg/ml.

Digoxin and quinidine have been used together for more than 60 years, yet it was not until 1978 that the significant interaction between the two was noted.[11] A clinical presentation such as that described in the previous case would have been attributed in past years to spontaneous changes in the severity of disease. With the availability of serum digoxin assays and the knowledge of how to conduct pharmacokinetic studies, we now know that quinidine, amiodarone, and some of the calcium entry blockers significantly influence digoxin elimination.

Digoxin is eliminated by both metabolism (about 40%) and renal excretion (about 60%). Metabolism of digoxin is inhibited by quinidine, verapamil, amiodarone, and possibly diltiazem and cyclosporine.[12–16]

There is controversy about whether nifedipine influences digoxin metabolism.[17,18] The effects of quinidine and quinine on hepatic clearance are mediated at least in part by inhibition of biliary clearance, owing to both reduced bile flow and reduced concentrations of digoxin in the bile.[19] Likewise, verapamil decreases biliary clearance of digoxin.[20] These same drugs, as well as spironolactone, inhibit tubular secretion of digoxin, resulting in reduced renal elimination as well.[21] Rifampin, in contrast, accelerates the elimination of digoxin, either by increased metabolism or by increased biliary secretion.[22] The magnitude of effect of drugs on digoxin elimination varies considerably from drug to drug and may be dose-related. Quinidine and spironolactone together have additive effects on digoxin elimination.[23]

Drug-related changes in hemodynamics such as in the therapy of patients with cardiac failure may influence digoxin renal excretion, possibly mediated by changes in renal blood flow. Hydralazine and nitroprusside acutely increase the filtration and secretion of digoxin,[24] although the relevance of this observation to long-term therapy is as yet undefined. In contrast, excessive diuresis results in reduced renal as well as nonrenal clearance of digoxin and may result in toxicity if the dose is not changed.[25]

Assuming an unchanged dosing regimen, changes in drug clearance or elimination rate result in a new steady-state concentration. This effect can result in toxicity as illustrated by the case example. There has been debate as to whether quinidine and other drugs might block the action of digoxin at the cardiac receptor. However, most animal studies and clinical observations indicate that quinidine and other drugs that increase digoxin levels may result in increased digoxin action and, presumably, toxicity. Therefore, adjustments should be made in the maintenance dose. For example, when adding quinidine to a stable dose of digoxin, a 50% reduction in clearance should be anticipated. Thus, the digoxin dose should be

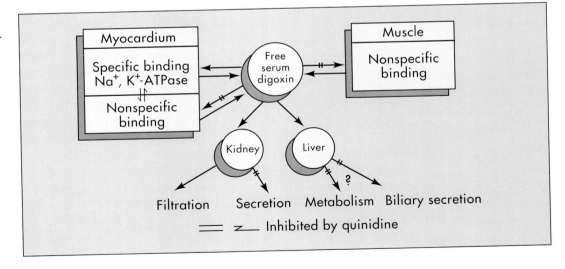

Figure 10.2 Mechanism of digoxin–quinidine interaction.

reduced by 50%. Because the magnitude of the effect is variable from person to person, final dose adjustments need to be made on the basis of repeated drug level determinations or on the basis of clinical responses, such as ventricular response rate in atrial fibrillation.

The time course of the rise of digoxin levels when clearance is reduced by an interacting drug needs to be considered in planning dosing. Because of the long half-life of digoxin, it takes at least 1 week and maybe as long as several weeks to reach a new plateau level. Patients need to be carefully monitored for development of toxicity during this period.

Whereas digoxin is primarily excreted by the kidney and secondarily metabolized, digitoxin is primarily metabolized. Metabolism of digitoxin is accelerated by drugs such as phenobarbital, phenytoin, rifampin, and phenylbutazone. Accelerated metabolism can reduce steady-state serum digitoxin concentrations, requiring increased dosage to maintain a desired level. Quinidine and verapamil inhibit digitoxin clearance.

PHARMACOLOGIC INTERACTIONS

Digitalis actions and toxicity are exaggerated in the presence of hypokalemia or hypomagnesemia. Deficiencies of both electrolytes may occur during treatment with diuretics. Serum potassium or magnesium levels do not necessarily reflect whole-body concentrations. For example, digitalis toxicity responsive to magnesium may occur in the presence of normal serum but reduced lymphocyte magnesium and potassium levels. Atrial fibrillation may be poorly responsive to digoxin in patients with hypomagnesemia.[26] Replacement of magnesium may therefore enhance the efficacy and decrease the toxicity of digitalis; however, guidelines for magnesium therapy in patients taking diuretics have not been established.

Case Example A 66-year-old man who had chronic heart failure, chronic obstructive lung disease, and a history of peptic ulcer disease and who was regularly taking digoxin and theophylline developed burning epigastric pain. Antacids and cimetidine were initiated, with relief of symptoms. Five days later he presented with atrial flutter with a rapid ventricular response rate. Theophylline was discontinued, and he was treated with extra doses of digoxin until the ventricular rate decreased. Three days later digitalis-toxic cardiac rhythms, including ventricular tachycardia, were noted. Theophylline and digoxin levels were 19.2 µg/ml and 3.4 ng/ml, respectively.

This case illustrates a complex but predictable sequence of pharmacodynamic drug interactions. Cimetidine inhibits theophylline metabolism (see the section on theophylline), which then resulted in theophylline toxicity. This was manifested as atrial flutter with a rapid ventricular response rate. Digoxin was used to treat this rhythm, although successful treatment required very high doses of digoxin. Digoxin toxicity was not noted despite high levels because of opposing effects of digoxin and theophylline on cardiac automaticity and conduction. However, the half-life of theophylline is much shorter than that of digoxin. As the toxic effects of theophylline resolved, digitalis toxicity became apparent. Similar pharmacologic interactions may be observed with digoxin and other sympathomimetic or anticholinergic drugs. Such an interaction is used to therapeutic advantage when digoxin is given before quinidine therapy in patients with atrial fibrillation, to prevent anticholinergic-mediated increases in the ventricular response rate.

Conversely, sympatholytic drugs, such as β-blockers, or drugs that depress cardiac conduction, such as calcium entry blockers, may interact with digitalis to produce additive atrioventricular block or bradyarrhythmias. Such interactions are used therapeutically when administered for control of ventricular response rate in atrial fibrillation. Adverse interactions due to combination therapy are discussed in later sections.

ANTIARRHYTHMIC DRUGS (FIGURES 10.3 AND 10.4)

LIDOCAINE

Case Example A 75-year-old woman with chronic congestive heart failure and peptic ulcer disease was admitted with dyspnea and somnolence. Chest films showed pulmonary edema. Drug treatment included oxygen, digoxin, furosemide, cimetidine, and intravenous theophylline. Eighteen hours after admission, she developed frequent premature ventricular beats. A 75-mg bolus of lidocaine was administered, followed by a 2 mg/min infusion. Twelve hours later she had generalized seizures. The following drug concentrations were noted: lidocaine, 14 µg/ml; theophylline, 17 µg/ml; and digoxin, 2.5 ng/ml.

Lidocaine is usually administered by bolus and then constant intravenous infusion. Slow distribution from the vascular system to tissues may result in unexpectedly high blood lidocaine concentrations and possibly toxicity in the few minutes after a bolus loading injection. The usual circumstance in which this occurs is severe cardiac failure or shock states. Slowed distribution to tissues is thought to be a consequence of intense sympathetic nervous stimulation and low cardiac output, resulting in reduced flow to organs such as muscle and adipose tissue, which are important reservoirs for lidocaine uptake. Although not well documented, coadministration of sympathomimetic drugs such as norepinephrine or dopamine could reduce the distribution volume of lidocaine.

Antiarrhythmic Drug	Interacting Drug	Change in Blood Level	Type of Interaction	Probable Mechanism	Comments
Lidocaine	Cimetidine	↑	Reduced clearance	Inhibits metabolism	Reduced lidocaine infusion rate; select another H$_2$-blocker
	Phenobarbital	↓	Increased clearance	Accelerates metabolism	Uncertain
	Propranolol (and other β-blockers except pindolol)	↑	Reduced clearance	Reduces liver blood flow; reduces rate of metabolism	Reduce lidocaine infusion rate
Quinidine	Antacids	↑	Reduced clearance	Alkalinizes urine, reduces renal clearance	Monitor quinidine levels; in some but not all patients dose may need to be reduced
	Amiodarone	↑	Reduced clearance	Inhibits metabolism	Reduce quinidine dose
	Cimetidine	↑	Reduced clearance	Inhibits metabolism	Reduce quinidine dose
	Phenobarbital (and other barbiturates), primidone	↓	Increased clearance	Accelerates metabolism	Increase quinidine dose; when these drugs are stopped, quinidine dose should be reduced
	Phenytoin	↓	Increased clearance	Accelerates metabolism	Increase quinidine dose; when phenytoin is stopped, quinidine dose should be reduced
	Rifampin	↓	Increased clearance	Accelerates metabolism	Increase quinidine dose; when rifampin is stopped, quinidine dose should be reduced
	Verapamil	↑	Reduced clearance	Inhibits metabolism	Reduce quinidine dose
Procainamide	Amiodarone	↑	Reduced clearance	Inhibits metabolism	Reduce procainamide dose, monitor levels
	Cimetidine, ranitidine	↑	Reduced clearance	Competes for tubular secretion	Monitor levels
	Trimethoprim	↑	Reduced clearance	Competes for tubular secretion	Monitor levels
Disopyramide	Phenytoin, rifampin	↑	Increased clearance; may also see enhanced anticholinergic toxicity	Accelerates metabolism	Active metabolite with more anticholinergic potency than disopyramide; may need to increase dose or select another antiarrhythmic drug
Mexiletine	Phenytoin	↓	Increased clearance	Accelerates metabolism	Increase mexiletine dose
	Rifampin	↓	Increased clearance	Accelerates metabolism	Increase mexiletine dose
Flecainide	Amiodarone	↑	Reduced clearance	Probably inhibits metabolism	Measure levels, decrease dose as necessary
	Cimetidine	↑	Reduced clearance	Probably inhibits metabolism	Measure levels, decrease dose as necessary
	Ammonium chloride	↓	Increased clearance	Decreased renal tubular reabsorption	Measure levels, decrease dose as necessary
	Sodium bicarbonate	↑	Decreased clearance	Increased renal tubular reabsorption	Measure levels, decrease dose as necessary
Encainide	Quinidine	↑*	Reduced clearance	Inhibits metabolism of encainide to active metabolites; in genetically extensive metabolizers only	*Encainide effects are due primarily to active metabolites. Quinidine may decrease the efficacy of encainide; avoid the use of quinidine in patients taking encainide
	Cimetidine	↑	Reduced clearance	Inhibits metabolism of encainide and metabolites	May enhance encainide effect due to accumulation of active metabolite; best to avoid use of cimetidine in patients taking encainide

The result could be toxicity following bolus injection of a usual dose of lidocaine. This type of interaction can be avoided by slowly administering loading doses.

During constant infusion, the level of lidocaine is determined primarily by clearance. Most drug interactions with lidocaine involve alterations in lidocaine clearance. Lidocaine is extensively metabolized, being extracted to a high degree by the liver. Clearance of lidocaine is approximately proportional to liver blood flow. Drugs such as β-blockers, which decrease liver blood flow, decrease clearance, and drugs such as isoproterenol, which increase hepatic blood flow, increase clearance of lidocaine.[25,27] In contrast to propranolol, pindolol, a β-blocker with sympathetic agonist activity that does not decrease

---

FIGURE 10.4 DRUG INTERACTIONS IN WHICH ANTIARRHYTHMIC DRUGS INFLUENCE OTHER DRUG ACTIONS

Antiarrhythmic Drug	Interacting Drug	Effect	Probable Mechanism	Comments
Lidocaine	Succinylcholine	Prolonged muscle paralysis and respiratory depression	Unclear	Intensively monitor respiratory function
Quinidine	Amiodarone, type I antiarrhythmic drugs	Marked QT prolongation, ventricular arrhythmias (torsades de pointes)	Additive slowing of repolarization	Use combinations cautiously
	Digoxin	Increased digoxin levels, digoxin toxicity	Quinidine reduces metabolism and renal excretion of digoxin	Reduce digoxin dose by 50%; monitor SDC
	Metoprolol	Increased metoprolol levels	Inhibits metabolism, in genetically extensive metabolizers only	May need to decrease dose
	Neuromuscular blocking agents (curare, succinylcholine, and others)	Prolonged muscle paralysis, postoperative respiratory arrest	Additive neuromuscular blockade	Intensively monitor respiratory function
	Verapamil (IV)	Hypotension	Additive α-adrenergic blocking effect	Use cautiously in combination
	Warfarin	Excessive anticoagulation, bleeding	Quinidine inhibits clotting factor synthesis, augments warfarin action	Reduce warfarin dose; monitor prothrombin time
Amiodarone	Digoxin	Increased digoxin levels	Reduces digoxin metabolism or renal excretion	Reduce digoxin dose; monitor SDC
	Phenytoin	Increases phenytoin concentrations, phenytoin toxicity	Inhibits phenytoin metabolism	Reduce phenytoin dose; monitor levels
	Procainamide	Increased procainamide levels, potential toxicity	Inhibits procainamide and N-acetyl procainamide (NAPA) metabolism	Reduce procainamide dose; monitor levels
	Quinidine	Increased quinidine levels, potential toxicity	Inhibits quinidine metabolism	Reduce quinidine dose; monitor levels
	Quinidine and other type I antiarrhythmic drugs	Ventricular arrhythmias (torsades de pointes)	Additive slowing of ventricular repolarization	Use cautiously in combination
	Warfarin	Excesssive anticoagulation, bleeding	Inhibits warfarin metabolism	Reduce warfarin dose; monitor prothrombin time
	Propranolol and other β-blockers	Hypotension, bradyarrhythmias, sinus arrest, asystole	Additive depression of myocardial contractility, sinus and AV node conduction	Use cautiously in combination, particularly in patients with cardiac failure or sinus/AV nodal disease
	Calcium entry blockers	Hypotension, bradyarrhythmias, sinus arrest, asystole	Additive depression of myocardial contractility, sinus and AV node conduction	Use cautiously in combination, particularly in patients with cardiac failure or sinus/AV nodal disease

SDC = Serum digoxin concentration; AV = Atrioventricular

cardiac output or presumably hepatic blood flow, does not affect lidocaine clearance.[28]

Alterations of intrinsic drug-metabolizing capacity may also influence lidocaine clearance. Phenobarbital accelerates and cimetidine reduces lidocaine clearance.[29] The effect of cimetidine on lidocaine clearance was considered at one time to be due to decreased liver blood flow; however, ranitidine, another H_2-blocker that also decreases liver blood flow, does not alter lidocaine clearance.[30] Thus, the action of cimetidine appears to be on drug-metabolizing enzymes. When there is a potential drug interaction it is prudent to adjust the lidocaine infusion by 25% to 50%. However, because there is considerable interindividual variability in lidocaine clearance and in the magnitude of effects of other drugs on lidocaine clearance, optimal doses for prolonged infusion therapy may require guidance from blood level monitoring.

The case example illustrates two possible adverse drug interactions. The patient was treated with intravenous theophylline for obstructive lung disease and with cimetidine for peptic ulcer disease. The patient ultimately had nearly toxic theophylline levels, which were probably the result of cimetidine inhibition of theophylline metabolism. For treatment of ventricular ectopy, which may have been related to theophylline toxicity, lidocaine infusion was started. However, in determining the dose of lidocaine that was given, the predictable effects of severe cardiac failure or of cimetidine on lidocaine clearance were not considered. Assuming multiplicative reductions of clearance by cardiac failure and cimetidine and assuming that the infusion should be reduced by 50% for each factor, then 25% of the usual dose, or 0.5 mg/min, would have been more appropriate. This dose reduction would have prevented the development of lidocaine toxicity with associated seizures. Lidocaine in high doses (repeated injection or sustained infusion) may enhance the neuromuscular blocking effect of succinylcholine, resulting in prolonged respiratory depression. A likely interaction is additive central nervous system toxicity with tocainide, a drug with similar pharmacologic and toxic actions.

Quinidine

Case Example A 38-year-old man with epilepsy and valvular heart disease was receiving long-term therapy with primidone. Because of recurrent atrial arrhythmias, he was begun on quinidine sulfate. Despite a quinidine dose of 300 mg every 4 hours, plasma levels were less than 1 µg/ml.[31]

Absorption of quinidine may be reduced by antacids and probably by drugs such as cholestyramine and colestipol. Such drugs should always be spaced at least an hour after the quinidine dose. As mentioned previously, quinidine may interact significantly with digoxin.

Quinidine is extensively metabolized. Several drugs have been shown to influence the rate of quinidine metabolism. Phenobarbital, phenytoin, and rifampin accelerate and cimetidine, amiodarone, and verapamil inhibit quinidine metabolism.[31–33] When these drugs are added to or deleted from a patient's drug regimen, the quinidine dose should be appropriately adjusted. In the illustrative case, phenobarbital, a major metabolite of primidone, accelerated the rate of quinidine metabolism threefold. Thus, much higher doses of quinidine were required to achieve therapeutic concentrations in this patient. Conversely, had the patient stopped his primidone but continued the quinidine dose, quinidine intoxication would be predicted.

Quinidine is excreted to a small degree (20%) unchanged by the kidneys. Because quinidine is a weak base, its renal excretion may be influenced by urinary pH. With alkaline urine, as might occur with intensive antacid therapy (such as might be used to treat quinidine-induced gastric upset), renal clearance will be reduced. For most patients, this will not have a significant effect on total clearance. Possibly in individual patients with relatively high renal and low metabolic clearance, such an interaction could result in quinidine toxicity.

Several pharmacodynamic interactions with quinidine have been described. Quinidine may increase the anticoagulant action of warfarin by direct inhibition of synthesis of clotting factors.[34] Hypotension has been described in patients receiving oral quinidine and intravenous verapamil.[35] This appears to be a result of additive α-adrenoceptor blocking actions. Quinidine weakly inhibits neuromuscular transmission. The duration of muscle paralysis after the use of curare or succinylcholine during anesthesia may be prolonged.[36] Quinidine and other type IA antiarrhythmic drugs slow ventricular repolarization associated with QT interval prolongation. This is occasionally associated with re-entry ventricular tachycardias of the polymorphous or torsades de pointes type. QT interval prolongation may be additive with other type IA antiarrhythmic drugs or amiodarone, resulting in an increased risk of torsades de pointes.[37] Similar interactions may occur with psychotropic drugs such as tricyclic antidepressants or phenothiazines. In management of poisoning involving the latter drugs, quinidine and other type I antiarrhythmics are absolutely contraindicated.

Procainamide

Procainamide and its active metabolite N-acetyl procainamide (NAPA) are excreted unchanged to a considerable extent (60% and 80%, respectively) by the kidneys. Renal excretion of these basic compounds is influenced by urinary pH. Clearance may be reduced when antacids or other drugs that alkalinize the urine are administered. The magnitude of the pH effect on renal clearance is small, suggesting that tubular secretion is the major determinant of renal clearance, with relatively little passive reabsorption.[38] Cimetidine, ranitidine, and trimethoprim, basic drugs excreted by renal tubular secretion, inhibit renal excretion of procainamide.[39,40] The mechanism is primarily competition for active secretion. The result is a 35% to 60% decrease in procainamide clearance. Reduction of glomerular filtration rate, which occasionally occurs during therapy with β-blockers or NSAIDs, is also expected to reduce the clearance of procainamide and NAPA. However, the clinically significant drug interactions involving changes in renal clearance are not well established. This is probably because of a relatively high toxic/therapeutic ratio, at least during short-term administration of procainamide.

Additive effects of procainamide and other type I antiarrhythmic drugs or amiodarone, as discussed with quinidine, are expected for procainamide.

Amiodarone

A number of significant interactions have been reported with amiodarone.[41] A major action of amiodarone is to reduce the rate of metabolism of other drugs. Amiodarone enhances the anticoagulant response to warfarin.[42] In anticipation of this effect, the warfarin dose should be halved. Onset of the inhibition of warfarin metabolism may be from 3 to 4 days up to several weeks, presumably reflecting the time required for buildup of amiodarone concentrations adequate to inhibit warfarin metabolism. Because amiodarone has an extremely long half-life, the effect on warfarin metabolism may persist for up to 4 months after amiodarone is discontinued.

Amiodarone consistently elevates digoxin concentrations, on average about twofold.[15] Amiodarone also elevates blood levels of quinidine, procainamide, N-acetyl procainamide, phenytoin, and flecainide.[33,41] These metabolic interactions plus the expected pharmacodynamic interaction with type I antiarrhythmic drugs may explain marked QT prolongation and the development of torsades de pointes observed after combined therapy with amiodarone and quinidine, disopyramide, propafenone, or mexiletine.[37]

Pharmacodynamic interactions have been reported between amiodarone and β-blockers or calcium entry blockers.[43,44] Amiodarone decreases sinus node automaticity, increases atrioventricular nodal refractoriness, and depresses myocardial contractility. Combining amiodarone with other drugs with similar effects may result in excessive bradycardia, sinus arrest, asystole, or low-output states. This is most likely to occur in patients with underlying sinus or atrioventricular node or myocardial disease. Because of the long half-life of amiodarone, such interactions might occur after treatment with β-blockers or calcium entry blockers weeks or even months after discontinuation of amiodarone.

Mexiletine and Tocainide

Mexiletine is extensively metabolized and is subject to the metabolic influences of other drugs.[45] Phenytoin and rifampin have been shown to accelerate mexiletine metabolism; phenobarbital would be expected to do so as well. Renal elimination of mexiletine is influenced by urinary pH. However, because only about 10% is excreted unchanged, changes in renal clearance have relatively little clinical significance.

Tocainide is both metabolized and excreted unchanged by the kidneys. Renal clearance is pH dependent, ranging from 35% to 40% of total clearance of uncontrolled or acid pH to 15% at alkaline pH.[46] Thus alkali therapy has the potential to significantly influence tocainide levels, although the clinical significance of this interaction is not established.

Flecainide, Encainide, and Propafenone

Flecainide is primarily metabolized, with variable renal excretion (10% to 50% of the dose), depending on urine pH. Acidification or alkalization of the urine can therefore enhance or diminish clearance and could influence blood levels. Amiodarone, cimetidine, and possibly propranolol increase levels of flecainide, presumably by inhibiting metabolism.

Encainide is in most people extensively metabolized with formation of active metabolites, O-desmethyl encainide (ODE) and 3-methoxy-O-desmethyl encainide (3-MODE). Most or all of the pharmacologic activity is due to the metabolites. The metabolism of encainide is genetically determined, and there are extensive and poor metabolizers (the latter in 10% of whites).

Quinidine inhibits the metabolism of encainide in extensive metabolizers and would be expected to reduce or abolish the pharmacologic effects of the drug.[47] However, cimetidine, which also inhibits the metabolism of encainide, appears to inhibit the metabolism of the metabolites to a greater extent, resulting in higher metabolite levels and potentially enhanced pharmacologic effects.[48]

Propafenone is extensively metabolized in most people, demonstrating genetically polymorphic metabolism similar to that of encainide. The main metabolites are active. Cimetidine increases blood levels of propafenone. Propafenone inhibits the metabolism of digoxin, warfarin, and metoprolol.

Additive pharmacodynamic effects between type IC antiarrhythmic drugs and type IA agents, β-blockers, amiodarone, and calcium entry blockers are expected.

β-Blockers (Figure 10.5)

Pharmacokinetic Interactions

Although many pharmacokinetic interactions involving β-blockers have been described, they are not perceived as creating a substantial therapeutic problem. This is because of difficulty in appreciating inadequate dosing in patients with dynamic diseases such as angina or hypertension, the high toxic:therapeutic ratio, and the intrinsic wide individual variability in the pharmacokinetics of many of the β-blockers. However, pharmacokinetic interactions can be of substantial magnitude and should be considered when there is toxicity or unexpected failure to respond.

β-Blockers fall into two broad pharmacokinetic classes. Propranolol and metoprolol are highly lipophilic and are rapidly and extensively metabolized. Absorption is complete, but bioavailability is relatively low owing to extensive first-pass metabolism. In contrast, atenolol, nadolol, and pindolol are less lipophilic and are eliminated primarily unchanged by the kidneys. Absorption may be incomplete, but because there is little first-pass metabolism, bioavailability is less variable than for the more lipophilic β-blockers.

Absorption of all β-blockers is potentially interfered with by coingestion of antacids or bile-acid-binding resins. Aluminum hydroxide antacids, cholestyramine, and colestipol have specifically been shown to decrease bioavailability of propranolol.

FIGURE 10.5 DRUG INTERACTIONS INVOLVING β-BLOCKERS

Drug	Interacting Drug	Effect	Probable Mechanism	Comments
All β-blockers	Verapamil and possibly other calcium entry blockers	Excessive bradycardia, complete heart block, asystole,* cardiac failure	Additive depression of myocardial conduction and contractility	Primarily seen in patients with pre-existing left ventricular dysfunction or conduction disturbance
	Amiodarone	Same as calcium entry blockers	Additive myocardial depressant and sympathetic blocking actions	
	Epinephrine, insulin, or oral hypoglycemic agents (hypoglycemia, epinephrine release)	Hypertension (stroke)	Unopposed α-adrenergic vasoconstriction	Primarily seen with nonselective β-blockers; possibly also with high doses of selective blockers
	Antacids, cholestyramine, colestipol	Reduced absorption	Binding in gut	Separate dosing by at least 1 hour
Nonselective β-blockers	Insulin or oral hypoglycemic agents	Prolonged hypoglycemia with masking of symptoms	Blunted β-adrenergic-mediated gluconeogenesis, antagonism of tachycardia and tremor	Use β-blockers with caution in patients treated with insulin or hypoglycemic drugs
Propranolol and metoprolol	Phenytoin, barbiturates, rifampin	Reduced bioavailability	Accelerated metabolism, increased first-pass metabolism	May need higher doses of propranolol or metoprolol
	Cimetidine	Increased bioavailability	Decreased first-pass metabolism	May need to decrease propranolol dose
	Hydralazine	Increased bioavailability; increased systemic clearance; variable effect on blood levels	Accelerated systemic metabolism; ? saturation of presystemic metabolism	Interaction is probably of hemodynamic nature; fixed relationship between propranolol and hydralazine dosing desirable
	Lidocaine	Propranolol may reduce lidocaine clearance, resulting in higher than expected levels	Reduced liver blood flow; ? direct inhibition of metabolism	Reduce lidocaine infusion rate; may occur with other β-blockers as well
Propranolol and pindolol	Indomethacin, possibly other NSAIDs	Reduced antihypertensive action of β-blockers	Inhibition of prostaglandin synthesis	Avoid combination if possible; if NSAIDS are necessary, monitor blood pressure closely
Metoprolol	Quinidine	Reduced clearance, increased levels	Inhibits metabolism; genetically extensive metabolizers only	May need to decrease dose of metoprolol

* After IV verapamil

For drugs with high presystemic (first-pass) metabolism, interacting drugs that affect rate of metabolism will influence both bioavailability and systemic clearance. When bioavailability is low owing to extensive first-pass metabolism, small changes in clearance may have large effects on bioavailability. For example, phenytoin, phenobarbital, and rifampin accelerate propranolol and metoprolol metabolism, resulting in reduced bioavailability.[49,50] Half-life after absorption may or may not be shortened owing to concomitant increase in systemic clearance. Conversely, cimetidine decreases the metabolism and increases the bioavailability of propranolol and metoprolol.[51] As a clinical consequence, excessive bradycardia associated with high levels of propranolol has been reported in a patient in whom cimetidine was added to propranolol therapy.[52] Quinidine inhibits the metabolism of metoprolol, resulting in a threefold increase in plasma levels. The effect is noted only in genetically extensive metabolizers of metoprolol (90% of whites), in whom quinidine transforms their metabolism to that of a slow metabolizer.[53]

Hydralazine has unusual effects on propranolol (and metoprolol) kinetics. Both systemic clearance and bioavailability increase.[54] Extraction of propranolol by the liver is high; therefore propranolol clearance is regarded as being dependent on hepatic blood flow. Hydralazine increases systemic clearance of propranolol by increasing cardiac output and hepatic blood flow. However, hydralazine may also increase bioavailability as a result of rapid delivery of drug to the liver and saturation of metabolic pathways. The magnitude of the increased bioavailability far exceeds the change in systemic clearance. As a result, propranolol (and metoprolol) levels increase in the presence of hydralazine (and presumably other vasodilators).

The magnitude of drug interaction effects on bioavailability of propranolol and metoprolol may be large, requiring substantial dosage adjustment to maintain constant blood levels or effects. For vasodilators the interaction appears to be of a hemodynamic nature, so the magnitude of effect may be related to the temporal relationship between dosing of the two drugs. To reduce dose-to-dose variability in blood levels of the β-blockers, vasodilators and propranolol should be given on a fixed relative dosing schedule.

The β-blockers that are eliminated by renal excretion are not subject to metabolic interactions but are sensitive to changes in renal function. Drugs that might affect renal function, such as NSAIDs, could therefore influence elimination rate.

β-Blockers can affect the pharmacokinetics of other drugs. Propranolol has been shown to reduce the clearance of antipyrine and may result in increased blood levels of chlorpromazine. The effect on antipyrine metabolism is a direct metabolic effect rather than a result of β-blockade. By reducing hepatic blood flow, β-blockers can slow the metabolism of other rapidly metabolized drugs, such as lidocaine and verapamil.

PHARMACODYNAMIC INTERACTIONS

Myocardial depression, cardiac failure, hypotension, bradycardia, and atrioventricular block are the most significant adverse effects of β-blockers as a drug class. Such adverse reactions generally occur in people who have underlying myocardial or conduction disease or who are taking other myocardial depressant drugs. Among these are the calcium entry blockers and type I antiarrhythmic drugs, particularly disopyramide. Of the calcium entry blockers, verapamil has been implicated in adverse interactions with β-blockers most often, presumably because it has the greatest myocardial depressant activity at usual therapeutic doses. Most instances of hypotension or asystole have occurred in patients on β-blockers following intravenous verapamil, possibly related to high circulating levels of verapamil after rapid administration.[55,56] Nifedipine and diltiazem combined with β-blockers are usually well tolerated. However, in patients with depressed cardiac function, hypotension or cardiac failure may occur with these combinations as well.[57,58] In high-risk patients on β-blockers, verapamil is best avoided; other calcium entry blockers should be administered initially in low doses and with careful observation. Amiodarone has sympathetic blocking activity and may also have additive myocardial depressant effects with β-blockers.[43]

All β-blockers inhibit reflex tachycardia. This property is used therapeutically in combining β-blockers with vasodilators in the therapy of hypertension. However, instances of profound hypotension in patients receiving β-blockers and then parenteral vasodilators, such as intravenous hydralazine or diazoxide, and potentiation of postural hypotension due to prazosin have been reported.

Case Example A 57-year-old woman taking propranolol, 60 mg/d, for palpitations visited an emergency room for treatment of urticaria. Two minutes after she received 0.3 ml 1:1000 epinephrine subcutaneously, her blood pressure rose from 120/70 to 220/110. The patient developed headache, right-sided weakness, and aphasia. Computed tomographic scan of the head showed a left parietal hematoma with associated subdural hematoma.[59]

Most β-blockers nonselectively antagonize; that is, they act on both cardiac and vascular β-adrenergic receptors. The cardioselective β-blockers such as metoprolol and atenolol are cardioselective only in low doses. At higher doses commonly used for many patients, cardioselectivity is lost. A consequence of mixed nonselective blockade is the epinephrine reversal phenomenon. In the absence of β-blockers, epinephrine increases systolic blood pressure slightly and decreases diastolic blood pressure. After pretreatment with propranolol, epinephrine produces marked systolic and diastolic hypertension.[60] Epinephrine alone constricts and dilates resistance blood vessels by stimulation of α_1- and β_2-receptors, respectively. These actions counterbalance each other. Blocking β_2-receptors, as occurs with nonselective β-blockade, results in unopposed α_1-stimulation and therefore hypertension. In patients receiving β-blockers, epinephrine administered therapeutically, such as in the case example, or released endogenously, as in association with insulin-induced hypoglycemia or an epinephrine-secreting pheochromocytoma, may result in severe hypertension with cerebrovascular accident or myocardial injury or infarction. Similar interactions between β-blockers and sympathomimetic drugs, which act by releasing catecholamines, might also be expected. Chronic β-blockade has been shown to increase twofold the pressor sensitivity to norepinephrine and angiotensin.[61] (See also the section on sympathomimetic and antihypertensive drugs.) The mechanism for this interaction has not been defined. The antihypertensive effects of β-blockers may be antagonized by addition of NSAIDs. This interaction is discussed in further detail in the section on NSAIDs.

CALCIUM ENTRY BLOCKERS (FIGURE 10.6)

PHARMACOKINETIC INTERACTIONS

Verapamil, diltiazem, and nifedipine are rapidly and extensively metabolized by the liver; thus, metabolism is dependent on liver blood flow.[62] Drugs such as β-blockers, which decrease liver blood flow, may decrease the clearance of verapamil, resulting in higher than expected verapamil concentrations during constant dosing. That interaction might aggra-

FIGURE 10.6 DRUG INTERACTIONS INVOLVING CALCIUM ENTRY BLOCKERS

Drug	Interacting Drug	Effect	Probable Mechanism	Comments
Verapamil (other calcium entry blockers possible but less likely)	β-Blockers	Heart block, cardiac failure, asystole (after IV verapamil)	Additive depression of AV conduction, myocardial contractility	Primarily seen with verapamil; should be used with caution in patients on β-blockers
	Digitalis (toxicity)	Aggravates heart block; asystole	Additive depression of cardiac conduction	Avoid use of calcium blockers in patients with digitalis toxicity
Verapamil Diltiazem	Propranolol	Reduced oral clearance with increased levels of propranolol	Inhibition of first-pass metabolism	Propranolol dose may need to be reduced
Verapamil Diltiazem	Digoxin	Reduced digoxin clearance, increased digoxin levels	Inhibition of metabolism and renal excretion of digoxin	Reduce digoxin dose after starting verapamil or diltiazem; monitor SDC
Verapamil Diltiazem	Cyclosporine	Increased cyclosporine levels	Uncertain	Reduce cyclosporine dose after starting verapamil or diltiazem; monitor cyclosporine level
Verapamil	Quinidine	Hypotension (after IV verapamil)	Additive α-adrenergic blockade	Use IV verapamil cautiously in patients taking quinidine or other drugs with α-blocking activity
Verapamil	Prazosin	Increased prazosin levels; greater hypotensive effect	Reduced clearance; additive α-blocking effect	Use combination cautiously; may need to decrease prazosin dose
Verapamil	Halothane	Bradycardia Hypotension	Additive depression of sinus node function and myocardial contractility	Avoid coadministration
Verapamil Diltiazem	Disopyramide Flecainide	Cardiac failure	Additive depression of myocardial contractility	Avoid use if possible, particularly in patients with impaired myocardial function
Verapamil Diltiazem	Amiodarone Flecainide	Sinus arrest Heart block	Additive depression of sinus node function and AV nodal conduction	Use combination with extreme caution
All calcium blockers	Cimetidine	Increased oral bioavailability of calcium blockers	Inhibition of metabolism; reduced presystemic metabolism	Reduce calcium entry blocker dose 30% to 40%
Verapamil	Rifampin Sulfinpyrazone	Reduced oral bioavailability of verapamil	Accelerated metabolism; increased presystemic metabolism	Increase verapamil dose; use alterative calcium blocker with less presystemic metabolism
Felodipine	Barbiturates Phenytoin Carbamazepine	Reduced plasma levels of felodipine	Accelerated metabolism; increased presystemic metabolism	Increase felodipine dose as necessary

AV = Atrioventricular; SDC = Serum digoxin concentration

vate the pharmacodynamic interaction between calcium entry blockers and β-blockers as discussed later. Verapamil, diltiazem, and nifedipine undergo considerable first-pass metabolism. Thus, the bioavailability of these drugs is relatively low (20% to 50%). Phenobarbital, phenytoin, and rifampin would be expected to accelerate the clearance and decrease the bioavailability of calcium entry blockers; conversely, cimetidine would be expected to decrease clearance and increase bioavailability.[63]

Verapamil and diltiazem reduce the metabolism or renal clearance of digoxin and cyclosporine, resulting in increased digoxin or cyclosporine levels and possibly toxicity.

Although not well studied, calcium entry blockers clearly have the potential to influence the disposition of other drugs by way of hemodynamic mechanisms. For example, these drugs decrease liver blood flow,[64] which could affect the rate of metabolism of drugs such as lidocaine or propranolol, whose metabolism is dependent on liver blood flow. Reversible deterioration of renal function following nifedipine treatment in patients with chronic renal insufficiency, presumably due to intrarenal hemodynamic effects, has been described.[65] Impaired excretion of other drugs could be a consequence.

PHARMACODYNAMIC INTERACTIONS

Case Example A 54-year-old man presented with new-onset angina. He had been treated with metoprolol, 100 mg twice a day for 16 days, without complete control of pain. Verapamil, 120 mg every 8 hours, was added. The following day the patient developed confusion, sweating, nausea, and vomiting, with findings of pulmonary edema, hypotension, and bradycardia with a junctional rhythm at 56 per minute. There were no electrocardiographic or enzyme changes indicating acute myocardial infarction. Medications were discontinued, and he recovered fully. Subsequent coronary angiography showed triple-vessel coronary disease with a normal ejection fraction.[56]

Cardiac toxicity from calcium entry blockers includes sinus bradycardia or arrest, high-grade atrioventricular block, asystole, hypotension, and cardiac failure.[66] These toxic reactions have occurred most often in patients receiving other drugs that depress cardiac conduction or contractility. For example, asystole following intravenous administration of verapamil has been seen in patients taking β-blockers or digitalis.[55,67] Excessive hypotension, worsening angina, or cardiac failure following administration of nifedipine has been observed in patients receiving β-blockers.[57,58,68] Verapamil, because it has the greatest effects on cardiac conduction and contractility, has been the most often implicated in such drug interactions. Nifedipine and diltiazem also depress myocardial function, but these drugs produce more vasodilation, activating sympathetic reflexes, so that heart rate, cardiac output, and atrioventricular conduction

are usually minimally affected. Blocking sympathetic reflexes with β-blockers may unmask the myocardial depressant actions of calcium entry blockers.

Identifying persons who are at risk for adverse drug interactions is important because combination therapy with calcium entry blockers and β-blockers is effective and often desirable therapy for anginal syndromes. Likewise, calcium entry blockers and antiarrhythmic drug combinations are often required for patients with coronary artery disease and chronic ventricular arrhythmias. Laboratory studies indicate that verapamil decreases cardiac performance in patients on β-blockers, but if left ventricular function is normal or only moderately depressed and if there are no conduction abnormalities, verapamil is well tolerated.[69,70] However, occasionally severe left ventricular dysfunction or conduction disease is not apparent on routine evaluation or, as in the case illustrated, patients may appear to have normal left ventricular function but are particularly sensitive to drug effects, and unpredictable interactions may develop. Because of its myocardial effects, it is most prudent (when possible) to avoid combining verapamil with β-blockers or antiarrhythmic drugs such as disopyramide, which strongly depress myocardial functions. Alternative calcium blockers should be selected. However, because of the unpredictability of interactions when starting any calcium blockers in patients taking β-blockers or antiarrhythmic drugs, the possible development of cardiac failure, hypotension, or bradyarrhythmias (including unexplained syncopal episodes) should be considered.

Verapamil and digitalis are frequently used together. The combination is tolerated well by most patients. However, there is concern about serious adverse interaction if digitalis toxicity develops. Patients have developed high-degree heart block or asystole after receiving intravenous verapamil with possible coexisting digitalis toxicity. Verapamil is contraindicated in the presence of digitalis toxicity. Caution is particularly necessary when adding verapamil (or diltiazem) to a stable digoxin regimen because these calcium blockers increase digoxin levels and could themselves induce digitalis toxicity, which would lead to a catastrophic drug interaction.

Case Example A 62-year-old man developed recurrent supraventricular arrhythmias following coronary artery bypass surgery. He was treated with digoxin and a quinidine gluconate, 320 mg three times a day. Four days later he developed atrial fibrillation with a ventricular rate of 140. Verapamil, 5 mg, was given by intravenous injection. Within 2 minutes his blood pressure fell from 130/70 to 80/50; his heart rate fell to 50. Two days later, after quinidine had been stopped, the patient was rechallenged with the same dose of verapamil without adverse consequence.[35]

In addition to direct effects on myocardial function or vascular tone, verapamil has α-adrenergic blocking activity. This is seen in concentrations associated with therapeutic use and is particularly evident after rapid intravenous injection when blood levels are high. The case example and other case reports describe hypotension following combination therapy with quinidine and verapamil, presumably due to additive α-blocking effects. Hypotension might also be anticipated after rapid injections of verapamil in any patient whose blood pressure is dependent on increased α-adrenergic tone or who is receiving other drugs, such as prazosin, with α-blocking activity.

Calcium may antagonize the action of calcium entry blockers. Calcium infusion has been used to manage overdoses and untoward cardiovascular reactions to calcium entry blockers.[71,72] Animal studies indicate that calcium will reverse negative inotropic effects and partially reverse depressed atrioventricular conduction but will not reverse sinus node depression or vasodilation.[73] Substantial increases in calcium levels are required to reverse calcium blocker effects; in most patients, oral calcium supplements or antacids are unlikely to raise calcium concentrations sufficiently to influence calcium blocker action.

Calcium entry blockers may inhibit glucose or sulfonylurea-induced insulin release by interfering with calcium entry into beta islet cells.[74] Deterioration of carbohydrate tolerance in diabetics may occur after calcium entry blockers are initiated,[75] although such effects are not consistently observed. Blood glucose should be monitored carefully when calcium blockers are given to diabetic patients. Doses of insulin or oral hypoglycemic drugs may need to be increased. Con-versely, when calcium blockers are stopped in patients under good control with hypoglycemic medications, the possible development of hypoglycemia should be anticipated.

DIURETICS

Pharmacokinetic interactions involving diuretics do not have major clinical significance. A few pharmacodynamic interactions can result in substantial changes in diuretic efficacy or toxicity (Fig. 10.7). The combination of loop and thiazide-type diuretics, used in some patients with refractory heart failure, may result in massive fluid and electrolyte losses and circulatory collapse.[76] The efficacy of loop diuretics in sodium-retaining states, such as severe cardiac failure, in which renal blood flow and glomerular filtration rates are depressed, is limited by avid distal tubular sodium reabsorption. Thiazide-type diuretics will inhibit distal tubular reabsorption of sodium, resulting in marked natriuresis and kaliuresis. This combination must be used judiciously, beginning with low doses of thiazide (2.5 mg of metolazone or 12.5 mg of hydrochlorothiazide), with careful monitoring for development of hypokalemia and azotemia. When diuresis is excessive, thiazide may be given every other day. Similarly, theophylline may act synergistically with loop diuretics, presumably by increasing renal blood flow and glomerular filtration rates.[77]

FIGURE 10.7 DRUG INTERACTIONS INVOLVING DIURETICS

Drug	Interacting Drug	Effect	Mechanism	Comments
Loop diuretics	Thiazides, metolazone	Marked natriuresis and diuresis	Inhibition of sodium reabsorption at multiple sites within nephron	May result in severe dehydration, circulatory collapse; start thiazide or metolazone at low doses
	Theophylline	Marked natriuresis and diuresis	Increased renal blood flow and GFR	Observe carefully when adding theophylline
	Indomethacin and other NSAIDs	Inhibition of diuretic and antihypertensive actions	Inhibition of prostaglandin-mediated renal vasodilation	Avoid NSAIDs or, if necessary, use lowest doses possible; may need to increase diuretics; monitor for ototoxity
	Aminoglycosides	Ototoxicity	Additive injury to vestibular or cochlear sensory cells	Use lowest possible dose of loop diuretics; monitor for ototoxicity
Thiazide diuretics	Sulfonylurea hypoglycemic agents	Hyperglycemia	Thiazides decrease insulin secretion and/or tissue sensitivity to insulin	Monitor blood glucose; may need higher doses of sulfonylurea
All diuretics	Digitalis	Ventricular arrhythmias	Potassium or magnesium depletion	Monitor potassium and magnesium levels; supplement as necessary
	Lithium	Increased lithium levels, lithium toxicity	Sodium depletion reduces renal clearance of lithium	Decrease lithium dose 25% to 50%; monitor lithium levels
	Angiotensin-converting enzyme (ACE) inhibitors	Hypotension	Inhibition of angiotensin II homeostatic response to volume contraction	Withdraw diuretics before initiating ACE inhibitors; begin with very low doses of ACE inhibitor

Natriuretic and antihypertensive actions of loop diuretics may be inhibited by indomethacin or other NSAIDs.[78] Loop diuretics appear to work in part by producing renal vasodilation by stimulation of renal prostaglandin synthesis, an effect that is blocked by indomethacin. Other adverse interactions involving the effects of diuretics and NSAIDs on renal function are discussed in the next section.

Ototoxicity is a well-described side-effect of loop diuretics. It most commonly occurs with high-dose administration in patients with diminished renal function. The risk of ototoxicity may be increased in patients receiving aminoglycoside antibiotics. Doses of loop diuretics should be kept to a minimum in such patients, and hearing should be appropriately monitored.

Diuresis itself may result in hemodynamically mediated changes in the elimination of other drugs. For example, tubular secretion and total renal clearance of digoxin may be reduced in patients who are diuresed to the point of prerenal azotemia in therapy of heart failure.[25] Any drug whose clearance is primarily by the kidney may be subject to similar interactions. A common diuretic–drug interaction is diuretic-induced hypokalemia or hypomagnesemia with digitalis, resulting in ventricular arrhythmias. This interaction was discussed in the section on cardiac glycosides.

Diuretic use, even without excessive diuresis, reduces the renal excretion of lithium, which may lead to lithium toxicity.[79] In a state of even mild sodium depletion, tubular reabsorption of lithium increases. Lithium dose should be reduced by 25% to 50% when diuretics are added, with the ultimate maintenance dose determined by serum level monitoring.

NONSTEROIDAL ANTI-INFLAMMATORY DRUGS

Case Example A 64-year-old man with a history of hypertension, angina, and hyperuricemia was taking Dyazide (25 mg of hydrochlorothiazide and 50 mg of triamterine), 3 per day, propranolol, and nitroglycerin. He was hospitalized for an acute myocardial infarction, which was uncomplicated. On the third hospital day, podagra of the right great toe developed, and the patient was treated with indomethacin, 50 mg every 6 hours, for seven doses. Within 12 hours of initiation of treatment, the patient became oliguric and subsequently anuric. His serum creatinine level rose from 1.1 to 14.0 mg/dl over 6 days, and intermittent hemodialysis was required. Sixty days later, renal function returned to normal.[80]

NSAIDs are among the most widely prescribed class of drugs, particularly in treatment of chronic arthritis in the elderly, a population with a high prevalence of heart disease. The potential for adverse drug interactions, although only recently recognized, is believed to be highly significant (Fig. 10.8). Pharmacokinetic interactions resulting in changes in

FIGURE 10.8 DRUG INTERACTIONS INVOLVING NONSTEROIDAL ANTI-INFLAMMATORY DRUGS

Drug	Interacting Drug	Effect	Probable Mechanism	Comments
Diflunisal	Warfarin	Transient excessive hypoprothrombinemia	Displacement from protein binding sites	Transient action—no dose adjustment necessary
Phenylbutazone	Warfarin	Excessive hypoprothrombinemia	Inhibition of drug metabolism	Reduce warfarin dose
All NSAIDs	Warfarin and other anticoagulants	Bleeding complications	Additive effects of hypoprothrombinemia and inhibition of platelet aggregation	Avoid combination when possible
All NSAIDs (except maybe sulindac)	Diuretics	Decreased creatinine clearance; acute renal failure (sodium-depleted patients)	Inhibition of prostaglandin-mediated vasodilation of renal blood vessels	Use NSAIDs cautiously in patients on diuretics (or in cardiac failure)
Indomethacin (? all NSAIDs)	Furosemide	Antagonizes diuretic action; worsening of heart failure; edema	Reduced renal blood flow, increased tubular reabsorption of sodium	Carefully monitor after adding NSAIDs
	Potassium supplements, potassium-sparing diuretics; captopril	Hyperkalemia	NSAIDs inhibit renin release and create a state of hyporeninemic hypoaldosteronism	Monitor potassium closely when using these combinations
	β-Blockers	Reverse antihypertensive actions; uncontrolled blood pressure	Unknown	Monitor blood pressure closely when using the combination
	Captopril	Reverse antihypertensive actions; uncontrolled blood pressure	Inhibition of prostaglandin-mediated vasodilator action of bradykinin	Monitor blood pressure closely when using the combination

blood levels of NSAIDs are not usually clinically significant. NSAIDs may influence the kinetics and effects of other drugs, particularly warfarin. For example, diflunisal, mefenamic acid, phenylbutazone, and possibly other NSAIDs, which are highly protein bound, displace warfarin from protein binding sites and transiently increase free warfarin concentrations and warfarin's hypoprothrombinemic effects. Conversely, when NSAID therapy is stopped, free warfarin levels and anticoagulant efficacy decrease. Phenylbutazone also inhibits warfarin metabolism, resulting in substantially and sustained increased anticoagulant action.[81] Ibuprofen, naproxen, and tolmetin appear not to affect the hypoprothrombinemic action of warfarin.

Indomethacin decreases renal clearance of lithium, resulting in 30% to 50% increased plasma lithium levels.[82] The mechanism of interaction is uncertain but may be linked to the increased sodium reabsorption associated with NSAID action on renal tubular function.

The most important interactions involving NSAIDs relate to their inhibition of cyclo-oxygenase and prostaglandin synthesis. Inhibition of prostaglandin synthesis in platelets results in a reduced platelet aggregation response. Hypoprothrombinemia, abnormal platelet function, and the potential for gastrointestinal irritation due to NSAIDs, in combination with warfarin or heparin therapy, predispose to hemorrhagic complications. Combined use of NSAIDs with anticoagulants is best avoided if possible. If NSAIDs are necessary in such patients, the safest are those that least potentiate warfarin action, as described above.

There has been much recent concern about adverse effects of NSAIDs on renal function. Renal effects are also a source of significant adverse drug interactions. Renal prostaglandins play an important role in autoregulation of renal blood flow and glomerular filtration rate, particularly in situations in which the renal circulation is threatened by hypovolemia, hypotension, or intrinsic kidney disease[83] (Fig. 10.9). Indomethacin, the prototypical NSAID, reduces renal blood flow and creatinine clearance in sodium-depleted persons but not sodium-replete healthy persons. Indomethacin reduces creatinine clearance and has resulted in acute renal failure in patients with hypovolemia, cardiac failure, cirrhosis, and intrinsic renal disease. Diuretic therapy is an important determinate of sodium and volume status. A person on diuretics, particularly if in treatment of congestive heart failure, is at risk for an adverse renal

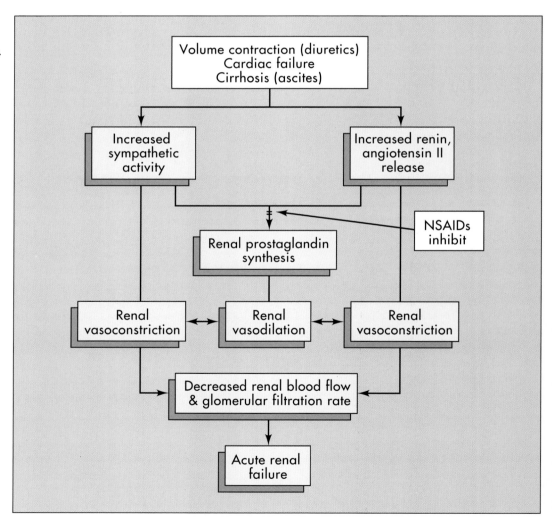

Figure 10.9 Mechanism of diuretic-cardiac failure-NSAID interaction therapy.

effect of NSAIDs, as illustrated in the case example. Although any diuretic that causes hypovolemia might increase the hazards of NSAIDs, triamterene in particular has been implicated in cases of indomethacin-induced acute renal failure.[80,84] Whether this is a coincidence or whether triamterene in particular presents a high risk for interactions with NSAIDs is not known. Aspirin has been shown to antagonize spironolactone-induced natriuresis in healthy volunteers; however, the clinical significance of this observation has not been established. It is prudent to monitor renal function carefully in any high-risk patient after initiation of NSAID therapy.

Case Example A 63-year-old man was treated for severe congestive heart failure with digoxin, furosemide, spironolactone, and isosorbide dinitrate. He developed acute gout, which was treated with indomethacin, 50 mg four times a day. Signs of cardiac failure increased, and he developed anasarca. The dose of furosemide was increased, with little improvement. The indomethacin was discontinued, and a brisk diuresis ensued. The cardiac failure resolved rapidly with a loss of 9 kg over 4 days.[85]

Renal prostaglandins play a role in sodium and water homeostasis. Prostaglandins increase renal blood flow and inhibit tubular reabsorption of sodium and chloride. Conversely, treatment with NSAIDs results in reduced renal blood flow and increased tubular reabsorption of sodium and chloride, resulting in reduced sodium excretion, sodium retention, and in some cases edema. These actions of NSAIDs directly oppose the therapeutic effects of diuretics. Experimental and clinical studies indicate that indomethacin antagonizes the natriuretic effects of furosemide and other diuretics.[86] The clinical consequence of such interactions may be the development or worsening of heart failure, as in the case example. Patients should be carefully monitored after initiation of NSAID therapy, and appropriate changes in NSAID or diuretic doses should be made if necessary.

Renal prostaglandins antagonize the effects of antidiuretic hormone and redistribute medullary blood flow such as to increase the ability of the kidney to produce dilute urine and excrete water. Therapy with NSAIDs results in impaired diluting ability and increased susceptibility to hyponatremia. Ibuprofen-induced hyponatremia in a patient with renal insufficiency has been reported.[87] One would predict a greater risk of hyponatremia in patients on combination therapy with NSAIDs and thiazides, because both drugs impair free water clearance.

Renal prostaglandins promote renin release and NSAIDs inhibit it. NSAID therapy may result in a state of hyporeninemic hypoaldosteronism. The consequence, particularly in diabetic patients or others with renal insufficiency, is impaired tolerance to potassium and increased susceptibility to hyperkalemia.[88,89] This represents a potentially serious drug interaction with potassium supplements, potassium-sparing diuretics, or captopril, the latter of which also inhibits angiotensin-mediated aldosterone release.

In view of the previous discussion, it is not surprising that NSAIDs may influence blood pressure control in patients treated for hypertension. The evidence concerning effects of indomethacin on blood pressure control in hypertensive patients is conflicting.[90] Several studies have found increased blood pressure; a few have found no effect. In addition to general effects on sodium balance and the renin-aldosterone system, indomethacin has also been reported to inhibit the blood-pressure-lowering effects of β-blockers and captopril.[91,92] The precise role of prostaglandins in the action of these drugs and the clinical significance of the interaction have not been established. One might expect that hypertensive patients whose hypertension is volume-dependent might experience worse hypertension with NSAIDs owing to sodium retention, but those with renin-dependent hypertension might have reduction of blood pressure due to suppression of renin.

In support of this concept is a recent study showing that aspirin reduced blood pressure in patients with hyperreninemia and renovascular hypertension but either had no effect or increased blood pressure in patients with essential hypertension.[93]

Although the response of hypertensive patients to NSAIDs is not at present predictable, the possibility of an interaction should be anticipated, and a patient's blood pressure should be monitored more frequently in the period after initiation of NSAID treatment. Because vasodilation with captopril is partly mediated by increased synthesis and release of vasodilator prostaglandins, dependent on angiotensin-converting enzyme inhibition, concomitant administration of indomethacin may curtail the beneficial effects of captopril in treatment of heart failure and hypertension.

Although all NSAIDs seem to act by inhibition of prostaglandin synthesis, they may differ in their risk of adverse effects on the kidney. Sulindac has been shown in several studies to have less effect on renal production of prostaglandin E_2 and renal hemodynamics in chronic renal disease, despite the same magnitude of inhibition of platelet cyclo-oxygenase as ibuprofen or indomethacin.[94,95] Sulindac may also be less likely to aggravate hypertension.[96] Sulindac itself is a pro-drug, which is converted from the inactive sulfoxide to the active sulfide, primarily in the liver.[97] The kidneys interconvert the sulfide and sulfoxide forms. On balance, the equilibrium favors the sulfoxide, so that in effect the kidneys are detoxifying the active sulfide. Because relatively little of the active sulfide is present in the kidney parenchyma, there is little inhibition of cyclo-oxygenase, and renal prostaglandin synthesis is minimally affected. Although experimental studies suggest that sulindac is the NSAID of choice in chronic renal failure and probably in cardiac failure, the safety advantage of sulindac over other NSAIDs in populations of high-risk patients remains to be demonstrated.

SYMPATHOMIMETIC AND ANTIHYPERTENSIVE DRUGS (FIGURE 10.10)

Sympathomimetic Drugs

Adverse reactions to sympathomimetic drugs resulting in excessive adrenergic stimulation usually occur as a consequence of unsuspected drug interactions. The epinephrine reversal phenomenon as discussed previously (see section on β-blockers) is an important example. Because so many people take propranolol and other nonselective β-blockers for therapy of hypertension, coronary heart disease, migraine headache, and other indications, the potential for an interaction involving epinephrine commonly arises in the therapy of anaphylactic or anaphylactoid reactions to drugs or insect bites. For such patients it is probably better to use β₂-agonists such as metaproterenol, terbutaline, or albuterol to treat bronchoconstriction and to titrate α-agonists such as dopamine or norepinephrine separately for management of vascular collapse. In people who have a history of anaphylactic reactions, it is best to use relatively cardioselective β-blockers, although in usual therapeutic doses cardioselectivity is only partial and epinephrine reversal might still be observed.

The pressor sensitivity to some sympathomimetic drugs is increased by other drugs that retard the removal of catecholamines from the circulation. Tricyclic antidepressants, guanethidine, and bretylium are examples of drugs that inhibit uptake of catecholamine by adrenergic neurons. The result is a significant increase in sensitivity to pressor effects of norepinephrine, epinephrine, and other direct-acting sympathomimetic drugs such as phenylephrine and phenylpropanolamine found in over-the-counter preparations.[98,99] If pressor drugs are required for such patients, therapy should be initiated with low doses and gradually increased to the desired end point. Patients taking inhibitors of catecholamine uptake should be advised about the risks of using over-the-counter sympathomimetic preparations.

Severe hypertension and other catastrophic reactions have occurred after the use of sympathomimetic drugs in patients receiving monoamine oxidase (MAO) inhibitors. These are discussed in the next section.

Hypertension has been reported in one patient following indomethacin ingestion during long-term therapy with phenylpropanolamine, taken as an appetite suppressant.[100] While taking phenylpropa-nolamine the patient was normotensive. Following ingestion of 25 mg of indomethacin, the patient's blood pressure rose to 200/150. The mechanism of this interaction is unknown but may represent prostaglandin synthesis as a homeostatic response in moderating phenylpropanolamine-induced vasoconstriction.

Vagal reflexes resulting in bradycardia represent another important homeostatic response to drug-induced hypertension. Atropine therapy doubles the pressor sensitivity to infused phenylephrine.[101] A number of over-the-counter antihistaminic and sedative drugs, as well as some tricyclic antidepressants, have strong anticholinergic activity, which could contribute to excessive hypertension following sympathomimetic drug treatment.

Anesthetic drugs, particularly cyclopropane and the halogenated anesthetics such as halothane, enflurane, and isoflurane, sensitize the heart to the arrhythmogenic actions of catecholamines. In experimental animals, the threshold dose of epinephrine required to induce ventricular fibrillation is lowered. Postoperative patients may be at risk for malignant cardiac arrhythmias during therapy with pressor drugs or bronchodilators that have significant β-adrenergic activity.

Monoamine Oxidase Inhibitors

Fortunately, very few patients are currently receiving MAO inhibitors for therapy of hypertension. However, these drugs are still widely used in psychiatric practice, particularly as the availability of electroconvulsive therapy for depression becomes more limited. Drug interactions involving MAO inhibitors continue to occur and should be understood by cardiologists. MAO is responsible for intraneuronal oxidation of amines. It is also present in the liver and the gastrointestinal tract, where it metabolizes amines before they reach the systemic circulation. The consequences of inhibition of MAO are to increase the neuronal content of catecholamines and serotonin and to reduce the presystemic metabolism of dietary amines such as tyramine. Sympathomimetic drugs such as amphetamines, ephedrine or pseudoephedrine, or phenylpropanolamine, which release catecholamines, can produce severe hypertension in persons taking MAO inhibitors.[102] Ingestion of foods high in tyramine content results in higher than usual blood levels of tyramine (because of reduced presystemic metabolism) and a greater magnitude of catecholamine release from neurons. As a result, hypertension, as well as flushing, headache, sweating, anxiety, and palpitations, occurs, presumably a combined effect of release of catecholamines, serotonin, and other vasoactive amines. Other drugs, such as meperidine and, rarely, tricyclic antidepressants, have been reported to cause a syndrome of excitement, delirium, hyperpyrexia, and convulsions, as well as hypertension. The mechanism of this interaction is unknown

Hypertension occurring in the context of MAO inhibitor drug therapy is catecholamine-mediated and is treated much like pheochromocytoma. α-Adrenergic blockers (such as phentolamine), combined α- and β-blockers (labetalol), or parenteral nitroprusside is most appropriate.

Antihypertensive Drugs

Drug interactions are commonly used therapeutically in combination antihypertensive drug regimens. These therapeutic interactions are not the focus of this chapter except to mention a few cases in which significant untoward reactions have occurred. For example, first-dose hypotension following prazosin or hypotension following intravenous diazoxide is more profound in patients who are hypovolemic as a result of prior diuretic therapy or who are receiving β-blockers, thereby blunting homeostatic responses. Tricyclic antidepressant therapy is associated with sig-

FIGURE 10.10 DRUG INTERACTIONS INVOLVING SYMPATHOMIMETIC AND ANTIHYPERTENSIVE DRUGS

Drug	Interacting Drug	Effect	Probable Mechanism	Comments
Epinephrine, indirect sympathomimetic agents	Propranolol and other nonselective β-blockers	Hypertension	Propranolol antagonizes β_2-vasodilation, leaving unopposed α-vasoconstriction	Particular problem in treating anaphylaxis. In patients on β-blockers, titrate β_1-bronchodilators and α-adrenergic vasoconstrictors separately
Epinephrine, norepinephrine	Chlorpromazine	Antagonism of pressor effects	Peripheral α-blockade	May require higher doses of pressor drugs
Sympathomimetic drugs (such as phenylephrine, phenylpropanolamine)	Tricylic antidepressants	Hypertension	Blockade of neuronal uptake of amines	Avoid these combinations; warn patients about over-the-counter sympathomimetics
	Anticholinergic drugs (including over-the-counter antihistamines)	Hypertension	Blunting of vagal reflex compensation for drug-induced vasoconstriction	Primarily of concern with excessive doses of sympathomimetic drugs; do not use atropine in such patients
Sympathomimetic pressor drugs (such as dopamine, norepinephrine)	Anesthetics	Arrhythmias	Sensitization of heart to actions of catecholamines	Use pressor drugs cautiously in postoperative patients; monitor heart rhythm
MAO inhibitors	Indirect sympathomimetic drugs	Hypertension	Excessive intraneuronal stores and release of catecholamines	Avoid the combination; warn patients about over-the-counter sympathomimetics
	Insulin	Potentiation of hypoglycemia	Stimulation of insulin release, inhibition of gluconeogenesis	Monitor blood glucose; adjust insulin dose as necessary
	Tyramine-containing foods	Hypertension	Decreased presystemic metabolism and increased bioavailability of tyramine	Avoid the combination; warn patients about tyramine-containing foods
	L-dopa	Hypertension	Inhibition of the metabolism of L-dopa-derived dopamine	Avoid the combination
	Meperidine; rarely tricyclic antidepressants	Hypertension, excitement, delirium, hyperpyrexia	Unknown	Avoid meperidine; begin tricyclics in low doses with careful monitoring
Methyldopa	Digoxin	Sinus bradycardia	Additive sympatholytic and vagal actions	Primarily seen in patients with sinus node disease
	Haloperidol	Delirium	Unknown	Unclear clinical significance
Clonidine, guanabenz	Propranolol, sotalol	Paradoxical hypertension, aggravated hypertension during clonidine rebound	Possibly due to unopposed α-vasoconstrictor action of clonidine	Uncommon, but should be considered as possible explanation for treatment failure
	Tricyclic antidepressants	Reversal of hypotensive actions	Blockade of central α-receptors	Avoid the combination
Guanethidine, bethanidine, debrisoquin, guanadrel	Tricyclic antidepressants, chlorpromazine, amphetamines	Reversal of hypotensive actions	Blockade of neuronal uptake of guanethidine and related drugs	Avoid the combination
	Catecholamines, direct sympathomimetic drugs	Hypertension	Increased adrenergic receptor sensitivity	Avoid over-the-counter sympathomimetics; begin pressor drugs in low doses
Captopril, enalapril, other ACE inhibitors	Potassium supplements, potassium-sparing diuretics, NSAIDs	Hyperkalemia	Inhibition of aldosterone release; inability to excrete potassium	Use potassium very cautiously; monitor potassium levels frequently
	Indomethacin (and possibly other NSAIDs)	Reversal of hypotensive action	Inhibition of kinin-mediated prostaglandin synthesis	Avoid combination if possible; if necessary, monitor blood pressure closely
	Diuretics	Hypotension	Inhibition of angiotensin II homeostatic response to diuretic-induced volume contraction	Withdraw diuretics before initiating ACE inhibitors; begin with very low doses of ACE inhibitors
	Lithium	Increased lithium levels, lithium toxicity	Unknown	Monitor levels; adjust lithium dose as necessary
Prazosin	Verapamil	Increased prazosin levels, greater hypotensive effect	Reduced clearance, additive α-blocking effect	Use combination cautiously; may need to reduce prazosin dose

nificant orthostatic hypotension. Compensation for orthostatic hypotension occurs in part by sodium and fluid retention. Patients on diuretics or other antihypertensive drugs are more likely to experience more severe orthostatic hypotension, which may result in vascular accidents, especially in the elderly.

A number of adverse interactions involving specific antihypertensive drugs have been described. Those involving diuretics and β-blockers are discussed in other sections.

METHYLDOPA AND CLONIDINE

Methyldopa has been associated with development sinus bradycardia in patients receiving digoxin.[103] This may occur, although rarely, even in patients with normal sinus node function, presumably on the basis of additive sympatholytic and vagal effects of the two drugs. Clonidine and other central-acting sympatholytic drugs would be expected to have similar interactions.

Clonidine has been reported to aggravate hypertension in some patients receiving propranolol or sotalol.[104,105] This is hypothesized to result from unmasking the intrinsic α-agonist vasoconstrictor activity of clonidine in the presence of β_2 (vasodilator) antagonism. Why this interaction occurs only rarely is unclear.

The antihypertensive action of clonidine is inhibited by prior treatment with tricyclic antidepressant drugs.[106] Clonidine exerts its hypotensive action by stimulating central nervous system α_2-receptors. Tricyclic antidepressants are α-adrenergic antagonists and by that mechanism antagonize the central actions of clonidine. Tricyclics do not inhibit the hypotensive action of methyldopa, which also acts on central system α-receptors. Maprotiline, a tetracyclic antidepressant, does not antagonize clonidine effects and may be used when antidepressant drug therapy is required in patients receiving clonidine.

GUANETHIDINE AND RELATED AGENTS

Case Example A 47-year-old man with chronic hypertension was taking guanethidine, 75 mg/d; methyldopa, 750 mg/d; and trichlormethazine, 8 mg/d. His blood pressure was 118/80 mm Hg supine and 118/96 mm Hg standing. Because of depression he was referred to a psychiatrist, who prescribed amitriptyline, 25 mg three times a day. One month later, his blood pressure was 190/122 mm Hg supine and 160/115 mm Hg standing.[107]

To exert their antihypertensive action, guanethidine and related compounds bethanidine, debrisoquin, and guanadrel must be taken up by adrenergic nerve terminals. Drugs that block uptake of amines inhibit the uptake and action of guanethidine and related drugs, resulting in loss of blood pressure control.[108] Many of the tricyclic antidepressants, as well as chlorpromazine, may reverse guanethidine action.[108,109] Tricyclic antidepressant reversal of guanethidine action occurs slowly, requiring more than 12 hours. In contrast, the reversal occurs quickly after bethanidine. The kinetics of the reversal are consistent with the idea that the rate of loss of antihypertensive action is related to rate of exit of drug from the neuron after reuptake is inhibited. Guanethidine

is slowly eliminated but bethanidine is rapidly eliminated from the neuron. Amphetamines and related over-the-counter sympathomimetic drugs may also reverse guanethidine action, both by blocking uptake and by causing release of intraneuronal guanethidine.[110]

Guanethidine competes with norepinephrine and related amines for neuronal uptake. Long-term therapy reduces endogenous adrenergic activity, resulting in enhanced receptor sensitivity. One or both of these actions may explain the pressor supersensitivity to exogenously administered or released norepinephrine in patients receiving guanethidine.[108] Similarly, hypertensive interactions are expected with over-the-counter sympathomimetic drugs. It is best to avoid the use of these drugs in patients taking guanethidine or related drugs.

CAPTOPRIL AND OTHER ACE INHIBITORS

Case Example A 58-year-old woman with ischemic cardiomyopathy was hospitalized for treatment of refractory cardiac failure. Therapy included digoxin, furosemide, hydrochlorothiazide, nitroglycerin ointment, and captopril. Admission electrolyte levels included sodium, 128 mEq/l; potassium, 3.0 mEq/l; chloride, 88 mEq/l; carbon dioxide, 26 mEq/l; blood urea nitrogen (BUN), 19 mg/dl; and creatinine, 0.7 mg/dl. Because of hypokalemia, potassium chloride, 40 mEq/d, was added. During the first 48 hours, the patient diuresed briskly, losing 4 kg in weight. She subsequently became oliguric. Her BUN and creatinine levels rose to 36 and 1.2 mg/dl, respectively. On the third hospital day, her serum potassium level was 4.9 mEq/l. On the fourth hospital day, 2 hours after the morning potassium dose, the patient had a cardiac arrest. The laboratory later reported that the serum potassium before the potassium dose had been 6.5 mEq/l.

This case illustrates the most important drug interaction involving captopril or other ACE inhibitors, that is, hyperkalemia during therapy with potassium or potassium-sparing diuretics. ACE inhibitors inhibit the formation of angiotensin II and therefore the release of renin and aldosterone. Inhibition of aldosterone release results in diminished potassium excretion and enhanced susceptibility to hyperkalemia. Patients are particularly susceptible when the glomerular filtration rate is reduced, as in patients with cardiac failure after vigorous diuresis. As in the case illustration, rapid and marked increases in serum potassium can be observed with even modest potassium supplementation. To avoid hyperkalemia, potassium supplementation should be ordered on a day-by-day basis after reviewing that day's potassium level.

Although the primary antihypertensive action of captopril appears to be by inhibition of angiotensin II, inhibition of metabolism of kinins also appears to contribute to captopril action. Kinins exert a hypotensive action in part by increasing prostaglandin synthesis. Indomethacin inhibits prostaglandin synthesis and antagonizes the antihypertensive actions of captopril.[92] Other NSAIDs, although not explicitly studied, could presumably interact in a similar fashion. For unknown reasons, indomethacin interacts with captopril but not with enalapril or lisinopril.[111]

THEOPHYLLINE

Case Example A 71-year-old woman had a history of chronic obstructive lung disease, coronary heart disease, and peptic ulcer disease. She was hospitalized for worsening of bronchospasm, for which she was treated with theophylline. On 300 mg every 6 hours, her serum theophylline level was 15 µg/ml. She developed midepigastric burning pain and was treated with cimetidine, 300 mg four times a day. Four days later, she experienced a grand mal seizure. Serum theophylline concentration 8 hours after the last dose was 29 µg/ml.

Theophylline is commonly prescribed to cardiac patients. It has a low toxic/therapeutic ratio and is one of the most common drugs causing adverse reactions. Many adverse reactions to theophylline occur because of interactions with other drugs (Fig. 10.11). Theophylline is almost exclusively (90%) metabolized. The rate of metabolism is variable and is influenced by age, liver disease, cardiac failure, smoking history, and diet. Most drug interactions are pharmacokinetic and as a consequence result in reduced or accelerated theophylline metabolism.[112]

Drugs that accelerate theophylline metabolism include phenobarbital, phenytoin, carbamazepine, rifampin, and sulfinpyrazone. Theophylline toxicity is observed when these drugs are stopped while the patient continues to take an unchanged dose of theophylline. Drugs that inhibit theophylline metabolism include erythromycin, triacetyloleandomycin (troleandomycin), cimetidine, oral contraceptives, and possibly allopurinol in high doses (600 mg/d). Commonly, adverse drug interactions occur when patients receiving theophylline for treatment of chronic obstructive lung disease develop a respiratory tract infection for which they are prescribed erythromycin, or when they develop abdominal symptoms (which may be a side-effect of theophylline itself) and are prescribed cimetidine. It is preferable in patients receiving theophylline to use antibiotics such as ampicillin or tetracycline or cephalosporins and to use antiulcer therapies such as famotidine, sucralfate, or antacids, which do not inhibit theophylline metabolism.

Influenza vaccination is given routinely to patients with severe cardiac and pulmonary disease. Vaccination results in formation of interferon, which potentially may inhibit cytochrome P-450 drug oxidation. Several reports have indicated an inhibitory effect of influenza vaccination on theophylline clearance, including a few cases of apparent clinical toxicity.[113] However, other researchers have not been able to confirm depression of theophylline clearance.[114,115] Although the clinical significance of this interaction is not confirmed, it is prudent to consider the possibility, particularly for patients whose usual theophylline concentrations are at the high end of the therapeutic range.

Pharmacodynamic interactions involving theophylline may occur in combination with diuretics, as discussed under Diuretics. Theophylline toxicity may

FIGURE 10.11 DRUG INTERACTIONS INVOLVING THEOPHYLLINE*

Interacting Drug	Serum Theophylline Concentration	Typical % Change in Clearance	Mechanism	Comments
Carbamazepine	Decreased	50	Acceleration of metabolism	When drugs are added to stable theophylline dose, monitor theophylline levels and increase dose as necessary.
Phenobarbital (and other barbiturates)	Decreased	30	Acceleration of metabolism	
Phenytoin	Decreased	40–70	Acceleration of metabolism	Discontinutation of interacting drug may lead to theophylline toxicity. Decrease theophylline dose when or before other drug is stopped.
Rifampin	Decreased	20	Acceleration of metabolism	
Sulfinpyrazone	Decreased	20	Acceleration of metabolism	
Allopurinol (high doses)	Increased	20	Inhibition of metabolism	When drugs are added decrease theophylline dose (in proportion to typical change in clearance), monitor levels to optimal dose.
Cimetidine	Increased	30–40	Inhibition of metabolism	
Ciprofloxacin	Increased	100	Inhibition of metabolism	
Erythromycin	Increased	20–30	Inhibition of metabolism	Discontinuation of interacting drugs may result in subtherapeutic levels and require an increased theophylline dose.
Interferon-α_{2a}	Increased	50	Inhibition of metabolism	
Mexiletine	Increased	50	Inhibition of metabolism	
Oral contraceptives	Increased	30	Inhibition of metabolism	
Triacetyloleandomycin	Increased	50	Inhibition of metabolism	

*Interactions in which there is on average at least a 20% change in theophylline clearance are listed. Many other drugs have been reported to interact with theophylline, in which cases the interaction is usually of lesser magnitude, although an occasional patient may have a more significant interaction with one of these drugs.

present as the development of tachyarrhythmias, the treatment of which with digoxin may result in subsequent digitalis intoxication, as described under Cardiac Glycosides.

When drug therapy that is known to change theophylline kinetics is required, dosage adjustments should be anticipated. However, because the magnitude of interaction is variable, adjustments should be guided by measurements of serum theophylline concentrations.

ANTICOAGULANTS

Case Example A 71-year-old man with an aortic valve prosthesis placed for rheumatic heart disease and coronary artery disease had been taking warfarin, 5 mg/d, for 10 years. Because of ventricular arrhythmias refractory to other medications he was begun on amiodarone, 600 mg/d. Two weeks later he presented with bruising and easy bleeding. Prothrombin time had gone from its usual 20 seconds to 85 seconds. On a warfarin dose of 2.5 mg/d, prothrombin time again returned to the therapeutic range.[42]

Oral anticoagulants are typically taken over long periods, and concurrent administration of cardiovascular and other drugs is common. Many drug interactions involving anticoagulants have been described and have been known to physicians for many years (Figs. 10.12 and 10.13).[81] Yet in most hospitals adverse drug interactions involving anticoagulants continue to occur. The consequences of such interactions, excessive bleeding or thrombosis, are potentially life-threatening. Nearly all are avoidable. Most of the interactions described in this section refer to warfarin (Coumadin). Pharmacokinetic interactions may not necessarily be the same for bishydroxycoumarin (dicumarol); pharmacodynamic interactions are similar.

Drugs That Enhance Responses to Oral Anticoagulants

Initiation of drugs that enhance responses to anticoagulants in patients who have been stabilized on a particular dose of an oral anticoagulant requires reduction in that dose; cessation of therapy requires increasing the anticoagulant dose to maintain the same degree of anticoagulation.

PHARMACOKINETIC INTERACTIONS

Pharmacokinetic interactions are those which result in increased concentrations of unbound warfarin in plasma. Most commonly the interacting drug slows the metabolism of warfarin. This type of interaction persists as long as the interacting drug is administered. Drugs that have been clearly shown to inhibit the metabolism of warfarin include allopurinol, chloramphenicol (inhibits dicumarol), cimetidine, disulfi-

ram, metronidazole, oxyphenbutazone, phenylbutazone, trimethoprim-sulfamethoxazole and other sulfonamides, and possibly amiodarone and erythromycin.[81,116] Warfarin is a racemic mixture of equal amounts of two optical isomers: S-warfarin is four times more potent than R-warfarin. This is significant because some warfarin-drug interactions involve stereoselective alterations in warfarin metabolism. Phenylbutazone, sulfinpyrazone, and metronidazole, as well as trimethoprim-sulfamethoxazole, primarily inhibit S-warfarin metabolism.

Warfarin is highly (99%) bound to plasma proteins, predominantly albumin. Drugs that displace warfarin from protein binding sites increase the unbound warfarin concentration and potentially cause a greater hypoprothrombinemic action. However, the unbound concentration also determines the rate of metabolism of warfarin. Increased unbound warfarin results in an increased rate of metabolism, which ultimately results in return of the unbound drug concentration to its original level, despite the persistence of the interacting drug. Thus, transient enhancement of anticoagulant action is observed. Because the unbound fraction is increased, but the steady-state concentration of the unbound drug is held constant by metabolism, the total plasma concentration of warfarin decreases. Chloral hydrate, diflunisal, mefenamic acid, oxyphenbutazone, phenylbutazone, and possibly clofibrate interact with warfarin by displacing it from plasma proteins.

The time course of drug interactions involving warfarin may be complex. It depends on the kinetics of the interacting drug, the kinetics of the interacting event, the kinetics of warfarin, and the kinetics of the clotting factors. For example, cimetidine has a half-life of 2 to 3 hours. With constant dosing, steady-state levels of cimetidine occur within 24 hours. Inhibition of metabolism occurs rapidly and becomes maximal in a day or two.[117] Increased prothrombin time is observed within 2 or 3 days. In contrast amiodarone has a half-life of a month or more. Two weeks of constant dosing may be necessary before amiodarone blood levels accumulate to the point where the maximal interaction occurs.[118] The effects of amiodarone on warfarin metabolism may persist for months after amiodarone is discontinued.

The half-life of warfarin averages 35 hours. If an interacting drug suddenly changes the rate of warfarin metabolism, it takes three half-lives, or 105 hours (longer if the half-life is prolonged), to reach a new steady-state level of warfarin. When a displacing drug is administered, there is an immediate change in protein binding, but the return to the original unbound concentration requires metabolism and the same 100 hours (three half-lives). Changes in the hypoprothrombinemic action of warfarin depend on changes in the synthesis of clotting factors, each of which has its own characteristic kinetics. The half-lives of factors VII, IX, X, and II are approximately 6, 20, 40, and 60 hours, respectively. Thus, it may take 180 hours, or a little more than 1 week, to reach a steady-state effect when the blood level of warfarin changes.

Because of the complexities of simultaneous kinetic processes it is impossible to predict exactly the time course of warfarin drug interaction effects on coagulation. For most drugs, interactions start and become manifest within 2 or 3 days and become maximal at 1 to 2 weeks. Drug displacement interactions are maximal at 3 to 5 days and return to baseline by 2 weeks.

PHARMACODYNAMIC INTERACTIONS

Drugs may enhance warfarin action by increasing the hypoprothrombic response to a given unbound warfarin concentration. This may occur by reducing the availability of vitamin K, by inhibiting the synthesis or accelerating catabolism of clotting factors, or by affecting nonprothrombin-dependent hemostatic mechanisms.

FIGURE 10.12 DRUGS INCREASING RESPONSES TO WARFARIN

Interacting Drug	Mechanism	Comments
Allopurinol Amiodarone Cimetidine Ciprofloxacin Dextrothyroxine Disulfiram Erythromycin Lovastatin Metronidazole Norfloxacin Oxyphenbutazone Phenylbutazone Propafenone Ranitidine Sulfinpyrazone Sulfonamides Trimethoprim-sulfamethoxazole	Inhibition of warfarin metabolism	Requires reduction in warfarin dose
Chloral hydrate Diflunisal Mefenamic acid Nalidixic acid	Displacement of warfarin from plasma proteins	Transient increase in hypoprothrombinemic action; warfarin dose does not need adjustment
Erythromycin, third-generation cephalosporin, and other broad-spectrum antibiotics	Reduction in vitamin K availability	Primarily in malnourished patients
Salicylate (high doses) Quinidine, quinine	Depression of clotting factor synthesis	May need to adjust warfarin dose
Thyroid hormones Clofibrate Anabolic steroids	Accelerated catabolism of vitamin K-dependent clotting factors	May need to adjust warfarin dose
Salicylates and other NSAIDs Carbenicillin Cefamandole Cefoperazone Moxalactam	Interference with platelet function	Avoid combination when possible; if necessary, monitor closely for bleeding complications

FIGURE 10.13 DRUGS DECREASING RESPONSES TO WARFARIN

Interacting Drug	Mechanism	Comments
Barbiturates Carbamazepine Glutethimide Griseofulvin Phenytoin Rifampin	Accelerated warfarin metabolism	Warfarin dose needs to be increased to maintain hypoprothrombinemic effect. Caution concerning excessive antiocoagulation when interacting drugs are discontinued—reduce warfarin dose at time of or before discontinuation of interacting drug.
Cholestyramine Colestipol	Decreased absorption; possibly interferes with enterohepatic recycling of warfarin	Warfarin dose needs to be increased to maintain hypoprothrombinemic effect. Caution concerning excessive anticoagulation when interacting drugs are discontinued—reduce warfarin dose at time of or before discontinuation of inter-acting drug.
Vitamin K	Antagonizes action of warfarin	Avoid combination.

Vitamin K is primarily obtained from food. Intestinal bacteria synthesize small quantities of vitamin K, which becomes important when dietary intake is poor. Sensitivity to warfarin is increased in patients who are deficient in vitamin K owing to starvation or malabsorption. In such patients therapy with antibiotics may result in a critical reduction in vitamin K availability, resulting in an enhanced warfarin response.[119]

Drugs that depress clotting factor synthesis include salicylate in high doses (>3 g/d) and quinidine. Accelerated catabolism of vitamin K-dependent clotting factors may be seen in treatment with thyroid hormones, clofibrate, and possibly anabolic steroids.

The most significant pharmacodynamic interactions involve additive effects of drugs that affect hemostasis by another mechanism. This may result in excessive bleeding without alteration in prothrombin time. Drugs such as salicylates and other NSAIDs, clofibrate, carbenicillin, some of the third-generation cephalosporins (cefamandole, cefoperazone), and moxalactam, which affect platelet function, or drugs such as heparin, which affect other clotting factors, are most commonly implicated. When possible, these drugs should not be administered in patients receiving oral anticoagulants.

Drugs That Decrease Responses to Oral Anticoagulants

Initiation of drugs that decrease responses to oral anticoagulants in patients stabilized on oral anticoagulants may result in inadequate anticoagulation and thrombosis. To avoid this possibility an increase in the anticoagulant dose should be anticipated. Cessation of therapy with the same drug may result in excessive anticoagulation if the dose of warfarin is not adjusted. The latter is the source of many adverse drug interactions.

PHARMACOKINETIC INTERACTIONS

Most drugs that antagonize anticoagulant responses to warfarin do so by decreasing warfarin concentrations. Several do so by accelerating warfarin metabolism. These include barbiturates, carbamazepine, glutethimide, griseofulvin, phenytoin, and rifampin. Other drugs, such as cholestyramine and colestipol, may decrease warfarin concentrations by binding warfarin in the gut. This is an obvious problem when the drugs are given in temporal proximity.

There may also be an element of enterohepatic recirculation of warfarin such that warfarin clearance is accelerated in patients taking repeated doses of cholestyramine.

PHARMACODYNAMIC INTERACTIONS

Pharmacodynamic interactions that antagonize the effects of warfarin include administration of vitamin K analogues (vitamin K_1 and vitamin K_2), which directly antagonizes the actions of warfarin, and the administration of oral contraceptives, which increases the synthesis of factors VII and X.

Heparin

Doses of heparin are generally adjusted according to the activated partial thromboplastin time (APTT), so drug interactions are not usually appreciated as a clinical problem. However, drug interactions may significantly affect the dose of heparin required for effective anticoagulation and may influence the risk of toxicity.

Intravenous infusion of nitroglycerin may interfere with the anticoagulant effect of heparin, so that higher doses of heparin are necessary to achieve a therapeutic APPT.[120] Conversely, discontinuation of nitroglycerin may result in excessive anticoagulation and bleeding due to heparin. The interaction seems to occur even if nitroglycerin is infused without propylene glycol, and one report indicates that the interaction is seen only with infusion rates of 350 µg/min or greater.[120,121] The mechanism of interaction has not been fully clarified, but appears to involve at least in part the functional antagonism of antithrombin III activity.

Aspirin and other NSAIDs inhibit platelet function and significantly increase the risk of bleeding during administration of heparin. While the use of once daily 320 mg aspirin along with heparin has become widespread in the treatment of cardiac ischemia, higher doses of aspirin and other NSAIDs should be avoided.

OTHER DRUGS
Cyclosporine

Heart and heart-lung transplantations have been performed with increasing frequency in recent years in the management of end-stage heart disease. Lifelong immunosuppression is required for all transplant patients, and cyclosporine (often in combination with predisone and azothioprine) is the mainstay of immunosuppressive therapy. Cyclosporine is extensively metabolized by liver enzymes, and is subject to a number of drug interactions involving its metabolism. Cyclosporine is incompletely and variably absorbed from the gastrointestinal tract, and is also subject to some drug interactions affecting absorption.

Maintenance of therapeutic blood levels of cyclosporine is important both to prevent rejection, which can occur as a result of subtherapeutic levels, and to avoid nephrotoxicity, which occurs with excessive blood levels of cyclosporine. Therefore, the anticipation and management of potential drug interactions with cyclosporine is critical for safe and effective management of transplant patients. Drug interactions involving cyclosporine are summarized in Figure 10.14.

Lovastatin and Other Hypolipidemic Drugs

The major drug interaction involving lovastatin involves an increased risk of severe myopathy and rhabdomyolysis; the latter can produce acute renal failure. Myalgia or myopathy is relatively uncommon, less than 0.2% of patients, when lovastatin is used alone. The incidence increases to 2% when lovastatin is co-administered with niacin, 5% with gemfibrozil, and up to 30% in patients receiving cyclosporine.[122,124] The mechanism of lovastatin-induced myopathy is unknown, but may be related to accumulation of active metabolites, the metabolism of which is inhibited by cyclosporine or other interacting drugs. Cases of lovastatin enhancing the hypoprothrombinemic effects of warfarin have been published, but this seems to be an uncommon interaction.[125]

FIGURE 10.14 DRUG INTERACTIONS INVOLVING CYCLOSPORINE

Interacting Drug	Plasma Cyclosporine Concentration	Mechanism	Comments
Diltiazem*	Increased	Inhibition of metabolism	Measure levels and adjust dose of
Ciprofloxacin	Increased	Inhibition of metabolism	cyclosporine when interacting drugs
Erythromycin	Increased	Inhibition of metabolism	are introduced or discontinued.
Fluconazole	Increased	Inhibition of metabolism	Excessive cyclosporine levels may
Ketoconazole	Increased	Inhibition of metabolism	result in nephrotoxicity; inadequate
Nicardipine	Increased	Inhibition of metabolism	rates may result in organ rejection.
Verapamil*	Increased	Inhibition of metabolism	
Metoclopramide	Increased	Increased absorption	
Carbamazepine	Decreased	Acceleration of metabolism	
Rifampin	Decreased	Acceleration of metabolism	
Phenytoin	Decreased	Decreased absorption	
Trimethoprim-sulfamethoxazole (IV)	Decreased	Unknown mechanism	If possible TMP-SMX should be avoided in patients taking cyclosporine;
Trimethoprim-sulfamethoxazole (oral)	Decreased	Increased risk of nephrotoxicity	if not avoidable, monitor levels and adjust dose as described above.

*Diltiazem and verapamil may also ameliorate cyclosporine-induced nephrotoxicity by preventing cyclosprine-induced reduction of renal blood flow.

REFERENCES

1. Koch-Weser J: Drug interactions in cardiovascular therapy. Am Heart J 90:93, 1975
2. Friedman HS, Bonventre MV: Erythromycin-induced digoxin toxicity. Chest 82:202, 1982
3. Manninen V, Melin J, Apajalahti A et al: Altered absorption of digoxin in patients given propantheline and metoclopramide. Lancet 1:398, 1981
4. Bjornsson TD, Huang AT, Roth P et al: Effects of high-dose cancer chemotherapy on the absorption of digoxin in two different formulations. Clin Pharmacol Ther 39:25, 1986
5. Lindenbaum J, Rund DG, Butler VP et al: Inactivation of digoxin by gut flora. N Engl J Med 305:789, 1981
6. Brown DD, Juhl RP, Warner SL: Decreased bioavailability of digoxin due to hypocholesterolemic interventions. Circulation 58:164, 1978
7. Caldwell J, Bushe A, Greenberger NJ: Interruption of the enterohepatic circulation of digitoxin by cholestyramine: II. Effect on metabolic disposition of tritium-labeled digitoxin and cardiac systolic intervals in man. J Clin Invest 50:2638, 1971
8. Lalonde RL, Deshpande R, Hamilton PP et al: Acceleration of digoxin clearance by activated charcoal. Clin Pharmacol Ther 37:367, 1985
9. Pond S, Jacobs M, Marks J et al: Treatment of digitoxin overdose with oral activated charcoal. Lancet 2:1177, 1981
10. Powell JR, Fenster PE, Hager WD et al: Quinidine-digoxin interaction. N Engl J Med 302:176, 1980
11. Leahy EB, Reiffel JA, Drusin RE et al: Interaction between quinidine and digoxin. JAMA 240:533, 1978
12. Hagar WD, Fenster P, Mayernsohn M et al: Digoxin-quindine interaction. N Engl J Med 300:1238, 1979
13. Klein HO, Lang R, Weiss E et al: The influence of verapamil on serum digoxin concentration. Circulation 65:998, 1982
14. Rameis H, Magometschnigg D, Ganzinger U: The diltiazem-digoxin interaction. Clin Pharmacol Ther 36:183, 1984
15. Moysey JO, Jaggarao NSV, Grundy GN et al: Amiodarone increases plasma digoxin concentrations. Br Med J 282:272, 1981
16. Dorian P, Strauss M, Cardella C et al: Digoxin-cyclosporine interaction: Severe digitalis toxicity after cyclosporine treatment. Clin Invest Med 2:108, 1988
17. Belz GG, Doering W, Munkes R et al: Interaction between digoxin and calcium antagonism and antiarrhythmic drugs. Clin Pharmacol Ther 33:410, 1983
18. Schwartz JB, Raizner A, Akers S: Effects of nifedipine on serum digoxin concentrations in patients. Am Heart J 107:669, 1984
19. Hedman A, Angelin B, Arvidsson A et al: Interactions in the renal and biliary elimination of digoxin: Stereoselective difference between quinine and quinidine. Clin Pharmacol Ther 47:20, 1990
20. Hedman A, Angelin B, Arvidsson A et al: Digoxin-verapamil interaction: Reduction of biliary but not renal digoxin clearance in humans. Clin Pharmacol Ther 49:256, 1991
21. Waldorff S, Andersen JD, Heebøll-Nielsen N et al: Spironolactone-induced changes in digoxin kinetics. Clin Pharmacol Ther 24:162, 1978
22. Gault H, Longerich L, Dawe M et al: Digoxin-rifampin interaction. Clin Pharmacol Ther 35:750, 1984
23. Fenster PE, Hagar WD, Goodman MM: Digoxin-quinidine-spironolactone interaction. Clin Pharmacol Ther 36:70, 1984
24. Cogan JJ, Humphreys MH, Carlson J et al: Acute vasodilator therapy increased renal clearance in patients with congestive heart failure. Circulation 64:973, 1981
25. Benowitz NL: Effects of cardiac disease on pharmacokinetics: Pathophysiologic considerations. In Benet LZ, Massoud N, Gambertoglio JG (eds): Pharmocokinetic Basis for Drug Treatment, p 89. New York, Raven Press, 1984
26. DeCarli C, Sprouse G, LaRosa J: Serum magnesium levels in symptomatic atrial fibrillation and their relation to rhythm control by intravenous digoxin. Am J Cardiol 57:956, 1986
27. Ochs HR, Carstens G, Greenblatt DJ: Reductions in lidocaine clearance during continuous infusion and by coadministration of propranolol. N Engl J Med 303:373, 1980
28. Svendsen TL, Tangø M, Waldorff S et al: Effects of propranolol and pindolol on plasma lignocaine clearance in man. Br J Clin Pharmacol 13:223S, 1982
29. Knapp AB, Maguire W, Keren G et al: The cimetidine-lidocaine interaction. Ann Intern Med 98:174, 1983
30. Jackson JE, Bentley JB, Glass SJ et al: Effects of histamine-2 receptor blockade on lidocaine kinetics. Clin Pharmacol Ther 37:544, 1985
31. Data JL, Wilkinson DR, Nies AS: Interaction of quinidine with anticonvulsant drugs. N Engl J Med 294:699, 1976
32. Twum-Barima Y, Carruthers SG: Quinidinerifampin interactions. N Engl J Med 304:1466, 1981
33. Saal AK, Werner JA, Greene HL et al: Effects of amiodarone on serum quinidine and procainamide levels. Am J Cardiol 53:1264, 1984
34. Koch-Weser J: Quinidine-induced hypoprothrombinemic hemorrhage in patients on chronic warfarin therapy. Ann Intern Med 68:511, 1968
35. Maisel AS, Motulsky HJ, Insel PA: Hypotension after quinidine plus verapamil. N Engl J Med 312:167, 1985
36. Argov Z, Mastaglia FL: Disorders of neuromuscular transmission caused by drugs. N Engl J Med 301:409, 1979
37. Tartini R, Steinbrunn W, Kappenberger L et al: Dangerous interaction between amiodarone and quinidine. Lancet 1327, 1982
38. Galeazzi RL, Sheiner LB, Lockwood T et al: The renal elimination of procainamide. Clin Pharmacol Ther 19:55, 1976
39. Somogyi A, McLean A, Heinzow B: Cimetidineprocainamide pharmacokinetic interaction in man: Evidence of competition for tubular secretion of basic drugs. Eur J Clin Pharmacol 25:339, 1983
40. Kosoglou T, Rocci M, Vlasses PH: Trimethoprim alters the disposition of procainamide and N-acetylprocainamide. Clin Pharmacol Ther 44:467, 1988
41. Marcus FI: Drug interactions with amiodarone. Am Heart J 106:924, 1983

42. Hamer A, Peter T, Mandel WJ et al: The potentiation of warfarin anticoagulation by amiodarone. Circulation 65:1025, 1982

43. Derrida JP, Ollagnier J, Benaim R et al: Amiodarone et propranolol: Une association dangereuse? Nouv Presse Med 8:1429, 1979

44. Lee TH, Friedman PL, Goldman L et al: Sinus arrest and hypotension with combined amiodarone-diltiazem therapy. Am Heart J 109:163, 1985

45. Bigger T: The interaction of mexiletine with other cardiovascular drugs. Am Heart J 107:1079, 1984

46. Lalka D, Meyer MB, Duce BR et al: Kinetics of oral antiarrhythmic lidocaine congener, tocainide. Clin Pharmacol Ther 19:757, 1976

47. Funck-Brentano C, Turgeon J, Woosley RL et al: Effect of low-dose quinidine on encainide pharmacokinetics and pharmacodynamics. Influence of genetic polymorphism. J Pharmacol Exp Ther 249:134, 1989

48. Quart B, Gallo D, Sami M et al: Drug interaction studies and encainide use in renal and hepatic impairment. Am J Cardiol 58:104, 1986

49. Wood AJJ, Feely J: Pharmacokinetic drug interactions with propranolol. Clin Pharmacokinet 8:253, 1983

50. Bennett PN, John VA, Whitmarsh VB: Effects of rifampin on metoprolol and antipyrine kinetics. Br J Clin Pharmacol 13:387, 1982

51. Heagerty AM, Donovan MA, Castleden CM et al: Influences of cimetidine on pharmacokinetics of propranolol. Br Med J 282:1917, 1981

52. Donovan MA, Heagerty AM, Patel L et al: Cimetidine and bioavailability of propranolol. Lancet 1:164, 1981

53. Leeman T, Dayer P, Meyer UA: Single-dose quinidine treatment inhibits metoprolol oxidation in extensive metabolizers. Eur J Clin Pharmacol 29:739, 1986

54. McLean AJ, Skews H, Bobik A et al: Interaction between oral propranolol and hydralazine. Clin Pharmacol Ther 27:726, 1980

55. Benaim ME: Asystole after verapamil. Br Med J 15:169, 1972

56. Wayne VS, Harper RW, Laufer E et al: Adverse interaction between beta-adrenergic blocking drugs and verapamil: Report of three cases. Aust NZ J Med 12:285, 1982

57. Anastassiades CJ: Nifedipine and beta-blocker drugs. Br Med J 281:1251, 1980

58. Opie LH, White DA: Adverse interaction between nifedipine and beta-blockade. Br Med J 281:1462, 1980

59. Hansbrough JF, Near A: Propranolol-epinephrine antagonism with hypertension and stroke. Ann Intern Med 92:717, 1980

60. van Herwaarden CLA, Fennis JFM, Binkhort RA et al: Haemodynamic effects of adrenaline during treatment of hypertensive patients with propranolol and metoprolol. Eur J Clin Pharmacol 12:397, 1977

61. Reeves RA, Boer WH, DeLeve L et al: Nonselective beta-blockade enhances pressor responsiveness to epinephrine, norepinephrine and angiotensin II in normal man. Clin Pharmacol Ther 35:461, 1984

62. McAllister RG, Hamann SR, Blouin RA: Pharmacokinetics of calcium entry blockers. Am J Cardiol 55:30B, 1985

63. Loi CM, Rollins DE, Dukes GE et al: Effect of cimetidine on verapamil disposition. Clin Pharmacol Ther 37:654, 1985

64. Hamann SR, Blouin RA, Chang SL et al: Effects of hemodynamic changes on the elimination kinetics of verapamil and nifedipine. J Pharmacol Ther 231:301, 1984

65. Diamond JR, Cheung JY, Fang LS: Nifedipine-induced renal dysfunction. Am J Med 77:905, 1984

66. Pearigen PD, Benowitz NL: Poisoning due to calcium antagonists—experience with verapamil, diltiazem and nifedipine. Drug Safety 6:408, 1991

67. Kounis NG: Asystole after verapamil and digoxin. Br J Clin Pract 34:57, 1980

68. Boden WE, Korr KS, Bough GW: Nifedipine-induced hypotension and myocardial ischemia in refractory angina pectoris. JAMA 253:1131, 1985

69. Reddy RS, Uretsky BF, Steinfield M: The hemodynamic effects of intravenous verapamil in patients on chronic propranolol therapy. Am Heart J 107:97, 1984

70. Packer M, Meller J, Medina N et al: Hemodynamic consequences of combined beta-adrenergic and slow calcium channel blockade in man. Circulation 65:660, 1982

71. Zoghbi W, Schwartz JB: Verapamil overdose: Report of a case and review of the literature. Cardiovasc Rev Rep 5:355, 1984

72. Morris DL, Goldschlager N: Calcium infusion for reversal of adverse effects of intravenous verapamil. JAMA 249:3211, 1983

73. Harriman RJ, Mangiardi LM, McAllister RG et al: Reversal of the cardiovascular effects of verapamil by calcium and sodium: Differences between electrophysiologic and hemodynamic responses. Circulation 59:797, 1979

74. Devis G, Somers G, VanObberghen E et al: Calcium antagonists and islet function: I. Inhibition of insulin release by verapamil. Diabetes 24:547, 1975

75. Bhatnagar SK, Amin MMA, Al-Yusuf AR: Diabetogenic effects of nifedipine. Br Med J 289:19, 1984

76. Oster JR, Epstein M, Smoller S: Combined therapy with thiazide-type and loop diuretic agents for resistant sodium retention. Ann Intern Med 99:405, 1983

77. Sigurd B, Olesen KH: The supra-additive natriuretic effect addition of theophylline ethylenediamine and bumetanide in congestive heart failure. Am Heart J 94:168, 1977

78. Chennavasin P, Seiwell R, Brater DL: Pharmacokinetic-dynamic analysis of the indomethacin-furosemide interaction in man. J Pharmacol Exp Ther 215:77, 1980

79. Himmelhoch JM, Poust RI, Mallinger AG et al: Adjustment of lithium dose during lithium-cholothiazide therapy. Clin Pharmacol Ther 22:225, 1977

80. McCarthy JT, Torres VE, Ramero JC et al: Acute intrinsic renal failure induced by indomethacin. Mayo Clin Proc 57:289, 1982

81. Koch-Weser J, Sellers EM: Drug interactions with coumarin anticoagulants. N Engl J Med 285:487, 1971

82. Frolich JC, Leftwich R, Ragheb M et al: Indomethacin increases plasma lithium. Br Med J 1:1115, 1979

83. Clive DM, Stoff JS: Renal syndromes associated with nonsteroidal antiinflammatory drugs. N Engl J Med 310:563, 1984

84. Lavre L, Glasson P, Vallotton MB: Reversible acute renal failure from combined triamterene and indomethacin. Ann Intern Med 96:317, 1982

85. Allan SG: Interaction between diuretics and indomethacin. Br Med J 283:1611, 1981

86. Favre L, Glasson PH, Riondel A et al: Interaction of diuretics and nonsteroidal antiinflammatory drugs in man. Clin Sci 64:407, 1983

87. Blum M, Aviram A: Ibuprofen induced hyponatremia. Rheumatol Rehabil 19:258, 1980

88. Berioniade.V, Corneille L, Haraoui B: Indomethacin-induced inhibition of prostaglandin with hyperkalemia. Ann Intern Med 91:499, 1979

89. Tan SY, Shapiro R, Franco R et al: Indomethacin-induced prostaglandin inhibition with hyperkalemia: A reversible cause of hyporeninemic hypoaldosteronism. Ann Intern Med 90:783, 1979

90. Gerber JG: Indomethacin-induced rises in blood pressure. Ann Intern Med 99:555, 1983

91. Durao V, Prata MM, Guncalves LMD: Modification of antihypertensive effect of beta-adreno-receptor-blocking agents by inhibition of endogenous prostaglandin synthesis. Lancet 2:1005, 1977

92. Moore TJ, Crantz FR, Hollenberg NK et al: Contribution of prostaglandins to the antihypertensive action of captopril in essential hypertension. Hypertension 3:168, 1981

93. Imanishi M, Kawamura M, Akabane S et al: Aspirin lowers blood pressure in patients with renovascular hypertension. Hypertension 14:461, 1989

94. Ciabattoni G, Cinotti GA, Pierucci A et al: Effects of sulindac and ibuprofen in patients with chronic glomerular disease. N Engl J Med 310:279, 1984

95. Berg KJ, Talseth T: Acute renal effects of sulindac and indomethacin in chronic renal failure. Clin Pharmacol Ther 37:447, 1985

96. Steiness E, Waldroff S: Different interactions of indomethacin and sulindac with thiazides in hypertension. Br Med J 285:1702, 1982

97. Miller MJS, Bednar MM, McGiff JC: Renal metabolism of sulindac: Functional implictions. J Pharmacol Exp Ther 231:449, 1984

98. Boakes AJ, Laurence DR, Teoh PC et al: Interaction between sympathomimetic amines and antidepressant agents in man. Br Med J 1:311, 1973

99. Muelheims GH, Entrup RW, Paiewonsky D et al: Increased sensitivity of the heart to catecholamine-induced arrhythmias following guanethidine. Clin Pharmacol Ther 6:757, 1965

100. Lee KY, Beilin LJ, Vandongen R: Severe hypertension after ingestion of an appetite suppressant (phenylpropanolamine) with indomethacin. Lancet 1:1110, 1979

101. Goldstein DS, Keiser HR: Pressor and depressor responses after cholinergic blockade in humans. Am Heart J 107:974, 1984

102. Cuthbert MF, Greenberg MP, Morley SW: Cough and cold remedies: A potential danger to patients on monoamine oxidase inhibitors. Br Med J 1:404, 1969

103. Davis JC, Reifeel JA, Bigger JT: Sinus node dysfunction caused by methyldopa and digoxin. JAMA 245:1241, 1981

104. Warren SE, Ebert E, Swerdlin A et al: Clonidine and propranolol paradoxical hypertension. Arch Intern Med 139:253, 1979

105. Saarimaa H: Combination of clonidine and sotalol in hypertension. Br Med J 1:810, 1976

106. Briant RH, Reid JL, Dollery CT: Interaction between clonidine and desipramine in man. Br Med J 1:522, 1973

107. Meyer JF, McAllister K, Goldberg LI: Insidious and prolonged antagonism of guanethidine by amitriptyline. JAMA 213:1487, 1970

108. Mitchell JR, Cavanaugh JH, Arias L, Oates JA: Guanethidine and related agents: III. Antagonism by drugs which inhibit the norepinephrine pump in man. J Clin Invest 49:1596, 1970

109. Stafford JR, Fann WE: Drug interactions with guanidinium antihypertensives. Drugs 13:57, 1977

110. Gulati OD, Dave BT, Gokhale SD et al: Antagonism of adrenergic neuron blockade in hypertensive subjects. Clin Pharmacol Ther 7:510, 1965

111. Breckenridge AM: Drug interactions with ACE inhibitors. J Human Hypert 3:133, 1989

112. Jonkman JHG, Upton RA: Pharmacokinetic drug interactions with theophylline. Clin Pharmacokinet 9:309, 1984

113. Renton KW, Gray JD, Hall RI: Decreased elimination of theophylline after influenza vaccination. Can Med Assoc J 123:288, 1980

114. Bukowsky M, Mont PW, Wigle R et al: Theophylline clearance: Lack of effect of influenza vaccination and ascorbic acid. Am Rev Respir Dis 129:672, 1984

115. Meredith CG, Christian CD, Johnson RF et al: Effects of influenza virus vaccine on hepatic drug metabolism. Clin Pharmacol Ther 37:396, 1985

116. Standing Advisory Committee for Haematology of the Royal College of Pathologists: Drug interaction with coumarin derivative anticoagulants. Br Med J 285:274, 1982

117. Serlin MJ, Mossman S, Sibeon RG et al: Cimetidine: Interaction with oral anticoagulants in man. Lancet 2:317, 1979

118. Kerin NA, Blevins RD, Goldman L et al: The incidence, magnitude, and time course of the amiodarone-warfarin interaction. Arch Intern Med 148:1779, 1988

119. Sato RI, Gray DR, Brown SE: Warfarin interaction with erythromycin. Arch Intern Med 144:2413, 1984

120. Habbab MA, Haft JI: Heparin resistance induced by intravenous nitroglycerin—a word of caution when both drugs are used concomitantly. Arch Intern Med 147:857, 1987

121. Becker RD, Corrao JM, Bovill EG et al: Intravenous nitroglycerin-induced heparin resistance: A qualitative antithrombin III abnormality. Am Heart J 119:1254, 1990

122. Cockburn ITR, Krupp P: An appraisal of drug interactions with Sandimmune. Transplant Proc 21:3845, 1989

123. Corpier CL, Jones PH, Suki WN et al: Rhabdomyolysis and renal injury with lovastatin use—report of two cases in cardiac transplant recipients. JAMA 260:239, 1988

124. Tobert JA: Efficacy and long-term adverse effect pattern of lovastatin. Am J Cardiol 62:28J, 1988

125. Ahmad S: Lovastatin-warfarin interaction. Arch Intern Med 150:2407, 1990

Index

pregnant patients and anticoagulant therapy, 9.32
Protein binding, 1.9–1.10, **1.9**
  concentration-dependent, **1.9**, 1.10
Protein C, 9.6, **9.6**
Prothrombin time, 9.15–9.16
Prourokinase. *See* Single-chain urokinase-type plasminogen activator
Proximal tubule, 2.7–2.8
Pulmonary hypertension:
  alpha-adrenergic blockers and, 5.5
  calcium channel blockers and, 6.23
  nitrates and, 4.14

Q T interval prolongation syndrome, 5.14
Quinidine, 3.21
  digoxin interaction mechanism, 10.4, **10.4**
  drug interactions of, 10.8
Quinidine effect, 5.11

R aynaud's phenomenon:
  alpha-adrenergic blockers and, 5.5
  beta-adrenergic blockers and, 5.15
  calcium channel blockers and, 6.24
Receptors, 1.3–1.4, **1.4**
Recombinant tissue-type plasminogen activators, 9.18–9.19
Renal clearance, 1.8–1.9
Renal disease:
  drug disposition and, 1.18
Renal failure:
  digitalis and, 3.18
Renal physiology, 1.8–1.9, 2.2–2.5

S albutamol, 3.32
Septic shock:
  inotropic agents and, 3.46
Serotonin, 9.4
Shear rate, 9.20
Shock:
  alpha-adrenergic blockers and, 5.5
Single-chain urokinase-type plasminogen activator (scu-PA), 9.19–9.20
Sinus node dysfunction, 5.15
Sinus tachycardia, 5.12
Sodium, 2.2–2.6, 2.10
Sodium nitroprusside, 7.8–7.10
  acute myocardial infarction patient and, 4.11
  hemodynamic effects of, 7.9, **7.9, 7.14–7.15**
  mechanisms of action, **4.2**

Solute diuresis, 2.5
Sotalol, 5.12, 5.17
Spironolactone, 2.6, 2.14, 2.15
  adverse reactions of, 2.17, 2.18
  for cirrhotic patient with ascites, 2.14
  mechanism of action, **2.7**, 2.8
Steady state, 1.13–1.14
Streptokinase, 9.18
Structure-activity relationships, 1.4–1.5
Sublingual isosorbide dinitrate, **7.6**
Sublingual nitrates, 4.17, 7.6
Sulfinpyrazone, 9.10
Sulindac, 10.17
Sulmazole, 3.43–3.44
Sympathetic nervous system, 3.8, 3.9
  nitrates and, 4.5–4.6, **4.5**
Sympathomimetic drugs:
  drug interactions, 10.18, **10.19**
  hemodynamic effects of, **3.26**

T A-064, 3.33
Terazosin, 5.6, 7.8
  adverse effects of, 5.6
  pharmacokinetics of, 5.3, **5.3**
  use in hypertension, 5.4
Tetralogy of Fallot, 5.14
Theophylline, 3.36–3.37
  drug interactions, 10.21–10.22, **10.21**
Therapeutic ratio, 1.5
Therapeutic window, 1.5, **1.5**
Thiazide diuretics, 2.14–2.16
  adverse reactions of, 2.17, 2.18
  drug interactions of, 10.14
  in essential hypertension, 2.15–2.16
Thrombin, 9.3, 9.5
  heparin as inhibitor of, 9.10–9.14
  peptide blockers of, 9.10
Thrombolytic agents:
  acylated plasminogen streptokinase activator complex, 9.19
  mechanism of action, 9.17
  recombinant tissue-type plasminogen activators, 9.18–9.19
  streptokinase, 9.18
  urokinase and single-chain urokinase-type plasminogen activator, 9.19–9.20
Thrombosis:
  endogenous inhibitors of, 9.5–9.6
  labile versus fixed, 9.20
  vascular injury and, 9.21–9.23
Thromboxane A$_2$ (TXA$_2$), 9.3–9.6
  blockers of, 9.8
  inhibitors of, 9.7–9.8
Thyrotoxicosis, 5.14–5.15
Ticlopidine, 9.9–9.10

Timolol, 5.17
  use in glaucoma treatment, 5.15
  use in myocardial infarction, 5.13
Tocainide, 1.18
  drug interactions, 10.9
Transdermal nitroglycerin patches, 4.18, 7.6
Transmucosal nitroglycerin, 4.17
Triamterene, **2.7**
  adverse reactions of, 2.17
Trimazosin, 5.3, **5.3**, 7.8
Tubular reabsorption, 1.9, 2.3–2.4
Tubular secretion, 1.8–1.9, 2.4–2.5

U D-CG 115, 3.44
UD-CG 212, 3.44
Unstable angina:
  anticoagulants for, 9.25
  aspirin therapy for, 9.25
  thrombolytic therapy for, 9.25–9.26
Urapadil, 5.3
Urokinase, 9.19–9.20

V ascular injury, **9.21**
  thrombosis and, 9.21–9.23
  types of, 9.20–9.23
Vasodilators:
  angiotensin-converting enzyme inhibitors, 7.10–7.12
  arteriolar, 7.3–7.6
  combination therapy, 7.12
  effects on left ventricular compliance, 7.12–7.13
  mechanical lesions and, 7.14–7.15
  mixed-effect drugs, 7.7–7.10
  pathophysiologic basis for, 7.2–7.3
  selection of in chronic congestive heart failure, 7.15–7.17
  venodilators, 7.6–7.7
Vasoselective calcium antagonists, 6.9–6.11, **6.10**
Vein graft disease:
  after bypass surgery, 9.28
  early occlusion, 9.28
  late occlusion, 9.28
  vascular injury as initiator of, 9.22–9.23
Venoconstriction, 7.2
Venodilation, 4.3–4.5
Venodilators, 7.6–7.7
  major drugs in class of, 7.6–7.7, **7.6–7.7**
Venous tone, 5.10
Verapamil, 3.21, 6.12, 6.5, 6.7–6.8
  adverse effects of, 6.25
  as alpha-adrenergic blocker, 5.3
  cardiac arrhythmias and, 6.19–6.20, **6.19**
  drug interactions of, 10.12–10.14